Population Health Analytics

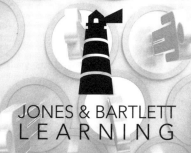

MARTHA L. SYLVIA, PHD, MBA, RN
President, ForestVue Healthcare Solutions
Associate Professor, Medical University
of South Carolina, College of Nursing

INES MARIA VIGIL, MD, MPH, MBA
Independent Physician Executive and
Leader in Population Health &
Advanced Analytics

JONES & BARTLETT
LEARNING

World Headquarters
Jones & Bartlett Learning
25 Mall Road, 6th Floor
Burlington, MA 01803
978-443-5000
info@jblearning.com
www.jblearning.com

Jones & Bartlett Learning books and products are available through most bookstores and online booksellers. To contact Jones & Bartlett Learning directly, call 800-832-0034, fax 978-443-8000, or visit our website, www.jblearning.com.

24272-0

Production Credits
VP, Product: Marisa Urbano
Director of Product Management: Matthew Kane
Product Manager: Sophie Fleck Teague
Content Strategist: Sara Bempkins
Project Manager: Jessica deMartin
Project Specialist: David Wile
Digital Project Specialist: Rachel DiMaggio
Senior Marketing Manager: Susanne Walker
VP, Manufacturing and Inventory Control: Therese Connell

Composition: Exela Technologies
Project Management: Exela Technologies
Cover Design: Briana Yates
Text Design: Kristin E. Parker
Media Development Editor: Faith Brosnan
Rights Specialist: Maria Leon Maimone
Cover Image (Title Page, Part Opener, Chapter Opener):
    © Franck-Boston/iStock/Getty Images.
Printing and Binding: McNaughton & Gunn

Library of Congress Cataloging-in-Publication Data

Names: Sylvia, Martha L., author. | Vigil, Ines, author.
Title: Population health analytics / Martha Sylvia, PhD, MBA, RN Ines Vigil, MD, MPH, MBA.
Description: First edition. | Burlington : Jones & Bartlett Learning, [2022] | Includes bibliographical references and index.
Identifiers: LCCN 2020058536 | ISBN 9781284182477 (paperback)
Subjects: LCSH: Medical informatics. | Medical care–Data processing. | Medical care–Information services. | BISAC: EDUCATION / General
Classification: LCC R858 .S94 2022 | DDC 610.285–dc23
LC record available at https://lccn.loc.gov/2020058536

6048

Printed in the United States of America
25 24 23 22 21   10 9 8 7 6 5 4 3 2 1

"I dedicate this book to my rock, my fun, my love, Michael."

—Martha Sylvia

"This book is dedicated to my family who to this day do not understand my profession, to the people who still call me friend after repeatedly not connecting during the creation of this book, to my husband Korey who politely asked for a one year advance notice before taking on another project of this magnitude in the future, and to our child Dean who will likely choose a different career and never read this, with love."

—Ines Maria Vigil

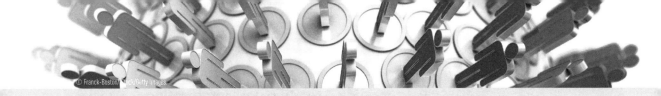

Brief Contents

SECTION VII Analytics Support for the Population Health Process   375

SECTION VIII Creating the Culture in Organizations   453

Contents

SECTION I Overview of Population Health Analytics   1

CHAPTER 1 Introduction to Population Health Analytics 3

Martha Sylvia

Ines Maria Vigil

CHAPTER 2 **Guiding Frameworks for Population Health Analytics** **15**

Martha Sylvia
Ines Maria Vigil

CHAPTER 3 **Medical Administrative Claims Data for Population Health Analytics** **29**

Martha Sylvia

SECTION III Data Contexualizers   123

CHAPTER 18 **Person Identity Management 289**

Martha Sylvia

SECTION VI **Analytic Methods**   **299**

CHAPTER 19 **Overview of Analytic Methods Used in Population Health Management 301**

Martha Sylvia

CHAPTER 20 **Epidemiological Methods 309**

Martha Sylvia

CHAPTER 21 **Risk Adjustment . . . 323**

Martha Sylvia

CHAPTER 22 **Predictive and Prescriptive Analytics** **331**

Martha Sylvia

CHAPTER 23 **Advanced Analytic Methods** **347**

Martha Sylvia

CHAPTER 24 **Run Charts and Statistical Process Control** **365**

Martha Sylvia

CHAPTER 29 **Storytelling with Data** 427

Mary Terhaar

SECTION VIII **Creating the Culture in Organizations** 453

CHAPTER 30 **Assessing Organizational Capabilities for Population Health Analytics** 455

Martha Sylvia

Evelyn Ann Borucki

CHAPTER 31 **Building a Team Culture for Population Health** . . . **475**

Ines Maria Vigil

CHAPTER 32 **Skills Assessment of Population Health Analysts** **501**

Elizabeth McCormick

CHAPTER 33 **Clinical Workflow Transformation** **511**

Ron Parton

Ines Maria Vigil

CHAPTER 34 **Ethical Principles for Population Health Analytics . . .523**

Martha Sylvia

Preface

Ines Maria Vigil, MD, MPH, MBA
Martha L. Sylvia, PhD, MBA, RN

*Tell me and I forget, teach me and I may
remember, involve me and I learn.*

—Benjamin Franklin

This book represents a labor of love, a passion, and a commitment to the discipline of population health. We have experienced firsthand both the challenges that organizations have when implementing population health concepts and analytic methodologies, as well as the benefits that this work can bring to improve health and well-being of populations and make health care more affordable. With more than 35 years of combined experience in implementing population health at healthcare organizations across the Unites States and in limited settings internationally, we are thrilled to share with you what we believe are the fundamental building blocks of population health analytics, their applications in healthcare settings, and learnings.

We set out to write this book with the intention of preparing and training analysts and data scientists to effectively work in the field of population health, providing them with a single and comprehensive source of information to support population health initiatives and activities. This textbook provides both the population health concepts as well as the practical elements needed to perform the analytics required to fully support any population health initiative. Understanding the data assets, their sources, and any calculations or transformations performed to ready the data for analytic use are important for analysts and data scientists working in population health to know,

along with the techniques and methods in which analytics can be used to identify opportunities to improve health and cost, determine health outcomes, and influence health determinants that define population health.

Sections and chapters most relevant to analyst and data scientists include Sections 1 through 4, Chapters 16 through 18, Sections 6 and 7, and Chapters 31, 32, and 34.

We also recognize population health analytics is most successful in a workforce culture that supports ongoing analytic learning and improvement, and analysts and data scientists need support from their leaders to successfully manage the analytic needs of an organization. As such, this textbook also provides leaders of analysts and data scientists a blueprint for supporting population health analytics, an overview of the data assets needed, and the analytic tools of the trade available in the market. Also woven throughout each chapter are the advantages and disadvantages of the various methods, tools, and techniques when applied to specific populations to help guide leaders of analysts and data scientists in the appropriate applications of descriptive, diagnostic, predictive, and prescriptive analytics when used to support population health. It is the opinion of the authors that clinical, business, and analytic leaders need to be fluent in how analytics that support population health are unique and different from other more traditional forms of analytics used to support health care. This differentiation requires a different level of support in the form of tools and their applications that are important for analytic leaders to know. Analytic leaders can then use this knowledge to help set expectations of organizational leaders for what level or maturity of analytics can and cannot be delivered, to advocate for additional learning and development of skill sets for their staff, and to work in partnership with their information technology colleagues to develop the data infrastructure needed to support a population health approach to data-driven decision-making.

Sections and chapters most relevant to analytic leaders include Sections 1, 3, and 4; Chapters 16 through 18; and Sections 6 through 8.

It is our firm belief that population health analytics cannot succeed without a strong data infrastructure. Several best practices included in this textbook are aimed at the data infrastructure and the partnerships required between analytic leaders and information technology leaders to build and maintain the environments needed to support and protect patient information required in the application of population health activities at the point of care. This information may appear prescriptive and is meant to impart our learnings to assist organizations in avoiding costly and detrimental investments in infrastructure that cannot support population health analytics. This information can be used by analytic and technology leaders to modernize existing analytic platforms, ensure that protected information is secure, integrate various analytic and technology solutions, and bring transparency to end users of calculations, completeness, timing, and the accuracy of data sources.

Sections and chapters most relevant to technology leaders include Sections 1 and 2, Chapter 8, Sections 4 and 5, Chapters 22 through 24, 30, 33, and 34.

An organizational culture of improvement and population health cannot be created by analytic tools and technology alone. Investments in talent, tools, and technology are not enough to ensure the successful implementation of population health at the organizational level.

Investments must also be made to improve the organization's structure and culture. Working in population health over the years, we have experienced the challenge of organizations who purchase tools and technology as population health solutions only to suffer from their lack of adoption and integration, mostly because of a lack of commitment and investment in also transforming the culture of the organization to adopt a new way of thinking and working. This textbook provides a wealth of information for clinical and business leaders to create a culture that supports data-driven decision-making and analytics for population health, strategies for involving frontline staff in the development of actionable analytics, and tactics for developing pathways to monitor the efficiency and effectiveness of population health interventions. This information can be used by organizational leaders as a road map not only for the talent, tools, and technology but also for the elements needed to ensure a successful and transformational experience for adopting population health across an organization.

Sections and chapters most relevant to clinical and business leaders include the Foreword, the Preface, Sections 1 and 3, Chapters 19 through 21, and Sections 7 and 8.

It is truly a pleasure and a humbling experience to bring this practical application of population health analytics to both existing and future healthcare workforces. Our goal of this textbook was to create a standard base of knowledge for population health analytics and a reference tool to leapfrog healthcare organizations into the future use of data and analytics to improve health. We look forward to the accomplishments and innovations this information can generate through existing and future healthcare workforces and hope you enjoy this textbook.

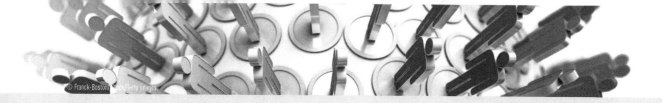

Reviewers

Kelli A. Barrieau, DNP, MBA, RN
College of Our Lady of the Elms
Chicopee, MA

Allysceaeioun D. Britt, PhD, MPH
Assistant Professor
School of Graduate Studies and Research,
  Division of Public Health Practice
Meharry Medical College
Nashville, TN

Jennifer Bueche, PhD, RDN, CDN
Distinguished Service Professor
Director, M.S. Nutrition and Dietetics Program
Department of Human Ecology
SUNY Oneonta
Oneonta, NY

Whende M. Carroll, MSN, RN-BC

Karen Jiggins Colorafi, PhD, RN
Assistant Professor
Gonzaga University School of Nursing and
Human Physiology
Spokane, WA

Lynda R Hardy, PhD, RN, FAAN
The Ohio State University, College of Nursing

Alice Kindschuh, DNP, APRN-CNS, CNE
Nebraska Methodist College
Omaha, NE

**Patricia Biller Krauskopf, PhD, FNP-BC,
  FAANP**
Professor
Shenandoah University
Winchester, VA

**Dorcas E. Kunkel, DNP, RN, CNE,
  PHNA-BC, CPHIMS**
Assistant Professor
Jacksonville University
Jacksonville, FL

Michelle A. McDonald, DrPH, MS
Chair, Population Health
Baptist College of Health Sciences
Memphis, TN

Mary A. Moore, PhD
CSU Global
Aurora, CA

**Edmund J. Y. Pajarillo, PhD, RN BC, CPHQ,
  NEA BC**
Associate Professor, Department Chair, Graduate
  Studies in Nursing & Director,
Nursing Education and Nursing Administration
  Tracks
Adelphi University
Garden City, NY

Erin M. Reynolds, PhD, MPH
Associate Professor
University of Southern Indiana
Evansville, IN

Cynthia Tomcanin Rost, DNP, RN, HFQE
Clinical Assistant Professor of Nursing
Duquesne University
Pittsburgh, PA

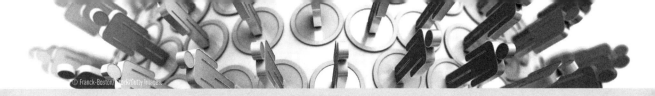
© Franck-Boston/iStock/Getty Images.

Contributors

Evelyn Ann Borucki, MHA
Program Coordinator
Department of Plastic Surgery
Boston Children's Hospital

Richa Bundy, MPH
Biostatistician
Department of Internal Medicine
Wake Forest Baptist Health
Winston-Salem, NC

Seray Gardner, BS
Product Architect
Johns Hopkins Healthcare Solutions
Baltimore, MD

Jonathan Goodhue, MS
Biostatistician

Gary Hinz
Regional VP of Sales
Lightbeam Health Solutions

Sarah Kachur, PharmD, MBA, BCACP
Executive Director, Population Health Analytics
Johns Hopkins
Baltimore, MD

Raj Lakhanpal, MD, FACEP
Founder & CEO
SpectraMedix
East Windsor, NJ

Donna Logan, MPH
Senior Analytics Advisor
Johns Hopkins HealthCare
Baltimore, MD

Yanyan Lu
Senior Business Intelligence Analyst
Johns Hopkins HealthCare, LLC
Hanover, MD

John W. Malone
Principal
Lumina Health Partners

Elizabeth McCormick, MBA

Shannon M. E. Murphy
Distinguished Biostatistician
Edwards Lifesciences
Irvine, CA

Ron Parton, MD, MPH
Chief Medical Officer Christus Population Health
  and Health Plans
Christus Health
Irving, TX

Mary Frances Terhaar, PhD, RN, ANEF, FAAN
Professor and Chair of Nursing, College of Public
  Health
Temple University
Philadelphia, PA

**Marisa L. Wilson, DNSc, MHSc, RN-BC,
  CPHIMS, FAMIA, FIAHSI, FAAN**
Associate Professor, Interim Chair, Family,
  Community and Health Systems, Director
  Nursing Health Services Leadership Pathways
The University of Alabama at Birmingham
  School of Nursing
Birmingham, AL

Timothy C. Zeddies, MHSA, PhD
Independent Consultant

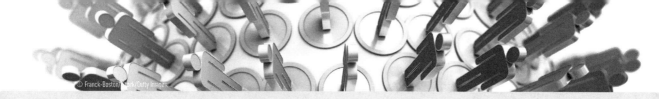

Foreword

Interest in *population health* is on the ascendency within the U.S. healthcare system. Decades of rising medical care costs in the face of poor health outcomes has led to the conclusion that health and well-being can best be achieved by a shift in focus. In addition to meeting the clinical needs of presenting patients, we must also consider a wide range of socioeconomic, behavioral, and environmental factors that impact the health of all persons in a community.

To accomplish this, medical care, public health and social service organizations need to become more fully integrated. Relevant to readers of this monograph, this must all be underpinned by robust information created by analyzing complex digital data derived from numerous secondary sources.

This foreword and most of the book was written in the midst of the COVID-19 pandemic of 2020. The Coronavirus threat has underscored the critical importance of cross-sector collaboration in the population health analytics domain. Specifically, this crisis has made it abundantly clear that the only way to mount an effective response to a major health threat is to apply surveillance and predictive modelling analytic tools based on timely, accurate, and multisector data sources.

The last decade has seen an unprecedented increase in the availability of electronic data enveloping most every aspect of medical care. And this health-related digital milieu is being extended further still as consumer and community-level data relevant to our day-to-day lives and found within commercial and government databases are being linked in. The strategic, technical, and ethical challenges involved in applying these "big data" to improve health and health care are numerous.

As this digital journey proceeds, medical and public health organizations will need a book like this one to help them manage and bridle this torrent of data. To date, most organizations have used data directly in their possession (e.g., insurance claims or electronic health records) mainly to support financial and patient care functions. And this has not been easy. But the technical and conceptual tasks that must be confronted as traditional and novel data sources are applied to population health will arguably be more difficult still. Addressing these expanded challenges in a proficient and comprehensive manner is precisely what this book so ably accomplishes.

As health organizations increasingly focus on the health of populations and social and behavioral factors affecting individuals, healthcare workers in the 2020s will all need some level of understanding of population health analytics. And this skill set must not be limited to so-called analysts or those specializing in *population health*. Each of us must achieve one of three levels of competency in this domain. Everyone will become involved in creating community-wide data assets as a by-product of the actions we take daily (e.g., seeing patients or processing bills). All of us will need to learn how to extract information from the cloud to do our jobs more effectively. This basic level of competency will be required of all clinicians, administrators, and executives.

A second group of specialists—often labeled as *analysts* or *information specialists*—will require an even higher level of competency. They will be responsible for collating, curating, and adding value to data in order to create information for the entire organization and society at large. They will support and train others.

In large organizations and among technology companies, academia, and government, there will also be the need for a subset of professionals at a third level of competency. These data science and informatics specialists will expand and improve the field of population health analytics by melding medical data and public health sciences to develop new tools, techniques, and knowledge across this growing interdisciplinary field.

Everyone across these three competency levels will need this book. Whether you are a general user, a specialist, or future leader, some—or all—of the knowledge contained here will be essential to you. For example, doctors, nurses, case managers, and executives wishing to succeed within *value-based* delivery systems such as patient-centered medical homes, accountable care organizations, or health maintenance organizations must apply the lessons in this book. Beyond that, any healthcare analyst—not just those with *population health* in their title—should fully embrace the teachings and guidance found in this book. Likewise, any public health or social service agency analyst or manager who envisions working closely with medical care systems will need this book.

This book should also be required reading for technology vendors and data scientists wishing to support the needs of the healthcare field. Because most of these individuals come from other disciplines, it will be essential for them to gain an appreciation for the many nuances in this complex, growing healthcare focus area.

This book should become required reading for all these parties, both currently employed, and in the training pipeline.

With its 34 chapters, this book becomes the most comprehensive and encyclopedic textbook on this topic ever written on its day of publication. For the reasons I have already outlined, this comes at a time when it is needed most. In addition to an extensive array of practical "nuts and bolts" that you, as a reader, can apply immediately, this book will also equip you to strategize and innovate and enlarge the tool kit. It will also help you more effectively and ethically apply the information unleashed by these expanded and linked databases to take action that will help people that you and your organization serve.

Drs. Sylvia and Vigil represent an ideal team to create this novel monograph. They are two extremely well trained and seasoned population health analytic professionals with extensive experience and advanced training in nursing, medicine, business management, public health, and data methods. They have worked in leading insurance, medical delivery, and academic organizations. Their professional journey has put them in the shoes of all three levels of their target audience: users, leaders, and innovators.

The field of population health analytics has never been more advanced. This has happened thanks to a huge public and private investment in data systems, increasing sophistication of measurement, risk- and predictive-modeling tools, financial and organizational innovation implemented by policy makers, and advances in the data, social, and public health sciences. That said, the field is not yet mature, and the challenges intrinsic within this domain are manifold. By interweaving the key threads of the field so effectively, and by offering the tool kits and roadmaps herein, this book will help you apply, expand, and extend population health analytics within your organization and beyond. In this way, I believe this book will play a substantial role in contributing to the health and well-being of communities across the nation and the globe.

Jonathan P. Weiner, DrPH
Professor of Health Policy and Management and of Health Informatics
Founder and Co-Director—The Center for Population Health Information Technology
Co-Developer and Scientific Director of the Johns Hopkins ACG© System
The Johns Hopkins Bloomberg School of Public Health
Baltimore, MD

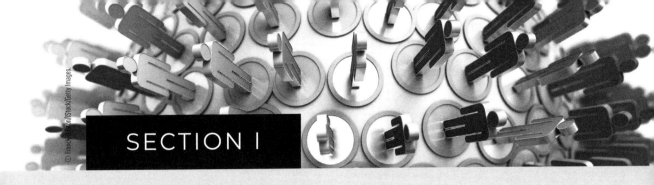

SECTION I

Overview of Population Health Analytics

CHAPTER 1

Introduction to Population Health Analytics

Martha Sylvia, PhD, MBA, RN
Ines Maria Vigil, MD, MPH, MBA

PERSPECTIVE AND CONTEXT

Population health is an evolving discipline, one that draws on the intersection of many fields of study, including public health and policy, medical and clinical care, economics, healthcare administration, biostatistics, environmental science, social and psychological sciences, and more. For the purposes of this textbook, *population health* is defined as the "distribution of health outcomes within a population, the health determinates that influence this distribution and the policies and interventions that affect the determinants" (Kindig & Stoddart, 2003).

Unlike other developed countries around the world, managing the health of the population in the United States is uniquely challenged by fragmented and disparate healthcare systems, misaligned profit incentives, and a focus on cost and utilization over improved health outcomes. As such, standardized healthcare data representing the entire U.S. population is either unavailable or difficult if not impossible to access. When accessible, publicly available population-based health and household data sets are often not generated at the person level and do not link to data derived from the healthcare marketplace. This set of challenges, combined with the potential solution of population health management, creates a unique opportunity to define a set of standards, protocols, and best practices for performing analytics to support population health management in the United States. This is the focus of this textbook.

This textbook outlines a structured process and standard approach to performing population health analytics that closely aligns with the delivery of evidence-based health care. This process is proposed through a series of phases, each phase contributing to the goal of simultaneously improving the health outcomes of the population and financial outcomes of health care providers. Each phase of the population health process outlined in this textbook includes the building blocks, options, advantages, disadvantages, and best practices to practically and successfully implement analytics to create information that can be used to drive decision-making, stimulate action, and achieve results in healthcare organizations. Also included are primary analytic techniques, methods, data outputs, and industry best practices used in health care and clinical analytics today.

This textbook focuses on the *practical application of population health analytics and is best applied in healthcare organizations currently managing healthcare cost by providing healthcare services in the form of population-based clinical interventions and programs.* Although applicable in many ways, this textbook is not targeting the audience of community health, public health, healthcare research, employer-based health care, or healthcare innovation. The goal of the editors and authors of this textbook is to share years of learnings from applying population health theory (as opposed to explaining it) and provide learnings from real-world practical experience to assist users in moving from population health theory to its application in analytics quickly and effectively. The information in this textbook is provided by leaders across the healthcare industry who have first-hand experience in working with healthcare data and population health management theory to improve health outcomes and lower its cost. At times, this book provides prescriptive actions for the user to take that stem from the learnings of the authors, and are meant to be used to avoid known pitfalls of applying population health theory to real patients in real clinical settings, to motivate action, and to leapfrog healthcare organizations into data-driven population health informed decision-making.

Population Health Analytics (PHA)

Effectively managing the health of any population is made possible by transforming data into information, gleaning insights from the information, and translating those insights into action. Data can be aggregated and used to support various clinical care processes in populations in the same way that a clinician's stethoscope is used to diagnose various health conditions in individual patients. Just as a clinician's stethoscope can detect individual sounds from different body parts at different times throughout a patient's lifetime to provide a diagnosis, individual data collected at multiple points of time and engagement with the healthcare system can be aggregated into actionable information that can be used to improve the health of an entire population. The distinction between a clinician's stethoscope and aggregated data insights is in their applicability. For instance, where an individual's heart sounds are used to determine the treatment and prescription for one patient, the range and mean of heart sounds in a population are used to determine evidence-based programs for groups of patients with heart conditions.

For the purposes of this textbook and to create a standard definition for healthcare, *population health analytics* (PHA) is defined as the following:

The systematic computational transformation of data into information to assess populations, identify health outcome determinants, predict and prescribe preventable health conditions and events,

drive decisions in the development, implementation and optimization of population-level interventions, and to monitor and evaluate results.

PHA requires the optimization of robust data sources; the application of business, clinical, and financial context and meaning to data; rigorous analytic and epidemiologic methods; an interdisciplinary approach; and a structure and process designed to meet the strategic objectives to improve the population's health and the financial performance of the healthcare organization.

This text is organized into an introductory section and eight sections that build on each other to achieve population health analytic objectives. Throughout the textbook there are "Applied Learning" case studies and use cases that provide the learner with opportunities to relate concepts to real-life scenarios. Case studies demonstrate concepts, whereas use cases present scenarios and ask the learner to respond to a set of questions.

Section I: Chapter 1: Introduction & Chapter 2: Guiding Frameworks for Population Health Analytics

The first section of the textbook covers the broader context of population health. Following this introductory chapter, Chapter 2 introduces the ForestVue Population Health Implementation and Analytics Framework, which serves as both a stepwise process to implement population health concepts and a guide for deploying analytics across the population health continuum. Incorporating leading definitions of population health, the Triple Aim, and evidence-based practice, this framework follows innovative scientific methods and provides a practical translation of these methods into a seven-phase process that carefully outlines the analytics needed at each step to successfully transform an idea to results. Also covered in this chapter are analytics capabilities needed to truly support population health management.

Section II: Data Sources

Population health management seeks to obtain person-level data from multiple data sources on an ongoing basis to develop evidence-based strategies directed at reversing negative trends in the health status of a defined population that have been shown in the health literature to lead to overall increased costs, inappropriate use of healthcare services, and overall decline in the health of the population.

Chapter 3: Medical Administrative Claims Data for Population Health Analytics

Medical claims data are generated when providers and healthcare facilities bill payers for the provision of healthcare services to patients. In this chapter, data structure, lineage, and coding systems are described. The value of medical claims data for use in population health analytics is expressed, and ways of using medical claims data to answer questions of importance to population health management are examined.

Chapter 4: Lab Data for Population Health Analytics

Clinical lab data reports the results of any type of test done on samples such as blood or tissue and are used to identify diseases or other conditions and can be used to monitor a person's overall health to cure, treat, or prevent disease. Lab data are one of the most complex sources of data to use in population health analytics because of the wide variation of data structures and reporting and lack of standardization. This chapter describes the sources and structures of lab data, describes techniques for transforming lab data into meaningful information, explains the value of lab data, and identifies ways to use lab data to answer questions of importance in population health.

Chapter 5: Pharmacy Data

Pharmacy data are derived through patient treatment encounters with the healthcare system, either those that result in a prescription being generated or those associated with filling a prescription. Medications that require a prescription from a healthcare provider or dispensing from a local pharmacy create administrative records that generate pharmacy data for analysis. This chapter describes common sources of pharmacy data used in population health analytics, including a description of how data sets may vary and be used differently based on source system. Common coding systems used for pharmacy data are described, along with applications of pharmacy data in analyses.

Chapter 6: Electronic Medical Record Data for Population Health Analytics

Data from electronic medical records (EMRs) are vast and varied and include any information that is collected to describe patients' health and treatment histories. EMRs are transactional systems containing data collected during healthcare delivery to patients and can be repurposed for population health analytics. This chapter describes the structure of an EMR database and provides examples of the types of data found, demonstrates how EMR data can be used to answer questions of interest in population health, and explains the advantages and disadvantages of using EMR data for population health analytics in comparison to other data sources.

Chapter 7: Social and Behavioral Data

Social determinants of health (SDOH) are the conditions in which people are born, grow, live, work, learn, worship, and play (World Health Organization, 2017). Given that the majority of healthcare organizations only have data related to the delivery of clinical care services, data about the SDOH are the most difficult to include in population health analytics. This chapter explores data sources that measure SDOH and ways in which to include these data in analyses used to understand the health of populations. Data structures and attempts at standardization are described and a case study is presented.

Section III: Data Contextualizers

Adding context to population health data can be an effective way of focusing analytic efforts to identify actionable opportunity to improve health and reduce unnecessary healthcare costs. Many methods exist to apply context by grouping data into discreet areas of opportunity. Applying context to population health data can be used to simulate the healthcare experience, provide decision support to clinicians at the point of care, and understand service patterns and trends. Section III of the textbook broadly introduces the use and application of data contextualizers and goes deeper into those contextualizers that are commonly applied in population health analytics.

Chapter 8: Grouping, Trending, and Interpreting Population Health Data for Decision Support

This chapter introduces the concept of grouping data into different focus areas of opportunity, provides a general overview and comparison of data groupers available in the marketplace, and highlights examples of how population health data with context can help aid executive strategic planning, business decision-making, and

clinical decision support. Data contextualizers are framed in the context of the Triple Aim of improving the health of populations, enhancing the experience and outcomes for populations, and reducing per capita cost of care (Berwick, Nolan, & Whittington, 2008). This chapter also reviews the cautions that must be considered when applying context by grouping population health data because the information from these data can easily be misinterpreted.

Chapter 9: Grouping, Trending, and Interpreting Population Health Data for Receptivity, Engagement, and Activation

Patient engagement is an important aspect of building impactful population health solutions. Combining demographic, consumer behavior, and health determinants with clinical and financial data can enable a deeper understanding of patient engagement and further the development of analytic models that predict a patient's willingness and readiness to participate in a particular clinical program or intervention. This chapter outlines how adding receptivity, engagement, and activation context to data can enhance patient relationships, promote personal responsibility, detect selection bias, and support planning, prioritization, and triage in the most effective program or intervention that can provide the most benefit. Also included in this chapter are examples of how data and analytics can align a patient's engagement with clinical and behavioral health-improvement programs, and clinically and financially impact monitoring and evaluation metrics to measure performance.

Chapter 10: Grouping, Trending, and Interpreting Population Health Data for Assessing Risk and Disease Burden

Robust clinical categorizations of clinical conditions are a staple of population health management and analytics. This chapter discusses the use of clinical, financial, health determinants, and supplementary data to assess and stratify populations into varying risk categories; identifying patients with understated, suspected, or rising risk that can lead to worsened health outcomes; and how to adjust for risk and disease burden when identifying patients for select clinical programs or interventions and in reporting outcomes. Additional information included in this chapter is the context that can be applied to data to identify coding patterns for suspected clinical conditions, verify patients' existing conditions, assess severity of illness, determine status of control of clinical indicators for illness, monitor morbidity and mortality trends, and predict future cost, utilization, and worsening health outcomes.

Chapter 11: Grouping, Trending, and Interpreting Population Health Data for Waste and Inefficiency

Variation in the provision of medical services is significant, and clinical and administrative reduction is a strong focus of many healthcare organizations seeking to reduce unnecessary services and waste in health care to achieve financial success and optimize health outcomes. This chapter looks at the ways data can be grouped into clinical episodes of care, evidence-based practice of medicine, and clinical and administrative care pathways to identify diagnostic and clinical errors, administrative and transactional waste, and promote cost-effective and cost-efficient programs and interventions.

Section IV: Creating the Population Health Data Model

Population health management is made possible through the translation of data into meaningful information. Aggregated data are used to carry out clinical processes of care in a population in the same way that the tools of the clinician are used in the clinical process of care for individual patients. Individual data collected at multiple points of contact within the care system are aggregated to understand the health of an entire population. The population health data model (PHDM) provides the necessary data infrastructure for readily assembling individuals into populations of interest, understanding health determinants and key drivers of outcomes, and measuring outcomes of the Triple Aim. This section is split into two chapters that describe the use-case–based approach for delivering incremental value in the PHDM, explains the process for developing the PHDM, and presents the core structure and components of the PHDM.

Chapter 12: Development of a Data Model

Data models in population health are complex and highly technical, requiring a prototyping approach to development where incremental executable portions of the model are delivered for use and acceptance. When done well, a strong data-modeling architecture is flexible because it can accommodate changes when business rules and clinical logic changes. The goal of data modeling in population health is to optimize the ability to perform the analytic functions in support of the population health process. This chapter describes key components of the approach to use when developing data models for population health management. A use-case–based approach is taken to help prioritize the layering of high value data assets into data model development. Agile project management supports the use of prototypes in developing population health data models. The process of moving from conceptual to physical to logical data models allows all stakeholders in the model the ability to actively participate, with all of them understanding the important roles they play in developing a high functioning data model.

Chapter 13: The Population Health Data Model

Although a population health data model is developed with specific organizational goals in mind, all population health data models share basic features. These features make up the core of the data model. At its core, the model has person-level observations from multiple data sources at equally distant points in time that can be aggregated to an entire population and segmented by smaller subgroupings. This chapter describes the core components and functionality of a population health data model, proposes a process for developing the model, and provides an example of a conceptual model. With these basic principles in mind, stakeholders and resources can be organized to develop a population health data model that is uniquely tailored to unique organizational strategy, data availability, and technical capabilities.

Section V: Data Infrastructure

Analytic infrastructure refers to tools, services, applications, and platforms that support analytic processes and the constellation of analytic products from simple reports to data models to estimating and validating models that diagnose conditions, predict adverse outcomes, or prescribe action. Databases, data warehouses, statistical and data-mining systems, scoring engines, grids (computers that interact to coordinate data processing) and clouds (Grossman, 2009). The best analytic infrastructure uses standards-based procedures for data processing; appropriately applies technology like grids and cloud-based services to support large volume, high-velocity, and variety of data; supports analytics for the entirety of the organization; is nimble in supporting new and innovative analytic undertakings; and fully integrates systems data (Grossman, 2009; Halper & Stodder, 2014). This section is split into five chapters that detail the process and options for data warehousing, describe data-preparation techniques, demonstrate methods for assessing the quality of data, and delineate a process for person-level identity management.

Chapter 14: Options for Warehousing Data for Population Health Analytics

A data warehouse environment is built to hold historical data integrated from several source

systems, often operational, in an organized manner. Operational systems are built for specific functions and traditionally are not built to serve the purpose of data analytics or data mining. To support the activities of population health analytics, new environments must be created to merge the population health data from these systems and other more traditional data sources into one central area called a *population health data warehouse system* for overall enterprise use. This chapter describes the ways in which a data warehouse supports population health analytics, identifies the components of and alternatives for a comprehensive data warehouse, identifies factors that affect the choice of a data warehouse, and analyzes the implications of this choice.

Chapter 15: Process for Warehousing Data for Population Health Analytics

This chapter describes the basic processes associated with building an effective data warehouse and the additional processes that are required to effectively support population health analytics and management. Resolving data inconsistencies, denormalizing, or normalizing data, and inserting frequently used calculations and definitions are critical aspects of the process for warehousing data to support population health analytics. This chapter also includes best practices to incorporate and pitfalls to avoid when optimizing the data to support a population health data model, framework, and the maturation of analytics over time.

Chapter 16: Data Management and Preparation

The majority of data used for population health analytics is secondary data, meaning that the data were collected for a purpose other than understanding the health determinants and outcomes for populations and subgroupings. As such, these data are rarely, if ever, fully prepared to answer questions of interest and execute on improving outcomes in population health. This chapter provides a broad overview of the ideal state of data preparation where robust master data management (MDM) processes are in place to manage person-level identification, linking of data files, and scouring of data fields for acceptable levels of data error. Absent MDM, the chapter describes a process to handle some of the most commonly found errors in data when performing population health analyses, offers methods for managing these issues, and encourages placing these methods into automated processes.

Chapter 17: Assessing Data Quality

Building a sustainable data infrastructure for population health requires an understanding and monitoring of the quality of data assets. Accurate measurement of health determinants and outcomes rely on the presence of high-quality data as does the decisions made to inform the financial viability of healthcare organizations using these data. This chapter defines the domains of data quality and their ability to assess the value of data in their entirety, demonstrating the ability of data points to represent their intended meaning completely and accurately in a timely manner. Emphasis is placed on a data profiling approach to data quality evaluation where proactive measures are put into place and regularly monitored, and results are used to improve data quality.

Chapter 18: Person Identity Management

Achieving the Triple Aim requires reduced waste and inefficiencies in the healthcare system. Because of poor patient-identity management, healthcare dollars are needlessly spent on duplicate testing, multiple submissions, and rejections to payers from providers; the wrong results given to the wrong person; and, much worse, wrong treatments are provided to patients. The importance of matching data at the person level for population health analytics and the enormity of the challenges in doing so cannot be understated. The methods of patient-identity management and master data management are used in this chapter to solidify the tenants by which unique person identification can be optimized and maintained for population health analytics.

Section VI: Analytic Methods

The population health process critically depends on the ability of analytics to inform each phase of the population health framework. When providing care to individuals, clinicians use data points about patients to make diagnoses and determine appropriate treatments. At the population level, data points that are aggregated into analyzable data structures are necessary to understand health determinants and determine the appropriate interventions for improving outcomes. Multiple analytic methods are applied to turn these data into information and insights. This section is presented in six chapters that provide an overview of analytic methods and detail the methodologies for epidemiological, risk adjustment, predictive analytics, prescriptive analytics, statistical process control, and other advanced techniques.

Chapter 19: Overview of Analytic Methods Used in Population Health Management

Each phase of the population health framework requires certain analytic methods to glean insight and understanding in executing during that phase. Analytic methods refer to the calculations, statistics, and models developed from data that facilitate the transfer of data to knowledge and wisdom. Although some methods can be used in multiple phases of the population health process, many are primarily used in specified phases and are key to gleaning the necessary insights within a phase. This chapter provides an overview of analytic methods commonly used to execute in each phase of the population health process. A description of the methods is provided and framed within the processes of population health.

Chapter 20: Epidemiological Methods

Epidemiological methods allow the ability to understand the "distribution of health outcomes" within a population, one of the main components of the definition of population health management (Kindig & Stoddart, 2003). In addition, epidemiologic methods form the basis of and are used to validate more complex analytic methods in population health, including risk adjustment and predictive modeling. This chapter focuses on the discipline of epidemiology and its analytics methods, which form the basis for answering questions of interest in population health management and is presented in a way that focuses on applications specific to population health analytics.

Chapter 21: Risk Adjustment

Risk adjustment is a way of controlling for observable differences between patients when paying for the health care of those patients and is widely used in population health management. Although used for many different purposes in the population health process, it is mainly used to set payments to health plans that reflect the expected cost of providing health insurance to their members. In other applications, governments, health plans, and other payers in health care will also apply risk adjustment when paying for value (versus paying for services rendered) when measuring outcomes and comparing health systems and providers and when measuring the impact of population health interventions (Schone & Brown, 2013; Schokkaert & Van de Voorde,

2009). This chapter introduces the concept of risk adjustment and important considerations for risk-adjustment methodology. A case study is used to apply these concepts in population health analytics.

Chapter 22: Predictive and Prescriptive Analytics

Using mathematical theory and data to estimate outcomes that cannot immediately be measured, predictive analytics is touted as one answer to addressing health needs in populations and improving outcomes when the need is to identify future beneficiaries (Brown, 2018). Similarly, prescriptive analytics—which moves the question of predictive analytics that is "what will happen" to "what should I do"—is seen as the pinnacle of analytic capabilities for which many healthcare organizations strive. This chapter identifies methods used in the development of risk prediction models and their validation, distinguishes between predictive and prescriptive modeling, describes applications of predictive and prescriptive modeling in population health, and summarizes key decision points for decisions around using these methods in practice.

Chapter 23: Advanced Analytic Methods

Advanced analytic methods have the potential to disruptively change the way health care is delivered. Advanced analytical techniques are applied to what is considered big data in terms of large volume, variety, velocity, and veracity through the process of knowledge discovery in databases (KDD). This chapter distinguishes between key terms used in pattern-based risk modeling, describes the KDD process, identifies common machine-learning techniques applied in population health analytics, and describes natural language-processing methods. Techniques are presented in terms of their applicability to population health analytics, and methods for assessing feasibility are presented.

Chapter 24: Run Charts and Statistical Process Control

Statistical process control (SPC) is a method used to understand when population health initiatives are stable in that they are running as planned and also to understand when intentional improvements are meeting set targets. A monitoring strategy using SPC as the methodology prepares the analysts and intervention leadership to make ongoing adjustments to improve or keep processes stable and informs business leaders about the value of investments. This chapter describes SPC methods and the ways in which they are used to monitor metrics of interest in population health and demonstrates the use of SPC in population health management.

Section VII: Analytics Support for the Population Health Process

Previous sections of this textbook outline the concepts, frameworks, assets, tools, methods, and processes that are needed to effectively perform population health analytics. This section focuses the reader on population health analyses that are commonly used in real-world healthcare administrative and clinical settings across the United States. Assessing the health, segmenting, monitoring, and intervening with populations is core to population health analytics and is discussed in the following four chapters. An additional important chapter included in this section focuses on the basic principles of using storytelling to effectively communicate population health analytic derived opportunity and urgency to a variety of clinical and nonclinical audiences.

Chapter 25: Assessing Populations

A population health assessment stems from the identification of problems in health care, many of which are complex and multifaceted.

U.S. healthcare delivery organizations, payers, governments, and other independent organizations regularly monitor pertinent health indicators and resource utilization. An unexpected rise or fall in these indicators often triggers the need to understand more deeply the unique characteristics of the affected population and the health determinants that impact care, cost, and utilization. This chapter outlines the process to identify the types of challenges in health care that lead to the need for a population health assessment, defines data and non-data elements necessary for the assessment, and details the process steps required to comprehensively assess a population's health to identify opportunities for health improvement. This chapter also introduces the concept of using person-centered analytics to assess the health of a population.

Chapter 26: Targeting Individuals for Intervention

The crux of improving health outcomes while reducing healthcare costs and utilization is being able to identify the small groups of high-needs patients and intervene to prevent superutilization and strive for a more normally distributed curve of healthcare spending. This chapter brings together an understanding of population health data sources and structures, risk-prediction modeling, population assessment, and linkages between health determinants and health outcomes to explain the application of identifying, stratifying, and segmenting populations for intervention.

Chapter 27: Analytics Supporting Population Health Interventions

A variety of analytic methods and techniques exist to support the development and application of cost-effective, cost-efficient, and evidence-based clinical and administrative interventions. This chapter outlines the elements of successful population health interventions using analytics and highlights several examples of how clinical and population health analytics can enhance the development and deployment of interventions across population subsets. Also included are approaches to developing effective population health interventions, best practices, and pitfalls to avoid when using analytics to develop and deploy interventions and additional resources for engaging clinicians and patients.

Chapter 28: Monitoring and Optimizing Interventions

As the intervention progresses from initiation to steady state, monitoring takes place to ensure that the intervention is being delivered as intended and that progress is being made toward achieving desired outcomes. During this phase, all stakeholders have a role in reviewing and interpreting reports about the interventions. This chapter describes the multiple vantage points for monitoring the results of population health interventions with examples of the types of reporting to meet the needs of each. Intervention monitoring is framed within the context of quality improvement and evidence-based practice processes. Process and outcome measures of interest to population health interventions are suggested along with a case study.

Chapter 29: Storytelling with Data

Those who practice in population health, including analysts, are endowed with an abundance of data. This chapter explains how one can surround data with compelling stories in service of impact and asserts that another set of tools, those of storytellers, strongly complement analytics. A well-crafted and well-told story has the capacity to extend the reach and the impact of science and analytics. Impactful stories seize and hold the attention of the target audience and bring that audience into the world of the characters. This chapter discusses the role of story in society, explains the ways storytelling affects the brain, introduces the basics of good story, describes the

best practices and devices of effective storytellers, explores the elements of effective stories and their ability to create credible narrative in population health, and applies storytelling to presentation of analytics and results.

Section VIII: Creating the Culture in Organizations

Integral to effectively managing the health of a population is the healthcare organization's commitment to the community of patients it serves; the accountability of the organization, its clinicians, and patients to mutually engage in preventing disease and unnecessary care; and the capability of the organization to provide the skills, tools, and services that enable a data, analytics, and information-driven organizational culture. This section establishes a proven method for assessing an organization's capabilities and readiness to adopt a culture of data-driven informed decision-making and proposes several best practices for organizing teams to lead the promotion and integration data and analytics across multiple disciplines, departments, and divisions within an organization. The section ties important concepts throughout the textbook together through clinical workflow transformation. The section and text conclude with one of the most important and least considered topics in population health analytics that are the ethical principles that guide this important work.

Chapter 30: Assessing Organizational Capabilities for Population Health Analytics

Utilizing a framework to assess an organization's population health analytic capabilities creates a standardized method to identify specific areas for improvement and potential future strategies.

This chapter describes a framework for assessing organizational capabilities to execute on population health analytic objectives and achieve desired results. Capabilities are described in terms of structure, process, and outcome according to the framework laid out by McDonald et al. (2007). Publicly available organizational assessments are explored, and an organizational assessment tool is proposed.

Chapter 31: Building a Team Culture for Population Health

Analytics to support population health cannot be developed properly without a team-based approach. Solutions built in isolation or from one person's expertise often cannot be generally applied to populations or scaled. Building a team for population health analytics is essential to ensure the success of the solution. This chapter outlines the importance of a team and its application to population health management and analytics, and it introduces the PopHealth Troika (PHT)™, a method for identifying the right team members, setting clear roles and expectations, realizing each team member's potential, building trust, creating shared understanding, and practicing open communication to transform the way health care is delivered to achieve extraordinary results. Also discussed are tactics to create a safe space for team members to simultaneously innovate and learn, set clear performance goals, define the scope of work and stick to it, and challenge one another's assumptions with respect to the betterment of desired results.

Chapter 32: Skills Assessment of Population Health Analysts

Analytics and analysts are central to success in population health analytics; therefore, an organization must identify, develop, and retain the talent needed to support this work using job descriptions and skills assessments to manage this critical function. Skills assessments are designed to provide a best practice methodology for measuring and understanding workforce skills. The process supports an effective skills-management practice, and the value is delivered through aligning a company's most important asset, its people, with its ability to deliver meaningful and targeted outcomes. This chapter focuses on three areas of the skills assessment process: (1) defining the components of a skills-assessment framework and process, (2) identifying the analytic and business skills that support population health analytics, and (3) how skills assessments can be implemented for success within organizations.

Chapter 33: Clinical Workflow Transformation

Population health management and analytics requires that a different approach be taken when delivering healthcare services to patients. Population health seeks to address the total cost and quality of care with a proactive approach to health optimization as opposed to a status quo reactive approach of symptom management and procedure-based care. At a system level, the way care is delivered becomes a fundamental building block to successful management of populations. Several considerations need to be clearly articulated to implement a population health approach, and few rise to the level of importance than transforming the clinical workflow. This chapter highlights examples of how organizations have incorporated best practice steps to transform the way healthcare services are delivered to a population. It seeks to describe the common elements and building blocks of clinical workflow transformation and discusses key issues, resource requirements, information technology, and data and analytics that can impact clinical workflow development. Additionally, it applies population health concepts and methods to clinical workflows to transform healthcare services.

Chapter 34: Ethical Principles for Population Health Analytics

Population health analytics makes data readily available at the person level to make inferences about the factors impacting health outcomes, determine which health interventions are best suited to healthcare needs in the aggregate, predict adverse outcomes, and make decisions about the allocation of healthcare resources. Data-driven decision-making in population health is plagued by restrictions in data availability at the person level, leading to a limited ability to understand the complexity of problems in health care, ensure the inclusion of diverse subgroups of populations, and measure a constellation of health determinants in addition to those that are clinical in nature. For these reasons, it is important to be intentional in addressing ethical concerns in population health analytics. This chapter focuses on the application of ethical principles to population health analytics, presents pertinent use cases, and suggests methods to incorporate ethical principles purposefully and regularly into population health analytic processes.

Conclusion

Population health is a dynamic and evolving field of study, and a career in population health analytics can be a fulfilling and powerful way to participate in developing insights and solutions to the challenges that exist in health care today as well as directly and positively impact the health and well-being of the population. This book was crafted with the learner in mind and is meant to expose students at every level of the discipline and relatively new practitioners in this field to learnings, experiences, challenges and successes from the practical application of population health concepts, methods, and principles on existing populations across the United States.

References

Berwick, D. M., Nolan, T. W., & Whittington, J. (2008). *The Triple Aim: Care, health, and cost*. Health Affairs, 27(3), 759–769. https://doi.org/10.1377/hlthaff.27.3.759

Brown, M. S. (2018). *Predictive analytics terms business people need to know*. Forbes. https://www.forbes.com/sites/metabrown/2018/07/30/predictive-analytics-terms-business-people-need-to-know-no-hype-allowed/#7f29de913d43

Grossman, R. L. (2009). What is analytic infrastructure and why should you care? ACM SIGKDD Explorations, 11(1). Chicago: University of Illinois and Open Data Group. https://www.kdd.org/exploration_files/p1V11n1.pdf

Halper, F., & Stodder, D. (2014). TDWI analytics maturity model guide. TDWI. https://www.tableau.com/asset/tdwi-analytics-maturity-model-assessment-guide?utm_campaign_id=2017049&utm_campaign=Prospecting-ALL-ALL-ALL-ALL-ALL&utm_medium=Paid+Search&utm_source=Google+Search&utm_language=EN&utm_country=USCA&kw=&adgroup=CTX-IT-Whitepaper-DSA&adused=DSA&matchtype=b&placement=&gclid=CjwKCAiAxKv_BRBdEiwAyd40N3pxun51dTgu4s7yjD_kogAFHxRwP3hJrOWJ_Krq7tF67TO5dk6DHxoCkEgQAvD_BwE&gclsrc=aw.ds

Kharrazi, H., Lasser, E. C., Yasnoff, W. A., Loonsk, J., Advani, A., Lehmann, H. P., . . . , Weiner, J. P. (2017). A proposed national research and development agenda for population health informatics: Summary recommendations from a national expert workshop. *Journal of the American Medical Informatics Association*, 24(1), 2–12. https://doi.org/10.1093/jamia/ocv210

Kindig, D. A., & Stoddart, G. (2003, March 1). What is population health? *American Journal of Public Health*, 93, 380–383. https://doi.org/10.2105/AJPH.93.3.380

McDonald, K. M., Sundaram, V., Bravata, D. M., et al. (2007, June). *Closing the quality gap: A critical analysis of quality improvement strategies*. Vol. 7: Care coordination. Agency for Healthcare Research and Quality. https://www.ncbi.nlm.nih.gov/books/NBK44008/

Schokkaert, E., & Van de Voorde, C. (2009). Direct versus indirect standardization in risk adjustment. *Journal of Health Economics*, 28(2), 361–374. https://doi.org/10.1016/j.jhealeco.2008.10.012

Schone, E., & Brown, R. (2013, July 1). Risk adjustment: What is the current state of the art and how can it be improved? The Synthesis Project, Robert Wood Johnson Foundation. https://www.rwjf.org/en/library/research/2013/07/risk-adjustment---what-is-the-current-state-of-the-art-and-how-c.html

World Health Organization. (2017). About social determinants of health. https://www.who.int/health-topics/social-determinants-of-health#tab=tab_1

CHAPTER 2

Guiding Frameworks for Population Health Analytics

Martha Sylvia, PhD, MBA, RN
Ines Maria Vigil, MD, MPH, MBA

The winds and the waves are always on the side of the ablest navigators.

—Edward Gibbon (n.d.)

EXECUTIVE SUMMARY

Effectively managing the health of any population is made possible by transforming data into information, gleaning insights from the information, and translating those insights into evidence-based action to improve patient experience, health, and cost. Analytics is a fundamental component of population health and is woven throughout many population health activities and certainly throughout the life cycle of any population health project. As teams form to solve complex population health challenges, it is important to guide the population health team with a framework by which to work and follow.

Several population health frameworks have been described in the literature (Institute for Healthcare Improvement, n.d.; Kindig & Stoddart, 2003; Population Health Alliance, n.d.). Many of these frameworks are meant to provide a way for population health teams to conceptualize population health concepts and methods, and they often stop short of describing practical ways of applying these concepts and methods in a phased manner to enable teams to progress in a structured way from an insight to results utilizing population health analytics, tools, and technology. This chapter introduces a new practical framework and stepwise process for the application of population health within organizations that draws on models used for evidence-based processes in health research, public health, quality, and safety improvement. This Population Health Implementation and Analytics Framework and stepwise process from ForestVue Healthcare Solutions, LLC, is meant to be used in the practical application of population health analytics. The framework and process can help guide population health project activities for a variety of healthcare organizations, particularly for those organizations currently managing healthcare cost by providing healthcare services in the form of population-based clinical interventions and programs.

The Population Health Implementation and Analytics Framework was developed with a special attention to the role that analytics plays in population health, including but not limited to the optimization of robust data sources; the application of business, clinical, and financial context and meaning to data; rigorous analytic and epidemiologic methods; an interdisciplinary approach; and a structure and process designed to meet the strategic objectives to improve the health of the population and the financial performance of the healthcare organization.

LEARNING OBJECTIVES

At the end of this chapter, the learner will be able to:

1. Understand the concepts of population health, the Triple Aim, and evidence-based practice (EBP).
2. Describe each process phase from ForestVue's Population Health Implementation and Analytics Framework.
3. Describe and apply the analytics needed to support each process phase from ForestVue's Population Health Implementation and Analytics Framework.

Introduction

Population health is commonly described in publications as a strategy or an approach (Kindig & Stoddart, 2003; Magnusson, Eisenhart, Gorman, Kennedy, & Davenport, 2019). It provides linkages between evidence-based information and practice, utilizes analytics to drive decision-making, and supports healthcare organizations in effectively managing the risk of their populations. It can be applied to the disciplines of clinical practice, public health, health policy, research, and more.

A review of the Internet and evidence-based literature drew more than a dozen different population health frameworks, with each tailoring the framework to their population of interest's specific needs such as children, adults, patients with diabetes, primary care clinicians, and the world (Berwick, Nolan, & Whittington, 2008; Initiative, n.d.; Kindig & Stoddart, 2003; NHS, n.d.; Population Health Alliance, n.d.).

This same review failed to locate a population health framework that both focuses on the process steps teams can take to ensure they are following evidence-based best practices in population health and where, when, and why to use certain analytics to support the management of risk across diverse populations.

This chapter introduces the ForestVue Population Health Implementation and Analytics Framework, which serves as both a stepwise process to implement population health concepts and a guide for deploying analytics across the population health continuum. Incorporating leading definitions of population health, the Triple Aim, and evidence-based practice, this framework follows innovative scientific methods and provides a practical translation of these methods into a seven-phase process that carefully outlines the analytics needed at each step to successfully transform an idea into results. Also covered in this chapter are analytics capabilities needed to truly support population health management.

What Is Population Health?

Population health is an emerging discipline that draws on the intersection between many fields, including public health and policy, medical and clinical care, economics, healthcare administration, biostatistics, environmental science, social and psychological sciences, and more. As a result, the definition of population health continues to evolve. For the purposes of this text, it is important to be grounded in common definitions as a reference point.

The most commonly accepted definition of population health was first introduced by David Kindig in 2003: the "distribution of health outcomes within a population, the health determinates that influence this distribution, and the policies and interventions that affect the determinants" (Kindig & Stoddart, 2003). When describing activities that are more focused on clinical populations and a narrower set of health outcomes, the term *population health management* is used because it implies that interventions will be used to mitigate the impact of health determinants on health outcomes (Kindig, 2015). The term refers to the process of improving clinical health outcomes of a defined group of individuals through targeted interventions supported by appropriate financial and care models (American Hospital Association, 2020).

Inherent in this definition of population health is that many sources of health determinants reflect the way that people live their lives and make choices and the systems, communities, and environments in which they live and grow. Health determinants are vast and include things such as individual characteristics and behaviors; social, economic, and environmental influences; access to health care; the quality and delivery of healthcare services; public health; and governmental policy and more. In fact, only an estimated 20% of health outcomes are impacted by clinical care; the remaining 80% are determined by factors other than healthcare delivery (Givens, Gennuso, Jovaag, van Dijk, & Johnson, 2019). Population health outcomes can be improved by understanding the determinants and working to mitigate their negative impact on health outcomes.

The Triple Aim

In a world of limited healthcare resources, a critical component of population health is understanding how the most health return can be produced from the next dollar invested such as expanding clinical services or enhancing health benefits (Kindig, 2015). The term *Triple Aim* refers to the simultaneous pursuit of improving the patient experience of care, improving the health of populations, and reducing the per capita cost of health care (**Figure 2.1**). The Triple Aim components are not interdependent and form a single

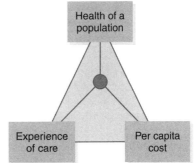

Figure 2.1 The Triple Aim.

The IHI Triple Aim framework was developed by the Institute for Healthcare Improvement in Boston, Massachusetts (www.ihi.org).

aim with three dimensions; changes in any one of the components can impact the other two negatively or positively (Berwick et al., 2008). The Triple Aim is achieved by providing care that is safe, effective, patient centered, efficient, timely, and equitable (Institute of Medicine, 2001).

Evidence-Based Practice (EBP)

Population health management follows a structured process that is built on an evidence-based practice (EBP) framework. Before describing the population health process, it is important to understand EBP's basic principles and process.

EBP is the conscientious, explicit, and judicious use of the best evidence available to make decisions about the care of patients and populations (Sackett, Rosenberg, Gray, Haynes, & Richardson, 2007). EBP follows a structured process whereby a question is asked of data in the form of an identified problem in practice or, in the case of population health, a determination of a health care need in a segment of the population. For example, a population health assessment may determine that there is a high prevalence of diabetes in a population with a subset of those with

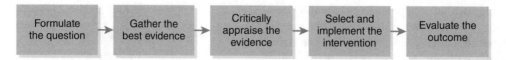

Figure 2.2 The EBP Process.

diabetes using more health care. The question asked of the data may be, "What are the drivers of high healthcare utilization in this subset of people with diabetes?" Data are analyzed to determine drivers, and the problem is identified. In this hypothetical example, the driver of high healthcare utilization is a subset of people with diabetes having hospital admissions for complications related to diabetes, including nonhealing foot ulcers and kidney failure.

Evidence is then gathered to address the problem by searching the literature for ways to prevent acute events in people with diabetic complications, determining clinicians' recommendations, and assessing patients' goals, needs, and receptivity to new ways of managing their illness. The accumulation of evidence is used to develop interventions and deliver them to targeted patients within the population. In this example, patients with diabetes who are at high risk for a future hospitalization may be segmented and encouraged to engage in appropriate interventions derived from the evidence-gathering process. The EBP process culminates in an evaluation of the outcomes in which the intervention was intended to impact.

Various models of EBP lay out similar processes for its execution. **Figure 2.2** shows one such step-by-step process for using EBP to improve patient outcomes.

The Population Health Process

Just as having a common definition of population health is important, it is also useful to follow a standardized process when approaching population health. Population health management is a structured and standardized process that aligns with an EBP approach. The process is followed through a series of phases that achieves the goal of improving outcomes. **Figure 2.3** summarizes the phase and milestones of the population health process.

Assess

The first phase of the process is *assess*. Understanding the health determinants that are impacting health outcomes is important. The assess phase begins with an exploration of the health determinants within a population from an analytical, clinical, and business perspective, also referred to as the PopHealth Troika (PHT)™ of the clinician, analyst, and business expert. See Chapter 31, "Building a Team Culture for Population Health," for details on PHT™. The end goal is to gain insights into the relationship between health determinants and health outcomes in a population of patients that can lead

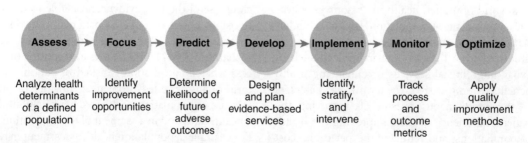

Figure 2.3 The Population Health Process.

© ForestVue Healthcare Solutions.

to opportunities to improve health and reduce poor health outcomes (Sylvia, 2020).

Focus

The next phase of the process is *focus* in which information from the assess phase is further synthesized by the PHT™ to identify impactful relationships between health determinants and health outcomes in smaller subgroupings of the population. More attention is given to cost and utilization drivers within the subgrouping and the relationship to health-improvement opportunities. The PHT™ works together in this phase to make recommendations for addressing identified opportunities in actionable subgroupings of the population. A comprehensive population health assessment is a written and oral presentation of the assess and focus phases using storytelling techniques to disseminate and gather stakeholder support for addressing these opportunities (Sylvia, 2020).

Predict

In the *predict* phase, a method of predicting the likelihood or the estimate of poor outcomes based on health determinants is identified. Predictive analytics use the insights from the assess and focus phases to determine the important predictor or explanatory variables that will be used to predict an unknown future adverse outcome like cost or utilization. For example, age, gender, geography, chronic conditions, frailty, and other health determinants could be used to predict the patient-level probability that a hospitalization will occur or the estimated costs per patient in an upcoming year. These patient-level estimates are applied in the intervention phase to create lists of patients who are amenable to intervention and prioritize them for action (Sylvia, 2020).

Develop

During the *develop* phase, interventions are created with the specific needs of the defined population in mind and informed by previous phases. Information about the drivers of outcomes is used to determine which intervention will be implemented and is usually determined by a team of stakeholders, including business, clinical, and analytic leaders. For example, to address the impact of medication adherence on healthcare costs, a medication therapy monitoring program may be developed to improve adherence and reduce costs. Once an intervention is chosen, development focuses on creating the workflow needed to implement this change and includes identification and targeting of patients; outreaching, enrolling, and engaging patients; executing intervention components; and developing monitoring metrics and outcomes along with target values for the results. Development also encompasses information technology systems. The developed workflow needs to be translated and configured into the systems that will be used to document and interact with patients (Sylvia, 2020).

Note that development encompasses all types of interventions—not only clinical interventions. For instance, in the medication adherence example, an intervention could be to simply amend a policy with the goal of removing the burden of patient copayments for important medications.

Implement

All of the work in the previous phases culminates in the *implement* phase, where interventions are put into action. The risk-prediction model is put into action, usually in the form of an algorithm, to identify and stratify and then to prioritize patients for intervention. During this phase, risk-prediction models and algorithms are made operational by integrating them into the systems where outreach and clinician transactions are taking place, which is often the electronic medical record. At the same time, workflows and intervention processes involving the interaction between staff and patients are also made operational. The beginning of the implement phase is considered a period of ramp-up, where it is expected that glitches in the transition from development to operations will need to be addressed. Fully functional operations may be realized anywhere from 3 to 9 months after interventions are initiated (Sylvia, 2020).

Monitor

As the intervention progresses from initiation to steady state, monitoring takes place to ensure that the intervention is being delivered as intended and that progress is being made toward achieving desired outcomes. During this phase, all stakeholders have a role in reviewing and interpreting reports about the interventions. Staff working on the frontlines of the intervention and directly with patients are monitoring reports focused on the numbers of patients who are receiving the intervention and whether the cohorts are directly responsible for receiving each component. Managers and directors are analyzing reports of the entire cohort eligible for the intervention to ensure that targets for enrollment and engagement are achieved and that patients, once engaged, are receiving the intended intervention components. Executive-level leaders are monitoring process and outcomes metrics on a regular basis for the overall intervention to ensure targets are achieved (Sylvia, 2020).

Optimize

Optimization in the population health process means achieving the best possible outcomes for a given population. Daily management is the overarching philosophy of quality improvement whereby optimization is achieved through incremental changes in the day-to-day work done to meet the needs of individuals and populations and consists of daily improvement and control. *Improvement* is the continuous quest of uncovering work process improvement opportunities to enhance effectiveness, efficiency, productivity, and timely services. *Control* involves using monitoring metrics and actively ensuring that the population health interventions are running as planned (Moran & Duffy, 2009). Desired outcomes are achieved when processes are optimized (Donabedian, 1980). Optimization is achieved through the collaboration of the multiple stakeholders monitoring population health interventions and working collectively to execute a program of daily management.

Population Health Analytics

Each phase of the population health process has a set of primary analytic techniques, methods, and outputs that are used to accomplish the stepwise goals. This section describes the analytics used for each phase of the population health process. **Figure 2.4** summarizes the analytics used in each phase.

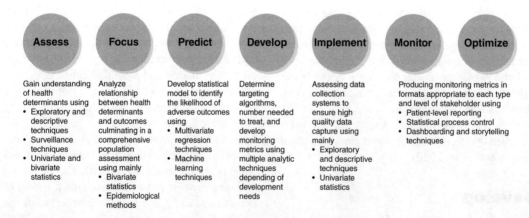

Figure 2.4 Analytic Support for the Population Health Process.

Assess Phase Analytics

Analytics in the assess phase are mainly exploratory at the onset and evolve into examining the relationship between health determinants and health outcomes of interest. The assess phase starts in a large population with an examination of available data points that represent determinants of health and include demographic variables such as age and geographic location; social and financial variables such as health insurance, employment, and financial status; clinical variables like chronic condition categorizations, medication adherence markers, or indicators of illness severity; health system and access variables such as site and providers of care; indicators of having received preventive care; healthcare utilization variables like hospitalizations, readmissions, and emergency department visits; and indicators of the quality of care. The exploration of these variables uses simple graphical display of distributions and reporting of percentages and averages and is reviewed by the triad of the analyst, clinician, and business team leading to interpretations about the relationship between health determinants and health outcomes.

The review of exploratory data leads to identifying smaller subgroupings of the larger population based on the findings within the larger population. At this point, the same exploratory variables are used to create the smaller subgroupings. Further analysis of variables is done in the smaller identified subgroupings and leads to opportunities to improve outcomes and into the next phase of population health analytics, which is *focus*. A substantial amount of time is spent in the assess phase of population health analytics to allow for multiple perspectives and examination of the data (Sylvia, 2020).

Focus Phase Analytics

Analytics in the *focus* phase examine the relationship between health determinants and health outcomes with the goal of settling on a set of recommendations based on the findings. At this point, the analysis is focused on a subgroup of interest and focusing on those indicators that have the most impact on utilization, cost, and quality and for which there are feasible interventions. To understand the magnitude and impact of these relationships, comparisons of determinants and outcomes can be made between similar subgroupings or the larger population.

In this phase, proportions and means between groups are compared and, when appropriate, statistical tests can be used to determine whether the differences are statistically significant. In addition, evidence from journals, professional and government organizations, and other sources is reviewed to put findings in context and determine feasible interventions.

All the analyses performed during this and the assess phase are reviewed for their relevance and ability to make the case for addressing opportunities recommended by the team triad. The chosen analyses culminate in the population health assessment that is used to disseminate the findings to a broader audience to get stakeholder and clinician buy-in for moving further through the population health process with identified opportunities (Sylvia, 2020).

Predict Phase Analytics

Analytics in the predict phase are focused on the development or selection of risk-prediction models that will ultimately be used in the intervention. The information gleaned during the assess and focus phases, which culminate in the population assessment, is used to create predictor and outcome variables that are tailored to the intervention. In this phase, analytic capability is required for population identification, development of prediction variables, longitudinal data analysis, complex statistical computations, model validation, and the ability to transition a developed model into operations. Whether developing in-house or using market solutions, the end result of this phase is a tested and validated risk-prediction model that can be used in the implementation phase to select and stratify patients who are appropriate for intervention (Sylvia, 2020).

Development Phase Analytics

During the development phase, analytic needs vary depending on the planned intervention, although all analytics that are performed support the development of the intervention. In this phase, analytics are used to support identification and targeting and include analyses to determine the number of people needed in the intervention to achieve the desired outcome in the entire population. Process and outcome metrics are also developed during this phase and are based on the ability of the intervention to improve health determinants and their impact on health outcomes identified in the assess and focus phases (Sylvia, 2020).

Implement Phase Analytics

Analytic functions during the *implement* phase are first focused on ensuring that the analytics that were made operational are working as intended. Identification and risk-stratification models are analyzed to ensure that the right patients are associated with the right interventions. Workflow is analyzed to determine whether the patient flow to interventions works in practice in the same way it did in the development phase. Another important analytic function in the implementation phase is the initial data collection for monitoring metrics. In the initial stages of implementation, analysts determine that timely, accurate, and complete data are collected to ensure that numerators and denominators for monitoring metrics are collected and designed in a way that makes them readily available for ongoing monitoring (Sylvia, 2020).

Monitor and Optimize Phase Analytics

Analytics during the *monitor* and *optimize* phases produce patient-level reporting and dashboards used to track key program process and outcome metrics defined in the development phase. The design for reporting metrics is tailored to the information needed at each level and type of stakeholder for the intervention. Patient-level reports, dashboards, run charts, statistical process control, and benchmarking are used for ongoing monitoring of population health intervention metrics. These methodologies allow for a continuous quality-management feedback loop where data are continuously analyzed, compared to expectations, and used by quality-improvement teams for continuous improvement of ongoing program processes (Sylvia, 2020).

Analytic Capabilities

In addition to framing analytics within a population health framework, it is important to be able to describe and demonstrate analytic capabilities within an organization and to be able to assess and understand the ability to operationally perform the required analytics for each phase of the population health process.

Using varied terminology like *analytic maturity*, *analytics adoption*, and *analytics ascendency*, multiple frameworks exist to define and measure analytic capacity within a healthcare organization. Although the frameworks have different names, the domains used to make a measured determination of capability are similar and include organizational culture, data content, infrastructure, processes, functions, and analytic products.

The impact of organizational culture on the extent of analytic capabilities cannot be understated. When organizations value data-driven decision-making, analytic capabilities naturally mature. Robust organizational culture with thriving analytic capabilities is evidenced by expectations for fact-based decision-making, an openness to poor and positive results, and ensuring analytic skill sets and knowledge in all employees from executives to frontline clinicians (Duncan & Howson, 2016). Organizations with high levels of analytic capabilities create and implement an analytic strategy that lays out the roadmap for decisions about how an organization uses its data to take action, including the selection of analytic opportunities and the integration of analytic operations, infrastructure, and models to achieve its mission and vision (Grossman, 2018).

Data content includes the extent to which the organization can integrate and capitalize on all the necessary and available sources of data for analytic purposes. This includes the ability to manage large volumes, high velocities, and numerous varieties of data (Halper & Stodder, 2014). Healthcare organizations that can use the data within all their internal transactional systems as well as bring in pertinent external sources of data and exchange data with partners have greater analytic capabilities.

Analytic infrastructure refers to tools, services, applications, and platforms that support analytic processes, supporting the constellation of analytic products from simple reports to data models, to estimating and validating models that diagnose conditions, predict adverse outcomes, or prescribe action. Examples of analytic infrastructure include databases, data warehouses, statistical and data-mining systems, scoring engines, grids (computers that interact to coordinate data processing) and cloud data storage (Grossman, 2009). The best analytic infrastructure uses standards-based procedures for data processing; appropriately applies technology like grids and cloud-based services to support large volumes, high velocities, and numerous varieties of data; supports analytics for the entirety of the organization; is nimble in the ability to support new and innovative analytic undertakings; and fully integrates systems data (Grossman, 2009; Halper & Stodder, 2014).

Analytic processes are used to build data infrastructure as well as create meaning from data and encompasses data-management functions of processing, storing, quality management, and access to data. Criteria used to measure capabilities include the extent to which processes are defined, standardized, and controlled; analytic needs and priorities are met; data-governance structure, policies, compliance, stewardship are developed and functioning; analytic project management is agile; metadata are robust and ensure accurate understanding; training is provided for data content, tools, and infrastructure;

and risks and opportunities are balanced when making decisions that impact analytic capabilities (Duncan & Howson, 2016; Halper & Stodder, 2014).

Capability Models

The most referenced analytic capability models measure analytic advancements in terms of the functional needs met by analytics and the analytic outputs or products that are possible, which incorporate aspects of organizational culture, data content, analytic infrastructure, and processes. The healthcare analytics adoption model is a framework for healthcare organizations to measure their progress toward analytic adoption, understand the level of analytics adoption in health care overall, evaluate vendor-based solutions, and most important for the purposes of this text, provide a reference point for presenting the many aspects of population health analytics.

The healthcare analytics adoption model consists of eight levels that progress from 0 (lowest) to 8 (highest) in terms of expanding data content, increasing data timeliness, broadening data governance, and sophistication and complexity of processes and outputs (Sanders et al., 2013). Note that even though analytic adoption is measured in a hierarchical fashion, it is commonly and well understood that healthcare organizations can demonstrate and even realize value at higher levels of the scale while still not yet achieving full capacity in lower levels of the scale. For example, a healthcare organization may be able to develop and use a predictive model based on electronic medical records even as data from the records are not yet organized in a data warehouse.

The Analytics Capabilities Model simplifies analytic capabilities into four advancing categories: descriptive, diagnostic, predictive, and prescriptive. Analytic capabilities advance as they move from measuring and describing what happened to diagnosing why something happened to predicting what is likely to happen to optimizing or prescribing what should happen (Sallam & Cearley, 2012). **Figure 2.5** describes the questions asked of the data in each layer

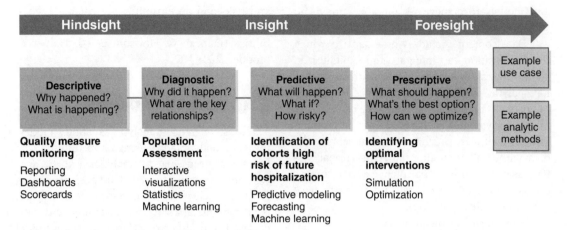

Figure 2.5 The Analytics Capabilities Model.

Data from Sallam, R. L., & Cearley, D. W. (2012). Advanced Analytics: Predictive, Collaborative and Pervasive. Gartner.

along with example methods and a population health-based use case. Like assessing capabilities in the healthcare analytics adoption model, healthcare organizations can be performing in all layers of the model without necessarily optimizing each layer. In addition, it is not required that organizations delay higher-level capabilities until achieving optimal performance in lower levels.

Conclusion

The goal of population health is to improve the overall health and well-being of populations. Population health frameworks assist in translating population health evidence-based concepts into easy-to-understand categories of stakeholders, activities, and methods. Across the frameworks called out in this chapter, analytics can be found within each and is often described as one of the most critical components of population health. However, the details of when, how, and why to use analytics to support population health projects is a gap. The ForestVue Population Health Implementation and Analytics Framework closes the analytic gap and provides a step-by-step process to guide population health teams to successfully identify opportunities and interventions that positively affect health outcomes.

The phases of assess and focus bring forward the opportunity for a variety of analytics to be performed, assisting the population health team in understanding the needs of their defined populations, assessing the magnitude of the healthcare problem to solve, and narrowing the opportunities identified into discrete actionable opportunities that can be addressed. The phases of predict and develop incorporate advanced analytic methodologies such as predictive analytics, machine learning, and big data. These phases enable population health and care teams to identify patients with rising and high risk with significant time in advance to intervene so as to avoid unplanned or unnecessary healthcare services. The implementation phase brings forward statistical rigor, data governance, and analytic methodologies that tailor the models and algorithms to best suit the care team, workflows, and patient behaviors. The monitor and optimize phases create the opportunity to track progress and convey results to individuals, management, executives, and the community and culminates in the analytic development of dashboards and metrics that incorporate data capabilities of data storytelling and visualization.

The healthcare analytics adoption model is provided to enable an analytics maturity journey for organizations and individuals seeking to deploy population health in their organizations and body of work. Meant to provide a set of expectations for organizations to guide their analytic advancement, the model also sets a standard for what is possible for organizations that may have not yet accomplished all capabilities listed.

Study and Discussion Questions

- Compare and contrast other population health frameworks to ForestVue's Population Health Implementation and Analytics Framework. What is similar? Different?
- Why is a population health framework for analytics important for advancing the discipline?

- What are examples of frameworks from other industries that rely on analytics, and how do they compare to the one outlined in this chapter?

Resources and Websites

DEEP. (n.d.). What is an analytic framework? https://deephelp.zendesk.com/hc/en-us/articles/360006969651-What-is-an-Analytical-Framework-

NHS Providers. (2019, June). Population health framework for healthcare providers. https://nhsproviders.org/population-health-framework

Sakrab, S., & Elgamma, A. (2016). Towards a comprehensive data analytics framework for smart healthcare service. *Big Data Research, 4*, 44–58. https://doi.org/10.1016/j.bdr.2016.05.002

References

American Hospital Association. (2020). Population health management. https://www.aha.org/center/population-health/population-health-management

Berwick, D. M., Nolan, T. W., & Whittington, J. (2008). The Triple Aim: Care, health, and cost. *Health Affairs, 27*(3), 759–769. https://doi.org/10.1377/hlthaff.27.3.759

Donabedian, A. (1980). *Basic approaches to assessment: Structure, process, and outcome.* Health Administration Press.

Duncan, A. D., & Howson, C. (2016). IT score for BI and analytics. Gartner Research. https://www.gartner.com/en/documents/3136418/itscore-overview-for-bi-and-analytics

Givens, M., Gennuso, K., Jovaag, A., van Dijk, J. W., & Johnson, S. (2019). 2019 county health rankings key findings report. University of Wisconsin Population Health Institute. www.countyhealthrankings.org

Grossman, R. L. (2009). What is analytic infrastructure and why should you care? *ACM SIGKDD Explorations Newsletter, 11*(1). https://doi.org/10.1145/1656274.1656277

Grossman, R. L. (2018). A framework for evaluating the analytic maturity of an organization. *International Journal of Information Management, 38*(1), 45–51. https://doi.org/10.1016/j.ijinfomgt.2017.08.005

Halper, F., & Stodder, D. (2014). *TDWI analytics maturity model guide.* Transforming Data with Intelligence. https://tdwi.org/whitepapers/2014/10/tdwi-analytics-maturity-model-guide.aspx

Institute for Healthcare Improvement. (n.d.). Pathways to population health framework. https://populationhealthalliance.org/research/understanding-population-health/

Institute of Medicine. (2001). *Crossing the quality chasm: A new health System for the 21st Century.* National Academy Press. https://pubmed.ncbi.nlm.nih.gov/25057539/

Kindig, D. A. (2015, April 6). What are we talking about when we talk about population health? Institute for Healthcare Improvement. http://www.ihi.org/about/news/Pages/WhatAreWeTalkingAboutWhenWeTalkAboutPopulationHealth.aspx

Kindig, D., & Stoddart, G. (2003). What is population health? *American Journal of Public Health, 93*(3), 380–383. https://ajph.aphapublications.org/doi/10.2105/AJPH.93.3.380

Magnusson, D. M., Eisenhart, M., Gorman, I., Kennedy, V. K., & Davenport, T. E. (2019). Adopting population health frameworks in physical therapist practice, research, and education: The urgency of now. *Physical Therapy, 99*(8), 1039–1047.

Moran, J. W., & Duffy, G. L. (2009). Daily management. Pp. 1–14 in R. Bialek & G. L. Duffy (Eds.), *The public health quality improvement handbook*. American Society for Quality.

Population Health Alliance. (n.d.). PHA framework. https://populationhealthalliance.org/research/understanding-population-health/

Sackett, D. L., Rosenberg, W. M., Gray, J. A., Haynes, R. B., & Richardson, W. S. (1996, February). Evidence based medicine: What it is and what it isn't. *Clinical Orthopaedics and Related Research, 455,* 3–5. https://pubmed.ncbi.nlm.nih.gov/8555924/

Sallam, R. L., & Cearley, D. W. (2012, February 16). *Advanced Analytics: Predictive, Collaborative and Pervasive.* Gartner Research.

Sanders, D., Burton, D. A., & Protti, D. (2013). *The healthcare analytics adoption model: A framework and roadmap* [White paper]. Health Catalyst. https://downloads.healthcatalyst.com/wp-content/uploads/2013/11/analytics-adoption-model-Nov-2013.pdf

Sylvia, M. (2020). Introduction to population health analytics. In *Population Health Management Learning Series.* ForestVue Healthcare Solutions.

SECTION II

Data Sources

CHAPTER 3

Medical Administrative Claims Data for Population Health Analytics

Martha Sylvia, PhD, MBA, RN

Administrative data related to health insurance claims [are] extremely powerful for driving improvements in population health to address issues related to cost, quality, and outcomes.

—National Rural Health Resource Center (2020)

EXECUTIVE SUMMARY

Medical claims data are among the earliest sources of healthcare data used for population health analytics and remain some of the most common sources for gaining a comprehensive, longitudinal view of the health status and outcomes of populations. Medical claims data are considered a secondary source of data for population health analytics because their primary purpose is to collect payment for medical services. However, such data are rich with information about the diagnoses assigned to patients, the healthcare services used for treatment of medical conditions, the providers of healthcare services, patterns of healthcare service use by patients and prescribed by providers, and costs. These data can be used in isolation or in combination with other data sources in an analytic program to support population health management.

LEARNING OBJECTIVES

At the end of this chapter, the learner will be able to:

1. Explain the value of medical claims data for population health analytics.
2. Compare and contrast coding systems used in billing for medical services.
3. Use medical claims data to answer questions of importance to population health management.

Introduction

Medical claims data are generated from the provision of healthcare services to patients seeking those services. Any service that is eligible to receive payment is billed by healthcare facilities and providers. In the United States, the major routes for people to receive health insurance is through employers or through government programs such as Medicare, Medicaid, and the Veterans Benefits Administration. Once a person has health insurance from one of these payers, the payer receives all of the medical claims data for that person as long as they remain insured. This results in a rich source of information about people and their health status over considerable time trajectories.

This chapter describes the life cycle of medical claims data from its origin at the site of care delivery to its ability to be used for population health analytics. The coding systems used in medical claims data are explained in the context of their purpose for understanding clinically related health determinants and outcomes. For the purposes of this textbook, *medical claims data* refer to that which is collected from the process of billing for virtually all medical healthcare services. In terms of population health analytics, medical claims data are considered secondary data with their intended primary purpose of use to bill payers for healthcare services.

Life Cycle of Medical Claims Data

Medical claims data go through a multitude of steps before they can become a source of data used for population health analytics. **Figure 3.1** depicts this process, which starts with a patient accessing

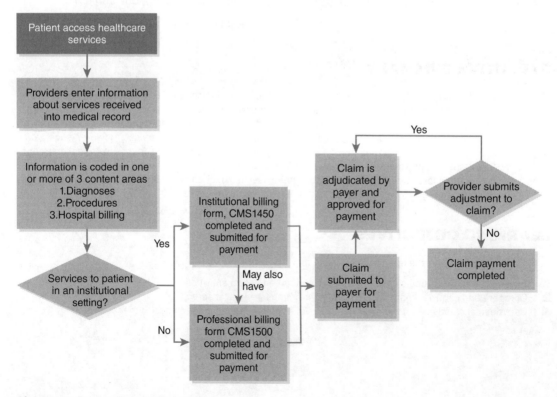

Figure 3.1 Medical Claim Billing Process.

some type of healthcare service administered by a healthcare provider who is authorized to receive payment from the Centers for Medicare and Medicaid Services (CMS) or a private insurer for the provided services. To bill for the services provided to the patient, a provider must document the diagnoses for which the patient was seen and the service that was provided. Provider documentation does not have to be in any format as long as it can be translated into one of the required coding systems. Healthcare organizations usually have staff who are trained in the compliant coding systems and will translate the provider and other documentation to the appropriate codes for diagnoses and procedures.

Two types of billing forms are submitted for payment, depending on where services are performed. An *institutional provider* refers to a hospital; skilled nursing facility; end-stage renal disease providers; home health agencies; hospice organizations; outpatient physical therapy, occupational therapy, and speech pathology services; comprehensive outpatient rehabilitation facilities; community mental health centers; critical access hospitals; federally qualified health centers; histocompatibility laboratories; Indian Health Service facilities; organ procurement organizations; religious nonmedical healthcare institutions; and rural health clinics (CMS, 2018b).

Institutional billing is completed using the CMS 1450 form (also known as the *UB04 form*). In addition to diagnoses and procedures, the institutional billing forms require hospital uniform billing codes. Services provided in noninstitutional settings or by noninstitutional affiliated providers within an institution use the professional billing CMS 1500 form. Form details and information contained within them are discussed in the next section.

Once the claim form is completed, it is submitted (usually electronically) for payment to the payer, usually CMS, a private health insurance company, a managed care organization, or an organization managing payments on the behalf of a self-insured company. Once received,

the payer decides to pay the claim by applying rules to the information contained in the claim form. These rules are based on compliance with healthcare regulations, benefit allowances, and others.

On occasion, a previously submitted claim for payment needs adjustment, especially when services are provided over multiple days in an institutional setting. For example, a patient may be in the hospital for a week, which may overlap a hospital billing cycle; in such a case, the same claim would have billing in two different time periods. In addition, when services are provided in an institutional setting, the claim is reviewed at the completion of services to ensure accuracy, with any changes resulting in an adjustment to the claims submission.

If there are no adjustments to the claim, it is considered completed. At this point, claims data reside in a transactional system and are not available for analysis. A process must be completed to move the data to a proper environment and model to facilitate analysis. This process of moving the data for analysis purposes is different and unique for each payer.

Although this process uses the framework of fee-for-service claims payment, a similar process is used when providers are paid under capitated arrangements or when one payment is provided for a group or bundle of services. In this scenario, claims are submitted in the same fashion but are not paid on an individual claim basis. These types of claims can be referred to as *encounters*.

Data Points Collected in Billing Forms

Two types of forms are used to submit bills for medical payment. The CMS 1450 or UB 04 form is used to submit for institutional services, and the CMS 1500 form is used to submit for professional billing. The forms contain a great deal of useful information used in population health (**Table 3.1**).

Table 3.1 Billing form Data Points Relevant for Population Health Analytics

Data Point	1430-UB04 Institutional	1500 Professional
Patient name, address, birthdate	X	X
Billing provider name, address, phone number, national provider identifier (NPI)	X	X
Attending provider name and identifiers using NPI	X	O
Other providers' names and identifiers using NPI	X	O
Rendering provider NPI	O	X
Type of bill code	X	O
Beginning and end service dates	X	X
Beginning and end admission and start of care dates and hour	X	O
Priority type for admission	X	O
Referral source for admission	X	O
Patient discharge disposition	X	O
Revenue code and description	X	O
Place of service	O	X
CPT and HCPCS code for outpatient ancillary services	X	X
Number of service units	X	X
Total charges	X	X
Principal diagnosis code using ICD-10-CM	X	X
Other diagnosis codes using ICD-10-CM	X	X
Admitting diagnosis code using ICD-10-CM	X	O
Principal procedure code using ICD-10-PCS	X	O

X = Data point is contained in the form.
O = Data point is not contained in the form.
Centers for Medicare and Medicaid Services. (2018b). Medicare billing: Form CMS-1450 and the 837 institutional print-friendly version. https://www.cms.gov/Outreach-and-Education/Medicare-Learning-Network-MLN/MLNProducts/Downloads/837I-FormCMS-1450-ICN006926.pdf

Coding Systems Used for Medical Claims Data

This section covers coding systems with medical billing that are often used to determine population health indicators and create analyses relevant to answering questions of interest in population health management. Diagnoses codes lead to an understanding of condition prevalence, illness burden, and expectation of health outcomes. Procedures performed help us to determine health system factors, such as appropriate and inappropriate treatment for certain conditions and whether conditions are left untreated. Determining the setting in which healthcare is delivered through revenue and place of service coding leads to initiatives that direct people to appropriate care settings. The type of bill is important to know because an analysis may or may not include certain types of claims such as voided or corrected claims.

International Classification of Diseases, 10th Revision, Clinical Modification (ICD-10-CM)

The *International Classification of Diseases*, 10th revision (ICD-10-CM), is a morbidity classification published in the United States for classifying diagnoses and reason for visits in all healthcare settings. The National Center for Health Statistics and CMS publish guidelines in how to use the ICD-10-CM for coding and reporting.

The ICD-10-CM coding system offers a deep understanding of the complexity of illness because it reveals the etiology or manifestation of the condition using inclusion and exclusion criteria, complications of a condition, whether a condition is acute or chronic, whether the condition is impending or threatened, sequela of a condition, and the body system that is affected. For instance, a skin infection can manifest from an insect bite, an abrasion injury, or another source and can occur on the back, leg, or other location. In addition, signs and symptoms and abnormal laboratory findings that are not yet a medical diagnosis can also be coded (CMS, 2019b).

There are more than 70,000 ICD-10-CM codes. Codes can be three to seven digits in length; if longer than three digits, a decimal point is added after the third digit. The first digit is alpha, the second is numeric, and digits 3 to 7 can be alpha or numeric. The first three digits refer to the category of the diagnosis; for

instance, *cardiomyopathy* is represented by the first three digits of "I42." The code "I42.0" represents "Dilated cardiomyopathy," thus digits 3 to 7 provide more detail by adding digits to the code. Detailed information for ICD-10-CM codes can be found on the CMS website (https://www .cms.gov/Medicare/Coding/ICD10/2020-ICD -10-CM.html). As many as 18 diagnosis codes per each 1450 billing form and 12 diagnosis codes per each 1500 billing form diagnosis can be submitted. The assignment of a diagnosis code is based on the provider's diagnostic statement that the condition exists. The code assignment is not based on clinical criteria used by the provider to establish the diagnosis (CMS, 2019b).

International Classification of Diseases, 10th revision, Procedure Coding System (ICD-10-PCS)

The *International Classification of Diseases*, 10th revision, *Procedure Coding System* (ICD-10-PCS) is a procedure classification published by the United States for classifying procedures performed in hospital inpatient healthcare settings. The Healthcare Common Procedure Code System (HCPCS) (described in the next section) are used for settings other than inpatient.

ICD-10-PCS codes are composed of seven characters with each character placement indicating an aspect of the procedure performed. One of 34 possible values can be assigned to each character placement in the seven-character code: the numbers 0 through 9 and the alphabet except for I and O. The spectrum of numbers and alphabet used varies, depending on the information provided in that placeholder. The meaning of any single value is a combination of its placement and dependency on the preceding values. See **Table 3.2**. **Figure 3.2** displays an example of ICD-10-PCS coding for a stomach bypass procedure.

Table 3.2 ICD-10-PCS Character Placement Descriptions

	Title	Description	Information About Possible Values
1	Section	The general type of procedure; e.g., medical and surgical, obstetrics, etc.	Values can be 0–9 or B, C, D, F, G, H, X
2	Body system	The system in the body in which the procedure takes place; e.g., endocrine, gastrointestinal	Dependent on value of Section; can be any combination of 0–9 or A–Z except for I and O
3	Root operation	The objective of the procedure; e.g., incision, insertion, inspection	Dependent on value of Section and Body system with 31 different possible values
4	Body part	The body part within a particular body system on which the procedure is performed; e.g., esophagus, stomach	Values represent different body parts dependent on the value of Section and Body system
5	Approach	Techniques used to reach the site of the procedure	Seven techniques are dependent on three components: (1) *Access location*—the external site through which an internal body part is reached. (2) *Method*—how the external access location is entered. (3) *Type of instrumentation*—specialized equipment used to perform the procedure.
6	Device	The devices that remain after the procedure is completed.	Four general types of devices remain after the procedure is completed: (1) *Grafts and prostheses* (2) *Implants* (3) *Simple mechanical appliances* (4) *Electronic appliances* No Device
7	Qualifier	Unique values used for individual procedures as needed.	

Centers for Medicare and Medicaid Services. (2020). ICD-10 procedure coding system (ICD-10-PCS): 2020 tables and index. https://www.cms.gov/Medicare/Coding/ICD10/2020-ICD-10-PC

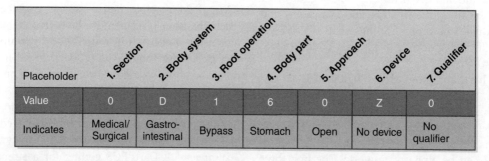

Figure 3.2 Example of ICD-10-PCS Code with Placeholder and Indicators of Values.

Healthcare Common Procedure Coding System (HCPCS)

The HCPCS is divided into two principal subsystems: level I and level II. Level I of the HCPCS is primarily a numeric coding system called *current procedural terminology* (CPT) and maintained by the American Medical Association (AMA). Identifying medical services and procedures by healthcare providers outside the hospital setting use the CPT (CMS, 2019a).

Level I HCPCS Codes

CPT codes fall into three categories. Category I are five-digit numerical codes that are reviewed annually and are mandatory to report for services and reimbursement. More than 7,000 codes with titles and modifiers range between values 00100 and 99499. Codes are selected based on a section such as "surgery," a subsection such as "cardiovascular system," and any provided guidelines for the section and subsection selection. In this example, codes 33010 to 37799 represent codes for "surgery" and "cardiovascular system," with selection of the specific code depending on provided guidelines (CMS, 2019a).

Category II CPT codes are in alphanumeric format with the letter "F" in the last position. These codes are optional and are for tracking performance measurements for CMS and other payer quality reporting programs. For example, the code 4013F indicates that a provider counseled a patient regarding statin therapy for coronary artery disease. This code would be submitted along with the appropriate level office visit category I CPT code 99211–99215. The AMA lists the criteria for these codes on its website: https://www.ama-assn.org/practice-management/cpt/category-ii-codes (American Medical Association [AMA], 2019).

Category III CPT codes are temporary codes for emerging technologies, services, and procedures created by the AMA with a "T" in the last position; they do not need to be reported with an additional category I code. For example, code 0559T is used to bill for a procedure to create a 3D-printed anatomic model. These codes are updated twice each year, and details can be found on the AMA website: https://www.ama-assn.org/practice-management/cpt/category-iii-codes.

Level II HCPCS Codes

Level II of the HCPCS is a standardized coding system documented by CMS that is used to bill for products, supplies, and services not included in the CPT code set; examples include ambulance services and durable medical equipment (DME), prosthetics, orthotics, and supplies when used outside of a provider's office. Level II codes comprise an alpha first digit and four following numerical digits. Level II HCPCS codes are considered temporary by CMS in that if another code becomes permanently available to represent the service, the existing temporary level II code is retired (CMS, 2018a).

"G" codes are an important set of codes to understand for use in population health analytics because they can be used to identify services that are often provided in population health management initiatives by ancillary care providers such as nurses and social workers. Examples include the codes G2001–G2013, which are used to represent varying degrees of postdischarge in-home visits, and G2014, which is used to represent the creation of postdischarge care plans.

"C" codes are used to bill for device categories, new technology, procedures, and drugs, biologicals, and radiopharmaceuticals that are not defined by other HCPCS codes. As an example, code C9756 was recently added to represent fluorescence mapping of lymph nodes. Other level II HCPCS codes created for use when another HCPCS code does not exist include "Q" codes for drugs, biologicals, and other medical equipment and services; "K" codes for durable medical equipment; "S" codes primarily used by private insurers to bill for drugs, services, and supplies; "H" codes used by state Medicaid agencies for mental health and alcohol and drug treatment services; and "T" codes, which are also used primarily by state Medicaid agencies (CMS, 2019a).

Updates of HCPCS level II codes are published quarterly by CMS: https://www.cms.gov /Medicare/Coding/HCPCSReleaseCodeSets/HCPCS -Quarterly-Update.html.

Revenue Codes

Revenue codes are used with procedure codes on medical bills for inpatient procedures to indicate where the procedure occurred or what type of procedure occurred. These codes are necessary because many services can happen in more than one setting. In addition, some revenue codes allow for greater specificity around the supply used or procedure performed when the ICD-10-PCS procedure code does not provide enough detail. The amount of payment for a claim depends on the appropriate revenue–procedure code combination.

The National Uniform Billing Committee (NUBC) maintains a list of approved revenue codes for the CMS1450 inpatient billing form. Revenue codes are four-digit numbers; the first digit is typically a zero and therefore ignored in data. The second two digits represent a broad heading such as "operating room services" with the digits of 36; a fourth digit provides more detail. In this example, the revenue code of 0361 represents "operating room services, minor surgery." There are multiple sources for looking up revenue codes electronically; one source is https://www.findacode.com/ub04-revenue/ub04 -revenue-cms-1450-codes-01-group.html (Medical Billing Answers, 2020).

Place-of-Service (POS) Codes

Place-of-service (POS) codes are two-digit codes maintained by CMS and used on professional claims to indicate where a service was performed. There are close to 100 POS codes and include clinical settings as well as nonclinical settings such as community settings, prisons, and schools. Place-of-service codes can be found at

https://www.cms.gov/Regulations-and-Guidance /Guidance/Manuals/Downloads/clm104c26.pdf (CMS, 2018a).

Type-of-Bill Codes

Type-of-bill codes are three-digit codes published by NUBC that describe the type of bill a provider is submitting on an inpatient billing form. The first digit refers to the type of facility such as hospital, skilled nursing, or home health. The second digit depends on the first and is a classification of the bill such as "Inpatient, Medicare Part A," "Inpatient Medicare Part B," or "Subacute Inpatient." The third digit indicates frequency such as "Admit Through Discharge Claim" or "Void or Cancel of Prior Claim or Corrected Claim" (Hicks, 2019).

Common Structure for Medical Claims Data

Once claims are processed for payment, most organizations who are performing population health management functions will transfer claims data from the transactional payment system to a data store. This data store varies, depending on the organization, and is different for each organization. Transactional claims payment systems usually have some sort of method for organizing claims data into a database. An organization that has advanced data warehousing capabilities will clean and arrange medical claims data so that it is accessible in a database with other data sources. At their best, claims data are organized in a data warehouse, integrated with other data sources, and easily accessible for analytics.

Medical claims data are usually organized from its raw form into a data table, with each row representing an individual claim. The data points in the data table are those that are on the billing form along with any additional descriptive information about the claim. There are many examples of data dictionaries for medical claims, and most have similar elements. **Table 3.3** is an example of a data dictionary for Medicare claims provided by CMS.

Table 3.3 Medical Claims Data Table Example

Field Short Name	Label	Description	Type	Length
DSYSRTKY	LDS beneficiary ID	This field contains the key to link data for each beneficiary across all claim files.	NUM	9
CLAIMNO	Claim number	The unique number used to identify a unique claim	NUM	12
THRU_DT	Claim through date (determines year of claim)	The last day on the billing statement covering services rendered to the beneficiary (also known as "Statement Covers Thru Date")	DATE	8
RIC_CD	National claims history near line record identification code	A code defining the type of claim record being processed	CHAR	1
CLM_TYPE	NCH claim type code	The code used to identify the type of claim record being processed in NCH	CHAR	2
DISP_CD	Claim disposition code	Code indicating the disposition or outcome of the processing of the claim record	CHAR	2
CARR_NUM	Carrier number	The identification number assigned by CMS to a carrier authorized to process claims from a physician or supplier. Effective July 2006, the Medicare Administrative Contractors (MACs) began replacing the existing carriers and started processing physician or supplier claim records for states assigned to its jurisdiction.	CHAR	5
PMTDNLCD	Carrier claim payment denial code	The code on a noninstitutional claim indicating to whom payment was made or if the claim was denied.	CHAR	2
PMT_AMT	Claim payment amount	The Medicare claim payment amount.	NUM	12
PRPAYAMT	Carrier claim primary payer paid amount	The amount of a payment made on behalf of a Medicare beneficiary by a primary payer other than Medicare, that the provider is applying to covered Medicare charges on a noninstitutional claim.	NUM	12
RFR_UPIN	Carrier claim referring physician unique physician identification number (UPIN)	UPIN of the physician who referred the beneficiary to the physician who performed the Part B services	CHAR	12

(continues)

Table 3.3 Medical Claims Data Table Example *(continued)*

Field Short Name	Label	Description	Type	Length
RFR_NPI	Carrier claim referring physician national provider identifier (NPI) number	The NPI number of the physician who referred the beneficiary or the physician who ordered the Part B services or durable medical equipment. NPIs replaced UPINs as the standard provider identifiers beginning in 2007. The UPIN is almost never populated after 2009.	CHAR	12
ASGMNTCD	Carrier claim provider assignment indicator switch	Variable indicates whether or not the provider accepts assignment for the noninstitutional claim.	CHAR	1
PROV_PMT	NCH claim provider payment amount	The total payments made to the provider for this claim (sum of line item provider payment amounts) Variable called LINE_PRVDR_PMT_AMT.	NUM	12
BENE_PMT	NCH claim beneficiary payment amount	The total payments made to the beneficiary for this claim (sum of line payment amounts to the beneficiary) Variable called LINE_BENE_PMT_AMT.	NUM	12
SBMTCHRG	NCH carrier claim submitted charge amount	The total submitted charges on the claim (the sum of line item submitted charges) Variable called LINE_SBMTD_CHRG_AMT.	NUM	12
ALOWCHRG	NCH carrier claim allowed charge amount	The total allowed charges on the claim (the sum of line item allowed charges). This variable is the beneficiary's liability under the annual Part B deductible for all line items on the claim; it is the sum of all line-level deductible amounts (variable called LINE_BENE_PTB_DDCTBL_AMT). The Part B deductible applies to both institutional (e.g., HOP) and noninstitutional (e.g., carrier and DME) services.	NUM	12
DEDAPPLY	Carrier claim cash deductible applied amount	The amount of the cash deductible as submitted on the claim. This variable is the beneficiary's liability under the annual Part B deductible for all line items on the claim; it is the sum of all line-level deductible amounts. (variable called LINE_BENE_PTB_DDCTBL_AMT). The Part B deductible applies to both institutional (e.g., HOP) and noninstitutional (e.g., carrier and DME) services.	NUM	12

HCPCS_YR	Carrier claim HCPCS year code	The terminal digit of HCPCS version used to code the claim	CHAR	1
RFR_PRFL	Carrier claim referring PIN number	Carrier-assigned provider ID number of the physician who referred the beneficiary to the physician that performed the Part B services	CHAR	14
PRNCPAL_DGNS_CD	Primary claim diagnosis code	The diagnosis code identifying the diagnosis, condition, problem or other reason for the admission, encounter, or visit shown in the medical record to be chiefly responsible for the services provided. These data also are redundantly stored as the first occurrence of the diagnosis code (variable called ICD_DGNS_CD1).	CHAR	7
PRNCPAL_DGNS_VRSN_CD	Primary claim diagnosis code diagnosis version code (ICD-9 or ICD-10)	Effective with version J, the code used to indicate if the diagnosis is ICD-9 or ICD-10.	CHAR	1
ICD DGNS CD1	Claim diagnosis code I	The diagnosis code identifying the beneficiary's principal or other diagnosis (including E code)	CHAR	7
ICD DGNS VRSN CD1	Claim diagnosis code I diagnosis version code (ICD-9 or ICD-10)	Effective with version J, the code used to indicate if the diagnosis code is ICD-9 or ICD-10	CHAR	1
ICD DGNS CD2	Claim diagnosis code II	The diagnosis code identifying the beneficiary's principal or other diagnosis (including E code)	CHAR	7
ICD DGNS VRSN CD2	Claim diagnosis code II diagnosis version code (ICD-9 or ICD-10)	Effective with version J, the code used to indicate if the diagnosis code is ICD-9 or ICD-10	CHAR	1
ICD DGNS CD3	Claim diagnosis code III	The diagnosis code identifying the beneficiary's principal or other diagnosis (including E code)	CHAR	7
ICD DGNS VRSN CD3	Claim diagnosis code III diagnosis version code (ICD-9 or ICD-10)	Effective with version J, the code used to indicate if the diagnosis code is ICD-9 or ICD-10	CHAR	1
ICD DGNS CD4	Claim diagnosis code IV	The diagnosis code identifying the beneficiary's principal or other diagnosis (including E code)	CHAR	7
ICD DGNS VRSN CD4	Claim diagnosis code IV diagnosis version code (ICD-9 or ICD-10)	Effective with version J, the code used to indicate if the diagnosis code is ICD-9 or ICD-10	CHAR	1

(continues)

Table 3.3 Medical Claims Data Table Example *(continued)*

Field Short Name	Label	Description	Type	Length
ICD DGNS CD5	Claim diagnosis code V	The diagnosis code identifying the beneficiary's principal or other diagnosis (including E code)	CHAR	7
ICD DGNS VRSN CD5	Claim diagnosis code V diagnosis version code (ICD-9 or ICD-10)	Effective with version J, the code used to indicate if the diagnosis code is ICD-9 or ICD-10	CHAR	1
ICD DGNS CD6	Claim diagnosis code VI	The diagnosis code identifying the beneficiary's principal or other diagnosis (including E code)	CHAR	7
ICD DGNS VRSN CD6	Claim diagnosis code VI diagnosis version code (ICD-9 or ICD-10)	Effective with version J, the code used to indicate if the diagnosis code is ICD-9 or ICD-10	CHAR	1
ICD DGNS CD7	Claim diagnosis code VII	The diagnosis code identifying the beneficiary's principal or other diagnosis (including E code)	CHAR	7
ICD DGNS VRSN CD7	Claim diagnosis code VII diagnosis version code (ICD-9 or ICD-10)	Effective with version J, the code used to indicate if the diagnosis code is ICD-9 or ICD-10	CHAR	1
ICD DGNS CD8	Claim diagnosis code VIII	The diagnosis code identifying the beneficiary's principal or other diagnosis (including E code)	CHAR	7
ICD DGNS VRSN CD8	Claim diagnosis code VIII diagnosis version code (ICD-9 or ICD-10)	Effective with version J, the code used to indicate if the diagnosis code is ICD-9 or ICD-10	CHAR	1
ICD DGNS CD9	Claim diagnosis code IX	The diagnosis code identifying the beneficiary's principal or other diagnosis (including E code)	CHAR	7
ICD DGNS VRSN CD9	Claim diagnosis code IX diagnosis version code (ICD-9 or ICD-10)	Effective with version J, the code used to indicate if the diagnosis code is ICD-9 or ICD-10	CHAR	1
ICD DGNS CD10	Claim diagnosis code X	The diagnosis code identifying the beneficiary's principal or other diagnosis (including E code)	CHAR	7
ICD DGNS VRSN CD10	Claim diagnosis code X diagnosis version code (ICD-9 or ICD-10)	Effective with version J, the code used to indicate if the diagnosis code is ICD-9 or ICD-10	CHAR	1
ICD DGNS CD11	Claim diagnosis code XI	The diagnosis code identifying the beneficiary's principal or other diagnosis (including E code)	CHAR	7

ICD DGNS VRSN CD11	Claim diagnosis code XI diagnosis version code (ICD-9 or ICD-10)	Effective with version J, the code used to indicate if the diagnosis code is ICD-9 or ICD-10	CHAR	1
ICD DGNS CD12	Claim diagnosis code XII	The diagnosis code identifying the beneficiary's principal or other diagnosis (including E code)	CHAR	7
ICD DGNS VRSN CD12	Claim diagnosis code XII diagnosis version code (ICD-9 or ICD-10)	Effective with version J, the code used to indicate if the diagnosis code is ICD-9 or ICD-10	CHAR	1
DOB_DT	LDS age category	The beneficiary's date of birth coded as a range	NUM	1
GNDR_CD	Gender code from claim	The sex of a beneficiary	CHAR	1
RACE_CD	Race code from claim	Race code from claim	CHAR	1
CNTY_CD	County code from claim—Social Security Administration (SSA)	The three-digit SSA standard county code of a beneficiary's residence	CHAR	3
STATE_CD	State code from claim (SSA)	The SSA standard two-digit state code of a beneficiary's residence	CHAR	2
CWF_BENE_MDCR_STUS_CD	Common working file (CWF) beneficiary Medicare status code	The CWF-derived reason for a beneficiary's entitlement to Medicare benefits as of the reference date (CLM_THRU_DT)	CHAR	2
CLM_BENE_PD_AMT	Carrier claim beneficiary paid amount	The amount paid by the beneficiary for the noninstitutional Part B (carrier or durable medical equipment regional carrier) claim	NUM	12
CPO_PRVDR_NUM	Care plan oversight (CPO) provider number	The NPI number of the home health agency (HHA) or hospice rendering Medicare services during the period the physician is providing CPO	CHAR	12
CPO_ORG_NPI_NUM	CPO organization NPI number	The NPI number of the HHA or hospice rendering Medicare services during the period the physician is providing CPO	CHAR	10
CARR_CLM_BLG_NPI_NUM	Carrier claim billing NPI number	The CMS NPI number assigned to the billing provider	CHAR	10
ACO_ID_NUM	Claim accountable care organization (ACO) ID number	The field identifies the ACO identification number	CHAR	10

Centers for Medicare and Medicaid Services. (2019). Standard analytical files (Medicare claims). https://www.cms.gov/Research-Statistics-Data-and-Systems/Files-for-Order/LimitedDataSets/StandardAnalyticalFiles.html

Advantages and Disadvantages of Medical Claims Data for Population Health Analytics

One main advantage of using medical claims data for population health analytics is that they represent a comprehensive view of all the diagnoses and procedures for a patient over the time period when their care is paid for by one insurer. In addition, medical claims data provide information about the locations where a patient seeks care, the constellation of providers delivering that care, the number of services used, and the costs associated with those services. This allows for patient, provider, health system information, usage, and cost information to be analyzed in one data source.

Medical claims data can be aggregated at the person level and further at subgrouping and population levels. For example, the entire population of Medicaid enrollees can be analyzed to determine the prevalence of a chronic condition; that population can then be segregated into children and adults and other subgroupings to start understanding the distribution of that prevalence.

Data can also be aggregated for certain episodes of care such as a knee or hip replacement. Under CMS's Bundled Payments for Care Improvement initiative, providers are paid for the services a patient receives during an episode of care with the idea that a more efficient episode of care with desirable cost and quality outcomes will result in value for the patient, provider, and payer. An *episode of care* may be defined as the entirety of an inpatient stay, include a period of time before and after an inpatient stay, or represent another time period of healthcare service delivery for a specific condition (Riley, 2009).

Medical claims data can also be aggregated and analyzed longitudinally over time for patients, subgroupings, and populations in order to analyze trends in healthcare outcomes, quality, cost and utilization. As an example, a provider who is at-risk for ensuring treatment adherence for people with ischemic heart disease at her practice can use medical claims data to identify everyone with ischemic heart disease in her practice every month and whether or not the treatment prescription was taken by the patient.

Because medical claims data are generated for transactional payment services, an important advantage for analysis is that definitions for standardized fields are the same across all payers. The coding systems reviewed in this chapter are standard across the country. The code for a diagnosis of congestive heart failure is the same whether the claims data are from Medicaid, Medicare, or a private insurer. This allows for sharing and comparing of data across payers and at local, state, national, and globally for certain coding systems.

Medical claims data are used in practically every data contextualizer used for population health analytics including the following products: Adjusted Clinical Groups, Episode Treatment Groupers, and Hierarchical Condition Categories for risk adjustment. Electronic medical record systems now facilitate claims data as part of their platforms, allowing for the integration of administrative and clinical data.

Despite the advantages of medical claims data, disadvantages remain. Because these data are collected primarily for payment services and not for population health analytic purposes, the coding is more closely related to billing for procedures and services as opposed to being reflective of the medical record. The provider documents in the medical record, but it is often the job of a "coder" to interpret the provider's notes and documentation into standard coding systems, which are inputted into a bill. This interpretation of clinical information into standardized coding systems causes gaps in information when going from a rich clinical note to a single code.

In addition, medical claims data may contain biases related to provider incentives to maximize payment in fee-for-service arrangements. For example, a provider may get higher payment by assigning a procedure code that indicates higher severity of illness for a patient even if that patient may not have higher severity or may be on the cusp (Riley, 2009).

Special Considerations for Medical Claims Data

One specific consideration for using medical claims data to analyze patient populations is understanding completeness of the data. One aspect of completeness can be understood by spending time reviewing the benefit structure within which the patients in a payer group receive services. Medicare managed care plans, for instance, have specific rules about which services can be offered in these health plans, and they may be services that are not covered by a private commercial insurer.

Another important point is to understand that patients may have a secondary source to pay for healthcare services. When analyzing the services that a patient receives under a certain payer, it is important to understand whether another payer is providing a portion of the services. For instance, a person who served in the military may receive medications and other services for free from the Veterans Benefit Administration but use a private insurer to cover other costs.

Carve-out services are designated services for which a government policy or a health plan subcontracts a set of benefits to another plan or network. When analyzing medical claims data, it is important to understand whether or not carved-out services are included in the data. For instance, many Medicaid managed care plans carve out substance use services, and usually those claims' information are not shared with the primary payer. In fact, when receiving claims from CMS for provider incentive and risk-based contracting, substance use and some mental health claims are automatically removed from the files.

Medical claims data often have different categories of cost fields. Understanding the meaning of these fields is important when performing an analysis because the amount paid to a provider depends on the contractual arrangement with individual providers and facilities. For the same diagnosis, procedure, and place of service, two providers may receive decidedly different payment amounts because of the contracts. This is why medical claims data usually have an "allowed amount," the amount a provider is allowed to bill; and a "paid" amount, the amount the provider is actually paid. Allowed amounts are better to use for comparison and directional purposes when performing population health analyses.

Applied Learning: Case Study

Using Medical Claims Data to Understand Clinical, Utilization, and Cost Indicators for a Population of Patients in a New Provider-Based Risk Contract.

Background

A large employer was considering becoming self-insured, which means the employer would take the risk by paying for all of the healthcare services for company employees. The employer had an idea of the total costs of the care for the population over the last 5 years from reports provided by the current health insurance plan but did not understand any details behind those costs or the employees' healthcare needs. The employer needed to get more of these details from multiple data sources and started with medical claims data. The employer hired an agency to perform an analysis with medical claims data and provide the results.

Some of the questions to be answered and the ways in which medical claims data can be used to answer them are shown in the following table.

(continues)

Applied Learning: Case Study *(continued)*

Question	Using Medical Claims Data
What is the distribution of employees and dependents?	The member ID on claims is coded in a way that distinguishes the employee from a spousal and a child dependent. Count the unique number of people in each category and keep them as a dataset to get other information.
What are the demographic characteristics?	The claim contains age and gender.
What is the prevalence of certain chronic conditions?	ICD-10-CM codes can be aggregated into certain chronic conditions by person. For instance, to determine the prevalence of asthma, any person with one of the following codes is included as having the condition: J45.2x, J45.3x, J45.4x, J45.5x, J45.90x (the x includes all categories).
What is the overall use and cost by certain place of service?	Use dates of service, place of service, and revenue codes to determine the admissions and visits for certain types of facilities. For instance, an emergency department visit is defined by using the range of revenue codes between 0450 and 0459.

Results

Membership Demographics	Health Coverage			
	Employees Only	*Dependent Spouses*	*Dependent Children*	*All Enrollees*
Total members	10,404	3,258	6,303	19,883
Mean age	41.00	47.00	8.90	32.56
Male (%)	30.71	59.39	50.80	41.74
Female (%)	69.29	40.61	49.20	58.26

Chronic Condition Prevalence Rates (%)	
	All Enrollees
Any chronic condition	18.73
Asthma	3.04
Adults	2.27
Children	0.77
Chronic obstructive pulmonary disease (COPD)	0.39
Congestive heart failure (CHF)	0.32

Coronary artery disease (CAD)	0.55
Hyperlipidemia	8.86
Diabetes	3.89
Hypertension	12.09

Claims Use by Place of Service

All Enrollees	Rate / 1000	Total Spent ($) / Admit or Visit
Inpatient facility admits	54.60	14,509.65
Inpatient professional visits	373.97	314.44
Outpatient visits	1,256.04	718.88
Outpatient surgery visits	142.98	3,296.30
Outpatient nonsurgery visits	1,096.73	369.97
ER visits	164.64	637.00
Office visits	5,625.27	117.76
Other visits	544.62	198.90
Prescriptions	10,321.08	116.97
Dental visits	1,326.28	85.82

Health Claims Costs

	Total Spent Per Member Per Year ($)			
	Employees Only	Dependent Spouses	Dependent Children	All Enrollees
Total Medical	2,790.54	3,770	1,614.39	2,570.75

Conclusion

Medical claims data, transformed into meaningful knowledge, provide a rich understanding of the health and needs of large populations. Coding systems used in medical claims data provide information about the constellation of illness, patterns of healthcare service use, and quality and cost outcomes.

Study and Discussion Questions

- How can medical claims data be used in a program of population health analytics?

- What types of populations and subgroupings can be defined using medical claims data?

- How could medical claims data be used to determine quality outcomes for populations?
- How could medical claims data be used to determine the use of appropriate treatment for certain health conditions?

- What types of comparisons can be made using medical claims data?
- How could medical claims data be combined with other data sources to perform population health analyses?

Resources and Websites

CMS has partnered with a research group to provide a set of realistic claims data for the 3-year period from 2008 to 2010. This is a great source of data to use for understanding the ways to use medical claims data.

Information and Data Sets

CMS 2008-2010 Data Entrepreneurs' Synthetic Public Use File (DE-SynPUF): https://www.cms .gov/Research-Statistics-Data-and-Systems /Downloadable-Public-Use-Files/SynPUFs/DE _Syn_PUF.html

Instructional Video

Acquiring Data from CMS DE-SynPU: Fhttps:// www.youtube.com/watch?time_continue =10&v=rs86OXHmVp4

Example Analysis Video

Analyzing SynPUF Claims Data: https://www .youtube.com/watch?time_continue=2&v =ZXOnbs2rAQ4

References

American Medical Association (AMA). (2019). CPT category II codes. https://www.ama-assn.org/system/files/2019-07/cpt -cat2-codes.pdf

Centers for Medicare and Medicaid Services. (2018a). Completing and processing form CMS-1500 data set transmittals for Chapter 26. In *Medicare Claims Processing Manual*. Centers for Medicare and Medicaid Services. www.cms.gov

Centers for Medicare and Medicaid Services. (2018b). *Medicare billing: Form CMS-1450 and the 837 institutional print-friendly version.* https://www.cms.gov /Outreach-and-Education/Medicare-Learning-Network -MLN/MLNProducts/Downloads/837I-FormCMS-1450 -ICN006926.pdf

Centers for Medicare and Medicaid Services. (2019a). *HCPCS general information.* https://www.cms.gov/Medicare/Coding /MedHCPCSGenInfo/index.html

Centers for Medicare and Medicaid Services. (2019b). *ICD-10-CM official guidelines for coding and reporting, FY 2019.* https://www.cms.gov/Medicare/Coding/ICD10 /Downloads/2019-ICD10-Coding-Guidelines-.pdf

Centers for Medicare and Medicaid Services. (2019c). ICD-10 Procedure Coding System (ICD-10-PCS). (2019). 2020 tables and index. https://www.cms.gov/Medicare/Coding /ICD10/2020-ICD-10-PCS.html

Centers for Medicare and Medicaid Services. (2020). *ICD-10-PCS official guidelines for coding and reporting 2020.* https://www.cms.gov/Medicare/Coding/ICD10 /Downloads/2020-ICD-10-PCS-Guidelines.pdf

Hicks, J. (2019). *Type of bill codes for the UB-04 form.* Verywell Health. https://www.verywellhealth.com/types-of-billing -codes-2317067

Medical Billing Answers. (2020). Revenue codes. http://www .medicalbillinganswers.com/revenuecodes.html

National Rural Health Resource Center. (2020). Using claims data. https://www.ruralcenter.org/population-health -toolkit/data/using-claims-data

Riley, G. F. (2009). Administrative and claims records as sources of health care cost data. *Medical Care, 47*(7) (Suppl. 1), S51–S55.

CHAPTER 4

Lab Data for Population Health Analytics

Seray Gardner, BS
Martha Sylvia, PhD, MBA, RN

It amounts to a truism to say that progress in the practical arts of medicine in any of its branches, whether preventive or curative, only comes from the growth of accurate knowledge as it accumulates in the laboratories and studies of the various sciences.

—Walter Fletcher (1929)

EXECUTIVE SUMMARY

In 2017, Medicare paid more than $7.1 billion for 433 million outpatient lab tests billed by more than 655,000 providers. Most of that spending was concentrated among a small set of tests and a small set of lab vendors. Overall, 64% of spending was for a set of 25 lab tests. The top 25 list contains lab tests that are commonly used to understand the health status of and outcomes within populations of interest, especially those with chronic conditions, including:

- hemoglobin A1c (HbA1c) testing for people with diabetes,
- lipid testing for people with cardiac conditions, and
- panels to understand the composition of blood that are used to determine organ damage resulting from chronic conditions and their complications (U.S. Department of Health and Human Services [DHS], 2018).

With more than 28 million Medicare beneficiaries receiving at least one test and an average of 16 individual tests per beneficiary, lab data represent a valuable data source to assist with achieving population health goals (DHS, 2018). Laboratory results provide the first indication of the onset of chronic illness and comorbidities and complications of chronic illness as well as complicating acute illnesses. Moreover, lab results are quantitative biological indicators with evidence-based parameters used to discover clinical abnormalities.

Despite its value, lab data remains a difficult source of data to incorporate into population health analyses because these data are incomplete and unstructured, have little standardization within and across vendors, and lack interoperability with the systems in which clinicians work and the data warehouses sourcing population health analytics (Hauser, Quine, & Ryder, 2018).

LEARNING OBJECTIVES

At the end of this chapter, the learner will be able to:

1. Explain the value of lab data for population health analytics.
2. Compare and contrast the sources of lab data.
3. Describe techniques for transforming lab data into meaningful information.
4. Identify ways to use lab data to answer questions of importance to population health management.

Introduction

Since the passing of the Affordable Care Act in 2010, the passage of new regulations for reporting lab results, the demand for lab result data by payers, the saturation of electronic medical records (EMRs) and their ability to integrate lab results into point-of-care (POC) decisions, and the expansion of population health analytics have all led to greater opportunities to use lab data to improve patient outcomes. The opportunities to use data come at a cost in terms of managing the complexity involved with deciphering meaning.

This chapter seeks to untangle the complexity associated with using lab data for population health analytics by explaining the policies and guidelines that impact the standardization and reporting of lab data, the origins and sources of lab data, methods for standardizing and organizing the structure of lab data for analytic purposes, and ways to exploit the value of lab data for population health.

Defining Lab Data

For the purposes of this chapter, *clinical lab data* is defined as data that report the results of any type of test done on samples such as blood or tissue that have been taken from the human body, which is referred to as *in vitro*. In vitro tests are used to identify diseases or other conditions and can be used to monitor a person's overall health to cure, treat, or prevent disease (U.S. Food and Drug Administration, 2019). This chapter and definition *do not* include pathological or cytological lab data used in vitro testing of tissue or cells to determine the cause of disease. Genotypic analysis, which uses DNA sequencing to study disease, is also excluded from the lab data chapter.

Clinical lab data fall into major specialty categories defined by the U.S. Food and Drug Administration (FDA) summarized here.

Urinalysis

A urinalysis consists of chemical tests such as *glucose* and *nitrites*, physical observations like *color* and *density*, and microscopic analyses to determine the presence of abnormal cells, crystals, and bacteria.

General Chemistry

Chemistry panels are groups of tests, typically performed on blood or urine samples, that may be used to help evaluate a person's health status. Assays (i.e., analyses done to determine the presence and amount of a substance) may target a specific organ such as kidney health with urea nitrogen and creatinine measurements, evaluate the risk of disease development using assays such as hemoglobin A1c for diabetes, or provide an overview of general metabolic health with panels of multiple tests.

General Immunology

Immunology is a broad category of testing that studies the functionality and disorders of the immune system. Measuring hepatitis C antibodies to determine exposure to hepatitis C antigens is an example of an immunological assay targeting a specific disease. Human leucocyte antigen typing is a type of immunological testing that applies to transplant organ compatibility or to autoimmune disease evaluation.

Hematology

Hematological assays study the blood and associated blood disorders. Routine counts of white blood cells or red blood cells and platelets in whole blood may provide early indication of infection, anemia, or clotting disorders. Microscopic examination of whole blood or bone marrow smears may further help the diagnosis of anemia or leukemia.

Immunohematology

Immunohematology, commonly referred to as *blood banking*, is the study of red blood cell surface antigens and blood antibodies pertinent to blood transfusion. Before a transfusion, to prevent blood-matching errors and potentially life-threatening situations, blood antigens and antibody testing must be performed in addition to the usual major human blood group and protein (ABO/rh) testing and typing.

Endocrinology

Endocrinology testing targets assays for hormones that control or affect bodily processes such as metabolism, growth, bone health, and reproduction. As an example, an insulin antibody assay will help determine whether a person diagnosed with diabetes produces antibodies against insulin so that an endocrinologist may design an appropriate course of treatment.

Toxicology and Therapeutic Drug Monitoring (TDM)

Therapeutic drug monitoring (TDM) measures the amount of specific prescribed drugs in an effort to maintain the optimal concentration of the drug in the bloodstream. Measuring levels of cardiac drugs such as digoxin or immunosuppressants such as cyclosporin help ensure proper treatment of a condition and also help avoid overdosing.

Microbiology

Microbiology is the study of microorganisms—bacteria and viruses—to help identify invasive species, diagnose diseases related to microorganisms that are not normal flora, and help control infectious diseases.

Infections from single-celled bacteria such as *Staphylococcus aureus* and *Streptococcus pyogenes* are identified, respectively, as the causative agent in conditions such as toxic shock syndrome and strep throat or so-called flesh-eating bacteria incidents. Measuring the sensitivity and resistance of infectious bacteria to panels of antibiotics is extremely important for determining the appropriate and specific antibiotic, strength, and administration route for treatment.

Virology, like bacteriology, is a category of microbiology that traditionally studies disease-producing viruses. Routine viral culturing to isolate viruses such as Herpes simplex are still performed, but molecular testing for viruses such as human immunodeficiency (HIV), influenza, human papilloma, and others is more common.

Mycobacteriology is the specialized field that focuses on studying the slow-growing bacterial genera of *Mycobacterium*. *Mycobacterium tuberculosis* is the causative agent of tuberculosis and *Mycobacterium leprae* is the causative agent of leprosy.

Parasitology

Parasitology in the clinical laboratory typically focuses on parasites of the gastrointestinal tract. *Entamoeba histolytica* and different *Giardia* species are common intestinal parasites associated with diarrhea and enteritis. Nonintestinal parasites such as the lung fluke *Paragonimus westermani* are uncommon in the United States.

Mycology

Clinical mycology is the study of fungal pathogens, both mold and yeast. Isolation, identification, and drug treatment susceptibility testing contribute to improved treatment of associated mycoses. Fungal infections range in severity from common

Candida albicans yeast infections of mucous membranes to central nervous system infections from mold species such as *Aspergillus* spp.

Cytology

Cytology testing examines cells from the body for indications of disease or infection. Many cancers, such as cervical cancer, may be diagnosed via cytological examination. Histological testing in which a thin slice of tissue is examined microscopically is also used in the diagnosis of cancer and other diseases associated with abnormal cell morphology. Cytology testing is advantageous in identifying and confirming conditions where the cost of treatment is high, such as hepatitis C and HIV. When these conditions are detected early, more costly treatment regimens resulting from disease progression can be avoided.

Oversight of Lab Collection and Testing

To collect a lab specimen, an order from a licensed provider must be generated. Collecting lab specimens is not the same as testing. The testing of lab specimens is controlled by the Clinical Laboratory Improvement Amendments (CLIA), which requires that facilities must be certified to perform testing. A facility is required to possess a CLIA certificate (number) to draw blood, but the facility also needs distinct CLIA certifications for any type of tests performed, even a finger stick for glucose. Testing is controlled by CLIA, but facilities that perform nonwaived and moderate or high-complexity testing may be accredited by one of seven organizations such as the College of American Pathologists or the Joint Commission, which have standards deemed equivalent to CLIA by the Centers for Medicare and Medicaid Services (CMS).

Three federal agencies are responsible for CLIA: the FDA, CMS, and the Centers for Disease Control and Prevention (CDC). Each agency has a unique role in ensuring quality laboratory testing (U.S. Food and Drug Administration, 2020). The FDA categorizes tests based on complexity,

reviews requests for waivers of CLIA policy by application, and develops rules and guidance for the organization of lab types into CLIA categories of complexity.

The CMS:

- issues laboratory certificates,
- collects user fees,
- conducts inspections and enforces regulatory compliance,
- approves private accreditation of organizations for performing inspections and state exemptions,
- monitors laboratory performance on proficiency testing (PT) and approves PT programs, and
- publishes CLIA rules and regulations.

The CDC:

- provides analysis, research, and technical assistance;
- develops technical standards and laboratory practice guidelines, including standards and guidelines for cytology;
- conducts laboratory quality-improvement studies;
- monitors PT practices;
- develops and distributes professional information and educational resources; and
- manages the Clinical Laboratory Improvement Advisory Committee (Centers for Medicare and Medicaid Services [CMS], 2019).

Origins and Sources of Lab Data

Lab data are generated when a result of a collected lab specimen is officially released or documented by the testing facility. Blood samples for clinical laboratory testing can be collected at various types of sites, including companies whose sole business is lab sample collection and testing, doctors' offices, hospitals, and other healthcare facilities. Lab data gathered from processing—testing and its results—are generated at the site where the specimen is analyzed. It is important to understand where the lab analysis takes place when using lab data for population health analytics because, based on the expertise and experience of the organization generating the analysis and data, the quality, accuracy, and completeness of the data may vary (explained in further detail in upcoming sections). For instance, the drawing of blood for hemoglobin A1c testing from a patient with diabetes may be performed in a provider's office but, depending on the resources of the provider, that specimen may be tested in the provider's office for an immediate result or sent to a separate laboratory for processing.

Centralized Testing Laboratories

Centralized testing laboratories, often referred to as *reference laboratories*, perform high-volume, moderate, and high-complexity laboratory testing across these FDA lab specialty categories, and testing is often focused on condition monitoring and screening assays. Testing facilities are centralized within a region or a state, where samples collected across the region are delivered for processing and testing. Some reference laboratories may also offer higher volume specialty testing. Quest Diagnostics and Laboratory Corporation of America (LabCorp) are well known examples of reference laboratories to whom providers "refer" their patients and samples for laboratory testing needs. Reference laboratories also include a limited number of facilities that perform low-volume, highly specialized testing such as adrenocorticotropic hormone and erythropoietin measurements and genetic biomarker tests. Specialty Laboratories, Inc., is an example of a highly specialized testing facility.

Lab data from centralized laboratories are sent as file feeds to payers, providers, and other contracted entities with patient care accountabilities.

Health System Laboratories

Health system laboratories (HSLs) are those that are located within the same systems in which patients receive healthcare services on an inpatient or outpatient basis. HSLs provide centralized testing but for a much more limited customer base: the patients of their health system. However, HSLs are likely to send low-frequency tests or time-intensive tests to a larger, centralized lab vendor. In the inpatient setting, lab tests are often time sensitive and require immediate results and action. HSLs are invaluable in this situation where the focus is on acute conditions rather than chronic condition management and monitoring. Tests performed in HSLs may fall into all categories: acute diagnostic and chronic condition monitoring, time sensitive or not.

The results of laboratory tests may be delivered as a file feed from the HSL but can also be found as a patient-reported result in the EMR.

Point-of-Care Testing

Decentralized laboratory services performed at the point of healthcare delivery are referred to as *point-of-care* (POC) lab testing and occur at the bedside in inpatient settings, in urgent care clinics, primary care settings, and more. They are considered valuable because of their reduced expense, ability to provide immediate results, and facilitation of immediate treatment decisions (Rohr et al., 2016). POC devices in a hospital can include dozens of blood-gas analyzers, urine chemistry and cardiac marker systems, and hand-held coagulation instruments, as well as hundreds of glucose devices. In the outpatient settings, devices and instant collection and testing kits are available for certain tests such as hemoglobin A1c testing for patients with diabetes. POC lab tests may or may not be waived from CLIA's certification requirements.

POC testing results are typically difficult to obtain in lab data feeds and ultimately for analytic purposes because documentation is often in disparate locations within the EMR.

POC testing also shows more direct lab-to-consumer testing, where consumers may access laboratory testing without a physician's order. Tests are now available in the home for patients to monitor their own chronic conditions, determine the presence of acute conditions, screen common metabolic systems, or detect the presence of a pathogen or antibody. These tests may or may not be contracted in coordination with a certified lab vendor, and the results are unlikely to be included in lab data sets.

Quality Differences Among Sources of Lab Data

The quality of lab results can differ based on the type of testing facility (POC versus HSL) or differences in quality standards of lab processes between laboratories performing testing within the same categories of test complexity. Lab analytical errors are divided into three categories based on the step in the lab collection and testing process where the error originates.

- The *pre-analytical phase* occurs first in the laboratory process and includes specimen collection and handling tasks. Pre-analytical test errors include ordering an incorrect test, misidentifying patients, and incorrectly collecting, transporting, or processing samples for testing.
- The *analytical phase* includes the actual laboratory testing or diagnostic procedures, processes, and products that produce the results. Errors during this phase can be random (poor precision) or systematic (poor accuracy). Random errors during the analytic phase include instrument maintenance problems; improper testing environments; unstable reagents, calibrators, or controls; operator handling or interpretation errors; and testing of inadequate samples. Systematic errors during the analytic phase are related to changes in lots of reagents or calibrators, instrument errors, and degradation of vital electronic instrument components.
- The *postanalytical phase* occurs after the value or result is produced. Errors in this phase can be internal or external to the laboratory and are often related to misinterpretation of results, inaccurate data entry, and delay in

communication or transmission of critical or noncritical results (Klatt, 2020).

Because of their depth of experience, knowledge and expertise, ability to perform highly complex tests, proficiency in testing requirements, standardized and automated processes, high volume of tests, and strong quality-control monitoring programs, inpatient labs and centralized testing laboratories produce the best quality of lab data with less random error, less systematic error, and less postanalytical error. In centralized testing facilities and inpatient labs, most of the errors are in the pre-analytical phase where there is little to no control over the involvement of persons external to the lab who collect specimens (Laczin, 2013; Simons & Capraro, 2019).

Outside of inpatient labs, other HSLs may have more errors in the pre-analytical period such as submitting the wrong sample, or poor collection techniques because of the complexity of events happening in the healthcare setting as well as varying levels of experience and expertise. The laboratories themselves have highly trained and experienced personnel, which results in fewer errors in the analytical and post-analytical phases of testing.

POC testing is prone to more errors than centralized collecting systems during the collection and testing processes (Mardis, 2017). POC testing has the potential for accuracy and precision issues because of a lack of quality control oversight, lack of consistency in testing kits, poorly understood or undocumented specimen acceptance and rejection criteria, and incorrect specimen types used for testing. In addition, there is variable accuracy, precision, and poor understanding of interfering substances. This is of particular concern for POC HbA1c testing, which is commonly used in population health programs to determine the health status of people with diabetes and even indicate the quality of healthcare services (Radin, 2013). A growing number of POC testing kits are waived from CLIA regulatory requirements, which suppose a potential for increased lab result errors.

Standardization of Lab Data

Despite the vast amount of lab testing performed in the United States, lab data remain largely unstandardized and without industry-wide requirements for test names, reference ranges for normal and abnormal results, formatting of results and associated units, and coding systems to identify labs. This causes inefficiencies and ambiguity in using lab data for population health analyses (Hauser et al., 2018).

Some of the benefits of standardization are:

- improved patient care,
- improved quality control,
- less testing redundancy,
- decreased turnaround time from lab data to insights, and
- improved analytical accuracy of long-term trending studies.

Standardization Guidelines and Policy

In 2018, CMS undertook a substantial revision to the way it pays for lab testing by establishing a national fee schedule called the Clinical Laboratory Fee Schedule. This only applies to labs that provide a substantial amount of lab services for Medicare beneficiaries. The new payment methodology also required certain information to be reported by laboratories, including the procedure code (Healthcare Common Procedure Code System—see Chapter 3), the volume per test type, and other payer and payment information. Unfortunately, the requirements are around billing and not the reporting of actual lab tests and apply to aggregate reporting submissions that are not at the individual test level.

The Meaningful Use (MU) program in the United States sets standards for interoperability with systems interfacing with electronic medical records. Current requirements for standardization of lab data focus on provider ordering of lab tests and reporting required lab results to public health agencies. In stage 2 of MU lab data was required to be exchanged in a structured electronic format. However, the definition of *structured* is limited to a requirement for discrete data within fixed fields and does not require any standardized vocabulary like the Logical Observation Identifiers Names and Codes (LOINC) (Swain & Patel, 2014; U.S. Department of Health and Human Services, 2015).

The Health Level Seven (HL7) International is a not-for-profit, accredited organization that originated in 1987 and sets standards for the exchange, integration, sharing, and retrieval of electronic health information that supports clinical practice and the management, delivery, and evaluation of health services. In 2018, HL7 released standards for the interface of lab results with a 2-year trial and evaluation period in preparation for approval by the American National Standards Institute in collaboration with the U.S. Standards and Interoperability Framework within the Office of the National Coordinator for Health Information Technology (ONC) (HL7 International, 2019). If approved, these standards will deliver requirements for standardized data structures and coding systems for all relevant laboratory data fields. Once approved, the standards will need to be incorporated into existing policy.

The International Consortium for Harmonization of Clinical Laboratory Results originated in 2010 with the goal of improving the harmonization of results from clinical laboratories and providing a resource center on global activities to harmonize and standardize clinical laboratory measurement procedures. Harmonization of methodology ensures that results from different labs and results interpretation are equivalent regardless of the method of analysis, instrumentation, and location of testing (Myers & Miller, 2018).

Level of Standardization in Lab Data Sets

To understand the status of standardization and data cleaning in lab data, a distinction is made between the data sets that are generated by labs and provided to requesting entities—*reported lab data*—and analytic lab data sets that are the result of processing of the reported lab data. Reported lab data lack standardization and data processing and may have one or more of the following issues:

- lack of filtering to
  - distinguish between final versus preliminary results,
  - identify invalid results (e.g., exclusion of HbA1c results where the sample was grossly hemolyzed, values below assay acceptance level, and urine creatinine reported as a blood creatinine measurement);
- lack of standardization for
  - identifying units of measurement (HbA1c reported as mmol/mol, or %),
  - reporting of the assay (also known as analytic procedure) name (glycated hemoglobin = glycosylated hemoglobin = glycohemoglobin = hemoglobin A1c = hemoglobin A1c = HbA1c = HgbA1c, etc.),
  - setting a reference range for normal versus abnormal results (e.g., abnormal high from lab 1 > 100 mg/dL, abnormal high from Lab 2 > 105 mg/Dl),
  - data formats within fields (e.g. < 50, 1020, or Not Tested)
- inclusion of assay results external to the assays of interest for the analysis;
- inclusion of results from assays performed outside the time period relevant to the analysis;
- varying processing methods;
- more than one row per person per assay;
- the use of free text for items such as indicators of sample integrity, sample site, and data-collection observations; and
- missing results within rows

Regarding varying processing methods, historic results in lab data may have been produced using methods that differ from current methods and may not be comparable; for example, glycohemoglobin results through the early 1990s may

have represented total glycosylated hemoglobin or hemoglobin A1 (HbA1a + HbA1b + HbA1c) or just HbA1c and now HbA1c.

An analytic lab data set is one that is processed from a reported lab data set where the data are cleansed and standardized. This process is usually undertaken by the organization receiving the reported lab data. This means that the same reported lab data are likely to be processed and standardized differently depending on the needs, understanding, skills, and expertise of each recipient organization. Ideally, an analytic data set has removed the issues found in reported lab data and:

- contains only final and valid results,
- applies conversions to standardize units of measurement and assay names,
- normalizes indications of results as compared to reference ranges (e.g. *Abnormal High*, *Low*, etc.),
- includes only the assay that fits the purpose and results from relevant time periods,
- excludes incompatible results intended to represent the same assay, and
- creates a data structure that is amenable to programmatic analysis with:
  - uniquely formatted data types within a single field;
  - discrete numeric values where a number is expected;
  - one row per subject per assay result;
  - appropriate application, interpretation, and standardization of result modifiers; and
  - exclusion of missing result values unless meaningful to the analysis.

The Process of Standardizing Lab Data

Ideally, standardization of lab data would take place before its release by the performing laboratory. This would require fewer resources across multiple healthcare organizations and would ensure consistency in interpreting the same set of lab results. However, standardization of lab data is usually undertaken by an analytic department within the same organization that uses the data for patient care or analytic purposes. Because of the enormous commitment of time and personnel required to standardize lab data by an individual healthcare organization, the value of lab data for population health analytics is often unrealized.

Using LOINC for Standardization of Lab Data

Logical Observation Identifiers Names and Codes provide a vocabulary that standardizes the names of tests, observations, panels, and assessments, with the overall scope being anything that can be tested, measured, or observed about a patient (Regenstrief Institute, 2015). Note that LOINC vocabulary is used for many other types of clinical outcomes; for the purposes of this chapter, however, the focus is on the LOINC vocabulary used for lab results. Mapping of lab data results to LOINC vocabulary harmonizes or normalizes data and allows for analysis across multiple lab providers as well as longitudinally over time (Diaz, 2014).

To create different codes for each test and measurement, the LOINC process distinguishes a given observation across six components:

- *component* (or *analyte*)—the substance or entity being measured;
- *property*—the characteristic or attribute of the analyte;
- *time*—the interval of time over which a measurement was made;
- *system* or *specimen*—the system or specimen on which the observation was made; and
- *method*—a high-level classification of how the observation was made; this is only needed when the technique affects the clinical interpretation of the results.

As an example, here are the component assignments for LOINC code 41995-2, hemoglobin A1c (mass/volume) in blood.

- component (analyte): hemoglobin A1c;
- property: mass concentration (MCnc);

- time: point in time (Pt);
- system and specimen: blood (Bld); and
- method: blank (Regenstrief Institute, 2015).

LOINC mappings are updated yearly in June and December and can be downloaded from the LOINC website (Search LOINC, 2020).

Although mapping with LOINC vocabulary goes a long way toward standardization, more than one appropriate LOINC code exists for any individual assay or test, resulting in varying standardization of the same lab results. **Table 4.1** shows the multiple LOINC codes that can be assigned for hemoglobin A1c results. Thus, it is important to work in analyst, clinician, or clinical lab expert teams when mapping lab data to LOINC codes.

Additional Standardization Techniques

In addition to LOINC, other standardization of lab data needs to take place to make it amenable for analytics, including:

- parsing of result fields (for example, >5 parsed into > and 5;
- standardizing units of measurement (the Unified Code for Units of Measure Standardization [Hauser, 2018] has been used as a way to standardize the units of measurement);
- unifying expected ranges for results;
- fixing typos;
- adjusting text numbers to Arabic numerals (e.g., "1" instead of "one");
- standardizing acronyms across lab vendors (e.g., ND = not done, or not detected);
- ensuring proper conversions between different units of measurement; and
- capturing relevant testing comments such as "gross hemolysis," "Results verified by repeat analysis," and "Incorrect sample submitted, test not performed" (Hauser et al., 2018).

Although it is ideal to normalize or harmonize lab data collected from different testing facilities to make results directly comparable, this is not always possible across all types of results.

Table 4.1 LOINC Codes for Hemoglobin A1c Results

Loinc Code	Long Name	Component
41995-2	Hemoglobin A1c in blood(Mass/volume)	Hemoglobin A1c
43150-2	Hemoglobin A1c measurement device panel	HbA1c measurement device panel
71875-9	Hemoglobin A1c/hemoglobin total in blood (Pure mass fraction)	Hemoglobin A1c/hemoglobin.total
86910-7	Hemoglobin A1c/hemoglobin in blood (Total goal)	Hemoglobin A1c/hemoglobin.total goal
4548-4	Hemoglobin A1c/hemoglobin in blood (Goal)	Hemoglobin A1c/hemoglobin.total
17855-8	Hemoglobin A1c/hemoglobin total in blood by calculation	Hemoglobin A1c/hemoglobin.total
4549-2	Hemoglobin A1c/hemoglobin total in blood by electrophoresis	Hemoglobin A1c/hemoglobin.total
17856-6	Hemoglobin A1c/hemoglobin total in blood by HPLC	Hemoglobin A1c/hemoglobin.total
59261-8	Hemoglobin A1c/hemoglobin total in blood by IFCC protocol	Hemoglobin A1c/hemoglobin.total
96595-4	Hemoglobin A1c/hemoglobin total in DBS	Hemoglobin A1c/hemoglobin.total
62388-4	Hemoglobin A1c/hemoglobin total in blood by JDS or JSCC protocol	Hemoglobin A1c/hemoglobin.total

This material contains content from LOINC (http://loinc.org). LOINC is copyright © 1995–2020, Regenstrief Institute, Inc. and the Logical Observation Identifiers Names and Codes (LOINC) Committee and is available at no cost under the license at http://loinc.org/license. LOINC® is a registered United States trademark of Regenstrief Institute, Inc.

Database and Data-Transformation Considerations

Because the onus of creating analytic lab data sets relies on the analysts in healthcare organizations, it is important to provide some detailed considerations for transforming raw lab result files into analytic lab databases. The analyst does not have control over typographical and other reporting errors but has to make decisions about how to handle them when standardizing lab data. These suggestions provide guidance, but it is important to also work through these decisions as part of an interdisciplinary team within the healthcare organization to ensure that the analytic data set meets organizational standards and needs.

When cleaning lab data in preparation for analysis, the multitude of possible data errors such as typos, missing data, and erroneous results, coupled with the lack of standardization, requires decisions be made that may result in eliminating complete or partial rows of data, removing fields, editing fields, or calculating new fields from existing information. For example, a serum creatinine of 115 mg/dL is likely a reporting error because human life is not sustainable with a serum creatinine value of 115 mg/dL. The outlier result should be considered for exclusion from the data set based on the possibility that a decimal point was eliminated (11.5 mg/dL), the sample tested was urine and not serum (115 mg/dL may be normal for urine), or an incorrect unit of mg/dL was applied instead of µmol/L (115 umol/L is a normal blood creatinine value.)

Database-Related Concerns to Be Aware of When Cleaning Data

Table 4.2 describes issues and problems with lab data with an example of the problem and recommendations for handling each case. This list of database and data-transformation considerations is not exhaustive but exemplifies how complicated the development of a valid lab results data set may be. A data dictionary for the source data and for the lab data extract is imperative to ensure a valid data set results from data-cleaning efforts.

It is imperative that all data transformations are well documented.

Common Structure of Lab Data

Table 4.3 shows the fields, descriptions, and typical field values of a lab data set and includes the use of each field for population health analytic purposes where appropriate. There is no requirement that these fields or coding systems be formatted for the fields.

Table 4.2 Example Lab Data Issues and Potential Solutions

Issue	Example Problem	Example Solution
Case sensitivity	IU/ML = IU/mL or MG/DL = mg/dL	Ensure case dependency is not enforced, units exactly match a crosswalk table, or transform into desired case.
Mixed quantitative, semiquantitative and qualitative results in the results field.	101, <4, Immune, >600,000, and TNTC present in results field and numeric lab results are required.	*Example solution 1*: Transform <4 into 3, 3.999, −99, etc., and document the transformation. *Example solution 2*: Depending on the input requirements, transform qualitative results into binary or integer results or fit to other results represented by the normal range specified in the application. Transform Immune, TNTC, or Positive to the numerical value 1 and transform Not immune or Negative to the numerical value 0. Transform results like Test Not Performed (TNP) or Invalid to the numerical value −1. *Example solution 3*: Parse the symbols of equality from the numerical values and ensure the parsed values are accurately represented within the normal values range. Parse > from the numerical value 600,000 and ensure the interpretation is not negatively impacted when compared to the normal range of <50.
Units present in the results field	6.6%	Parse the units and the results into separate fields. Example, parse 6.6% into a numeric results field with 6.6 and an alphanumeric units field of %.

(continues)

Table 4.2 Example Lab Data Issues and Potential Solutions   *(continued)*

Issue	Example Problem	Example Solution
Commas or periods present when not expected	Values such as 7,1 or 2,000 present when numeric, decimal values are expected.	Remove the comma or transform to a decimal point where appropriate. Examine the assay and normal ranges before removing any commas. It may be appropriate to remove the comma from 2,000 to create a numeric input value of 2000; however, if the 7,1 value was reported in an international format, the transformation from 7,1 to 7.1 would be appropriate and removing the comma to create a value of 71 would be incorrect.
Unclear identifier	LOINC missing but assay name is present yet unclear. Example: Assay name (may be common name in electronic medical record [EMR] = Creat.) (1) Does Creat represent Creatine or Creatinine? (2) Is the sample blood or urine? (3) If urine, what type of urine creatinine assay—24 hour, random, or clearance?	Determining acceptable versus unacceptable results based on assay name is most difficult. Enlisting input from an individual familiar with the nuances of clinical laboratory science and results reporting is recommended. The assay name, result, normal ranges, ranges of clinically realistic results, specimen type, units, patient demographics, and the testing facility must all be considered when extracting laboratory results from a data warehouse where explicit identifiers are missing. If at all possible, it is best to exclude ambiguous results.
Incomplete lab data extract: missing results and results qualifiers may or may not be present	Comments such as "Grossly hemolyzed," "Preliminary result," "Site not specified," or "Assay verified by repeat analysis" are not present in an extract. Comments are extremely important to results interpretation and when deciding the validity of any assay result. If a sample is hemolyzed, triglyceride and glucose results may be affected. As another example, if conflicting HgbA1c results (4.0% and 7.1%) exist for a single patient where the assays were performed on two different samples drawn 1 week apart, one sample may be invalid and one sample with a comment of "Assay verified by repeat analysis" may be valid.	*Example solution 1*: If a comments field in not present within a lab data extract, verify the location of the field within the data warehouse and ensure it is included in the extract. The possibility exists that the data warehouse has failed to include a comments field. If a comments field is not available, then invalid lab results may be included in the data set. *Example solution 2*: If all comments are missing and a comments column is present in an extract, verify that no comments exist in the source data. It is unusual to see no comments in a lab results data set. *Example solution 3*: Exclude any results that are questionable.

| Incomplete lab data extract: sample collection and assay descriptors missing. | Lab sample collection and assay descriptors such as sample type, draw date or time and assay run time are important when considering appropriateness and validity for inclusion of any assay in a data set. Excluding consideration of such descriptors may mean that inappropriate or invalid results are included in a data set. For instance, a red-top tube drawn for a blood glucose assay may not be appropriate if too much time has lapsed between the time the sample was drawn and when serum was separated from the cells. Glycolysis will lower the glucose value by approximately 5% per every hour the serum is in contact with the red blood cells. A normal fasting serum glucose value obtained using serum from a red-top tube instead of a serum separator tube (SST) may or may not be accurate and may actually represent a prediabetic value. | If sample type, draw date, draw time, sample receipt time at the lab, and time of assay result are available, include those fields in the lab data extract. Depending on the assay, develop a set of acceptance criteria and exclude invalid results. |

Table 4.3 Common Structure for Lab Data

Field Name	Field Description	Typical Field Values and Format	Typical Use In Population Health Analytics
Unique patient identifier	An identifier that may be used as a primary key to identify a discrete patient. May be a medical record number, Medicare Beneficiary Identifier, deidentified, identifiable, or system generated.	003563388 CZ789UM892Q uidxx469c58bdkgz876 A1	Compute frequencies by patient. Track changes over time.
Patient age	Age at sample collection; may require parsing if <, >, or + included. Age band may be represented.	009; 09; 9; 100; 48; <1; >85; 85+ 0 – 17; 18 – 54; 55 – 85; 85+	

(continues)

Table 4.3 Common Structure for Lab Data *(continued)*

Field Name	Field Description	Typical Field Values and Format	Typical Use In Population Health Analytics
Gender	Patient gender. Biological gender is preferable as identifiable gender may misrepresent result interpretation.	M, F, U Male, Female, Other, Unknown, blank	
Specimen collection date and time	The date and time the specimen was collected. Only date without time may be available.	Datetime 2020-05-01 14:02.00.000 2020-05-01, 05/01/2020	Exploratory data analysis (EDA) Time tracking Longitudinal analysis Data quality evaluation
Specimen arrival at lab	The date and time the specimen was received at the testing laboratory. Only date without time may be available.	Datetime 2020-05-01 14:02.00.000 2020-05-01, 05/01/2020	Data quality evaluation
Sample type	The sample or draw type used for the assay	Alphanumeric Fasting SST, random urine, WB red top	EDA Data quality evaluation
Performing laboratory	Name of the laboratory that performed the assay	Alphanumeric Quest Diagnostics Incorporated 5th Floor ####	Look up test parameters in catalog Data quality evaluation
Laboratory type	Type of testing facility May not be known—especially from EMR	Alphanumeric Reference Point of care Hospital stat lab Unknown	Data quality evaluation
Result report date	The date and time the result was finalized by the laboratory. Only date may be available.	Date and time 2020-05-01 14:02.00.000 2020-05-01, 05/01/2020	Time tracking Longitudinal analysis Data quality evaluation
Test performed	The specific assay performed by the laboratory. Standardized LOINC result code is preferred. CPT or SNOMED codes may exist.	Alphanumeric 2161-8 Blank	EDA Standardizing or normalizing lab results Data quality evaluation
Common assay name	Common assay name. LOINC result code name is preferred. The laboratory order code name is often used.	Alphanumeric Creatinine, Urine Creatinine, 24-Hour Urine	EDA Standardizing or normalizing lab results Data quality evaluation

Laboratory order code	The internal order code unique to the laboratory	Alphanumeric 003042	EDA Standardizing or normalizing lab results Data quality evaluation
Assay sample type	The exact sample that was used to perform the assay. An SST may have been drawn, but the assay was performed on serum.	Alphanumeric Serum EDTA plasma NaF whole blood urine	EDA Data quality evaluation
Result	The exact result before transformation as reported by the laboratory.	Alphanumeric >100,000 1.2, <4 , 8.4%, 220 Immune, Positive Not detected, TNP, TNTC, blank	EDA Data quality evaluation Analytical comparisons and evaluation
Result modifier 1	Result qualifiers where the reported result is beyond assay detection limits, is semiquantitative or qualitative. May also represent a symbol referencing a comment.	< > * Blank	EDA Data quality evaluation Analytical comparisons and evaluation
Numeric result value	The numeric portion of the result stripped of any modifiers if present	100,000 1.2, 4 , 8.4, 220	EDA Data quality evaluation Analytical comparisons and evaluation
Reported units of measure	The units of measure associated with the result reported by the laboratory	mg/dL, MG/DL, mg%, µg/dL g/L, RU, mmol/L, %, copies per mL, cfu/mL	EDA Data quality evaluation Analytical comparisons and evaluation
SI units of measure	The SI units of measure are specific per LOINC/ assay.	g/L, units/mL, mmol/L, etc.	EDA Data quality evaluation Analytical comparisons and evaluation
Conventional to SI conversion	The conversion factor to transform conventional units to SI units—multiply by. Unique per lab and assay .	0.01 (mg/dL * .01 = g/L)	EDA Data quality evaluation Analytical comparisons and evaluation
Result modifier 2	Often the result comment	Gross hemolysis, QNS, verified by repeat analysis, 3+ lipemia, preliminary	EDA Data quality evaluation Analytical comparisons and evaluation

(continues)

Table 4.3 Common Structure for Lab Data *(continued)*

Field Name	Field Description	Typical Field Values and Format	Typical Use In Population Health Analytics
Reference range	Reference range as reported by the laboratory performing the test. May be present in 1 to 4 columns. Varies by assay, laboratory, region, gender, age.	Creatinine | Age	Male (mg/dL)	Female (mg/dL)
≤2 days	0.79–1.58	0.79–1.58
20–49 years	0.60–1.35	0.50–1.10		EDA Data quality evaluation Analytical comparisons and evaluation
Out-of-range flag, laboratory result interpretation	Out-of-range or other results interpretations provided by the laboratory	High, Normal, Panic Low, Moderately High, H, L	EDA Data quality evaluation
Specimen quality	Information related to specimen collection, transportation, and processing	Specimen broken in transit Wrong specimen type Specimen too old Nonfasting sample	EDA Data quality evaluation

Example Lab Data Sets

Recall that a distinction is made between the data sets generated by laboratories and provided to requesting entities, referred to as *reported lab data* and *analytic lab data sets*, that result from the processing of reported lab data. **Figure 4.1** displays an example of a reported lab data set, and **Figure 4.2** shows the analytic data set derived from Figure 4.1.

Laboratory Test Results Commonly Used in Population Health Analytics

The results of laboratory tests can be used in multiple ways for population health analytics. Lab values are used to understand and monitor health status and prevent adverse outcomes for people with chronic illness. When added to risk-prediction and prescription models, lab data add to the accuracy and predictive power of these models (Barda, Ruiz, Gigliotti, & Tsui, 2019). As part of quality-monitoring programs, the existence of lab results indicates that preventative maintenance has taken place and results are used to understand the quality of healthcare services through programs such as the Healthcare Effectiveness Data and Information Set (HEDIS) and CMS value-based programs. Lab results can be part of the guidelines used to optimize pathways that minimize waste and inefficiency in health care as in the Choosing Wisely campaign and in other types of care pathway optimization. **Table 4.4** describes lab tests commonly used in population health analytics along with more information about each test.

Patient_id	Testing facility	LOINC	Test_Name	Result	Numeric Result	Units	Normal Range	Comments	Result_date
aaaaaaa	Ref Lab 1	4548-4	HgbA1c	<4.0%	4	%	4.8%–5.60%		12/31/2019
aaaaaaa	Ref Lab 1	4548-4	HgbA1c	9.4*	9.4	%	4.8%–5.60%	Result repeated	1/15/2020
bbbbbbb	Ref Lab 1	2093-3	Total cholesterol	233	233	mg/dL	<200 mg/dL	Moderate hemolysis	2/2/2019
ccccccccc	Internal	2345-7	Glucose	98	98	mg/dL	74–106	Fasting	12/31/2019
dddddd	POC	3094-0	BUN	33	33	MG/DL			6/4/2020
eeeeeee			FBS	128					4/6/2020
fffffff	Ref Lab 1	2571-8	Triglycerides	313	313	mg/dL	<150	1+ lipemia	8/30/2020
ggggggg	Ref Lab 2	14956-7	Microalbumin	30	30	mg/L	<30 mg/L	24 hour	2/22/2020
hhhhhhh	POC		Creatinine	115	115	mg/dL			7/4/2020
iiiiiii	Lab 3		Glycosolated hemoglobin	53	53	mmol/mol	26–41	NaF	7/4/2020

Figure 4.1 Reported Lab Data Set Example.

Advantages and Disadvantages of Lab Data for Population Health Analytics

One main advantage of using laboratory data with medical claims data for population health analytics is that they add biomedical markers that can provide early detection of undocumented or unidentified conditions across large populations of patients. With this added information, healthcare organizations can plan and intervene to mitigate the impact of poor indictors before they result in irreversible disease. For instance, by identifying the numbers, geographic location, and primary care providers of patients with diabetes who have high hemoglobin A1C levels, an accountable care

Patient_id	Testing facility	LOINC	Test_Name	Result	Numeric Result	Units	Normal Low	Normal High	Comments	Result_date
aaaaaaa	Ref Lab 1	4548-4	HgbA1c	9.4*	4	%	4.8	5.6	Result repeated	1/15/2020
bbbbbbb	Ref Lab 1	2093-3	Total cholesterol	233	233	mg/dL		199	Moderate hemolysis	2/2/2019
ccccccccc	Internal	2345-7	Glucose	98	98	mg/dL	74	106	Fasting	12/31/2019
dddddd	POC	3094-0	BUN	33	33	MG/DL				6/4/2020
eeeeeee			FBS	128						4/6/2020
fffffff	Ref Lab 1	2571-8	Triglycerides	313	313	mg/dL		149	1+ lipemia	8/30/2020
ggggggg	Ref Lab 2	14956-7	Microalbumin	30	30	mg/L		29	24 hour	2/22/2020
iiiiiii	Lab 3		Glycosolated hemoglobin	7	7	%	4.8	5.6	NaF	7/4/2020

Figure 4.2 Example Lab Data Set Post-transformation and Cleansing.

Table 4.4 Lab Tests Commonly Used in Population Health

Laboratory Test Result	Source	Description	Typical Use in Population Health Analytics	A Common LOINC and Link (U.S.)	Info Link
Hemoglobin A1c	Whole blood	Hemoglobin A1c, also called *A1c* or *glycated hemoglobin*, is hemoglobin with glucose attached. The A1c test evaluates the average amount of glucose in the blood over the last 2 to 3 months by measuring the percentage of glycated hemoglobin in the blood.	Quality measurements Monitor ng diabetes Prediabetes identification	4548-4	https://labtestsonline .org/tests/hemoglobin -a1c
Fasting serum glucose	Serum	A fasting blood glucose (FBG) is a measurement of the serum concentration of glucose. Glucose is a simple monosaccharide and provides energy for cellular processes and aids metabolism within the body.	Diabetes screening Hypo- or hyperglycemia	2339-0	https://labtestsonline .org/tests/glucose-tests https://loinc.org/2339-0/
Creatinine	Serum Urine	Creatinine is a waste product produced by muscles from the breakdown of a compound called *creatine*. Creatinine is removed from the body by the kidneys, which filter almost all of it from the blood and release it into the urine. This test measures the amount of creatinine in the blood or urine or both.	Kidney function assessment Kidney disease monitoring	Serum creatinine 38483-4 24-hr urine creatinine 20624-3 Creatinine clearance 12195-4	https://labtestsonline .org/tests/creatinine
Blood, urea, nitrogen (BUN)	Serum	Urea is a waste product formed in the liver when protein is metabolized into its component parts (amino acids). Sometimes a BUN-to-creatinine ratio is calculated to help determine the cause of elevated levels.	Kidney function assessment Kidney disease monitoring Liver disease, malnutrition indicator	3094-0	https://labtestsonline .org/tests/blood-urea -nitrogen-bun

Microalbumin	Urine	Albumin is a major protein normally present in blood, but virtually no albumin is present in the urine when the kidneys are functioning properly. However, albumin may be detected in the urine even in the early stages of kidney disease.	Early indicator of kidney disease, possibly resulting from diabetes or high blood pressure. Indicator of increased cardiovascular risk	14957-5	https://labtestsonline.org/tests/urine-albumin-and-albumin-creatinine-ratio https://www.ncbi.nlm.nih.gov/pmc/articles/PMC3100287/
High-density lipoprotein (HDL)	Serum or fingerstick for point of care (POC)	High-density lipoprotein (HDL cholesterol, HDL-C) is one of the classes of lipoproteins that carry cholesterol in the blood. It is considered to be beneficial because it removes excess cholesterol from tissues and carries it to the liver for disposal.	Quality measures Cardiovascular disease (CVD) risk assessment	2085-9	https://labtestsonline.org/tests/hdl-cholesterol
Low-density lipoprotein (LDL)	Serum calculation	LDL cholesterol (LDL-C) is one type of lipoprotein that carries cholesterol in the blood. LDL-C is considered to be undesirable and is often called *bad cholesterol* because it deposits excess cholesterol in blood vessel walls and contributes to hardening of the arteries and heart disease. Most often this test involves using a formula to calculate the amount of LDL-C in blood based on results of a lipid profile. Occasionally, LDL-C is measured directly.	Quality measures CVD risk assessment	2089-1	https://labtestsonline.org/tests/ldl-cholesterol https://labtestsonline.org/tests/direct-ldl-cholesterol
Total cholesterol	Serum or fingerstick for POC	Cholesterol is a substance (a steroid) that is essential for life. The test for cholesterol measures total cholesterol that is carried in the blood by lipoproteins. Extra cholesterol in the blood may be deposited in plaques on the walls of blood vessels.	Quality measures CVD risk assessment	2093-3	https://labtestsonline.org/tests/cholesterol
Triglycerides	Serum	Triglycerides are a form of fat and a major source of energy for the body. Most triglycerides are carried in the blood by lipoproteins called *very low-density lipoproteins* (VLDL). High levels of triglycerides in the blood are associated with an increased risk of developing CVD, although the reason for this is not well understood.	CVD risk assessment	2571-8	https://labtestsonline.org/tests/triglycerides

organization can target specific interventions to prevent further diabetes complications like skin ulcers and kidney disease.

Incorporating lab values into the analytic tools of population health on an operational level in risk-prediction models, segmentation models, clinical pathway automation, and prescriptive analytics strengthens models and processes and also ensures that this additional information is informing all aspects of clinical programs. In addition, the use of lab values can improve targeting criteria and result in better resource allocation for clinical programs because fewer patients are falsely identified for a program and the patients that are identified for inclusion are more likely to meet criteria (higher true-positive and lower false-positive rates).

Lab values are an important component of value-based payment programs. They provide an objective, well-accepted, rigorously generated indicator of the quality of healthcare services, a critical piece of the Triple Aim. Government, regulatory, and private organizations depend on the measurement and monitoring of important lab-based indicators to improve healthcare delivery.

To benefit from lab data, healthcare organizations must be willing to invest time and resources. The use of lab data in population health analytics requires clinical and analytical expertise and familiarity with lab data and the time for experts to convene and create and review the rules that will be applied to raw claims data sets. In addition, poor data cleansing and standardization may result in inaccurate conclusions and misinterpretation, turning an advantage into a disadvantage.

Despite best efforts, lab data are not always readily available for population health analytics because of regulatory and privacy concerns and poor interoperability. The Health Insurance Portability and Accountability Act contains strict provisions regarding the rules for sharing lab data with healthcare entities. Because of these restrictions and patient privacy concerns, lab data are sometimes difficult to obtain by the organizations performing population health analytics. Lab data also suffer from issues of interoperability when they are incorporated into the

population health analytic data infrastructure. Because of the regulatory and privacy issues and problems with interoperability, lab data often are deprioritized as a prominent data source for population health analytics.

Special Considerations for Lab Data

In addition to the information provided in this chapter, there are other considerations that are worth mentioning that influence the use of lab data. The first consideration is the desire to match lab tests in administrative claims data to lab vendor data. When health payers are using lab data for analytics, one way they attempt to validate the volume and tests seen in lab data is to compare lab vendor data to the billing for lab services in administrative claims data. In addition, some quality measures that are based on the occurrence of lab tests use administrative claims data for the calculation instead of lab vendor data. For instance, HEDIS measures for frequency of HbA1c testing in patients with diabetes and relies on billing for these tests in administrative claims data. Unfortunately, it is difficult, if not impossible, to link billing data for labs to clinical data for labs because administrative claims data may not be inclusive of all performed lab tests for a patient. They represent the transformation of lab testing results and adhere to different standards for reporting.

When multiple results exist for the same test within a measurement time period, a decision must be made about which value to use for the measure at hand. This determination will depend on the purpose of the measure. For instance, a time-based measure looking for the occurrence of a value within a certain time frame may use the most recent value, whereas a criterion-based measure may use the "best" value during the time period.

Another consideration is the use of LOINC codes. If these codes are present in clinical lab data, then it is beneficial to download and use a LOINC crosswalk as a reference when standardizing, cleaning, and performing analytic methods with the data.

Lastly, when using lab data it is important to consider the data origin, including the country, vendor lab, electronic medical record, level of transformation, population inclusion and distribution, the purpose of data set, the data-collection time frame, and completeness of data.

Applied Learning: Case Study

More than 20 million Americans have chronic kidney disease (CKD), with more than half a million suffering from end-stage renal disease (ESRD). CKD is most commonly a complication of hypertension and diabetes and is preventable when these conditions are well managed (Drawz & Rahman, 2015). Population health management programs provide services to people with hypertension and diabetes with the aim of preventing complications like ESRD.

ESRD occurs when CKD progresses to a point where the kidneys can no longer function without support and is diagnosed based on laboratory values, specifically the level of serum creatinine (a by-product of muscle breakdown in the blood) and albuminuria (protein in the urine). Higher levels of these two constituents, along with other factors, indicate ESRD is present. Renal replacement therapy, accomplished through the process of dialysis, mechanically removes toxins from the blood when used on a regular basis (multiple times per week or by a continuous process) to treat ESRD (Drawz & Rahman, 2015).

The National Kidney Foundation's Kidney Disease Outcomes Quality Initiative (KDOQI) provides evidence-based guidelines for the management of ESRD and specifically provides targets for certain lab values in patients undergoing dialysis treatment. As part of their contract with health insurers, a large provider of dialysis services across the United States is incentivized to keep key kidney function indicators below the rates in the entire United States for all people with ESRD. Specifically, they are provided incentives when more than 80% of their dialyzed patients meet the KDOQI guidelines for all of these anemia indicators:

Ferritin indicates the amount of stored iron in the body. Iron is required for the production of red blood cells to prevent anemia. A low ferritin can deplete adequate red blood cell production and cause anemia.
Hematocrit indicates the total volume of red blood cells in the total volume of whole blood.
Hemoglobin indicates the oxygen-carrying capacity of the red blood cell, the red blood cells' chief job.

Figure 4.3 displays the monthly monitoring of the anemia indictors for this dialysis provider across all centers in one region of the country over a year. This analysis was undertaken by the health insurer in

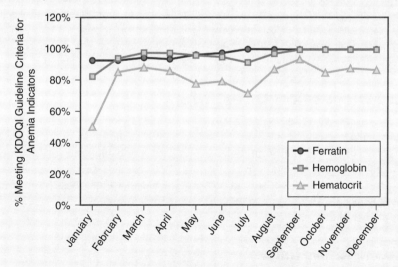

Figure 4.3 Monitoring of Anemia Indicators by Month.

(continues)

Applied Learning: Case Study   *(continued)*

the region who is providing the incentive payment. These providers from the regional centers perform well but are having difficulty adequately maintaining the hematocrit measure.

The following steps were taken to derive these monthly indicators:

- The raw lab value data set was exported to the health plan for analysis.
- Analysts at the health plan reviewed the raw lab data with a nephrologist to determine which tests, values, and ranges would be needed in a final analytic data set.
- The final analytic data set was created using rules from the previous step and included the variables needed for monthly monitoring including:
  - patient ID,
  - month,
  - serum ferritin value using the last value for the patient in the month,
  - serum hemoglobin value using the last value for the patient in the month, and
  - serum hematocrit value using the last value for the patient in the month.
- The KDOQI cutoff values for ferratin, hemoglobin, and hematocrit were compared to the patient-level test values, and an indicator was created for each patient that determines whether the value for the patient was above or below the cutoff.
- The percentage of the entire set of patients in each month that met the cutoff value was determined.

Conclusion

Lab data provide an opportunity to enhance population health analytics in every phase of the process from assessment to optimization by adding to the understanding of clinical conditions and their sequelae, enhancing risk-prediction and prescription models, determining impactful interventions, and improving the measurement of quality. Lab data originate from completed lab testing vary from large, experienced organizations to provider offices to individuals performing at-home testing. The variety of lab data sources, regulations, and standardization lends itself to a great deal of complexity when attempting to include lab results into population health analytics. This means that trade-off decisions must be made by individual healthcare organizations between the value of adding lab data and the resources and time necessary to make the data usable.

Study and Discussion Questions

- What are the barriers to standardizing clinical laboratory data?
- What challenges exist with transforming lab data that might make interpretation of clinical laboratory data difficult? What should be done with these results with respect to inclusion in the analytical data set?
- Considering analytical resources available at your facility, what might be the most important population health analytical initiatives that would incorporate lab data and that would have the most positive impact on the Triple Aim?

Resources and Websites

American Association for Clinical Chemistry: https://www.aacc.org/

Learning resources on LOINC site: https://loinc.org/learn/

LOINC search: https:// loinc.org

International Consortium for Harmonizing of Clinical Laboratory Results: http://www .harmonization.net/

Lab tests online for understanding lab tests: https://labtestsonline.org/#

Internet Pathology Laboratory for Medical Education: https://webpath.med.utah.edu/webpath.html

References

Barda, A., Ruiz, V., Gigliotti, T., & Tsui, F. (Rich). (2019). An argument for reporting data standardization procedures in multi-site predictive modeling: Case study on the impact of LOINC standardization on model performance. *JAMIA Open*, *2*(1), 197–204. https://doi.org/10.1093 /jamiaopen/ooy063

Centers for Medicare and Medicaid Services (CMS). (2019). How to obtain a CLIA certificate. Clinical Laboratory Improvement Amendments (CLIA). https://www.cms.gov /Regulations-and-Guidance/Legislation/CLIA

Diaz, B. (2014). Data normalization use case: Mapping disparate labs to LOINC. Wolters Kluwer Health Language Blog. https://blog.healthlanguage.com/data-normalization -use-case-mapping-disparate-labs-to-loinc

Drawz, P., & Rahman, M. (2015, June 2). Chronic kidney disease. *Annals of Internal Medicine, 162*(11), ITC1–ITC14. https://doi.org/10.7326/AITC201506020

Fletcher, W. M. (1929, November 30). Norman Lockyer lecture on medical research: The tree and the fruit. *The British Medical Journal, 2*(3595), 995.

Hauser, R. G., Quine, D. B., & Ryder, A. (2018, February). LabRS: A Rosetta Stone for retrospective standardization of clinical laboratory test results. *Journal of the American Medical Informatics Association, 25*(2), 121–126. https:// doi.org/10.1093/jamia/ocx046

HL7 International. (2019). HL7 standards product brief— C-CDA (HL7 CDA R2 implementation guide: Consolidated CDA templates for clinical notes—US realm). http:// www.hl7.org/implement/standards/product_brief.cfm ?product_id=492

Klatt, E. C. (2020). The Internet pathology laboratory for medical education. University of Utah. https://webpath .med.utah.edu/webpath.html

Laczin, J. A. (2013). The shift to a centralized lab approach. *Applied Clinical Trials*. https://www.appliedclinicaltrials online.com/view/shift-centralized-lab-approach

Mardis, C. (2017, October 24). Keeping up with POCT regulatory compliance. Medical Laboratory Observer. https://www.mlo-online.com/information-technology /lis/article/13009284/keeping-up-with-poct-regulatory -compliance

Myers, G. L., & Miller, W. G. (2018). The roadmap for harmonization: Status of the International Consortium for Harmonization of Clinical Laboratory Results [Opinion paper]. *Clinical Chemistry and Laboratory Medicine, 56*(10), 1667–1672. https://doi.org/10.1515/cclm-2017-0907

Radin, M. S. (2013, September). Pitfalls in hemoglobin A1c measurement: When results may be misleading. *Journal of General Internal Medicine, 29*, 388–394. https://doi .org/10.1007/s11606-013-2595-x

Regenstrief Institute. (2015). Quick start guide for mapping to laboratory LOINC. https://loinc.org/guides/quick-start/

Rohr, U. P., Binder, C., Dieterle, T., Giusti, F., Messina, C. G. M., Toerien, E., . . . , Hendrikschäfer, H. (2016, March 4). The value of in vitro diagnostic testing in medical practice: A status report. *PLoS ONE, 11*(3). https://doi.org/10.1371 /journal.pone.0149856

Search LOINC. (2020). https://loinc.org/guides/quick-start/

Simons, C. C., & Capraro, G. A. (2019, July 3). The pros and cons of centralizing microbiology services. American Association for Clinical Chemistry. https://www.aacc.org /publications/cln/articles/2019/julyaug/the-pros-and -cons-of-centralizing-microbiology-services

Swain, M., & Patel, V. (2014, February). Health information exchange among clinical laboratories. Office of the National Coordinator for Health Information Technology (ONC). Data Brief No. 14. https://www.healthit.gov/sites/default /files/onc-data-brief-14-testresultexchange_databrief.pdf

U.S. Department of Health and Human Services (DHS). (2015). 2015 edition health information technology (health IT) certification criteria, 2015 edition base electronic health record (EHR) definition, and ONC health IT certification program modifications; final rule. *Federal Register, 80*(200). https://www.govinfo.gov/content/pkg /FR-2015-10-16/pdf/2015-25597.pdf

U.S. Department of Health and Human Services (DHS). (2018, September). Medicare payments for clinical diagnostic laboratory tests in 2017: Year 4 of baseline data. https:// oig.hhs.gov/oei/reports/oei-09-18-00410.pdf

U.S. Food and Drug Administration. (2019). In vitro diagnostics. https://www.fda.gov/medical-devices/products-and -medical-procedures/vitro-diagnostics

U.S. Food and Drug Administration. (2020). Clinical laboratory improvement amendments (CLIA). https:// www.fda.gov/medical-devices/ivd-regulatory-assistance /clinical-laboratory-improvement-amendments-clia

CHAPTER 5

Pharmacy Data

Sarah Kachur, PharmD, MBA, BCACP

When summed at an individual or population level, pharmacy data provides vast insight into medication usage, disease burden, comorbidity, patient needs, and clinical and financial outcomes.

—Sarah Kachur

EXECUTIVE SUMMARY

Pharmacy data are a complete and accurate reflection of the medications a patient receives to treat acute and chronic conditions in the inpatient and outpatient settings. Although the primary purpose of these data is to maintain prescribing and dispensing records and to facilitate payment, pharmacy data are a critical resource for population health analytics. Pharmacy data may be used to understand the disease burden within a population, quantify treatment rates and medication adherence, establish medication-safety patterns in quality measure calculations, and in pharmacoeconomic studies. Pharmacy data are most commonly sourced from electronic medical records (EMRs) or administrative claims and may be used alone or in combination with other data sources to compile an understanding of the population's disease burden, predicted future risk, health needs, and outcomes.

LEARNING OBJECTIVES

At the end of this chapter, the learner will be able to:

1. Describe common sources of pharmacy data used in population health analytics.
2. Understand the structure of pharmacy data and data variables pertinent to analytics.
3. Understand common groupers and coding systems associated with medications and pharmacy data.
4. Use pharmacy data to define population characteristics and operationalize interventions to improve medication use and health of a population.

Introduction

Pharmacy data provides a wealth of information about the health of individuals and populations when used alone or more often in conjunction with other sources of health data. Pharmacy data can be used to understand drug utilization within a population, to discern clinical conditions and primary concerns, for safety surveillance, and to improve medication use.

Pharmacy data are generated through patient treatment encounters with the healthcare system, either those that result in a prescription being generated or those associated with filling a prescription. In most countries, many medications require a prescription from a healthcare provider and dispensing from a local pharmacy, and it is these administrative records that generate pharmacy data for analysis.

This chapter will describe common sources of pharmacy data used in population health analytics, including a description of how data sets may vary and be used differently based on the source system. Common coding systems used for pharmacy data are described, along with applications of pharmacy data in analysis.

Defining Pharmacy Data

Pharmacy data are records of medication history generated through patient treatment encounters. These data serve as the source of truth for medications that a patient was prescribed and received. Data may be generated at the time of prescribing during a provider office visit or at the time of filling a prescription at the pharmacy. Pharmacy data typically contain data elements pertinent to the patient, prescriber, pharmacy, and specific medication. Pharmacy data are commonly available in the format of one record per prescription or one record per fill and are tied specifically to each patient's record and dispensing pharmacy.

Sources of Pharmacy Data

The majority of pharmacy data available for population health analytics originate from two sources: prescribing records and administrative payment records. Prescribing data from the EMR contains details of medications ordered for a patient during encounters with the healthcare system, including medication, dosage, frequency (e.g., twice/day), and refills. EMR-sourced pharmacy data may be used as a reflection of the entire current and past medication list of the patient within the practices and prescribers using that EMR. Administrative payment records, also known as *claims*, originate from billing encounters between an outpatient pharmacy and a payer. These records consist of much the same data points as EMR-sourced pharmacy records, with the addition of related financial variables such as total medication cost and patient cost share. Pharmacy claims data contain a record of all medications reimbursed by a specific payer, regardless of prescriber or outpatient pharmacy used. These data sources often have overlap and similar advantages, but limitations should be considered carefully when developing an analysis. **Table 5.1** summarizes these sources and their application in population health analytics.

Within the United States, transfers of pharmacy data between entities (see **Figure 5.1**) are governed by standard file formats defined by the National Council for Prescription Drug Programs (NDPCP). The NDPCP defines and maintains file formats used for transferring pharmacy data between payers and pharmacies, standardizing dosage units for patient safety, using pharmacy data to meet EMR Meaningful Use standards, transmitting pharmacy data between EMRs, and sharing billing and financial records for prescriptions (National Council for Prescription Drug Programs, n.d.). These standards facilitate rapid, accurate interchange of prescription information between healthcare entities.

Organizations will often keep database records of these electronic standard transactions for a variety of administrative, clinical, and regulatory purposes. Healthcare providers will retain the record of EMR prescriptions generated to ensure the accurate population of each patient's medication list and prescription activity that resulted from a healthcare system encounter. Likewise, pharmacy benefit managers (PBMs) and health plans retain a data set of paid pharmacy claims for financial reconciliation and analysis purposes. Finally, pharmacies and clinics are required to hold records of prescriptions dispensed to satisfy regulatory requirements. Regardless of the rationale, the administrative needs just described will

Table 5.1 Application of Outpatient Pharmacy Data in Population Health Analytics

Type of Outpatient Pharmacy Data	Underlying Population	Level of Data	Common Types of Analysis	Limitations
EMR prescribing records	Patients of the provider office or health system	One record per prescription	Prescribing patterns by medication and medication class Frequency of drugs on med list Adherence to organizational formulary or care pathways	Does not support adherence calculations No record of prescriptions from "outside" providers May not indicate if prescription was ever filled No information about cost to patient or, often, system
Pharmacy claims data	Insured population	One record per dispensing event (multiple refills of one prescription)	Expenditures by medication and medication class Pharmacoeconomic and budget impact modeling Medication adherence Polypharmacy Unsafe medication use Pharmacy quality measures Detection of fraud or abuse	No record of prescriptions not covered by insurance plan Diagnosis information must be inferred or linked from medical claims data
Medication dispensing events	Pharmacy or clinic patients	One record per dispensing event (multiple refills of one prescription)	Medication utilization and trends Medication-safety studies Pharmacoeconomic and budget impact modeling	No record of prescriptions from other pharmacies Diagnosis information must be inferred or linked from clinic EMR

result in the organization housing and maintaining a longitudinal database of pharmacy data.

EMR Prescribing Records

Pharmacy data in the electronic medical record reflects the historic and current medication list of a patient. These data reflect the entirety of the prescribing record by providers within the practices using the relevant EMR. Depending on the scope of the EMR implementation, the medication list may be populated by a combination of electronically prescribed (e-prescribed) outpatient prescriptions, orders for inpatient or infused products, medication records obtained through a national or local health information exchange, or manual entry by office staff or patients.

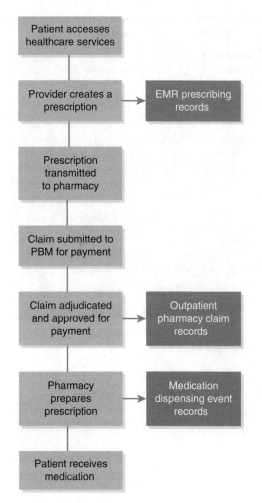

Figure 5.1 Generation of Outpatient Pharmacy Data.

The most common of types of EMR pharmacy data are inpatient orders and outpatient prescriptions. Inpatient orders are those prescriptions generated during the time an individual is a patient in a hospital, emergency room, or institution. They are intended to be administered by institutional staff and are often dispensed by a single organizational pharmacy. By contrast, outpatient prescriptions are intended for patient self-administration of medications in the home setting. They are generated within the EMR, sent electronically to the outpatient pharmacy of a patient's choosing, and filled as a take-home supply—often one month or more for medications for chronic disease.

Because of the limited nature of inpatient encounters (days to weeks) and the acute needs

of patients during that time, inpatient medications are frequently quite different than outpatient medications taken longitudinally by the general public. For that reason, most population health analyses rely on outpatient pharmacy data. Inpatient pharmacy data are more commonly used for specific inpatient-setting medication use evaluations, which are beyond the scope of this chapter. Resources for inpatient medication use evaluations are available from the Academy of Heath-Systems Pharmacy (American Society of Health-System Pharmacists, 1996).

As mentioned, EMR pharmacy data are the outpatient prescription records most commonly used for population health analytics. These records are generated through the activity of medication prescribing during a point-of-care encounter such as a provider office visit or discharge from an emergency department or hospital. Historically, prescriptions were handwritten by providers, but in the past decade evolving technology has resulted in most prescriptions being generated and transmitted electronically. Such e-prescribed medications are accurate and error free and are sent directly from the point of care to the pharmacy, resulting in fewer medication errors, increased patient safety, and a complete record of prescribed medications. Although not statutorily required in the United States, federal payment incentives beginning in 2009 coupled with state incentive and technology advancements have driven widespread adoption of e-prescribing by almost all outpatient pharmacies and more than 75% of physicians (Centers for Medicare and Medicaid Services [CMS], n.d.; Surescripts, 2018). Maintenance of an electronic medication list is required of EHRs certified for ambulatory use in the United States (Office of the National Coordinator, 2015). It is this e-prescribing activity that populates the medication list and results in data that may be secondarily used for analytic purposes.

Pharmacy Administrative Claims Data

Administrative pharmacy claims data may be used as a source for population health analytics. In the United States, most people obtain prescription drugs through health insurance provided by their employer or a government program. If this health insurance includes prescription drug coverage, billing activity for the prescription will generate records known as *prescription drug claims*. Prescription drug claims data are records of all prescriptions paid for by an individual's health plan. Because of the high cost of prescription drugs and the advent of Medicare Part D coverage for seniors, less than 10% of prescriptions in the United States are paid for without the use of insurance benefits (National Council for Prescription Drug Programs, 2009).

Prescription drug claims result from adjudication of these outpatient billing events by PBMs. These entities provide information systems and administrative support to manage prescription drug benefits for health plans, employers, and other plan sponsors (Pharmacy Benefit Management Institute, n.d.). Most health plans contract with PBMs to manage prescription drug benefits, with the PBM responsible for prescription drug claim processing, maintaining pharmacy networks, formulary administration, and price negotiation (Fox, 2003). As shown in Figure 5.1, these PBMs serve as clearinghouses for pharmacies to submit electronic bills for payment to various health plans.

Most organizations, either their health plans or their PBMs, will retain data sets of prescription drug claims internally. Although the primary purpose of these data is for billing and financial reconciliation, they may be used secondarily to understand disease burdens, quantify drug utilization, maintain safety surveillance, and develop and drive population-level interventions to improve medication use.

Individual Pharmacy or Clinic Data

Finally, an individual dispensing pharmacy will keep records in electronic format of all medications dispensed to relevant patients. These records are similar to prescription drug claims in that they represent individual dispensing events, but in this case for customers of a specific pharmacy or clinic. These records may be retained centrally if a pharmacy has multiple locations or kept onsite for pharmacies at a single location. Although narrowly representative when including data from a single pharmacy, these records are critically important in select settings where a single pharmacy or clinic setting may be serving the primary health needs of patients such as a student health clinic, infectious disease clinic, residential facility, or employer-based or occupational health clinic.

Common Structure for Pharmacy Data

As mentioned, because of electronic transaction standards and medical and pharmacy record retention requirements, healthcare organizations store records of medications prescribed and prescriptions filled. Once this information is finalized and processed, it is transferred from a transactional system (EMR or claims payment platform) into a data store that is updated regularly. More mature organizations will include pharmacy data as part of a data warehouse with linkages to other frequently used data points (patient demographics, prescriber information, and medical claims) that can be accessed by analytic staff.

Within a data table, pharmacy data is stored at the level of the individual transaction. For EMRs, that means one record for each prescription issued by a prescriber or medication dispensing event. For claims data and pharmacy and clinic dispensing, that results in one record per dispensing event. **Table 5.2** shows variables commonly found in pharmacy data. Often the pharmacy data tables in an organization's data warehouse will be similar or identical to the NDPCP transmission standards used between entities with substantial granularity that describes prescriber, prescription, patient, and billing attributes.

Note that for chronic medications that are refilled routinely, a single prescribing event can result in multiple dispensing events: one for each refill.

Pharmacy Coding Systems

This section covers coding systems and information that are commonly present within pharmacy claims data. These data points from

Table 5.2 Common Variables Found in Pharmacy Data

Variable Name	Variable Description	Typical Variable Values and Format	Typical Use in Population Health Analytics
Patient identifier	The patient identifier indicates the recipient of the medication.	Organizationally defined alphanumeric identifier For claims data, often health plan identifier. For EMR data, often organizational patient ID.	Aggregating all prescriptions a patient has received. Linking with other sources of data within the enterprise, including EMR records, medical claims, lab data, and ad-hoc data sets.
Prescriber identifier	This is the unique identification code for the prescriber of each prescription; commonly a physician, nurse practitioner, physician assistant, or other healthcare practitioner with local prescribing authority.	Commonly prescriber NPI number May also be organizationally defined prescriber identifier such as an internal physician ID.	Identifies the prescriber responsible for each prescription. Used to identify a treating relationship between prescriber and patient.
Medication identifier: National Drug Code (NDC)	Indicator of specific drug product. Most granular identification code for each drug.	11 digit numeric	Identifies the exact medication dispensed to the patient. Understanding drug strength, dosage form, and route of administration (i.e., 10-mg oral tablet).
Medication identifier: SNOMED Clinical Terms (CT) Code	Indicator of drug name and formulation	9 digit numeric	Most common in EMR data; not used in claims. Identifies drug prescribed or administered to patient.
Medication name	Contains the active ingredient name, strength, and dosage type of the mediation the patient was prescribed.	Text	Understand the medication ingredient, strength, and dosage type prescribed to the patient.
Medication class	Medication grouping information by type of drug	Text or numeric	Understand the type of medication, maintained grouper for analytic purposes.
Quantity	Amount of medication doses patient received	Numeric	Understand the number of doses given to the patient (e.g., 30 tablets, 200 mL).

Days supply or duration	Amount of time patient should take a medication	Numeric	Understand the duration of treatment (e.g., 30 days, 5 doses). With other variables, quantify medication adherence and treatment gaps.
Date	Date medication is dispensed or administered, may also include time.	System-specific date format	Identify dates medication are provided to the patient.
Filling pharmacy*	Pharmacy that dispensed the medication	System-specific text format; may include numeric identifier in some data sets.	Identify pharmacy dispensing the medication. Quantify pharmacy locations that population uses frequently.
Medication cost*	Total cost of dispensed medication	Dollars	Describes total billed cost for each dispensed prescription. Use in pharmacoeconomic studies and formulary management.
Patient cost share*	Portion of medication cost paid by patient	Dollars	Reflective of patient's copayment or coinsurance amount. Understand financial burden for patients, especially those with multiple chronic medications.

*Administrative claims data only

pharmacy data are often used within population health to create relevant analyses either alone or in combination with other data sources. Medication information can be used to understand condition prevalence, adherence to prescribed treatments, and drug safety concerns, as well as drive formulary management and decision-making. Drug-specific information can be used to discern dosage patterns, including under- and overuse, and specialized administration needs such as injection support. Prescriber information helps the analyst understand which providers and specialty types are being commonly used within the population. Finally, pharmacy data often include an indication of dispensing pharmacy.

Medication Identifiers in Pharmacy Data

At the most granular level, pharmacy data will contain the name, strength, unit, and formulation of the product dispensed and often a numeric National Drug Code (NDC) identifier. These individual drug products must be used in population health analyses, for example, to identify patients taking medications for a particular condition or taking a potentially unsafe medication.

Depending on the structure of the data, the drug name, strength, and formulation may be a single text string or three independent variables. *Drug name* indicates the product name prescribed for a particular patient and may include a brand name, a generic name, or both. The *strength* indicates the amount of active ingredient included in each dose, often described in metric units. Finally, the *formulation* indicates how the drug is delivered. Common oral formulations taken by mouth include tablets, capsules, or liquids. Products may also be formulated as injections; inhalations; ear, eye, or nose drops; or other less common routes of administration. An example of these variables is shown in **Table 5.3**.

In population health analyses, attention should be paid to the formulation when identifying drugs for inclusion in a data set because the same drug name may be used for different conditions in various healthcare settings. As shown in **Table 5.4**, ciprofloxacin, a commonly used antibiotic, is available in multiple formulations for both inpatient and outpatient use. An analysis of pediatric ear-infection medications would need to reference different products for inpatient intravenous utilization.

NDC Number

In addition to drug name and strength labeling, the U.S. Food and Drug Administration (FDA) requires all pharmaceutical products to be assigned a National Drug Code (NDC) identifier (U.S. Food and Drug Administration, 2019). The NDC number is an 11-digit numeric identifier that is specific to each unique drug product. Within the 11 digits are three segments that provide information about the product: XXXXX–XXXX–XX. The first segment, five digits, represents the drug manufacturer and may have leading zeros dropped. The second segment which is four digits is the product code and provides information about the strength and dosage form of the product. Finally, the last two-digit segment is an indicator of package size.

A current listing of drug products approved for sale in the United States and an accompanying data dictionary are available publicly from the FDA by accessing its National Drug Code Directory website (https://www.fda.gov/drugs/drug-approvals -and-databases/national-drug code-directory).

As demonstrated in **Table 5.5**, a given medication may have multiple NDCs based on its manufacturer, its strength, and the package size used for dispensing. As an example, one single

Table 5.3 Common Drug Name Variables

Drug Name	Strength	Unit	Formulation
Lipitor	10	mg	Tab
Atorvastatin	40	mg	Tab

Table 5.4 Example Healthcare Settings and Populations

Drug Label Variables	Primary Use	Population	Common Healthcare Setting
Ciprofloxacin 3 mg/mL ophthalmic solution	Eye infection	Pediatric and Adult	Outpatient
Ciprofloxacin 500 mg tablet	Systemic infection	Adult	Outpatient
Ciprofloxacin 2 mg/mL injection	Serious systemic infection	Adult	Inpatient or home health care
Ciprofloxacin 2 mg/mL otic suspension	Ear infection	Pediatric	Outpatient

IBM Watson Health, n.d.

Table 5.5 Medication Identifiers and NDC Codes

Product Trade Name	Drug Name	Strength	Package Size	Manufacturer	NDC
Lipitor	Atorvastatin	10 mg	90 tablets	Parke-Davis	00071-0155-23
Lipitor	Atorvastatin	40 mg	90 tablets	Parke-Davis	0071-0157-23
Lipitor	Atorvastatin	40 mg	500 tablets	Parke-Davis	0071-0157-73
Atorvastatin Calcium (generic)	Atorvastatin	40 mg	90 tablets	Teva	0093-5058-98
Atorvastatin Calcium (generic)	Atorvastatin	40 mg	500 tablets	Mylan	0378-3952-05

product, the common cholesterol-lowering medication atorvastatin, has multiple strengths, manufacturers, and package size. At the time of writing, atorvastatin has more than 50 active manufacturers and more than 300 unique NDC numbers.

SNOMED CT

SNOMED Clinical Terms (SNOMED CT) codes make up a healthcare terminology code set that is used to describe clinical conditions and treatment concepts (SNOMED International, n.d.) (see **Table 5.6**). SNOMED CT includes more than 300,000 clinical concepts, including nomenclatures for diseases, results, procedures, and medications. Also used in EMR systems, SNOMED CT contains a numeric identifier for each medication active ingredient. Similar to NDC, the SNOMED CT identifier is uniquely linked to an individual drug. However, NDC is specific to manufacturer and packaging size, whereas SNOMED is specific to ingredient only.

Unlike other nomenclature systems, SNOMED CT provides standardized language to identify medication allergies. These codes are separate and distinct from the identifiers for medications themselves and should be considered in a nuanced analysis of population-level or clinical data. For example, an analysis of patients prescribed a medication to manage high cholesterol may wish to exclude patients with a documented allergy to these medications. Alternately, these codes may be used to understand the burden of medication allergies within the population.

Medication Groupers in Pharmacy Data

When using pharmacy data for population health analytics, the frequency of new products, revised dosage forms, and changing manufacturers and package sizes all contribute to challenges in using an indicator of this granularity. The FDA

Table 5.6 SNOMED CT Medication and Medication Allergy Codes

Medication	SNOMED CT Code	SNOMED CT Allergy Code
Atorvastatin	373444002 Atorvastatin (substance)	13221000122100 Allergy to atorvastatin (finding)
HMG CoA reductase inhibitors	372912004 Substance with 3-hydroxy-3-methylglutaryl-coenzyme A reductase inhibitor mechanism of action (substance)	294970008 Allergy to 3-hydroxy-3-methylglutaryl-coenzyme A reductase inhibitor (finding)

website listing is updated daily with new products, manufacturers, strengths, and package sizes. In addition, an individual may receive a different manufacturer's product with each refill, depending on pharmacy stock. An analysis based on an incomplete or out-of-date medication names, SNOMED CT codes or the NDC list may inadvertently underrepresent medication use within the population by excluding new medications or manufacturers from the analysis. As a result, the analyst must account for the rapidly changing nature of pharmaceutical products, SNOMED CT, and NDC codes when using pharmacy data for population health analyses. If NDC, SNOMED code, or drug name is the only medication indicator available within the data set, the analyst should consider quarterly updates to the drug list to ensure new products and formulations are included.

To overcome this challenge and provide a more comprehensive approach, the analyst may choose to use medication data groupers to simplify analysis. Broadly, medication groupers map NDCs and SNOMED granular concepts into more usable categories that are clinically relevant and analytically simplified. A typical grouping arrangement will organize multiple medications into hierarchical categories of drug name and strength combination, ingredient, and therapeutic class level. A therapeutic class is a group of medications that have similar biochemical structures and are used to treat the same condition. An example of a typical pharmacy grouping is shown in **Figure 5.2**.

Publicly available and privately licensed drug classification systems can augment existing data sets and be used as groupers within large scale and recurrent analyses. The anatomical therapeutic chemical (ATC) drug classification is a drug grouping system developed and maintained by the World Health Organization (n.d.). The ATC is a five-level structured classification system. The highest level consists of 14 categories of pharmacological and anatomical groups, with levels 2, 3, and 4 providing additional granularity of subgroups. The ATC fifth level classification is at the drug name level. For ease of use, each seven-digit ATC code confers meaning, allowing various levels of granularity to be included in an analysis. See **Table 5.7**.

Similar to the NDC, the SNOMED CTs provide a grouper level inherent with their medication concepts. Unlike ATC and other commercially available groupers, SNOMED CT codes do not infer meaning inherent within digits and must be individually investigated using the publicly available lookup tool. However, they do provide granularity by mechanism of action and therapeutic use; as shown in **Figure 5.3**, they can be used within analyses of EMR data as groupers.

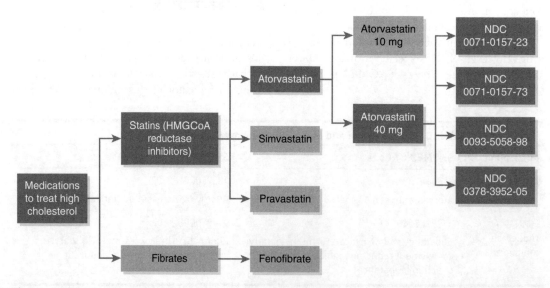

Figure 5.2 Medication Grouper Example.

Table 5.7 ATC Category Examples

ATC Category Level	Level 1	Level 2	Level 3	Level 4	Level 5
Format	Single letter	2 numeric digits	Single letter	Single letter	2 numeric digits
Example 1: Verapamil (World Health Organization, 2020)	C (cardiovascular)	08 (calcium channel blocker)	D (selective channel blocker)	A (phenylalkylamine derivative)	01 (verapamil)
Example 2: Atorvastatin (World Health Organization, 2019)	C (cardiovascular)	10 (lipid modifiers)	A (lipid modifiers, plain)	A (HMGCoA reductase inhibitors)	05 (atorvastatin)

RxNorm Data Set

In the United States, medication name, strength, and dosage naming conventions are standardized by the RxNorm data set, a service of the National Library of Medicine (National Library of Medicine, 2020). RxNorm establishes standard names to allow pharmacy systems and databases to list active medications for prescribing and communicate between each other in a uniform format. These functions are critical for e-prescribing systems and pharmacy dispensing systems to share information accurately when transmitting prescription data between systems because inaccurate transmission can result in a medication error and patient safety risk. Therefore, to ensure

quality of data transfer between systems, RxNorm naming conventions are a certification requirement for EMRs and dispensing systems within the United States (CMS, 2020a).

In addition to terminology and patient safety features, RxNorm provides a crosswalk of commonly used medication groupers, including the ATC and SNOMED CT groupers previously described. Additional commercially available and public groupers supported within RxNorm include First Databank, Multum, and the Veterans Health Administration National Drug File. A mapping and lookup function of publicly available classifications is available via the RxNorm web lookup feature: https://mor.nlm.nih.gov/RxClass/

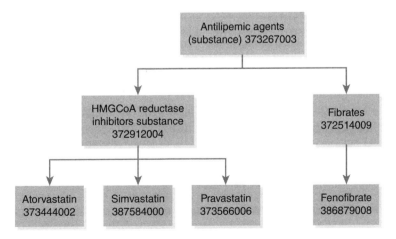

Figure 5.3 Hierarchy of SNOMED CT for Select Antilipid Medications.

Prescriber Identifiers in Pharmacy Data

Pharmacy data typically include an indicator of the healthcare provider responsible for generating each prescription, whether in the EMR or from pharmacy administrative claims. This indicator is the unique identifier for the prescriber of each prescription, commonly a physician, nurse practitioner, physician assistant, or other healthcare practitioner with local prescribing authority. Maintenance of the prescriber data for each prescription is a regulatory requirement for EMRs and dispensing pharmacies.

Within the United States, the National Provider Identifier (NPI) number represents the standard identifier for prescribers. The NPI was established nationally in 2004 for billing and regulatory purposes and is required for use by healthcare entities when transmitting data or billing the federal government for services (U.S. Department of Health and Human Services, 2004). The NPI is a 10-digit numeric identifier that is assigned to each healthcare provider by the National Plan and Provider Enumeration System (NPPES), which also maintains a publicly available lookup table and provides downloadable file of provider data (National Plan and Provider Enumeration System, n.d.). Within pharmacy data, the NPI number associated with each prescription may be used to establish and identify a treating relationship between prescriber and patient. In combination with other data such as provider type and specialty obtained from NPPES download files, it may also be used to understand the use of various specialties within a population, identify cases of duplicate prescribing or medication-safety issues, or understand "doctor shopping" behaviors.

Medication list and e-prescriptions in EMR data may include an organizationally defined prescriber identifier such as an internal provider identification number. If the organization maintains complete provider records, ideally the data warehouse will contain additional information about these internal provider identifications such as a crosswalk to NPI number, specialty, and provider department.

Advantages and Disadvantages of Pharmacy Data for Population Health Analytics

As described in this chapter, pharmacy data contain detailed and accurate records of medications that a patient was prescribed and received during his or her course of disease treatment. EMR-sourced pharmacy data will identify at granular level the medications an individual patient is prescribed and administered in an inpatient or outpatient clinic setting. Likewise, pharmacy administrative claims data provide exhaustive detail on prescriptions that patients received at an outpatient pharmacy. Together or separately, they represent a reasonably accurate and complete picture of an individual patient's prescribed medications and when those medications were received. When summed at an individual or population level, pharmacy data provide vast insight into medication usage, disease burden, comorbidity, patient needs, and clinical and financial outcomes.

In administrative settings, pharmacy data may be the nearest time data available to represent patient disease burden and morbidity. As described in Chapter 3, medical claims go through a lengthy payment process before being finalized in a data set for analysis. These medical claims may not represent a full reflection of utilization until up to 3 months after the patient has received service. By contrast, pharmacy claim processing is electronic and instantaneous. Payment records are generated instantaneously on request by a filling pharmacy, usually flowing into a database for analysis within 2 weeks of activity. This makes pharmacy administrative claim data a preferable near-time data source for understanding disease burden and utilization patterns.

By virtue of that same automated payment process and standardized electronic submission format, pharmacy administrative data contain a robust and accurate set of financial indicators associated with each dispensing event. For example, the Medicare Part D Prescription Drug Event file layout contains indicators of total medication cost, dispensing fee (amount paid to pharmacy as a service fee), sales tax, patient copay, amount of low-income subsidy applied, health plan paid amount, and additional indicators of patient and plan liability calculations (CMS, 2006). These indicators may be aggregated at the drug, drug therapy class, disease state, and patient levels to understand medication costs at various levels within the population.

One substantial drawback of pharmacy data is that individual sources do not reflect the entire clinical status of the patient and may have unknown gaps in comprehensiveness. As discussed, EMR prescription data reflects medications that are *prescribed* for the patient to take in the outpatient setting, whereas administrative claims data reflect medications that are *filled* at an outpatient pharmacy. Primary nonadherence is the gap that occurs if a medication is prescribed by the physician but unfilled by the patient. Literature suggests that rates of primary nonadherence are approximately 25%, depending on the type of medication (Park, Yang, Das, & Yuen-Reed, 2018). Understandably, this would result in different results if EMR data or administrative claims data were studied for the same patient.

This lack of specific clinical status also creates challenges in understanding specific disease conditions using pharmacy data as a standalone source. Pharmacy data alone, particularly administrative claims data, require that the disease condition be imputed from the drug type rather than more specifically known from ICD-10-CM or other diagnostic codes in the medical claims data (see Chapter 3). Analysts must use caution when imputing diagnoses at the patient level based on pharmacy data alone. For example, the generic drug metformin is commonly used for diabetes but rarely for polycystic ovarian syndrome and other infertility challenges. A population analysis using only pharmacy data could misidentify infertile women as having diabetes. Likewise, such an analysis could not indicate the severity level of diabetes (i.e., does the patient have complications?). This drawback may be overcome by using

a combined data set of administrative medical and pharmacy claims or by using a full suite of data tables generated by a robust EMR.

Special Considerations for Pharmacy Data

Pharmacy data used as a standalone analytic source have benefits and drawbacks that the analyst should consider when designing and conducting an analysis. Failing to consider these factors may lead the analyst to draw incorrect conclusions based on a lack of understanding of the underlying data set.

Similar to medical claims data, a primary consideration is the content of the data set being used. In general, pharmacy administrative claims include prescriptions intended for use in the outpatient setting that require a prescription and were submitted to a healthcare payer for reimbursement. Therefore, pharmacy claims data are reflective only of those medications prescribed and covered by the health plan. Typically, over-the-counter products and herbal remedies are not included in administrative claims. Likewise, payer-specific drug exclusions would not be reflected in administrative data—for example, drugs used for weight loss, cosmetic purposes, or nonmedical indications (CMS, 2016). Finally, drugs provided via manufacturer samples, direct programs for low-income individuals, or retail store generic drug discount programs may not be processed through the payer and thus would not be included in administrative claims data set (see **Table 5.8**) (Law, Chan, Harrison, & Worthington, 2019; Munigala, Brandon, Goff, Sagall, & Hauptman, 2019; Tungol et al., 2012).

A pharmacy administrative claims data set may have unique inclusion criteria for high-cost specialty drugs or medications administered in the provider clinic. A *specialty drug* is defined by the Centers for Medicare and Medicaid Services (CMS) as an outpatient prescription drug product that costs $670 or more per month, requires special handling or training (such as self-injection at home), or other unique handling requirements. Specialty drugs represent 1% or less of

Table 5.8 Common Products Excluded from Pharmacy Administrative Claims

- Noncovered medications such as those used for cosmetic purposes
- Over-the-counter products
- Herbal and vitamin supplements
- Office samples or trial supplies provided at no cost by manufacturer
- Drugs provided at direct discount by the retail pharmacy and bypassing payer

prescriptions in the United States but may skew cost analyses within the population (CMS, 2015). Special handling requirements may limit the types of pharmacies that can dispense these medications, and health plans often monitor utilization using tools such as prior authorization, restricted quantities and days supply, and limited distribution channels (AMCP, 2019; Mullins, Lavallee, Pradel, DeVries, & Caputo, 2006; Patel & Audet, 2014). As a result, these medications may not be included in an administrative claims data set or included within typical data variables.

Similarly, medications administered in a provider clinic setting are typically billed through the medical benefit using a Healthcare Common Procedure Coding System (HCPCS) code as described in Chapter 3. HCPCS codes with starting letter C or J are used to indicate office-administered injectables. Examples of such medications are chemotherapy and other injectable medications that require IV infusion in a physician's office rather than self-injection at home. Payer-specific coverage and billing guidance will determine inclusion of these products in medical claims versus pharmacy administrative claims. For example, CMS defines medical benefit drugs as "injectable and infusible drugs that are not usually self-administered and that are furnished and administered as part of a physician service" (CMS, 2006) (see **Table 5.9**). Select medications may be covered under the medical benefit in some situations and the pharmacy benefit in others, making a combined data set a necessity to understand the full utilization of these products. When completing analyses on patients or populations who may be using these medications, the analyst should be attentive to how these medications are reflected in their data set.

Finally, compounded products, mixtures of drug products that are formulated by pharmacists when a commercially available formulation is not available, may likewise be excluded or reflected in nonstandard variable layouts.

Table 5.9 Medicare Coverage Status for Select Injectable Products

Medication	Medical Benefit Coverage (Medicare Part B)	Pharmacy Benefit Coverage (Medicare Part D)
IV chemotherapy	Yes	No
Sumatriptan self-injectable	No	Yes
Epoetin	All patients with end-stage renal disease Other diagnoses when administered in physician office	Other diagnoses when self-injected at home
Insulin	When administered through infusion pump	When self-injected

Data from Medicare Rights Center (2015). Medicare Drug Coverage: Part D vs. Part B. https://www.medicareinteractive.org/wp-content/uploads/2015/08/B-vs-D-chart.pdf

Example Data Sets

The example data sets in **Tables 5.10** and **5.11** show typical data variables and formats for EMR and administrative claims data for a single patient. In this example, patient Jane Doe saw Dr. Smith on March 2, 2020. As reflected in the EMR data, Dr. Smith prescribed atorvastatin 40 mg to treat high cholesterol. Doe revisited Dr. Smith on May 12 and was prescribed an additional medication, fenofibrate 145 mg, as a second cholesterol medication.

Following her physician office visits, Doe visited the pharmacy on March 12, April 20, and May 26 to fill her prescriptions.

CMS provides a freely accessible file of synthetic pharmacy claims that is a good resource to practice using administrative claims data: https://www.cms.gov/Research-Statistics-Data-and-Systems/Downloadable-Public-Use-Files/BSAPUFS/BSA_PDE_PUF

Using Pharmacy Data for Population Health Analytics

In certain analytic situations, pharmacy administrative claims data may be the only clinical data available for a given population, such as in pharmacoeconomic analyses, PBM-centric analyses of medications or specialty drug usage, or Medicare Part D plans. In others, it may be combined with other data sources such as EMR data, medical claims, or other records to create a more complete picture of patient and population utilization and health status.

Medication Adherence

Pharmacy data may be used to identify opportunities to improve medication use among patients with chronic disease. Medication adherence, sometimes called *compliance*, is defined as the extent to which patients take medication as prescribed by their doctors with particular focus on doses taken and duration (Cramer et al., 2008). Medication adherence may be measured via metrics such as Medication Possession Ratio

(MPR), Proportion of Days Covered (PDC), and Medication Gaps (Sikka, Xia, & Aubert, 2005; Steiner & Prochazka, 1997).

Medication adherence measures are commonly used measures of medication-taking behavior within a population. Generally, MPR and PDC values are considered optimal to adequately treat a disease if a patient takes 80% or more of prescribed doses. **Table 5.12** shows commonly used medication adherence metrics and their definitions.

Population health analyses may seek to quantify medication adherence at a patient or population level as one indicator of the health of a population and its ability to self-manage chronic disease. Once suboptimal adherence is identified as a challenge, the analysis may further seek to understand and quantify population-level reasons for noncompliance such as high cost share for medications to treat chronic disease or requirement to take multiple medications in a complex regimen (known as *polypharmacy*) (Elliott, Shinogle, Peele, Bhosle, & Hughes, 2008).

Such analyses may be used to support population health interventions to improve health status and reduce utilization and costs associated with chronic disease. Case-management programs may aim to reduce barriers to obtaining medications among high-risk patients. A pharmacist-led medication therapy management program is a requirement of Medicare prescription drug plans and aims to improve therapeutic outcomes for targeted beneficiaries through improved medication use (CMS, 2020). At the population level, copay reduction programs and other incentives may reduce barriers to medication use within the population.

Interventions to improve medication adherence and other population-level programs to improve medication use may be measured using a framework implemented with pharmacy administrative claims alone or in combination with medical claims. The framework in **Figure 5.4** includes layers of metrics to identify process measures, intermediate outcomes, and ultimate utilization and cost improvements at the population level as a result of an intervention to improve medication use (Perlroth et al., 2013).

Table 5.10 Example EMR Data Set

Patient Identifier	Prescriber Identifier	SNOMED CT Code	Medication Name	Medication Class	Quantity	Instructions	Refills	Date
Jane Doe	Dr. Smith	373444002	Atorvastatin 40 mg	372912004	30	1 tab daily	6	3/2/2020
Jane Doe	Dr. Smith	386879008	Fenofibrate 145 mg	372514009	30	1 tab daily	6	5/12/2020

Table 5.11 Example Administrative Claims Data Set

Patient Identifier	Prescriber Identifier	NDC Code	Medication Name	Medication Class	Quantity	Days Supply	Date	Filling Pharmacy	Medication Cost ($)	Patient Cost Share ($)
Jane Doe	Dr. Smith	0071-0157-73	Atorvastatin 40 mg	C10AA05	30	30	3/12/2020	Fred's Drugs	13.45	10.00
Jane Doe	Dr. Smith	0071-0157-73	Atorvastatin 40 mg	C10AA05	30	30	4/20/2020	Fred's Drugs	13.45	10.00
Jane Doe	Dr. Smith	0093-5058-98	Atorvastatin 40 mg	C10AA05	30	30	5/26/2020	Green's Pharmacy	14.23	10.00
Jane Doe	Dr. Smith	0074-3173-90	Fenofibrate 145 mg	C10AB05	30	30	5/26/2020	Green's Pharmacy	62.58	20.00

Table 5.12 Common Medication Adherence Metrics

Adherence Metric	Definition
Medication Possession Ratio (MPR)	Total number of days for which medication is dispensed (excluding final prescription) divided by the total number of days between the first and last prescription. If a patient is on multiple medications for a single condition, the day's supply and prescribing days are totaled across all and averaged.
Proportion of Days Covered (PDC)	Ratio of day's supply divided by days between first prescription fill and end of observation period.
Number of Gaps	Count of occurrences where the time interval between the end of supply of one prescription and the onset of the next prescription for the same medication (active ingredient) is more than the grace period.

Reproduced from The Johns Hopkins University. (2018). The Johns Hopkins ACG® system version 12.0 user documentation. https://www.hopkinsacg.org/documents/system-documentation

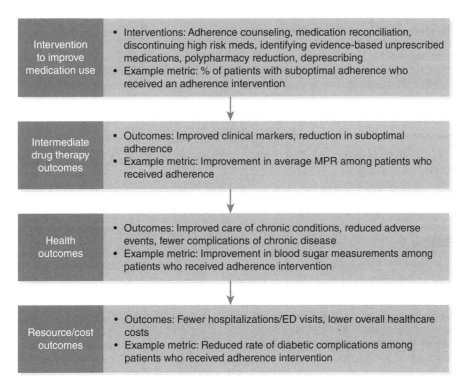

Figure 5.4 Framework to Improve Medication Adherence and Use.

Data from Perlroth, D., Marrufo, G., Montesinos, A., Lewis, C., Dixit, A., Li, B., Rusev, E., Ghimire, E., Packard, M., Olinger, L., Fair, S., Mercincavage, L., & Stratos, S. (2013). Medication therapy management in chronically ill populations: Final report. https://innovation.cms.gov/files/reports/mtm_final_report.pdf

Conclusion

Pharmacy data contain accurate, detailed medication-related information specific to patients and medications. The data include medications from multiple prescribers or specialists the patient has encountered, thus providing a more complete record of medications than that available from a single prescriber's perspective. This comprehensive view allows for improved patient safety and identification of drug interactions when integrated in front-end applications such as EMRs and retail pharmacies. Likewise, the data can be used as an accurate reflection of medications that a patient is taking, and they are often used to draw conclusions about patients' morbidity and predicted risk of adverse health events, as well as to improve use of medication within a healthcare setting or population.

Study and Discussion Questions

- How can pharmacy data be used within population health analysis?
- What are some challenges with using administrative pharmacy claims in population health analytics?
- Study the example EMR and administrative claims data sets. Calculate the MPR for Ms. Doe's atorvastatin prescription. Is the MPR optimal? What are some factors that may have contributed to her medication filling patterns? What was Ms. Doe's monthly medication cost during May 2020?

Resources and Websites

RxNorm Crosswalk lookup: https://mor.nlm.nih.gov/RxNav/

U.S. FDA NDC lookup and National Drug Code directory: https://www.fda.gov/drugs/drug-approvals-and-databases/national-drug-code-directory

SNOMED CT Code lookup: https://browser.ihtsdotools.org/

ATC therapy class lookup: https://www.whocc.no/atc_ddd_index/

Using Pharmacy Data in Economic Evaluations (ISPOR): https://www.ispor.org/

Using Pharmacy Data for Medication Use Evaluations (ASHP): http://www.ashp.org

NPI lookup and crosswalk: https://npiregistry.cms.hhs.gov/

Pharmacy benefits: AMCP: http://www.amcp.org

References

Academy of Managed Care Pharmacy. (2019, July 18). Specialty pharmaceuticals. https://www.amcp.org/about/managed-care-pharmacy-101/concepts-managed-care-pharmacy/specialty-pharmaceuticals

American Society of Health-System Pharmacists. (1996). ASHP guidelines on medication–use evaluation. *American Journal of Health-System Pharmacy, 53,* 1953–1955. https://pubmed.ncbi.nlm.nih.gov/8862210/

Centers for Medicare and Medicaid Services. (n.d.). Electronic prescribing (eRx) incentive program. https://www.cms.gov/Medicare/Quality-Initiatives-Patient-Assessment-Instruments/ERxIncentive/index.html

Centers for Medicare and Medicaid Services. (2006). Medicare drug coverage under Part A, Part B, and Part D. https://www.cms.gov/Outreach-and-Education/Outreach/Partnerships/Downloads/determine.pdf

Centers for Medicare and Medicaid Services. (2015, April 7). Medicare Part D specialty tier. https://www.cms.gov/medicare/prescription-drug-coverage/prescriptiondrugcovgenin/downloads/cy-2016-specialty-tier-methodology.pdf

Centers for Medicare and Medicaid Services. (2016). Chapter 6—Part D drugs and formulary requirements. Medicare prescription drug benefit manual. https://www.cms.gov/medicare/prescription-drug-coverage/prescriptiondrugcovcontra/downloads/part-d-benefits-manual-chapter-6.pdf

Centers for Medicare and Medicaid Services. (2020a). Medicare and Medicaid promoting interoperability program basics. CMS.gov. https://www.cms.gov/Regulations-and-Guidance/Legislation/EHRIncentivePrograms/Basics

Centers for Medicare and Medicaid Services. (2020b). Medication therapy management. Woodlawn, MD: Centers for Medicare and Medicaid Services. https://www.cms.gov/Medicare/Prescription-Drug-Coverage/PrescriptionDrugCovContra/MTM

Cramer, J. A., Roy, A., Burrell, A., Fairchild, C. J., Fuldeore, M. J., Ollendorf, D. A., & Wong, P. K. (2008, January–February). Medication compliance and persistence: Terminology and definitions. *Value in Health, 11*(1), 44–47. https://pubmed.ncbi.nlm.nih.gov/18237359/

Elliott, R. A., Shinogle, J. A., Peele, P., Bhosle, M., & Hughes, D. A. (2008). Understanding medication compliance and persistence from an economics perspective. *Value in Health, 11*(4), 600–610.

Fox, P. D. (2003, Winter). Prescription drug benefits: Cost management issues for Medicare. *Health Care Finance Review, 25*(2), 7–21. https://www.ncbi.nlm.nih.gov/pmc/articles/PMC4194804/

IBM Watson Health. (n.d.). Ciprofloxacin hydrochloride. In IBM Micromedex® DRUGDEX® [Electronic version]. https://www.ibm.com/watson-health/about/micromedex

Johns Hopkins. (n.d.). ACG® system version 12.0 user documentation. https://www.hopkinsacg.org/documents/system-documentation/

Law, M. R., Chan, F. K., Harrison, M., & Worthington, H. C. (2019, November). Impact of brand drug discount cards on private insurer, government, and patient expenditures. *Canadian Medical Association Journal, 191*(45), E1237–E1241. https://pubmed.ncbi.nlm.nih.gov/31712357/

Medicare Rights Center. (2015). Medicare drug coverage: Part D vs. Part B. https://www.medicareinteractive.org/wp-content/uploads/2015/08/B-vs-D-chart.pdf

Mullins, C. D., Lavallee, D. C., Pradel, F. G., DeVries, A. R., & Caputo, N. (2006, September–October). Health plans' strategies for managing outpatient specialty pharmaceuticals. *Health Affairs, 25*(5), 1332–1339. https://pubmed.ncbi.nlm.nih.gov/16966730/

Munigala, S., Brandon, M., Goff, Z. D., Sagall, R., & Hauptman, P. J. (2019, November–December). Drug discount cards in an era of higher prescription drug prices: A retrospective population-based study. *Journal of the American Pharmacists Association, 59*(6), 804–808. https://pubmed.ncbi.nlm.nih.gov/31422026/

National Council for Prescription Drug Programs. (n.d.). Standards and more. https://www.ncpdp.org/Standards-and-More.aspx

National Council for Prescription Drug Programs. (2009). Pharmacy: A prescription for improving the healthcare system, version 1.0.

National Library of Medicine. (2020). RxNorm overview. https://www.nlm.nih.gov/research/umls/rxnorm/overview.html

National Plan and Provider Enumeration System. (n.d.) National Provider Identifier Registry public search; https://npiregistry.cms.hhs.gov/

Office of the National Coordinator. (2015). Medication list, version 1.1. https://www.healthit.gov/test-method/medication-list

Park, Y., Yang, H., Das, A., & Yuen-Reed, G. (2018). Prescription fill rates for acute and chronic medications in claims-EMR linked data. *Medicine, 97*, 44.

Patel, B. N., & Audet, P. R. (2014, November). A review of approaches for the management of specialty pharmaceuticals in the United States. *Pharmacoeconomics, 32*(11), 1105–1114. https://pubmed.ncbi.nlm.nih.gov/25118989/

Perlroth, D., Marrufo, G., Montesinos, A., Lewis, C., Dixit, A., Li, B., Rusev, E., Ghimire, E., & Stratos, S. (2013, August). *Medication therapy management in chronically ill populations: Final report.* Acumen LLC. https://innovation.cms.gov/files/reports/mtm_final_report.pdf

Pharmacy Benefit Management Institute. (n.d.) Terminology glossary.

Sikka, R., Xia, F., & Aubert, R. E. (2005, July 1). Estimating medication persistency using administrative claims data. *American Journal of Managed Care, 11*, 449–457. https://www.ajmc.com/journals/issue/2005/2005-07-vol11-n7/jul05-2085p449-457

SNOMED International. (n.d.). http://www.snomed.org

Steiner, J. F., & Prochazka, A. V. (1997, January). The assessment of refill compliance using pharmacy records: Methods, validity, and applications. *Journal of Clinical Epidemiology, 50*(1), 105–116. https://pubmed.ncbi.nlm.nih.gov/9048695/

Surescripts. (2018). 2018 National progress report. https://surescripts.com/news-center/national-progress-report-2018/

Tungol, A., Starner, C. I., Gunderson, B. W., Schafer, J. A., Qiu, Y., & Gleason, P. P. (2012, November–December). Generic drug discount programs: Are prescriptions being submitted for pharmacy benefit adjudication? *Journal of Managed Care & Specialty Pharmacy, 18*(9), 690–700. https://pubmed.ncbi.nlm.nih.gov/23206212/

U.S. Department of Health and Human Services. (2004, January 23). HIPAA administrative simplification: Standard unique health identifier for health care providers: Final rule. https://www.cms.gov/Regulations-and-Guidance/Administrative-Simplification/NationalProvIdentStand/downloads/NPIfinalrule.pdf

U.S. Food and Drug Administration. (2019). National drug code directory. https://www.fda.gov/drugs/drug-approvals-and-databases/national-drug-code-directory

World Health Organization. (n.d.). Essential medicines and health products: Classification principles and challenges. https://www.who.int/medicines/regulation/medicines-safety/toolkit_atc_principles/en/

World Health Organization. (2019). Lipid modifying agents. Collaborating Centre for Drug Statistics Methodology. https://www.whocc.no/atc_ddd_index/?code=C10AA05

World Health Organization. (2020). Essential medicines and health products toolkit. https://www.who.int/medicines/regulation/medicines-safety/toolkit_about/en/

CHAPTER 6

Electronic Medical Record Data for Population Health Analytics

Richa Bundy, MPH

By computerizing health records, we can avoid dangerous medical mistakes, reduce costs, and improve care.

—President George W. Bush (2004)

EXECUTIVE SUMMARY

The electronic medical record (EMR) is a collection of digital charts that describe the health and treatment history of patients. An essential function of the EMR is to compile patient charts in an organized, secure, and consistent manner that supports coordinated clinical care delivery. The expansive and dynamic data housed in EMRs can also be repurposed for conducting population health analytics (Friedman et al., 2013). Demographic, socioeconomic, clinical, and behavioral data elements collected through patient care can be used alone or in conjunction with external data sources to compile longitudinal and comprehensive clinical assessments of populations.

Using EMR data for population health comes with unique benefits and challenges. The primary advantages include the timeliness, variety, and rich detail of EMR data. Without the EMR, data elements such as clinical markers and social and medical histories would require vast resources to compile. Another distinctive benefit is the potential for interventions to be implemented within the same system that the EMR data comes from through EMR engineering. Still EMR data present challenges, including a potential lack of generalizability, missing data, interoperability issues, and messy data. Knowing the potential benefits and implications of EMR data is imperative to recognize when to use EMR data and how to use it effectively in population health analysis.

LEARNING OBJECTIVES

At the end of this chapter, the learner will be able to:

1. Describe the structure of an EMR database and list examples of types of data found in the EMR.
2. Explain the advantages and disadvantages of using EMR data for population health analytics in comparison to other data sources.
3. Demonstrate how EMR data can be used to answer questions regarding population health.

Introduction

Before the advent of electronic medical records (EMRs), healthcare providers recorded patient information on paper, resulting in scattered, unsecure, and inconsistent patient health documentation. Aggregating information from paper charts required manual data abstraction, which is both time consuming and laborious. Although the first EMR was introduced in the 1960s as a basic digital transcription of paper charts, the rapid and widespread adoption of EMRs followed the introduction of the Health Information Technology for Economic and Clinical Health Act in 2009 (Center for Surveillance, Epidemiology, and Laboratory Services, 2019). Since then, EMRs have significantly changed the dynamics of how clinicians deliver care and how healthcare systems monitor patient outcomes.

EMRs track everything about patients and their hospital visits from admission to discharge, including patient demographics, vital signs, laboratory results, medications, procedures, progress notes, discharge notes, and billing information. The data entered into an EMR are transmitted to a relational database through an extract, transform, and load (ETL) process, which can be configured by a health system to occur on a regular basis. A relational database is a set of tables, organized in columns and rows, that are joined by a common unique identifier. A relational data model allows for large amounts of data to be stored in separate tables, which can then be joined using structured query language. The combination of a regular ETL process and relational database model provides health systems with an extremely rich and up-to-date data source that can support population health analytics (see Chapter 15). EMR data can be used to evaluate population health as well as assess areas where the health of the population can be improved. This chapter will elaborate on the components and structure of the EMR and present the advantages and challenges of using EMR data for population health analytics. In addition, real-world case studies are provided as examples of how to use EMR data for population health analytics.

Defining EMR Data for Population Health

The aim of using EMR data for population health is to gather a comprehensive clinical care view of a population. The vast EMR database aggregates a wide range of information on populations, including demographics, socioeconomic factors, disease status, clinical markers, and social history. Connecting these data elements allows health systems to conduct robust population health studies that aim to define a population, understand the drivers of poor health, and discover opportunities to improve patient experience, quality of care, and cost outcomes.

Processes for Applying EMR Data to Support Population Health Analytics

The application of the population health approach using EMR data is similar to that of other data sources. As with these other sources, EMR data can be used to define a population, analyze the population, and target subpopulations for an intervention. A distinctive feature of using EMR data is in the level of detail (using diagnoses, demographic, socioeconomic, and clinical data) that can be gathered in the analysis portion of a population health study (Cole, Stephens, Keppel, & Estiri, 2016). Another unique aspect of involving EMR data is that interventions can be set up within the EMR, allowing for seamless data collection of intervention outcomes. For example, a population health analysis with the aim of addressing smoking outcomes in young adults may use birth date data to define the population as patient ages 18 to 25 and use behavioral history data to define a cohort of smokers and nonsmokers. The analysis could then use other types of EMR data, including age, sex, race, hospital visits, insurance status, and ZIP Code to create a complete clinical assessment of each cohort. Comparing smokers and nonsmokers in this scenario could lead to findings on predictors of smoking habits. In addition, this analysis could also produce a targeted group for a potential smoking cessation intervention using EMR-based flagging mechanisms. Program involvement and health outcomes such as continued smoking status as well as healthcare utilization can also be found in the EMR. Therefore, it is possible for an entire population health analysis to be embedded within an EMR, allowing for integrated population health-improvement initiatives.

Advantages and Disadvantages of EMR Data to Support Population Health Analytics

There are multiple data sources for population health analytics beyond EMR data such as health insurance claims data, consumer or marketing data, and publicly available government data. Therefore, it is important to recognize when EMR data can be superior or inferior to other data sources.

Advantages of EMR Data

- EMR data are usually extracted on a daily schedule and do not encounter the same time lags that claims data do. Thus, population health analyses requiring timely data are best suited to use EMR data as opposed to other data sources.
- The EMR is a particularly favorable data source for healthcare provider organizations because the data infrastructure already exists for providing clinical care. In addition, it may not be practical for these organizations to acquire external data such as administrative claims from multiple insurers in a timely manner for their entire patient population. Therefore, EMR data extend population health analyses from beyond payer and public health organizations to healthcare provider organizations (Kharrazi et al., 2017).

- EMRs offer a wide variety of data, including diagnoses, demographics, behavioral and social history, laboratory results, procedures, vital signs, progress notes, medications, allergies, and immunizations. This remarkable level of patient detail is not available through other data sources, adding to the unique advantages of EMR data.
- Another exclusive benefit of using EMR data for population health analytics is in the ability to use informatics tools to integrate interventions back into the EMR. Furthermore, intervention process and outcome metrics can also be tracked using the EMR. For example, risk-prediction scores have been integrated into the EMR to stratify and intervene with high-risk patients. These data can also be extracted and analyzed to assess the health outcomes associated with interventions using the risk-prediction score.

Disadvantages of EMR Data

- Often a health system will only have access to the EMR data that are housed in their databases. In other words, a given EMR only contains data for patient visits that happened within a specific health system. This results in incomplete patient diagnosis and utilization data, especially for specialized or urgent services in which patients received care at another health system. For instance, Kharrazi et al. (2017) found outpatient EMR data was particularly less reliable than administrative claims data for diagnoses of cancer and depression. Therefore, EMR data can underestimate the level of healthcare severity and utilization of a population unless an EMR is fully interoperable with other healthcare provider organizations.
- Population health analyses using EMR data exclude patients who have not interacted with the health system. This is imperative to determine whether extrapolating results to the entire clinic population or the panel of patients for a provider. For example, those who interact with the health system regularly

may be sicker than the patients who do not. Therefore, certain characteristics of a population defined by EMR data may not match those of the same population defined by a health insurance or government data source, for instance.

- In the case where health systems agree to coordinate EMR data across sites of care and multiple EMR brands, interoperability issues may arise. Each unique EMR can have different database structures, creating inconsistencies between data derived from each database. Combining data from multiple EMRs usually requires the additional effort of data transformation and patient matching (Cole et al., 2016). However, efforts have been made to standardize healthcare information for improved data sharing. For example, Rosenbloom et al. (2017) describe examples of advanced efforts to combine disparate EMR data through the development of common data models and Health Level Seven international standards for data exchange.

- As opposed to relatively clean, well defined, and organized administrative claims data, EMR data are notoriously inconsistent in terms of data quality and accuracy (Diamond, Mostashari, & Shirky, 2009). EMR data should be assessed, scrutinized, and cleaned before they are applied to analyses. In addition, data elements such as free text notes require more data processing than other straightforward discrete data elements. The data-cleaning process can be laborious and time consuming, which should be accounted for when planning a population health analysis.

Common Structure for EMR Data

EMR data are vast and diverse and can therefore be extracted into hundreds of tables organized in a relational database structure. Each table contains a defined set of associated information from the health record. For example, a visit table may contain all encounters and information regarding that visit such as the date of the visit, the patient, the clinician providing care, and the location of the visit. The data structure also allows tables to be bridged together using a common unique identifier. For instance, a visit table may be joined to a patient table as well as a diagnosis table using unique common patient and diagnosis identifier fields found in both tables (**Figure 6.1**).

The primary attributes and associated tables that are necessary for population health analytics include demographics; healthcare utilization; procedures; laboratory results and vital signs; medications; immunizations; medical, behavioral, and social histories; and cost and billing.

Demographics

Patient demographics in EMR data include date of birth, primary address, race, ethnicity, sex, gender, marital status, language, and insurance status. These fields are essential for describing and contrasting the characteristics of populations. They are also important pieces of information for adjusted analyses because these individual and socioeconomic factors often introduce bias and confounding in population health analyses.

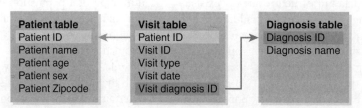

Figure 6.1 A simple example of a relational data model in which unique identifiers (PatientID and VisitDiagnosisID) in the visit table are used to gather additional information from related tables.

Healthcare Utilization

Healthcare utilization refers to the volume of emergency, inpatient, outpatient, and ambulatory visits. The EMR records and categorizes the type of each visit. Utilization data is an important health outcome metric used to track the success of population health interventions. Theoretically, if appropriate preventative care is provided, populations will not need to utilize the healthcare system as widely and as intensely However, the limitation to using EMR data, as opposed to administrative claims data, is that EMRs do not capture all patient visits external to the health system in which they were captured. This can lead to an underestimation of true healthcare utilization of a population because individuals may visit multiple health systems.

Diagnoses

Diagnosis information, which is coded using the *International Classification of Diseases, 10th Revision, Clinical Modification* (ICD-10-CM), is essential for defining a population of interest and for assessing incidence (the number of new people diagnosed with a condition) and prevalence (the number of people diagnosed with a condition). Diagnoses can be linked to a patient chart, visit, or medication order. A diagnosis tied to a patient chart typically includes the diagnosis and the date that it was noted. A visit diagnosis indicates that a patient was seen for a reason relating to that diagnosis. A medication diagnosis indicates that a patient has received a prescription for a drug to treat a specific health problem. Each of these diagnostic sources can be used in conjunction or separately to answer specific population health questions (see Chapter 3 for more information). For example, all three sources can be queried to create a sensitive set of inclusion criteria for a population definition. Alternatively, an analysis can also assess the discrepancy between patients with a diagnosis for a condition in their patient charts and those who have a visit or medication related to that condition in order to find potential gaps in care. For instance, the presence of a diabetes diagnosis on the patient chart but no record of any visit or medication diagnoses for diabetes could indicate that a patient is not receiving adequate management of his or her diabetes.

Procedures

Because of billing and reimbursement purposes, all procedures provided to patients must be documented in the EMR. Procedures are coded using current procedural terminology (CPT) or *International Classification of Diseases, 10th Revision, Procedure Coding System* (ICD-10-PCS). Procedures can be used in population health analytics to define a population or track outcomes. For instance, procedure codes can be used to define a population of patients who received a hip replacement in order to track postsurgery outcomes (see Chapter 3 for more information).

Laboratory Results and Vital Signs

A distinct advantage of using EMR data over other data sources is in the level of detailed clinical information in laboratory and vital signs data. Laboratories can be performed either on site or by external vendors. On-site laboratory orders and results are typically integrated within the EMR, whereas vendor labs are electronically transmitted between a laboratory information system and EMR. Although most laboratory results are entered into the EMR electronically, some instances require manual entry, which can result in limitations to data accuracy and completeness (Perrotta & Karcher, 2016). Laboratory results include various clinical markers that detect patient health and disease progression. For example, the combination of creatinine, albumin, and glomerular filtration rate results inform clinicians about kidney disease progression. Similarly, cholesterol and blood pressure are important markers in assessing cardiovascular health (see Chapter 4 for more information). Vital signs are measured at most ambulatory visits and on a regular cadence in the inpatient setting. These data elements include blood pressure, heart rate, temperature, and respiratory rate. In population health analyses, these labs and vital signs data are important for segmenting populations with abnormal laboratory results and vital signs or for tracking these clinical markers as health outcomes.

Medications

Medications prescribed by clinicians and administered during hospital stays are both documented in the EMR. Medication data can be used in conjunction with diagnosis data to determine if a patient is being prescribed treatment for a specific disease. The limitation of EMR medication data is that prescription dispensing data are often tracked outside of the EMR. Therefore, even though EMR medication data can provide information regarding medications that were prescribed, EMR data alone cannot provide information about whether the prescriptions were filled. Combining EMR prescribing data with claims pharmacy data would complete the clinical picture by providing important information on whether patients are taking medications as prescribed, also known as *medication adherence* (see Chapter 5 for more information).

Immunizations

Immunization data are recorded in EMRs either directly or indirectly via immunization reconciliation. Vaccine administration can be recorded directly in an EMR at the point of care by the healthcare provider. Immunization records can also be transmitted electronically to an EMR from state-level public health immunization registries. Immunization reconciliation occurs when healthcare providers save the vaccination history from the immunization registry to the patient's chart in the EMR. Immunization data are useful for tracking vaccination levels in a population and targeting populations that could benefit from immunization to prevent disease.

Medical, Behavioral and Social History

Medical history refers to the clinical disease history of a patient and his or her family. *Behavioral history* refers to the past and present health-related social habits of patients, including the use of tobacco, alcohol, and illicit drugs and sexual activity. *Social history* includes information on social determinants of health such as food, housing, and transportation insecurities. Medical, behavioral, and social indicators are important to understand in a population health study because ignoring these factors can result in the failure of health-improvement initiatives (see Chapter 7 for more information). However, because of the sensitive nature of social and medical history, these data elements are often underreported or not reported at all. Therefore, these data for population health analysis must be used cautiously.

Cost and Billing

Cost and billing data are recorded in the EMR for operational and reimbursement purposes. EMR billing data include line-by-line charges submitted to insurers for payment, such as procedures, supplies, medications, professionals, and facilities. Diagnosis, cost, and place of service information are also incorporated. Therefore, it is possible to aggregate billing data to assess utilization and disease prevalence. Although cost is provided, there is often a discrepancy between billed and paid amounts. Therefore, administrative claims data are more reliable for assessing the true cost of care (see Chapter 3 for more information).

Table 6.1 describes fields that are commonly found in the electronic health record.

Special Considerations When Using EMR Data

There are many considerations to make when using EMR data for population health analysis. A primary concern is data accuracy and completeness. Many types of data may be entered into the EMR, but this does not mean that these data are populated regularly. The amount of missing data in the EMR may require analysts to seek other sources of population health data. In addition, analysts must perform a great amount of data cleaning and transformation before applying the data for analysis. For example, analysts must look for outliers

Table 6.1 Common EMR Fields and Values with Definitions

Table	Field Name	Field Description	Typical Field Format	Typical Use in Population Health Analytics
Patient	Patient_ID	Unique patient identifier	Numeric	Describing a population
	Street_Address	Patient home address	Varchar*	Analyzing socioeconomic determinants of health
	Zipcode	Residential ZIP Code	Numeric	
	DOB	Date of Birth	Date	
	Marital_Status	Marital Status	Varchar	
	Insurance	Payor category	Varchar	
	Language	Preferred patient language	Varchar	
	Race	Patient Race	Varchar	
	Ethnicity	Patient Ethnicity	Varchar	
Healthcare utilization	Patient_ID	Unique patient identifier	Numeric	Assessing healthcare utilization
	Visit_ID	Unique healthcare visit identifier	Numeric	Targeting patients who require more or less utilization (i.e., reduce emergency department utilization and increase preventative visit utilization)
	Visit_Type	Type of healthcare visit (i.e., outpatient, inpatient)	Varchar	
	Visit_Admit_Date	Visit admission date	Date	
	Visit_Discharge_Date	Visit discharge date	Date	
	Department_ID	Visit department unique identifier	Numeric	
Vital signs	Patient_ID	Unique patient identifier	Numeric	Describing a population
	Visit_ID	Unique healthcare visit identifier	Numeric	Analyzing clinical determinants of health
	Height	Patient's height at visit	Numeric	
	Weight	Patient's weight at visit	Numeric	
	Pulse	Patient's heart rate at visit	Numeric	
	Temperature	Patient's temperature at visit	Numeric	
	Diastolic_BP	Patient's diastolic blood pressure at visit	Numeric	
	Systolic_BP	Patient's systolic blood pressure at visit	Numeric	

(continues)

Table 6.1 Common EMR Fields and Values with Definitions   *(continued)*

Table	Field Name	Field Description	Typical Field Format	Typical Use in Population Health Analytics
Diagnoses	Patient_ID	Unique patient identifier	Numeric	Defining a patient population by disease cohort
	Diagnosis_ID	Unique diagnosis identifier	Numeric	
	Diagnosis_Name	Name of diagnosis	Varchar	Assessing incidence and prevalence of diseases
	IDC10_Code	ICD10 diagnosis code	Varchar	
	Dx_Noted_Date	Date diagnosis was noted	Date	
Procedures	Patient_ID	Unique patient identifier	Numeric	Defining a patient population by procedure cohort
	Procedure_ID	Unique procedure identifier	Numeric	
	Procedure_Name	Name of procedure	Varchar	Assessing healthcare quality by tracking outcomes related to procedures
	CPT_Code	CPT code	Varchar	
	ICD10_PCS	ICD10 procedure code	Varchar	
	Procedure_Date	Date of procedure	Date	
Laboratory Results	Patient_ID	Unique patient identifier	Numeric	Analyzing clinical determinants of health
	Lab_ID	Unique lab identifier	Numeric	
	Lab_Name	Name of lab	Varchar	
	Lab_Result	Lab result value	Varchar	
	Lab_Result_Date	Date of lab result	Date	
Medications	Patient_ID	Unique patient identifier	Numeric	Defining a patient population by disease cohort
	Med_ID	Unique medication identifier	Numeric	
	Med_Generic_Name	Generic name of medication	Varchar	Assessing healthcare quality by tracking medication prescribing habits
	Med_Brand_Name	Brand name of medication	Varchar	
	Pharm_Class	Pharmaceutical class of medication	Varchar	Targeting patients missing appropriate medication prescriptions
	Route	Route of administration	Varchar	
	SIG	Instructions for taking medication	Varchar	
	Dosage	Medication dosage	Varchar	
	Med_Order_Date	Date of medication prescription or administration	Date	
	Med_Order_Type	Outpatient or inpatient medication order	Varchar	

Immunizations	Patient_ID	Unique patient identifier	Numeric	Assessing healthcare quality by tracking immunization practices
	Imm_ID	Unique immunization identifier	Numeric	
	Imm_Name	Immunization name	Varchar	Targeting patients for immunization interventions
	Imm_Date	Date of immunization administration	Date	
	Imm_Dose	Immunization dose	Varchar	
	Imm_Route	Route of immunization administration (ie. oral, nasal, intramuscular)	Varchar	
	Imm_Lot	Lot number of vaccine	Varchar	
Medical history	Med_Hx_ID	Unique	Numeric	Assessing clinical risk factors for disease
	IDC10_Code	ICD10 diagnosis code	Varchar	
	Med_Hx_Date	Date of medical history information	Varchar	
Behavioral history	Patient_ID	Unique patient identifier	Numeric	Assessing behavioral-based determinants of health
	Visit_ID	Unique healthcare visit identifier	Numeric	
	Tobacco_Status	Tobacco use status (ie. Never, Current, Former)	Varchar	Targeting populations for interventions to modify high-risk behaviors
	Tobacco_Years	Number of years of cigarette smoking	Numeric	
	Tobacco_PPD	Number of cigarette packs smoked per day	Numeric	
	Alcohol_Status	Alcohol consumption status (ie. Never, Yes, No, Former)	Varchar	
	Alcohol_Oz	Average ounces of alcohol consumed per week	Numeric	
	IV_Drug_Status	Intravenous drug use status (ie. Never, Current, Former)	Varchar	
	Sexual_Activity	Sexual activity status (ie. Yes, No)	Varchar	
	Exercise_Days	Number of days a week that patient exercises	Numeric	
	Exercise_Minutes	Number of minutes patient exercises on the days they exercise	Numeric	
	Education_Level	Highest level of education obtained	Varchar	

*Varchar = variable character field

in lab and vital sign data to ensure that values are clinically reasonable and exclude or impute any extraneous values. Population health analyses should recognize and plan for the time, effort, and data limitations associated with using EMR data.

For select population health analyses, EMR data alone may not be enough to complete an entire analysis. In these cases, one might want to combine EMR data with external data such as administrative claims or public health data to produce a more complete analysis of population. However, there are analytical and practical challenges that must be considered when combining data sources. For example, it is difficult to produce a 1:1 population match between claims and EMR data sets because of the differences in how each data source defines an attributed population. There may also be discrepancies in unique patient identifiers that impede a full data set match. In addition, challenges in analytic methodology may also arise, particularly when attempting to combine group-level public health data with individual-level EMR data. It is important to exercise caution and understand how to avoid the biases that may come up in such analyses (Haneuse & Bartell, 2011). Although combining EMR data with other population health data sources can be beneficial, it also comes with additional analytic complexities to consider.

Although the majority of this chapter describes structured data elements in the EMR, there is also great value in existing unstructured data. These data include free text in the form of discharge and progress notes that elaborate on a patient's disease progression and plans of care. Using unstructured data requires skills in advanced natural language processing (see Chapter 23 for more information). In addition, the medical lexicon used in these free text elements adds another layer of complexity for non-clinical analysts. Therefore, it is important to consider unstructured data in population health analytics with the understanding that this also adds a significant level of complexity.

Applied Learning: Case Study

Using EMR Data to Support Type 2 Diabetic Population A1c Control

Background

A large health system would like to understand their diabetic population and their management of care, as well as determine areas in which they can improve care delivery. After conducting a population health analysis, the health system created an intervention to reach out to patients with poorly managed A1c. This intervention was evaluated by assessing pre- and postintervention outcomes in the population cohort.

Question	Using EMR Data
What is the prevalence of diabetes in our health system?	Count the number of patients with type 2 diabetes ICD-10-CM diagnosis codes (E11.xx).
What are the demographic and socioeconomic characteristics of the patients with diabetes?	The health record includes the following information: age, race or ethnicity, sex, and insurance.
How well are the patients with diabetes controlling their disease?	Extract HbA1c and glucose measurements as well as diabetic medications prescribed in the previous year.
What is the healthcare utilization distribution of patients with diabetes?	Aggregate the number of primary care, endocrinologist, inpatient, and emergency visits in the previous year.

What are the modifiable risk factors of the patients with diabetes?	Gather social history data on tobacco, alcohol, and exercise behaviors.
What are the nonmodifiable risk factors of the patients with diabetes?	Gather medical history and diagnosis information on the population's other chronic conditions.
Which patients with diabetes should be targeted for intervention?	Filter the previously gathered data to groups with high emergency and inpatient utilization, low primary care and endocrinology utilization, poor diabetes control, and modifiable risk factors to generate an intervention population.
How can the intervention success be determined?	Track the clinical markers of diabetes and healthcare utilization for one year after the intervention to analyze whether clinical markers improved and healthcare utilization decreased.

Results

Population Demographics

	HbA1c Controlled Population*	HbA1c Uncontrolled Population
Age (Years)	45	51
Sex, % Female	52	47
Race or Ethnicity		
% white, non-Hispanic	78	65
% black, non-Hispanic	12	22
% Hispanic	6	10
% other	4	3
Insurance		
% commercial	50	35
% public	48	64
% other	2	1

*Diabetes controlled is defined as HbA1c < 7% and prescribed appropriate antidiabetic medications.

Resource Utilization

	HbA1c Controlled Population	HbA1c Uncontrolled Population
Primary Care	250 visits per 100 patients	150 visits per 100 patients
Endocrinology Specialist	51 visits per 100 patients	32 visits per 100 patients
Inpatient	4 visits per 100 patients	10 visits per 100 patients
Emergency	18 visits per 100 patients	30 visits per 100 patients

Targeting Population for Intervention

Patient ID	Age	Sex	A1c	On Diabetes Medication	Comorbidities	Tobacco Use	Exercise Level
xxx	36	F	9	N	HTN	Y	Low
xxx	53	M	7.6	Y	None	N	Moderate

Outcome Evaluation

	Preintervention	Postintervention
% on Diabetes Medication	10	33
% A1c < 8	7	15
Inpatient Utilization	10 visits per 100 patients	7.5 visits per 100 patients
Emergency Utilization	30 visits per 100 patients	26 visits per 100 patients
Endocrinologist Utilization	32 visits per 100 patients	38 visits per 100 patients
Primary Care Utilization	150 visits per 100 patients	200 visits per 100 patients

Conclusion

The rich, abundant, and up-to-date information collected in EMRs has the potential to substantially improve our understanding of population health. These data are ideal for the longitudinal assessment of the clinical and socioeconomic determinants of health, as well as the examination of healthcare resources utilized by populations. Challenges with regard to incomplete and untidy data in EMRs, however, must be acknowledged and mitigated. Nevertheless, EMR data will continue to be important components of the population health data model to complete the diagnostic, clinical, and social picture of population health.

Study and Discussion Questions

- Describe a population health analysis in which EMR data would be ideal. Conversely, describe a scenario in which EMR data would not be ideal.

- Select a population and describe how you would use EMR data to improve health outcomes in that population. List the EMR data elements that you would use in the process.

Resources and Websites

AHRQ Digital Healthcare Research. (2013, March 22). Health IT success: Using electronic health records to improve colonoscopy quality. [YouTube video]. AHRQ. Retrieved from https://www.youtube.com/watch?v=G4wF0DF1TXw

AHRQ-Funded Projects. (n.d.). AHRQ. Retrieved from https://digital.ahrq.gov/ahrq-funded-projects/

References

Bush, G. W. (2004). State of the Union address. https://georgew
bush-whitehouse.archives.gov/news/releases/2004
/01/20040120-7.html

Center for Surveillance, Epidemiology, and Laboratory
Services. (2019). Meaningful use. https://journalofethics
.ama-assn.org/article/hitech-act-overview/2011-03

Cole, A. M., Stephens, K. A., Keppel, G. A., & Estiri, H. (2016).
Extracting electronic health record data in a practice-based
research network: Lessons learned from collaborations
with translational researchers. eGEMs (Generating
Evidence & Methods to improve patient outcomes), 4(2).
http://doi.org/10.13063/2327-9214.1206

Friedman, D. J., Parrish, R. G., & Ross, D. A. (2013, August 7).
Electronic health records and US public health: Current
realities and future promise. *American Journal of Public
Health, 103*(9), 1560–1567. https://ajph.aphapublications
.org/doi/full/10.2105/AJPH.2013.301220

Haneuse, S., & Bartell, S. (2011). Designs for the combination
of group- and individual-level data. *Epidemiology, 22*(3),
382–389. https://pubmed.ncbi.nlm.nih.gov/21490533/

Kharrazi, H., Chi, W., Chang, H., Richards, T. M., Gallagher,
J. M., Knudson, S. M., & Weiner, J. P. (2017). Comparing
population-based risk-stratification model performance
using demographic, diagnosis and medication data
extracted from outpatient electronic health records versus
administrative claims. *Medical Care, 55*(8), 789–796.
https://pubmed.ncbi.nlm.nih.gov/28598890/

Perrotta, P. L., & Karcher, D. S. (2016). Validating laboratory
results in electronic health records. *Archives of Pathology &
Laboratory Medicine, 140*(9), 926–931. https://doi.org
/10.5858/arpa.2015-0320-CP

Rosenbloom, S. T., Carroll, R. J., Warner, J. L., Matheny,
M. E., & Denny, J. C. (2017, August 26). Representing
knowledge consistently across health systems. Yearbook
of Medical Informatics, 26(1), 139–147. https://pubmed
.ncbi.nlm.nih.gov/29063555/

CHAPTER 7

Social and Behavioral Data

Marisa L. Wilson, DNSc, MHSc, RN-BC, CPHIMS, FAMIA, FIAHSI, FAAN
Martha Sylvia, PhD, MBA, RN

To achieve health equity, barriers must be removed so that everyone has a fair opportunity to be as healthy as possible.

—Centers for Disease Control and Prevention (2020b)

EXECUTIVE SUMMARY

It is not hard to uncover evidence that factors of our daily lives in terms of our environments, the behaviors in which we engage, and the social structures in which we develop and grow all directly impact our health. The ability to access high-quality education, nutritious food, safe housing, reliable transportation, culturally sensitive healthcare providers, health insurance, and clean air and water are just some of the factors that determine health outcomes. Consider the following staggering statistics.

- The rate of death during pregnancy is three times higher for African American women compared to White women (Petersen et al., 2019).
- The rate of death for African American infants is 2.5 times the rate of death for White infants (Centers for Disease Control and Prevention, 2019).
- The proportion of COVID-19 cases in the United States is astonishingly higher for people of color with the ratios by racial or ethnic group reported as:
  - 4.4 for Hispanic or Latino,
  - 2.3 for Black or African American,
  - 4.2 for American Indian and Alaska Native,
  - 2.9 for Asian, and
  - 8.5 for Native Hawaiian and Pacific Islander (Moore et al., 2020).
- Lesbian, gay, bisexual, and transgender people are at greater risk of behavioral and mental health issues, including suicide, mood disorders, anxiety, eating disorders, and substance abuse (Cigna, 2017).
- In an inner-city neighborhood where 88% of the population are people of color, the overall mortality rate is 30% higher and with a 20-year disparity in life expectancy when compared to surrounding areas (Berkowitz et al., 2016; Blum, 2017).
- The development of obesity in young adults is significantly related to ZIP Code, with equal contributions from genetics and the environment (Lakhani et al., 2019).

The impact on healthcare costs attributable to these factors is unsustainable. An estimated 26% of healthcare costs are associated with modifiable health risks (O'Donnell, Schultz, & Yen, 2015). Smoking-related illnesses alone cost $170 billion each year in direct medical costs (Centers for Disease Control and Prevention, 2020a). For homeless patients, the median length of hospital stay is 1.8 times higher than for those with secure housing; $155 billion is attributable to food insecurity; and for those with English as a second language, there is a 60% risk of an emergency department visit (Sullivan, 2019). One of the largest studies to link the impact of the environment to healthcare costs found that the combination of having a condition like diabetes and the environment in which people live accounts for 60% of healthcare costs (Lakhani et al., 2019).

Optimizing the use of data in population health analytics to intentionally seek out and understand how social determinants of health are impacting the populations served can turn what seems like a dire situation into enormous opportunity for health improvement. Studies show that when social needs are identified and met, significant improvements in health outcomes and reductions in health expenditures can be realized (Johnson, 2018; Pruitt, Emechebe, Quast, Taylor, & Bryant, 2018).

LEARNING OBJECTIVES

At the end of this chapter, the learner will be able to:

1. Explain the value of social and behavioral data for population health analytics.
2. Compare and contrast the sources of social and behavioral data.
3. Translate social and behavioral data coding systems into meaningful information.
4. Use lessons from the social and behavioral sciences to answer questions of importance to population health management.

Introduction

The Affordable Care Act (ACA) was enacted to bring about a decrease in the number of uninsured Americans, demonstrate an improvement in the quality of care received, and reduce the overall cost of health care by increasing patient access to preventive services. The primary goals of the ACA were to improve the overall health of the country, improve the quality of life of the nation, and contain the ever-increasing cost of health care (Office of the Legislative Council, 2010). The ACA proposed that hospitals, aligned clinics, and affiliated clinicians would have the responsibility for collaborating to improve health care delivery and overall population health. This necessitated collaboration between stakeholders, patients, families, and community organizations. Given that approximately 80% of health is driven by factors outside of clinical care, it is essential to understand the ways in which data can be used to identify and determine the impact of nonclinical factors on the health of populations (Givens, Gennuso, Jovaag, Van Dijk, & Johnson, 2019).

With clinical care accounting for only 10% to 20% of health outcomes, successful population health innovation must consider much more than the data derived from transactions between healthcare providers and patients. Multiple data sources are used to expand the understanding of individuals beyond the clinic walls and into the home, community, and environment. This multifaceted analysis allows a comprehensive understanding what is driving health and what population health initiatives must do improve it.

Given that the majority of healthcare organizations only have data related to the delivery of clinical care services, data about social and behavioral determinants are perhaps the most difficult to include in population health analytics. This chapter explores data sources that measure social and behavioral factors and ways in which to include these data in analyses used to understand the health of populations. Data structures and attempts at standardization are described and a case study is presented.

Defining Social and Behavioral Determinants of Health

Social determinants of health (SDOH) are the conditions in which people are born, live, learn, work, play, worship, and age, and they affect a wide range of health, functioning, and quality-of-life outcomes and risks (World Health Organization, 2020a). The county health rankings provides a structure for understanding health determinants and their contribution to outcomes. **Figure 7.1.** shows the driver diagram based on a model of community health that emphasizes the many factors that influence how long and how

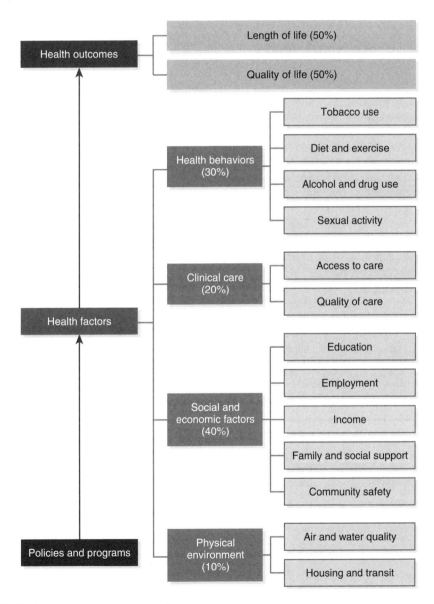

Figure 7.1 Factors Accounting for Health Outcomes.

well we live. Based on years of research, the diagram shows length of life and quality of life as outcomes at the top, and on the side it reports the percentage contribution of each factor to those outcomes. Social determinants of health focus on the social, economic, and environmental factors accounting for 50% of health outcomes, and health behaviors contribute an additional 30% of the impact to these indicators.

Social and Behavioral Data

For the purposes of this chapter, social and behavioral data are defined as

> any nonclinical information that could be used by a health system or other organization to better understand the needs of the patient population they are responsible for and can include demographics, behavioral or socioeconomic factors, or characteristics that describe the natural or built environment of the geographic area in which the patient resides. (Predmore, Hatef, & Weiner, 2019)

In its description of the determinants of health, the World Health Organization (WHO) includes forces and systems that shape the conditions in which people live their daily lives. Furthermore, the WHO includes economic policies, development agendas, social norms, social policies, and political systems. Within this framework, determinants of health are broadly conceptualized as inclusive of all domains, including inherent, health system, behavioral, social, economic, or environmental factors (Benach et al., 2010). **Table 7.1** lists the WHO health determinants.

The Institute of Medicine (IOM, 2014) culled the WHO domains into three categories—social, psychological, and behavioral—and aligned the definitions of the data elements with others widely used in other health and social care domains. Criteria used to determine the final list included the strength of association with health outcomes, clinical and population health relevance, and research usefulness. The list was then further refined based on readiness with a standard measure, feasibility of collection, usefulness for inclusion in an electronic health record (EHR), and committee judgement. In phase 2 of this work, the IOM then explored and recommended specific data elements and methods for collection (IOM, 2014). The final list of identified specific domains and core measures that capture targeted social and behavioral factors were intended to be included in EHRs as part of phase 3 of meaningful use.

Table 7.2 describes the final domains and their measures. Note that all measures are self-reported. If a measure has a list of response choices, then only the question is included in this table for informational purposes because

Table 7.1 World Health Organization Determinants of Health

Social Environment	Education	Transport
Economic environment	Social support	Food and nutrition
Individual characteristics	Genetics	Water
Behaviors	Culture	Waste and pollution
Income	Access and use of service	Radiation
Social status	Gender	Housing
Race or ethnicity		

World Health Organization. (n.d.). Social determinants of health. Retrieved August 17, 2020, from https://www.who.int/social_determinants/en

Table 7.2 Institute of Medicine Recommended Core Domains and Measures

Domain	Measure
Alcohol use	Three questions from the Alcohol Use Disorders Identification Test-C (AUDIT-C) (Bush, Kivlahan, McDonell, Fihn, & Bradley, 1998): 1. How often do you have a drink containing alcohol? 2. How many standard drinks containing alcohol do you have on a typical day? 3. How often do you have six or more drinks on one occasion?
Race and ethnicity	Two questions from U.S. Census categories: Question 5: Is the person of Hispanic, Latino, or Spanish origin? Question 6: What is the person's race? Mark one or more races to indicate what this person considers [him- or herself] to be.
Residential address	Reporting of address or derived from existing data
Tobacco use and exposure	Two questions from the National Health Interview Survey (Adsit & Fiore, 2013): Have you smoked at least 100 cigarettes in your entire life? Do you *now* smoke cigarettes every day, some days, or not at all?
Census track median income	Census track neighborhood and community compositional characteristic (derived from census track data and applied at address level)
Depression	Two questions from the Patient Health Questionnaire-2 (PHQ-2) (Kroenke, Spitzer, & Williams, 2003) Frequency with which there is: ■ Little interest or pleasure in doing things ■ Feeling down, depressed, or hopeless
Education	Two questions on educational attainment: 1. What is the highest level of school you have completed? 2. What is the highest degree you earned?
Financial resource strain	One question on overall financial strain (Kahn & Pearlin, 2006): 1. How hard is it for you to pay for the very basics like food, housing, medical care, and heating?
Intimate partner violence	Four questions from Humiliation Afraid Rape Kick (HARK) (Sohal, Eldridge, & Feder, 2007): 1. Within the last year, have you been humiliated or emotionally abused in other ways by your partner or ex-partner? 2. Within the last year, have you been afraid of your partner or ex-partner? 3. Within the last year, have you been raped or forced to have any kind of sexual activity by your partner or ex-partner? 4. Within the last year, have you been kicked, hit, slapped, or otherwise physically hurt by your partner or ex-partner?
Physical activity	Two questions from exercise vital signs (Coleman et al., 2012): 1. On average, how many days per week do you engage in moderate to strenuous exercise (like walking fast, running, jogging, dancing, swimming, biking, or other activities that cause a light or heavy sweat)? 2. On average, how many minutes do you engage in exercise at this level?

(continues)

Table 7.2 **Institute of Medicine Recommended Core Domains and Measures** *(continued)*

Domain	Measure
Social connections and social isolation	Four questions from National Health and Nutrition Examination Survey III (NHANES III) (Pantell et al., 2013): 1. In a typical week, how many times do you talk on the telephone with family, friends, or neighbors? 2. How often do you get together with friends or relatives? 3. How often do you attend church or religious services? 4. How often do you attend meetings of the clubs or organizations you belong to?
Stress	One question associated with indicators of health and psychosocial work characteristics (Elo, Leppänen, & Jahkola, 2003): Stress means a situation in which a person feels tense, restless, nervous, or anxious or is unable to sleep at night because his or her mind is troubled all the time. Do you feel this kind of stress these days?

Institute of Medicine. (2014). Capturing social and behavioral domains and measures in electronic health records: Phase 2. The National Academies Press. https://doi .org/10.17226/18951

instruments and questions evolve over time. If using these domains and measures, it is best to seek out the most up-to-date questionnaire before implementing and to ensure implemented processes allow for regular updating.

The IOM made several recommendations to the Office of the National Coordinator for Health Information Technology related to the potential inclusion of these SDOH domains and data elements in EHRs. Two of the recommendations were:

1. The certification process for EHRs should include the standard measures for four social and behavioral domains that are already collected (race or ethnicity, tobacco use, alcohol use, and residential address).
2. The certification process for EHRs should include the standard measures for the other eight recommended domains (educational attainment, financial resource strain, stress, depression, physical activity, social isolation, intimate partner violence, and neighborhood median income).

Standardization of the data elements within each selected domain has facilitated the development of products by vendors of health information systems that ease the acquisition, storage, transmission, and download of self-reported data pertinent to gathering social and behavioral data. Standardization allows for sharable, comparable data across all phases of care as well as within locations and systems of care. The goal is to advance understanding of the contributions of behavioral and social factors in the management of health to improve outcomes and quality while reducing costs of care.

Sources of Social and Behavioral Data

Given the importance of and focus on social and behavioral factors in individual and population health, many healthcare systems have begun to explore ways to integrate these data with patients' clinical data. Medicaid and the Children's Health Insurance Program payment reform projects are providing financial incentives for bringing the issue of SDOH data collection to a broader audience of providers beyond the community health centers and safety net providers who have traditionally worked to meet these needs among their high-risk populations

(Cantor & Thorpe, 2018). EHR vendors have begun to develop tools within their EHRs to capture and store social and behavioral data. Vendors are developing tools that use these data for individual risk assessment, referral, and population health management. However, this work does not necessarily follow a recommended strategy or use standard questions and answers or uniformly coded data elements, which ultimately thwarts attempts at transmission and analysis.

Community-Level Data: Community Indicators

Geography is one of the most prominent determinants of health. Where people live and the resulting consequences create barriers to care and exacerbate disparities. Health and longevity are greatly influenced by ZIP Code, which can be a stronger predictor of health than other factors such as race and genetic code (Graham, Ostrowski, & Sabina, 2015). With this in mind, it is important to consider the utility of data generated external to a healthcare system. Community-level social and behavioral data are useful for population assessment, can enhance performance of predictive models, can inform risk-adjustment models, and aid understanding of the impact of population health interventions.

Use of community-level data requires the involvement of community members for collaboration in measure development and use cases, particularly when the end product is a publicly available community comparison tool. Open source and publicly available data sets reflective of community-level social and behavioral indicators can be used to create single data sets that are mapped using an address at the census track level for analysis. Sources of these data include those available from the U.S. Department of Agriculture, the Centers for Disease Control and Prevention, the American Community Survey of the U.S. Census Bureau, and other private organizations. **Table 7.3** lists a selected few of the sources of community-acquired social and behavioral data.

Table 7.3 Select Sources of Community-Level SDOH Data

Organization	Title	URL
American Association of Retired Persons (AARP)	AARP Livability Index	https://livabilityindex.aarp.org
Brookings	Metro Monitor	https://www.brookings.edu/research/metro-monitor-2017/
Centers for Disease Control and Prevention (CDC)	Behavioral Risk Factors Data	https://chronicdata.cdc.gov/browse?category=Behavioral+Risk+Factors
CDC	Chronic Disease Indicators	https://www.cdc.gov/cdi/index.html
CDC	Sources for Data on Social Determinants of Health	https://www.cdc.gov/socialdeterminants/data/index.htm
CDC	National Center for HIV and AIDS, Hepatitis, STD, and TB (NCHHSTP AtlasPlus)	https://www.cdc.gov/nchhstp/atlas/index.htm
CDC	Social Vulnerability Index	https://www.atsdr.cdc.gov/placeandhealth/svi/index.html

(continues)

Table 7.3 Select Sources of Community-Level SDOH Data   (continued)

Organization	Title	URL
Community Commons	Community Health Needs Assessment	https://www.communitycommons.org/board/story/2019/03/04/chna/
Department of Population Health, New York University	City Health Dashboard	https://www.cityhealthdashboard.com/
Reinvestment Fund	PolicyMap Data Solutions	https://www.policymap.com/data/
RHIhub	Rural Health Information Hub	https://www.ruralhealthinfo.org/toolkits/sdoh/4/assessment-tools
University of Wisconsin Population Health Institute	County Health Rankings	https://www.countyhealthrankings.org/explore-health-rankings/measures-data-sources/county-health-rankings-model?componentType=health-factor&componentId=25
University of Wisconsin School of Medicine and Public Health	Neighborhood Atlas and the Area Deprivation Index	https://www.neighborhoodatlas.medicine.wisc.edu/mapping
U.S. Census Bureau	U.S. Census	https://www.census.gov
U.S. National Library of Medicine	Community Health Maps	https://communityhealthmaps.nlm.nih.gov

Although visualizing or analyzing these data may not be easy, in 2019 the Agency for Healthcare Research and Quality launched an application challenge to advance visualization resources of community-level social and behavioral data. The goal of the challenge was to support the development of tools that allow the visualization of data clusters to enhance research and analysis of community-level health services (see https://www.ahrq.gov/sdoh-challenge/about.html). This challenge opened the door to additional tools for evaluating community-level data.

Individual-Level Data

Social and behavioral data can also be collected directly from an individual, allowing a person-level linkage between nonclinical and clinical health determinants. This can be accomplished through electronic screenings, checklists, surveys, or even by using paper versions of surveys. Collection can be done at the point of care, through a portal or personal health record, or on a tablet or kiosk. An important consideration for collecting self-reported data is that the tool incorporates standardized terminology and data modeling and that data elements are encoded to ensure interoperability that will facilitate exchange of health information between sites of care.

With the onslaught of value-based care programs and pay for quality and outcomes, health information technology companies serving as EHR vendors are increasingly adding SDOH screenings into EHRs based on the Institute of Medicine recommendations; these include assessments of intimate partner violence, social isolation, alcohol and tobacco use, depression, financial resources, food, transportation, and housing insecurity. EHR vendors want to use standardized and structured tools and are doing so whenever possible, although there is variation of tools across health care settings because of differences in the populations being served, requests for customization, and a lack of common screening requirements across different federal or state programs (Freij et al., 2019). When analyzing social and behavioral data collected through the EHR, care must be taken to ensure that these screening tools incorporate reliable and valid tools and that the data elements are standardized and encoded. If these requirements are not ensured, then interpretation of results must be carefully scrutinized.

There are examples of individual-level tools that are valid, reliable, and standardized, but these may not be included or may only be partially included in organizational EHRs. A compilation of valid, reliable, and standardized individual-level social and behavioral data-collection tools can be found in the Social Interventions Research and Evaluation Network (SIREN) supported by the University of California, San Francisco (https://sirenetwork.ucsf.edu/tools-resources). SIREN catalyzes and disseminates research to advance efforts to address SDOH and houses an evidence library, tools, reports, and resources. The SIREN site also documents the various data elements used for each tool and provides detail on the definitions. The Protocol for Responding to and Assessing Patients' Assets and Experiences (PRAPARE) developed by the National Association of Community Health Centers is one such tool (http://www.nachc.org/research-and-data/prapare/about-the-prapare-assessment-tool/). PRAPARE is an SDOH assessment tool but also includes an implementation and action toolkit.

Comparison of SDOH Individual-Level Tools

When selecting a tool to use as an integrated screen within an EHR or as separate data-collection process outside of the EHR, a few considerations will impact that choice. It is important to decide the intended population. Is this screening for adults, children, pregnant women, everyone? What is the setting in which these data will be collected? What domains will be covered? It may not be best to screen for everything if the organization is only focusing on addressing food insecurity, for example. Is the tool valid and reliable? What is

the reading level? What is the average completion time? (This will impact workflow.) Is there a cost to using the tool? SIREN and PRAPARE offer insights to tool selection that are important to consider.

When using a tool that has already been built within an EHR, the analyst should conduct due diligence and determine the source of the questions and the standardization of the answers.

Common Structure for Social and Behavioral Data

To address common structures of social and behavioral data is not a simple process. At this time, there is a national collaborative working to advance interoperable SDOH data with common structures and definitions. Funded by the Robert Wood Johnson Foundation in partnership with SIREN, this project is titled the Gravity Project (SIREN, 2019). The Gravity Project focuses on three priority social domains identified based on recommendation, supported by literature, and demonstrated by projects: food security, housing stability, and transportation access.

These and all other areas of interest are currently being compiled and are listed in detail through the Compendium of Medical Terminology Codes for Social Risk (see https://sirenetwork.ucsf.edu/tools-resources/mmi/compendium-medical-terminology-codes-social-risk-factors) (Arons, DeSilvey, Fichtenberg, & Gottlieb, 2018). Using common structures for these data allows for these concepts to be included in code sets such as the *International Classification of Diseases* (10th revision) *Clinical Modification* (ICD-10-CM), Systemized Nomenclature of Medicine (SNOMED), and Logical Observations Identifier Names and Codes (LOINC). SNOMED focuses on data-gathering tools, LOINC focuses on responses and observables, and ICD-10-CM focuses on output. **Tables 7.4** and **7.5** list the current ICD-10-CM and LOINC social and behavioral codes, respectively. Additional details on all tools, domains, and subdomains, along with panel names, screening

Table 7.4 ICD-10-CM Codes Supporting Social and Behavioral Data Collection

Domain	Name
Educational circumstances	Z55.0 Illiteracy and low-level literacy
	Z55.1 Schooling unavailable and unattainable
	Z55.2 Failed school examinations
	Z55.3 Underachievement in school
	Z55.4 Education maladjustment and discord with teachers and classmates
	Z55.8 Other problems related to education and literacy
	Z55.9 Problems related to education and literacy, unspecified
Effects of work environment	Z56.0 Unemployment, unspecified
	Z56.1 Change of job
	Z56.2 Threat of job loss
	Z56.4 Discord with boss and workmates
	Z56.89 Other problems related to employment
	Z56.9 Unspecified problems related to employment
Foster care	Z62.822 Parent–foster child conflict
	Z62.21 Child in welfare custody
Homelessness and housing	Z59.0 Homelessness
	Z59.1 Inadequate housing
	Z59.2 Discord with neighbors, lodgers, and landlord
	Z59.8 Other problems related to housing and economic circumstances
	Z60.2 Problems related to living alone
Inadequate resources	Z59.4 Lack of adequate food and safe drinking water
	Z59.5 Extreme poverty
	Z59.6 Low income
	Z59.7 Insufficient social insurance and welfare support
	Z59.8 Other problems related to housing and economic circumstances
	Z59.9 Problems related to housing and economic circumstances, unspecified
	Z75.3 Unavailability of, and inaccessibility to, healthcare facilities
	Z75.4 Unavailability of, and inaccessibility to, other helping agencies
Other social factors	Z60.4 Social exclusion and rejection
	Z60.8 Other problems related to social environment
	Z60.9 Problems related to social environment, unspecified
	Z71.3 Dietary counseling and surveillance
	Z71.6 Tobacco abuse counseling
	Z71.82 Exercise counseling
	Z71.89 Other specified counseling
	Z71.9 Counseling, unspecified

	Z72.0 Tobacco use
	Z72.4 Inappropriate diet and eating habits
	Z91.82 Personal history of military deployment
Parent, child, family	Z62.810 Personal history of physical and sexual abuse in childhood
	Z62.820 Parent-biological child conflict
	Z63.4 Disappearance and death of family member
	Z63.8 Other specified problems related to primary support group

Table 7.5 LOINC Codes Supporting Social and Behavioral Panels

Panel	Tools
802167-5	2015 Health IT Certification Criteria
	Patient Health Questionnaire (PHQ-2)
	Alcohol Use Disorder Identification Test—Consumption (AUDIT-C)
	Humiliation, Afraid, Risk, and Kick (HARK)
	National Health and Nutrition Examination Survey (NHANES)
82152-0	Adverse Childhood Events (ACE)
	Behavioral Risk Factor Surveillance System (BRFSS)

questions, and codes for question panels can be found on the SIREN Compendium at https://sirenetwork.ucsf.edu/tools-resources/mmi/compendium-medical-terminology-codes-social-risk-factors.

Advantages and Disadvantages of Social and Behavioral Data for Population Health Analytics

With all of the evidence for the impact of social and behavioral factors on health outcomes and costs, the idea that these determinants must be considered in programs of population health seems straightforward. However, this is quite complex. In collecting, aggregating, and modeling data for population health analytics, there are several methods for gathering social and behavioral data. Each method comes with different advantages and disadvantages. The purpose of the analysis must be considered when determining which source to use. For example, "Is the purpose to understand a community and describe the social needs risks of that community or to gather patient-specific data for analysis?"

For analysis, social and behavioral data can be downloaded from publicly available community-level data sources and ascribed to an individual patient or they can be obtained directly from patients at the time of healthcare interactions and applied to only them. Population health programs could use community-level data to describe, prioritize, and plan for risks within a targeted area and then use these identified community-level risks to create or verify the use of a tool to collect individual data from a patient during healthcare encounters to determine an individual's social needs.

However, in the process of determining which data to use, the issues related to each have to be considered. This is not a straightforward or simple process. Community-level data come with varying levels of granularity and are collected at different times and by different organizations. Individual-level SDOH are gathered electronically or in person, may or may not be standardized to the recommended codes, and have varying levels of completeness. Before engaging in an analysis, all of the risks, processes, and data specifics must be considered.

Issues Related to Collection of Community-Level Data

Community-level social and behavioral data are often openly available for public use. The analyst would need to consider how to access the data and, more importantly, how to ascribe these data to an individual. Little of these data are found in an EHR. Much consideration must be made to the risk of attributing a factor to any one individual within a community. Consider that an individual can reside in the same census track or neighborhood as others but not be experiencing the identical risk of a neighbor. The lowest level of measurement also has to be considered. Are only state data or city data available, or can data at the level of census track or neighborhood be used? Consider how far down into the data we can delve without violating confidentiality. Some conditions like hemophilia may be relatively rare in a community, so there may be a risk of identifying a subject inadvertently.

To use publicly available data, an analyst will need to secure these data and other information describing them. The analyst would need to consider the temporal relevance of data by noting the date the dataset was created. In addition, the analyst may also need to consider his or her skill with big data techniques as these may be required because the velocity, volume, value, variety, and veracity of the data must be accounted for before processing and storing. The analyst may also need to learn about and use new tools to make sense of community-level data such as predictive and visual analytics tools, geocoding, and heat mapping.

Issues Related to Collection of Individual-Level Data

Just as there are issues related to the use of community-level social and behavioral data, there are issues to consider with individual-level data collection and use. Data collection can be problematic. Gathering social and behavioral data can be encumbered by documentation burden, workflow challenges, lack of clinician engagement in the process, patient refusal to answer, difficulty in language translation, training needs, operational challenges, and a lack of a closed loop between collection of data, risk calculation, and referral to a community-based resource (Gold et al., 2018). All of these issues affect the accuracy and completeness of social and behavioral data.

In 2015, the Office of the National Coordinator pushed for standardization of SDOH data in the EHR, but the accompanying certification requirements related to the collection of SDOH data were optional, resulting in a lack of standardization and interoperability. Interoperability, the physical location of the data in the EHR, and the lack of a complete standardized data set challenges the ability of population health programs to analyze the data and for clinicians to glean insights to improve care delivery (Sokol, 2020). In addition, lack of standardized screening tools, reliance on staff to screen and document, and the lack of ability to easily link diagnostic codes to social and behavioral data also prevent the collection of social and behavioral data during healthcare encounters (Olson, Oldfield, & Navarro, 2019). Capture and exchange of interoperable standardized data allows providers to share specific information with health plan payers and other population health programs that need to aggregate and analyze population health data for the purposes of stratifying risk and enabling data-driven models of care.

Applied Learning: Case Study

A group of health care providers in two counties in South Carolina have decided to join forces and form an accountable care network to take on risk with healthcare payers for the populations they serve in these two different counties, Colleton and Charleston. To create a strategy for managing health outcomes and cost, the providers need to know more about the population. The provider group has access to summary information from the health plan, which includes demographic information, prevalence of certain conditions, access to care, utilization of health services, and annual costs per year. The providers also have some information from their EHR, including demographics, prevalence of conditions, appointments, and clinical indicators such as height, weight, and blood pressure readings. The providers do not currently collect data about social and behavioral health determinants in the EHR, so they would like to explore external sources of data to understand the impact of these health determinants on the populations for which they plan to take on a risk contract.

As a first step, the County Health Rankings were accessed to determine county rankings for health factors (or health determinants) and health outcomes. The maps in figure 7.2 display the results. Charleston County (CH) and Colleton County (CL) are in the Southeast corner of the state. The county health rankings are based on a model of community health that emphasizes the many factors that influence how long and how well we live. The rankings use more than 30 measures that help communities understand how healthy their residents are today (health factors) and their health impacts (health outcomes). **Figure 7.2** shows that Charleston County ranks in the top 12 counties in the state for both health factors and outcomes (1st is best, 46th is worst), and Colleton County ranks in the bottom 12 counties.

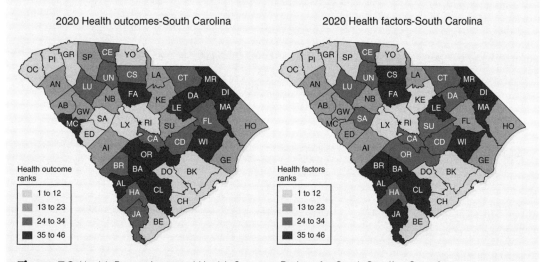

Figure 7.2 Health Determinant and Health Outcome Ratings for South Carolina Counties.

(continues)

Applied Learning: Case Study *(continued)*

To learn more about the factors impacting health in Colleton and Charleston counties, the provider group analyst looked to the detailed data behind the rankings and data from the local health department as well as from the U.S. Census Bureau and compiled the information in **Table 7.6**.

Table 7.6 Factors Impacting Health in Colleton and Charleston SC Counties

Factor	Charleston	Colleton	South Carolina
White (%)	65	60	64
Black (%)	26	37	27
Hispanic or Latino (%)	5	3.3	6
Current cigarette smoker	17	31	19
Adults with obesity (%)	27	42	33
Excessive drinking (%)	23	15	17
Teen birth rate	18/1000	45/1000	27/1000
Infant mortality rate	6.2/1000	11.7/1000	7.3/1000
Low birth weight rate	8.7/1000	12.4/1000	9.9/1000
Receiving adequate prenatal care (%)	75.3	77.0	73.9
With Medicaid coverage for birth (%)	31.9	72.0	50.8
Living in poverty (%)	14.2	20.0	15.3
Owner-occupied housing (%)	61	76	69
Median value of owner-occupied housing ($)	295,600	85,100	154,800
Households with a computer (%)	91	86	86
Households with broadband Internet (%)	77	76	75
High school graduate (>25 yrs old) (%)	92	87	87
Bachelor's degree (>25 yrs old) (%)	43	15	27
Firearm fatality rate	18/1000	33/1000	17/1000
Air pollution and particulate matter (avg. daily PM2.5)	8.9	10.0	10.2
Drinking water violations	No	Yes	
Median income ($)	61,028	36,276	51,015
Life expectancy male–female	74.9/80.5	69.2/77.6	74.1/79.8

Data from The Local Health Department and The U.S. Census Bureau.

The information gleaned from gathering outside data about nonclinical indicators in Colleton and Charleston counties is instrumental in forming the strategy to provide services to improve health in each of the counties. Considerations include the following:

- There are health disparities in Colleton County that need to be considered, including the overall worse infant mortality, life expectancy, and the larger portion of the population that is reliant on public health insurance (Medicaid).
- Cigarette smoking and obesity are a bigger problem in Colleton County, but alcohol overuse is more prevalent in Charleston County.
- Colleton County will benefit from targeted services around pregnancy and postpartum services for women because birth outcomes are worse in the county.
- Educational attainment is lower in Colleton County, which may impact health literacy.
- Colleton and Charleston counties have comparable access to computers and Internet services that will make streamlining delivery mechanisms for interventions more efficient (e.g., telehealth services can equitably be distributed for both counties).

The information gleaned from this assessment of community and national-level social and behavioral data will be added to the population assessment undertaken by the provider group.

Conclusion

Nonclinical health determinants that drive up to 80% of health outcomes include the constellation of forces and systems that shape the conditions in which people live their daily lives. These factors are critical to include in population health analyses in support of improving outcomes. However, acquiring, linking, and analyzing these data is uniquely difficult mainly because of the disjointed way in which they are collected and the lack of standardization. The Institute of Medicine and initiatives like SIREN are working to improve standardization and structuring of social and behavioral data, but this requires diligence from everyone involved in population health management to push for standards.

Study and Discussion Questions

- What do you think are the top areas of impact to consider when developing an analytics plan for a population health program?
- What recommendations would you offer as a program develops a process for collecting social and behavioral data?

- Explain the strengths and weaknesses of using social and behavioral data from an external source and an internal source.

Resources and Websites

American Planning Association: https://www.planning.org/policy/guides/

Community Tool Box: https://ctb.ku.edu/en/table-of-contents/overview/models-for-community-health-and-development/social-determinants-of-health/main

National Academies of Medicine: https://www.nationalacademies.org/our-work/educating-health-professionals-to-address-the-social-determinants-of-health

National Association of Community Health Centers (NACHC) PRAPARE: http://www.nachc.org/research-and-data/prapare/

Office of Disease Prevention and Health Promotion: https://www.healthypeople.gov

Social Interventions Research and Evaluation Network (SIREN): https://sirenetwork.ucsf.edu

References

Adsit, R., & Fiore, M. C. (2013). Assessing tobacco use. *The national landscape*. University of Wisconsin School of Medicine and Public Health Center for Tobacco Research and Intervention.

Arons, A., DeSilvey, S., Fichtenberg, C., & Gottlieb, L. (2018). Compendium of medical terminology codes for social risk factors. Siren, University of California, San Francisco. https://sirenetwork.ucsf.edu/tools-resources/mmi/compendium-medical-terminology-codes-social-risk-factors

Benach, J., Friel, S., Houweling, T., Labonte, R., Muntaner, C., Schrecker, T., & Simpson, S. (2010). *A conceptual framework for action on the social determinants of health*. World Health Organization. https://www.who.int/sdh conferencez/resources/Conceptualframeworkforactionon SDH_eng.pdf

Berkowitz, S. A., Brown, P., Brotman, D. J., Deutschendorf, A., Dunbar, L., Everett, A., Hickman, D., Howell, E., Purnell, L., Sylvester, C., Zollinger, R., Bellantoni, M., Durso, S. C., Lyketsos, C., & Rothman, P. (2016, December). Case study: Johns Hopkins Community Health Partnership: A model for transformation. *Healthcare, 4*(4), 264–270. https://doi.org/10.1016/j.hjdsi.2016.09.001

Blum, K. (2017). Improving community health, reducing health disparities. Johns Hopkins Medicine. https://www.hopkinsmedicine.org/news/articles/improving-community-health-reducing-health-disparities

Bush, K., Kivlahan, D. R., McDonell, M. B., Fihn, S. D., & Bradley, K. A. (1998). The AUDIT alcohol consumption questions (AUDIT-C): An effective brief screening test for problem drinking. *Archives of Internal Medicine, 158*(16), 1789–1795. https://doi.org/10.1001/archinte.158.16.1789

Cantor, M. N., & Thorpe, L. (2018). Integrating data on social determinants of health into electronic health records. *Health Affairs, 37*(4), 585–590. https://doi.org/10.1377/hlthaff.2017.1252

Centers for Disease Control and Prevention. (2019). Infant mortality. https://www.cdc.gov/reproductivehealth/maternal infanthealth/infantmortality.htm

Centers for Disease Control and Prevention. (2020a). Economic trends in tobacco. https://www.cdc.gov/tobacco/data_statistics/fact_sheets/economics/econ_facts/index.htm

Centers for Disease Control and Prevention. (2020b). Health equity considerations and racial and ethnic minority groups. https://www.cdc.gov/coronavirus/2019-ncov/community/health-equity/race-ethnicity.html

Cigna. (2017, February). LGBT health disparities. https://www.cigna.com/individuals-families/health-wellness/lgbt-disparities

Coleman, K. J., Ngor, E., Reynolds, K., Quinn, V. P., Koebnick, C., Young, D. R., Sternfeld, B., & Sallis, R. E. (2012). Initial validation of an exercise "vital sign" in electronic medical records. *Medicine and Science in Sports and Exercise, 44*(11), 2071–2076. https://doi.org/10.1249/MSS.0b013e3182630ec1

Elo, A. L., Leppänen, A., & Jahkola, A. (2003). Validity of a single-item measure of stress symptoms. *Scandinavian Journal of Work, Environment and Health, 29*(6), 444–451. https://doi.org/10.5271/sjweh.752

Freij, M., Dullabh, P., Lewis, S., Smith, S. R., Hovey, L., & Dhopeshwarkar, R. (2019, April–June). Incorporating social determinants of health in electronic health records: Qualitative study of current practices among top vendors. *Journal of Medical Internet Research, 21*(6). https://doi.org/10.2196/13849

Givens, M., Gennuso, K., Jovaag, A., Van Dijk, J. W., & Johnson, S. (2019). 2019 county health rankings key findings report. www.countyhealthrankings.org

Gold, R., Bunce, A., Cowburn, S., Dambrun, K., Dearing, M., Middendorf, M., Mossman, N., Hollombe, C., Mahr, P., Melgar, G., Davis, J., Gottlieb, L., & Cottrell, E. (2018, September). Adoption of social determinants of health EHR tools by community health centers. *Annals of Family Medicine, 16*(5), 399–407. https://doi.org/10.1370/afm.2275

Graham, G., Ostrowski, M., & Sabina, A. (2015, August 6). Defeating The ZIP Code Health Paradigm: Data, technology, and collaboration are key. Health Affairs Blog. https://www.healthaffairs.org/do/10.1377/hblog201 50806.049730/full/

Institute of Medicine (IOM). (2014). Capturing social and behavioral domains and measures in electronic health records: Phase 2. National Academies Press. https://www.ncbi.nlm.nih.gov/books/NBK268995/pdf/Bookshelf_NBK268995.pdf

Johnson, S. R. (2018, August 25). In depth: Hospitals tackling social determinants are setting the course for the industry. Modern Healthcare. https://www.modernhealthcare.com/article/20180825/NEWS/180809949/in-depth-hospitals-tackling-social-determinants-are-setting-the-course-for-the-industry

Kahn, J. R., & Pearlin, L. I. (2006, April). Financial strain over the life course and health among older adults. *Journal of Health and Social Behavior, 47*, 17–31. https://www.researchgate.net/publication/7195790_Financial_Strain_Over_the_Life_Course_and_Health

Kroenke, K., Spitzer, R. L., & Williams, J. B. W. (2003, November). The patient health questionnaire-2: Validity of a two-item depression screener. *Medical Care, 41*(11), 1284–1292. https://journals.lww.com/lww-medicalcare/Abstract/2003/11000/The_Patient_Health_Questionnaire_2__Validity_of_a.8.aspx

Lakhani, C. M., Tierney, B. T., Manrai, A. K., Yang, J., Visscher, P. M., & Patel, C. J. (2019, January 14). Repurposing large health insurance claims data to estimate genetic and environmental contributions in 560 phenotypes. *Nature Genetics, 51*(2), 327–334. https://www.nature.com/articles/s41588-018-0313-7

Moore, J. T., Ricaldi, J. N., Rose, C. E., Fuld, J., Parise, M., Kang, G. J., Driscoll, A. K., Norris, T., Wilson, N., Rainisch, G., Valverde, E., Beresovsky, V., Brune, C. A.,

Oussayef, N. L., Rose, D. A., Adams, L. E., Awel, S., Villanueva, J., Meaney-Delman, D., & Honein, M. A. (2020, August 21). Disparities in incidence of COVID-19 among underrepresented racial/ethnic groups in counties identified as hotspots during June 5–18, 2020—22 states, February–June 2020. *Morbidity and Mortality Weekly Report, 69*(33). https://doi.org/10.15585/mmwr.mm6933e1

O'Donnell, M. P., Schultz, A. B., & Yen, L. (2015). The portion of health care costs associated with lifestyle-related modifiable health risks based on a sample of 223,461 employees in seven industries: The UM-HMRC Study. *Journal of Occupational and Environmental Medicine, 57*(12), 1284–1290. https://doi.org/10.1097/JOM.0000000000000600

Office of the Legislative Council. (2010). Compilation of patient protection and Affordable Care Act, including patient protection and Affordable Care Act health-related portions of the Health Care And Education Reconciliation Act of 2010. Pub. L. No. Public Law 111–148.

Olson, D. P., Oldfield, B. J., & Navarro, S. M. (2019, March 18). Standardizing social determinants of health assessments. Health Affairs. https://www.healthaffairs.org/do/10.1377/hblog20190311.823116/full/

Pantell, M., Rehkopf, D., Jutte, D., Syme, S. L., Balmes, J., & Adler, N. (2013). Social isolation: A predictor of mortality comparable to traditional clinical risk factors. *American Journal of Public Health, 103*(11), 2056–2062. https://ajph.aphapublications.org/doi/10.2105/AJPH.2013.301261

Petersen, E. E., Davis, N. L., Goodman, D., Cox, S., Syverson, C., Seed, K., Shapiro-Mendoza, C., Callaghan, W. M., & Barfield, W. (2019, September 6). Racial/ethnic disparities in pregnancy-related deaths—United States, 2007–2016. *Morbidity and Mortality Weekly Report, 68*(35), 762–765. https://www.cdc.gov/mmwr/volumes/68/wr/mm6835a3.htm?s_cid=mm6835a3_w

Predmore, Z., Hatef, E., & Weiner, J. P. (2019). Integrating social and behavioral determinants of health into population health analytics: A conceptual framework and suggested road map. *Population Health Management, 22*(6), 488–494. https://doi.org/10.1089/pop.2018.0151

Pruitt, Z., Emechebe, N., Quast, T., Taylor, P., & Bryant, K. (2018). Expenditure reductions associated with a social service referral program. *Population Health Management, 21*(6), 469–476. https://doi.org/10.1089/pop.2017.0199

SIREN. (2019). The gravity project. San Francisco, CA: University of California, San Francisco. https://sirenetwork.ucsf.edu/TheGravityProject

Sohal, H., Eldridge, S., & Feder, G. (2007). The sensitivity and specificity of four questions (HARK) to identify intimate partner violence: A diagnostic accuracy study in general practice. *BMC Family Practice*, no. 8. https://bmcfampract.biomedcentral.com/articles/10.1186/1471-2296-8-49

Sokol, E. (2020). Integrating social determinants of health into the EHR. HER Intelligence. https://ehrintelligence.com/features/integrating-social-determinants-of-health-into-the-ehr

Sullivan, D. (2019). Population health advisor social determinants of Health 101: Addressing patients' non-clinical risk factors in ongoing management.

United Healthcare. (2019). 2019 Social Determinants of Health ICD-10 Codes ICD-10 Codes to Identify SDOH. https://www.uhcprovider.com/content/dam/provider/docs/public/resources/other-resources/2019-SDOH-ICD-10-Codes.pdf

University of Wisconsin Population Health Institute. (2020). 2020 county health rankings. https://www.countyhealthrankings.org/

World Health Organization. (2020a). About social determinants of health. http://www.who.int/social_determinants/sdh_definition/en/

World Health Organization. (2020b). Social determinants of health. https://www.who.int/social_determinants/en/

SECTION III

Data Contexualizers

CHAPTER 8

Grouping, Trending, and Interpreting Population Health Data for Decision Support

Ines Maria Vigil, MD, MPH, MBA

Data are just summaries of thousands of stories – tell a few of those stories to help make the data meaningful.

—Chip & Dan Heath

EXECUTIVE SUMMARY

Adding context to population health data can be an effective way of focusing analytic efforts to identify actionable opportunity to improve health and reduce avoidable and unnecessary healthcare costs. Several methods exist to apply context by grouping and trending data into discreet areas of opportunity. Strategically, grouping and trending data can derive meaning from what can otherwise be considered unusable data and can help to optimize strategic planning and population health clinical decision-making. Applying context to population health data can simulate the healthcare experience, provide decision support to clinicians at the point of care, and help users understand service patterns and trends. It can also be used to identify and track engagement, the risk of poor health outcomes, and healthcare waste and inefficiency. Many infrastructure benefits exist by adding context to data through grouping and trending, including speeding up the time from population health data set development to analytic insight, bringing several related data together in a logical way, and allowing for the addition of clinical and business acumen into the build of the data, thereby aiding in the interpretation of the data. These *data contextualizers* can be used in combination with one another or in isolation, and it will be important for analysts and analytic leaders to apply and interpret them appropriately in support of population health management planning and activities.

LEARNING OBJECTIVES

At the end of this chapter, the learner will be able to:

1. Describe the ways in which data can be placed into context.
2. Compare and contrast the uses of data with context commonly used in population health analytics.
3. Identify the appropriate data contextualizer for a given population health use case.
4. Recognize the pitfalls of interpreting contextualized data incorrectly.

Introduction

Healthcare data have grown exponentially since 2010 and are expected to grow by another 36% by 2025, outpacing data in financial, media, and entertainment industries (Reinsel, Gantz, & Rydning, 2018). The growing availability, type, volume, and sources of data in combination with the fast-paced need for decision-making among patients, clinicians, and healthcare executives make applying context to data a necessary component of any population health analysis.

This chapter will introduce the concept of grouping data into different focus areas of opportunity, provide a general overview and comparison of data groupers and data-classification systems available in the marketplace, and highlight examples of how population health data with context can help aid executive strategic planning and clinical and business decision-making (decision support). This chapter will also review the cautions that must be used when applying context to population health data because the information from these data can easily be misinterpreted.

Options for Applying Context to Data for Decision Support

Adding context by grouping and trending data into discreet areas of opportunity starts with a clear understanding of the healthcare challenge to be solved. For the purposes of this chapter, population healthcare challenges will be aligned with one or more of the goals of the Institute for Healthcare Improvement in achieving the Triple Aim: simultaneously enhancing the experience and outcomes of the patient or member, improving the health of the population, and reducing per capita cost of care for the benefit of communities (Berwick, Nolan, & Whittington, 2008). When used in isolation, context applied by grouping and trending population health data can be effective in serving up data insights to achieve one of the three aims. When used in combination with one another, use of these same data can be an effective way to achieve two or more aims simultaneously.

Options exist for applying context to data to *enhance the experience and outcomes of the patient/ member*, including grouping and trending into the types of population health data summarized in **Table 8.1**. Insights and patterns can be inferred from self-reported, consumer, social media, and health determinants data as they relate to how open and activated a person may be to new ideas, participating in or leading activities or events, engaging in health content, or being self-motivated. This information can then be translated into content, programs, and interventions that are tailored to patients' degrees and types of receptivity, levels of engagement, and abilities and willingness to self-motivate to take action to improve their health and experience. In addition, a wealth of information exists in the clinical evidence base just waiting to be translated into clinical, administrative, and patient decision support such as the development of clinical care pathways and cost-comparison tools. Clinical care pathways can be developed for both clinicians and patients to assist in identifying where a

Table 8.1 Applying Context to Data to Enhance the Experience and Outcomes of the Patient or Member

Use Case	Description	Example
Receptivity	A person's openness to new ideas, activities, participation	*Likelihood to participate*: Measures a person's likelihood to participate in certain types of events, wellness programs, care-management interventions. Uses encounter, activity, likes, dislikes, and consumer types of data. *Mode of communication*: Measures a person's preferred method of communication such as face-to-face, telephonic, e-mail, chat, or text messaging. Uses demographic, consumer, and engagement types of data. *Direct messaging*: Measures a person's interaction with automated messaging delivered through chat bots, automated telephonic decision trees, e-mails, and Internet website use. Uses demographic, self-reported, consumer, and social media types of data.
Engagement	A person's participation in ideas, activities, programs, interventions	*Meaningful encounter*: Measures a person's participation in certain activities, programs, interventions such as the number of visits, the activities or goals set and completed. Uses encounter, activity, goal setting, and event types of data. *Touchpoints*: Measures the number and type of interactions with patients across an activity, intervention, program, organization, or system such as the number of health outreach communications made each year. Uses encounter, activity, communications, marketing, self-reported, consumer, social media, and event types of data.
Activation	A person's level self-confidence, motivation, and ability to set and accomplish tasks and goals to get results	*Readiness to take action*: Measures the self-confidence, motivation, comprehension, and ability to set and accomplish tasks and goals such as the self-assessment results of a person who is motivated to lose weight to reduce the risk of diabetes, including the person's perceived ability to exercise. Uses activity, tasks, goals, and self-reported types of data. *Level of activation*: Measures the change in the level of self-confidence, motivation, comprehension, and ability to set and accomplish tasks and goals such as the self-assessment results over time of a person who initially was motivated to lose weight and then participated in weight-loss activities to lose a total of 30 pounds. Uses activity, tasks, goals, and self-reported types of data over time.
Clinical decision support	Information used by clinicians at the point of care and business stakeholders in administration to assist in data-driven decision-making	*Appropriateness of care*: Measures whether a given service, encounter, activity, or event follows a standard of care, clinical care guidelines, or the evidence-based medical literature recommendations such as the appropriateness of having standard orders for lab tests that may be unnecessary and costly to the health system and patients. Uses administrative medical claims, EMRs, care guidelines, care pathways, and supplemental types of data.

(continues)

Table 8.1 Applying Context to Data to Enhance the Experience and Outcomes of the Patient or Member *(continued)*

Use Case	Description	Example
		Member benefit eligibility: Measures whether a health plan member is currently a member of the health plan, the duration of the membership, and the health insurance product such as a member enrolled in a type of insurance that provides a care-management program.
		Uses administrative enrollment and benefit types of data.
		Site of service: Measures the various locations that like services are provided such as dialysis centers, ambulatory surgical centers, and primary care outpatient practice locations.
		Uses demographic, geographic, provider network, provider credentialing, administrative medical claims, and supplemental types of data.
		Preauthorization and authorization criteria: Measures the utilization management functions of a clinician or health system's request for authorization of services for benefit eligible services based on the type of insurance of the patient or member and the clinical evidence-based literature such as the request for a genetic test to identify a genetic cause for a clinical set of symptoms or disorder.
		Uses self-reported clinician or health system requests for services, administrative claims, medical policies, evidence-based medical literature, administrative enrollment, and benefit types of data.
		Shared decision-making: Measures the presence of a conversation, event, or services where options for care exist for patients and are used to inform treatment decisions where patient preferences exist.
		Uses self-reported, encounter, event, activity, and evidence-based medical literature types of data.
		Referral networks: Measures the activity across a provider network of referrals for adjunct services or care such as a referral from an in-network primary care provider to an out-of-network specialty care provider for the advanced treatment of heart failure.
		Uses administrative medical claims, provider network, and EMR referral types of data.
		Postacute care: Measures the encounters, activities, and events surrounding a hospital admission such as acute rehabilitation, skilled nursing, and home health care. Can include patient assessments of progression of disease and activities of daily living.
		Uses encounter, activities, events, administrative claims, EMR referral, and self-reported data.
Patient decision support	Information used by patients to assist in data-driven decision-making for point-of-care services and treatments	*Cost calculator*: Measures and provides information for patients to view costs of services and treatments across multiple provider networks, geographic regions, in- and out-of-network services and benefits such as cost comparisons for an MRI scan or the patient or member's cost share for a knee-replacement surgery.
		Uses demographic, administrative claims, benefit, provider network, provider credentialing, and geographic types of data.

Member benefit cost share: Measures and provides information for patients to view their health plan type benefits such as deductibles, copays, cost share, co-insurance, and out-of-pocket maximum.

Uses demographic, administrative claims, benefit, eligibility, and enrollment types of data.

Member benefit eligibility: Refer to "Clinical decision support" in the left column of this table. An example of a patient decision support use case is the number of outpatient physical therapy sessions allowed under the health plan type benefit before a different cost share, copay, or co-insurance is applied.

Site of service: Refer to "Clinical decision support" in the left column of this table. An example of a patient decision support use case is the location of several facilities that provide the service, all of which are geographically close to the patient's home.

Quality of care: Measures the level of value assigned to care provided in an encounter, service, or treatment according to a clinical evidence base, clinical pathways, care guidelines such as measuring the presence of retinal eye exams in patients with diabetes to screen for and prevent advanced severity of disease.

Uses administrative medical claims data, EMRs, pharmacy, laboratory, imaging, and safety types of data.

Shared decision-making: Refer to "Clinical decision support" in the left column of this table. An example of a patient decision support use case is the development of patient education materials that provide information on two or more options for treatment such as an advance directive to assist in planning for end-of-life care.

patient is in his or her care journey, the various risk factors and disease burden that may lead to significant unplanned utilization of healthcare services if left unmanaged, and avoidable costs to the health system and patients. Transactional data used by health insurance plans can also be used to bring transparency of healthcare service and pricing options to patients, enabling patients to make prudent healthcare decisions when choices are available to minimize their cost burden and assist health insurers in avoiding unnecessary costs and generate savings that can be provided back to communities in the form of reduced health insurance premiums, enhanced benefits, and lower cost shares, deductibles, and co-insurance.

Table 8.1 outlines the examples of existing use cases where analytics can support clinical and administrative initiatives and decision-making to *enhance the experience and outcomes of the patient*

or member. More information on how to develop the data in a population health data model can be found in Chapter 12, "Development of a Data Model."

Options exist for applying context to data to *improve the health of the population*, including grouping and trending into the types of population health data summarized in **Table 8.2**. Insights and patterns can be inferred from demographic, administrative claims, EMR, laboratory, imaging, pharmacy, social and health determinants, and other supplemental data as they relate to tracking and trending the presence, severity, underlying causes, contributing factors, and risk of disease and disease burden across populations. This information can then be translated into content, programs, and interventions that target the diseases underlying causes and contributing factors to improve the health of populations across diverse characteristics and geographic

Table 8.2 **Applying Context to Data to Improve the Health of the Population**

Use Case	Description	Example
Presence of diagnoses or disease	Presence or absence of a specified health condition or disease	*Diagnoses*: Measure the presence or absence of a specified health condition, set of conditions, or disease such as diabetes, degenerative joint disease (DJD), and breast cancer. Uses administrative medical claims data, EMR, laboratory, imaging, pharmacy, ancillary or durable medical equipment (DME), self-reported, and health determinant types of data.
Progression of diagnoses or disease	Worsening or advancement of a specified health condition or disease over time	*Related diagnoses*: Measures the presence or absence over time of comorbidities, complications, gaps in medications, and health determinants such as patients with diabetes and depression, patients with DJD and morbid obesity, and patients with invasive breast cancer. Uses administrative medical claims data, EMRs, laboratory, imaging, pharmacy, ancillary and DME, self-reported, and health determinant types of data.
		Level of severity: Measures the presence or absence over time of comorbidities, complications, gaps in medications, and health determinants within a categorical designation of severity such as patients whose diabetes is unmanaged secondary to untreated depression, patients whose pain associated with DJD is worsened by the wear and tear caused by morbid obesity, and patients with breast cancer that has metastasized to other organs. Uses administrative medical claims data, EMRs, laboratory, imaging, pharmacy, ancillary and DME, self-reported, and health determinant types of data.
Care or treatment pathways	A documented set of standards of care, care guidelines, care pathway that indicates a disease's life cycle from risk factors to symptoms, diagnosis, morbidity, treatments, and death	*Related diagnoses*: Refer to "Progression of diagnoses or disease" in the left column of this table. An example of a care or treatment pathway's use case is the translation and incorporation of the 2020 American Diabetes Association's set of clinical guidelines to treat patients with diabetes in a health system's EMRs (American Diabetes Association Primary Care Advisory Group, 2020). *Level of severity*: Refer to "Progression of diagnoses or disease" in the left column of this table. An example of a care or treatment pathway's use case is the identification of patients who are along the care pathway or the time and way in which a patient deviates from a care pathway or care guideline to alert clinicians to make adjustments to their care or treatment plan.
Risk or presence of worsened or poor health outcomes	The presence or absence of often clinical or health determinant indicators that categorize a patient as having poor health or an adverse event that has significant impact on their day-to-day activities and well-being	*Related adverse outcomes*: Measures the presence or absence over time of comorbidities, complications, gaps in medications, health determinants, and harm of patients within a categorical designation of outcomes such as patients with diabetes that have been unmanaged over time and resulted in kidney failure requiring dialysis. Uses administrative medical claims data, EMRs, laboratory, imaging, pharmacy, ancillary or DME, self-reported, and health determinant types of data.

Related procedures: Measures utilization of specified surgical and pharmacy procedures such as patients with diabetes that have been unmanaged over time and resulted in multiple leg amputations because of poor wound healing and blood circulation complicated by multiple wound infections.

Uses administrative claims, EMR, and imaging types of data.

Related events: Measures utilization of specified hospital-based emergency department, admission, and readmission events such as recurring admissions of patients with congestive heart failure with volume or fluid overload.

Uses administrative claims and EMR types of data.

Quality of care: Refer to the section in Table 8.1 titled "Patient decision support." An example of a risk or presence of worsened or poor health outcome use case is the harm caused to a patient who had an allergic reaction to a medication that resulted in a loss of hearing.

Related diagnoses: Refer to "Progression of diagnoses or disease" in the left column of this table. An example of a risk or presence of worsened or poor health outcome use case is the presence of pneumonia in a patient with severe asthma and an inpatient hospitalization to assist the patient to breathe using supplemental oxygen and inhaled steroid medication.

Level of severity: Refer to "Progression of diagnoses or disease" in the left column of this table. An example of a risk or presence of worsened or poor health outcome use case is the patient with severe asthma complicated by pneumonia being treated in a hospital who worsens and requires mechanical ventilation to breathe.

Adherence: Measures a patient's actions in following a given care plan, medication regimen, or treatment such as a patient with hypertension who suffers a heart attack from years of not following a heart-healthy lifestyle and not consistently taking blood pressure medication.

Uses self-report, administrative claims, benefits, EMR, pharmacy, laboratory types of data.

Factors influencing health status: Measures a patient's social and behavioral factors that influence health such as a patient with severe asthma who lives in a geographic region with significant air pollution and requires a hospital admission to treat an asthma attack.

Uses demographic, geographic, social determinants, administrative medical claims, EMR, and laboratory types of data.

---

regions. As with improving experience, a wealth of information exists in the clinical evidence base just waiting to be translated into clinical, administrative, and patient decision support such as the prevention of disease and lowered disease burden through innovative distribution channels of wearable technology, applications, and lifestyle programs.

Presence or absence of disease can be detected, along with the tracking of data over time, to identify patterns in disease burden and progression of disease in populations. As with using data to improve experience, clinical care pathways can be developed for both clinicians and patients to assist in identifying where a patient is in his or her care journey, the various risk factors and disease burden that may lead to significant unplanned utilization of healthcare services if unmanaged, and avoidable cost to the health system and patients. Pharmacy data can be used to track and monitor the cost of medications over time, medication side effects, the occurrence of adverse health events, medication adherence, and medication persistence to effectively treat disease, reverse harmful risk, and prevent the development of disease. Adjusting data for risk can be represented in many use cases, and more detailed information can be found in Chapter 21, "Risk Adjustment."

Table 8.2 outlines the examples of existing use cases where analytics can support clinical and administrative initiatives and decision-making to *improve the health of the population.*

Options exist for applying context to data to *reduce per capita cost of care for the benefit of communities,* including grouping and trending into the types of population health data summarized in **Table 8.3**. Insights and patterns can be inferred

Table 8.3 Applying Context to Data to Reduce per Capita Cost of Care for the Benefit of Communities

Use Case	Description	Example
Cost or price	The costs and prices associated with the delivery of clinical and administrative healthcare services	*High cost*: Measures the costs associated with the delivery of clinical and administrative healthcare services such as the total cost of care of a patient with lung cancer or the cost per member per month of a patient with hepatitis C.
		Uses demographic, administrative claims, administrative, EMR, and other supplemental types of data.
		Risk of future high cost: Measures the predicted costs associated with the delivery of clinical and administrative healthcare services such as the average total predicted cost for caring for patients with Congestive Heart Failure.
		Uses demographic, administrative claims, administrative, EMR, and other supplemental types of data.
Utilization or volume	The utilization and volume of clinical and administrative healthcare services	*High volume*: Measures the volume of clinical and administrative healthcare services delivered such as the average number of chemotherapy medication infusions for a patient with lung cancer.
		Uses demographic, administrative claims, administrative, EMR, and other supplemental types of data.
		Risk of future high volume: Measures the predicted volume of clinical and administrative healthcare services estimated to be delivered in the future such as the total number of patients with diabetes that involves the kidneys that will likely require dialysis.
		Uses demographic, administrative claims, administrative, EMR, and other supplemental types of data.
Point-of-care events or service types	Information that describes the qualitative aspects of an event or service	*Lower level of care*: Measures the activity of appropriately moving a person from a higher level of care to a lower level of care such as movement from a hospital ICU bed type to a medical bed type when his or her care needs decrease.
		Uses demographic, administrative medical claims, EMR, laboratory, imaging, and pharmacy types of data.

		Appropriateness of care: Refer to the section in Table 8.1 titled "Clinical decision support." An example of a point-of-care events or services type use case is the consideration of a surgery in an ambulatory surgical outpatient center for procedures that can be safely performed with less need for high-acuity services such as those provided by a hospital.
		Uses administrative medical claims, EMR, care guidelines, care pathway, and supplemental types of data.
		Outcomes-based care: Measures effectiveness or efficiency of an event or service to achieve a specified health or financial outcome such as a technology company receiving payment for use of its medical device only when a patient achieves an improved health outcome as a result of a clinical response to treatment with the medical device.
		Uses administrative claims, EMR, laboratory, imaging, pharmacy, and other supplemental types of data.
Procedures	Information that describes a service that is meant to diagnose or treat and can be invasive (an operation) or noninvasive (changing a dressing on a wound)	*High cost*: Refer to "Cost or price" in the left column of this table. An example of an invasive procedure use case that is high cost and invasive is the placement of a pacemaker device in a patient with a heartbeat irregularity or arrhythmia.
		Uses demographic, administrative claims, administrative, EMR, and other supplemental types of data.
		High volume: Refer to "Utilization or volume" in the left column of this table. An example of a noninvasive procedure use case that is high volume is the use of electrocardiography to monitor heart rate, rhythm, and function in patients with cardiovascular disease or symptoms of disease.
		Uses demographic, administrative claims, administrative, EMR, and other supplemental types of data.
		Appropriateness of care: Refer to the section in Table 8.1 titled "Clinical decision support." An example of a procedure use case is the decision to perform highly invasive life-sustaining procedures such as cardiac defibrillation in a patient who has significant morbidity and has designated his or her end-of-life care as Do Not Resuscitate (DNR).
		Shared decision-making: Refer to the section in Table 8.1 titled "Clinical decision support." An example of a procedure use case is the different treatment options for male patients with prostate cancer, including an invasive operation and noninvasive radiation-based treatments.
Variation in care	Differences in cost and volume of services across providers, facilities, geographic regions, services, ancillary services or DMEs, imaging, laboratory, pharmacy, and so on	*High cost*: Refer to "Cost or price" in the left column of this table. An example of a variation in care cost-use case is the differences in cost across provider networks of the delivery of medication regimens to treat a specified type of lung cancer.
		Uses demographic, administrative claims, administrative, EMR, and other supplemental types of data.
		High volume: Refer to "Utilization or volume" in the left column of this table. An example of a variation in care volume use case is the differences in volume across provider networks of the use of CT scan imaging studies in the management of a specified type of lung cancer.
		Uses demographic, administrative claims, administrative, EMR, and other supplemental types of data.

(continues)

Table 8.3 Applying Context to Data to Reduce per Capita Cost of Care for the Benefit of Communities *(continued)*

Use Case	Description	Example
Inefficient or unnecessary care (waste or harm)	Avoidable encounters, events, services, procedures, tests, treatments that are not needed to diagnose, treat, or manage health	*Appropriateness of care*: Refer to the section in Table 8.1 titled "Clinical decision support." An example of an inefficient or unnecessary care use case is a laboratory test for vitamin D deficiency when it is suspected as the treatment with supplements or sunlight with recovery is appropriate and low harm.
		Defensive medical decision-making: Measures the overutilization of services to rule out a variety of conditions performed with the motivation to protect the clinician or health system from malpractice litigation.
		Uses administrative claims, EMR, laboratory, imaging, pharmacy, and other supplemental types of data.
		Fraud and abuse: Measures the overuse and inappropriate utilization of services for financial gain or some other personal reward such as billing CMS for home healthcare visits to patients that were never performed for financial gain.
		Uses administrative claims, EMR, laboratory, imaging, pharmacy, and other supplemental types of data.
		Avoidable medical errors: Measures the level of value assigned to care provided that causes harm to patients such as the wrong medication being delivered to a patient in the hospital.
		Uses administrative medical claims data, EMR, pharmacy, laboratory, imaging, and safety types of data.

from demographic, administrative claims, EMR, laboratory, imaging, pharmacy, social and health determinants, and other supplemental data as they relate to tracking and trending cost, utilization, events, services, and procedures. This information can then be translated into insights that can support financial planning, financial analyses, underwriting, and the allocation of scarce resources for populations to identify areas of opportunity to reduce unplanned cost and inappropriate utilization. As with improving experience and improving health, a wealth of information exists in the clinical evidence base just waiting to be translated into clinical, administrative, and patient decision support such as variation in cost and utilization driven by economics and can be corrected for in the market through proper management of the pricing and volume of healthcare services.

Often this is done through the contracting process and is the basis for many healthcare entities that bear risk through alternative financial payment models such as bundled payments or accountable care organizations (ACOs). Combining and contrasting multiple data types can be used to identify unnecessary variation in care and volume, and inappropriate care that is wasteful to the health system and harmful to patients. Various analyses of the location of services and the ancillary services that are provided to patients can also identify inefficiencies in the administration of healthcare services, allowing healthcare organizations to reallocate resources to reduce administrative burden.

Table 8.3 outlines the examples of existing use cases where analytics can support clinical and administrative initiatives and decision-making to *reduce per capita cost of care for the benefit of communities.*

More detailed information on specific data sources can be found in Section 2, "Data Sources," of the textbook. More definitions and examples can be found throughout Section 3, "Data Contextualizers."

Process for Applying Context to Data for Decision Support

Before grouping or trending data, a multitude of steps must be taken to ready the data for use in any one or more of the options listed previously; more specific information on how to ready the data for analytic use can be found in chapters throughout this book. It is important to validate the level of completeness, accuracy, and timeliness for each data type used before conducting any type of analysis. This assessment is critical to articulating limitations of the analysis, which can have a significant downstream effect on the ability to complete the following:

- draw meaningful conclusions, insights, and opportunities to improve;
- develop practical and actionable solutions that drive results; and
- deliver timely lists of members or patients identified for any opportunity.

The general process outlined in the following text can be followed when working to build a population health data set with context for any of the options listed previously. For those population health data sets that are identified to be built, consider a use-case and team-based approach to

ensure success. For more information on a use-case–based approach, refer to Chapter 12; for more information on a team-based approach, refer to Chapter 31. See also **Figure 8.1**.

Several tools exist in the analytic marketplace that apply context to data. The advancement of healthcare data since 2010 has focused many analytic and technology companies to build out solutions that make analyzing population health data for trends simple and effective. These tools often include the term *Grouper* in their names or are defined as a *classification system* and provide ready data for one or more of the use cases listed previously. **Table 8.4** is a sample list of healthcare data Groupers and classification systems available for free or for purchase, along with a general overview of their functions. Please note that the list provides examples and is not exhaustive. Other market solutions for adding context to data exist, and many are embedded within existing analytic and technology platforms or health-risk assessment tools. In many of the solutions available for purchase, the calculations and groupings of data are proprietary. It is important to request information on how the calculations and groupings are made to ensure they are used appropriately and as intended by the design. In addition, many of the tools described perform multiple functions and are organized by their primary grouping method.

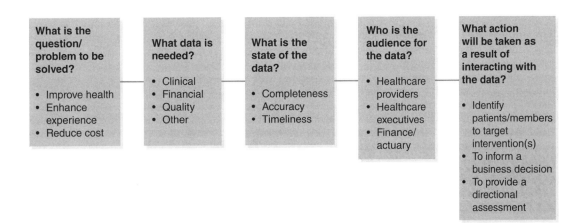

Figure 8.1 Applying Context to Population Health Data Process.

Table 8.4 Adding Context to Data: Market Solutions Available for Free or for Purchase

Receptivity, Engagement, Activation

Market Solution	Company	Description
Welltok	Welltok	Uses consumer and provider data to identify a patient's activation, engagement, and likelihood to disenroll. Predicts receptivity to enroll in programs and communication channel preference to personalize outreach (Welltok, n.d.).
LIWC	Receptiviti	Linguistic inquiry and word count (LIWC) measures revenue, retention, engagement, risk mitigation, compliance and defection using natural language from individual communications (Receptiviti, n.d.).
PAM-13	Insignia Health	Patient activation measure (PAM-13) maps consumer health characteristics to patient activation levels to predict avoidable healthcare cost and utilization (Insignia Health, n.d.; Patient Activation Measure, n.d.).
CG-PAM	Insignia Health	Caregiver patient activation measure (CG-PAM) assesses caregiver knowledge, skills, and confidence in caring for an individual's health and healthcare (Insignia Health, n.d.; Patient Activation Measure, n.d.).

Diagnoses, Treatments, Risk Profile, Risk Prediction

Market Solution	Company	Description
ACG	Johns Hopkins ACG System	Adjusted clinical grouper (ACG) models and predicts health over time, stratifies risk, forecasts health care cost and utilization for medical services and pharmacy, and identifies patients suitable for care management interventions (Johns Hopkins ACG System, n.d.).
CRG	3M CRG	3M™ Clinical Risk Grouping (3M™ CRG) assesses individual patient's risk of illness and severity and forecasts future medical cost and utilization. (n.d.-a, n.d.-b, 2018)
CCHGs	Milliman (n.d.)	Chronic Conditions Hierarchical Groups (CCHGs) identifies cost-trend drivers and identifies and stratifies patients suitable for care-management interventions (MedInsight, n.d.; Milliman, n.d.)

Medical Episodes, Surgical Episodes, Provider Profiling, Cost and Utilization Variance

Market Solution	Company	Description
Cave Grouper	Cave Consulting Group Cave Grouper	Cave Grouper identifies clinical categories of diagnoses and episodes, provider variation in cost and utilization, and provider variation in quality (Cave Consulting Group, n.d.).
CCGroup Efficiency Care	Cave Consulting Group Efficiency Care	CCGroup Efficiency Care identifies variation in and efficiencies of cost and utilization of healthcare services and episodes of care across provider peer groups (Cave Consulting Group, n.d.).
CCGroup BullsEye	Cave Consulting Group BullsEye	CCGroup BullsEye identifies underservice and overservice, procedure, and episode utilization, upcoding, and unbundling of healthcare costs (Cave Consulting Group, n.d.).
MEG	IBM Watson Health	Medical episode grouper (MEG) identifies episodes of care for all medical services for one diagnosed medical condition for one patient (IBM Watson Health, n.d.).

ERG	Optum Symmetry	Episode Risk Groups (ERG) assesses current and predicts future healthcare risk in individuals and populations. Identifies patients suitable for care-management interventions using episode-based diagnoses (Optum, 2011, 2018a, 2020).
ETG	Optum Symmetry	Episode Treatment Groups (ETG) identifies clinical episodes of illness and measures cost and utilization of specific disease categories and related services (Optum, 2012).
PEG	Optum Symmetry	Procedure Episode Groups (PEG) assesses risk, measures quality, and identifies cost trend drivers of surgical procedures (Optum, n.d., 2018b, 2018c).

Risk-Adjustment and Payment Classification Systems

Market Solution	Company	Description
Hierarchical condition categories	CMS	HCCs identify the level of severity and profile of risk for an individual based upon diagnoses and demographic information and stratifies patients by high and low cost. Used to risk adjust prospective payments from CMS (CMS, n.d.-b).
MDC and MS-DRG	CMS, 3M	Major diagnostic category (MDC) and Medicare severity diagnosis related group (MS-DRG) are classification systems for inpatient discharges that use weighting factors such as diagnoses and inpatient procedures to adjust payment under the Medicare inpatient prospective payment system (IPPS) (Centers for Medicare and Medicaid, n.d., MS-DRG classifications).
AP-DRG	CMS	All patient diagnosis related group (AP-DRG) is based on the MS-DRG and identifies non-Medicare patient populations, including pediatric populations and women's health (Centers for Medicare and Medicaid, n.d., MS-DRG classifications).
APR-DRG	3M APR-DRG	All Patient Refined DRGs (APR-DRG) are based on the MS-DRG and AP-DRG and identify non-Medicare patient populations, including pediatric populations and women's health, also adds categories for severity of illness and risk of mortality (3M, n.d.-a; Shafrin, 2012).
APC	CMS, HHS	Ambulatory payment classification (APC) is a classification system for outpatient ambulatory services that uses weighting factors such as diagnoses to adjust payment under the Medicare Outpatient Prospective Payment System (OPPS) (CMS, n.d.-c), CY, 2016, 2020).

Cost and Utilization Benchmarks, Waste, and Inefficiency

Market Solution	Company	Description
Health Cost Guidelines—Grouper (HCG)	Milliman Grouper	These HCGs analyze and benchmark cost and utilization data by hospital, surgical, medical, and other service categories (Milliman Grouper, n.d.).
Health Waste Calculator	Milliman (n.d.); VBID Health	Health waste calculator identifies healthcare waste and inefficiency using guidelines developed by the Choosing Wisely campaign and the U.S. Preventive Services Task Force. Wasteful and inefficient categories include inappropriate or avoidable lab testing and imaging studies (Milliman, n.d.; Milliman Grouper, n. d.).

(continues)

Table 8.4 Adding Context to Data: Market Solutions Available for Free or for Purchase   *(continued)*

Cost and Utilization Benchmarks, Waste, and Inefficiency

Market Solution	Company	Description
nH Predict	naviHealth	nH Predict identifies patients most likely to need post–acute care services and predicts risk of future post–acute care needs (NaviHealth, n.d.).
nH Perform	naviHealth	nH Perform identifies providers and provider networks that perform well in cost and utilization, particularly in patients who require post–acute care (NaviHealth, n.d.).

Build versus Buy Decision-Making: Contextualized Data

When making the decision to build or buy contextualized data, several considerations must be made. Adding context to data requires both business and technical acumen. For example, defining an episode of care requires knowledge of not only the clinical condition driving the episode but also the related pre- and post-medications and primary, specialty, and ancillary care services. The pre- and post-medications and services often follow a specified sequence. In the case of an episode of degenerative joint disease of the knee that requires a knee replacement, there may be therapeutic services such as physical therapy in conjunction with medications such as steroids or opioids before the surgical procedure. These same services may be appropriate to include after the surgical procedure, along with same-cause hospitalizations, infections, and complications. Each episodic condition warrants a thorough review of the care pathways and clinical guidelines to determine the costs or services that are appropriate to include in an episode of care.

In addition, adding context to data by grouping and trending data into discreet areas of opportunity requires the integration of multiple varying data types, often sourced from disparate locations. Developing a contextualized population health data set will likely require data architecture, data science, data engineering, and data visualization skill sets to build out the needed data infrastructure and governance that a contextualized population health data set requires. An assessment to determine the availability of these skill sets relative to the time frame within which results are expected will assist in making the decision to build versus buy contextualized data solutions.

The decision to build versus buy may also be influenced by the availability for purchase, or lack thereof. New and emerging evidence base and data types may drive the need for a contextualized population health data set that may not yet be available as a purchased tool. An assessment of the organization's strategic roadmap and the data needed to support the analytics will assist in determining which population health contextualized data sets to purchase and which population health contextualized data sets to build. Some examples of hard-to-find population health contextualized data for purchase include the following:

- national, regional, and local benchmark comparison data for non-Medicare beneficiaries;
- service events such as observations stays;
- site-of-service care such as retail clinics;
- emerging technologies such as wearable devices;
- care and treatment pathways;
- social determinants;
- ancillary care and services;
- disease-specific risk modeling and scoring;
- employee, spouse, and dependents; and
- parents and infants.

Applying Population Health Contextualized Data to Clinical and Business Decision-Making Support

A use-case and team-based approach is best when applying population health data to clinical and business decision-making. Building on the general process to apply context to population health data outlined in Figure 8.1, applying a use-case and team-based approach assumes the data used in the analysis have been tailored to the problem; contain the information needed to solve the problem; are complete, accurate, and timely; have a known audience; and actions to take as a result of interacting with the data and required to change the outcome are understood. Often, speed to insight or action is desired by both the clinicians and the business. It is important to note that much of the work will go to ensure all of the needed data elements are included in the data set, and that the data are complete, accurate, and timely and can be completed ahead of any analysis, particularly when using a population health data model as a comprehensive data source for analytics. The time saved by using a population health data model as a data source can be used to generate more and timelier analyses to assist clinicians and the business in decision-making.

More detailed information on a use case–based approach can be found in Chapter 13, "The Population Health Data Model," and a team-based approach in Chapter 31, "Building a Team Culture for Population Health."

A few of the most important elements to consider in any population health analysis are timing, types and quality of data needed, and the risk associated with the decision being made using information from data. Timing the analysis to meet the clinical and business decision timeline can be in the form of identifying the best time to intervene on a patient or informing him or her about the development of a new strategy for the organization. Before performing the analysis, take the time to understand the timetable

given to perform the analysis and to set time-to-completion expectations with the requester. Data often are not in a state that can be easily analyzed, particularly if not using a population health data model. Many factors can delay an analysis, such as server processing speed, storage capability, coding errors, and data-refresh delays. These factors must be taken into consideration when developing a time-to-completion estimate.

Types and the quality of the data needed also must be a factor considered when applying contextualized data to clinical and business decision-making. The familiar computer science adage "garbage in, garbage out (GIGO)" is directly applicable to using data to make business decisions and can lead to poor or wrong decisions being made (Techopedia, n.d.) Challenges in the quality of the data, the types of data used, or the quality of the analysis can lead to incorrect conclusions, patterns, and insights being drawn. These factors must be taken into consideration by developing a confidence estimate of the analysis (low, medium, high). A vote of low confidence indicates that a challenge exists in data accuracy, integrity, or analysis. A vote of high confidence indicates any challenges have been removed and the analysis, insights, and conclusions can be applied with high confidence.

Lastly, understanding the risk associated with the decision being made using information from data is an important element to consider when determining what data to use and what level of analysis to perform. Not every data set needs to be perfect to help make business decisions, and not every data set can be used to make clinical decisions.

An example of a low-risk decision can be described in health insurance. Many employer-based, commercial health plans offer health-risk assessments to employees purchasing their products. It is common for these health insurers to use the results from the employees' health-risk assessment to tailor wellness offerings. Because wellness offerings can change over time and are often optional for employees, it is a low-risk decision. The data can be imperfect and still contribute to the decision of which wellness products to offer. An example of a high-risk decision can be described in the clinical setting of care. When using data to identify patients to be eligible for a select service or procedure, patient-level detail data are needed, and accuracy of the data is of most importance. An incorrect diagnosis, risk profile, or identification too early or too late can have significant negative downstream consequences for that patient and even be fatal. Because patient care depends on accuracy, integrity, and judgement, it is a high-risk decision. The data must be of the right type and quality and be at the most granular level of patient-level detail.

Applying population health contextualized data to support clinical and business decision-making can also be thought of in terms of the type of decision the process is meant to support. Examples of types of decisions that can be supported by population health analytics include informing an organization or strategy, developing initiatives, or bringing forth a specific action within a discreet time period. Grouping population health data to support the following clinical and business decisions can add significant value at the system, practice, and individual levels.

Setting Direction

The natural course of disease is to progress in severity over time, and the health status of a given population can look different, depending on the makeup of the population and the speed at which disease is progressing. Patients can also move in and out of different geographic coverage areas, changing the demographic of a given population. As the population's severity of disease and demographics change over time, so does its needs. Using population health contextualized data can help medical and financial leaders understand the severity of disease of the population and how that severity, along with demographic information, can impact an organization financially over time. Population health data can be used to inform the development of public health policies and health insurance products such as the Affordable Care Act and state health policy (Kominski, Nonzee, & Sorensen, 2017; National Academy for State Health Policy, n.d.).

An example of applying context to population health data to set direction can be achieved when grouping data into cohorts by age and social and behavioral demographics. Social determinants data such as age, demographics, insurance history, and access to care can be used to highlight the needs of varying subpopulations and predict their future utilization and cost. Han, Zhu, and Jemal (2016) studied the subpopulation of young adults on their parents' insurance plans and concluded, based on their age, demographics, behaviors, and historical patterns of utilization when accessing healthcare services, that there would be little expected increase in cost and utilization relative to their respective insurance premium. This type of information is particularly applicable to health plans and government programs that can use these findings to design new benefits and to determine what services to cover.

Often health insurance companies compete for members by offering desirable benefits or services. Population health data can inform the direction of new products and benefits by providing an understanding of the population's needs now and in the future. Creating benefits and services that are tailored to the population's health needs increases the likelihood of members selecting the insurance product and can lead to membership growth for the health plan. In this example, a direction taken by a health plan applying this knowledge of young adults on their parents' insurance can be to invest in raising awareness of this subgroup to the no-cost preventive services available to them through their insurance plan and product.

Informing Strategy

Population health data can be applied to assist an organization in developing its 1-, 3-, 5-, and 10-year strategies by providing an overall understanding of the health and disease status of the populations it serves. Using population health data to inform health management strategies is becoming an important way for both providers and payers to effectively address the various determinants and behaviors that negatively affect health. In addition, as the industry moves toward financing value-based care as opposed to process and procedure-based care, population health data can be used to effectively identify opportunities to increase value (Sokol, n.d.).

For example, grouping population health data into discreet clinical episodes can help identify the clinical episodes that are most prevalent and costly. Adult type 2 diabetes is often identified as a clinical episode that drives significant cost. Understanding the total number of patients with diabetes and the rate at which new patients are identified can provide information on the magnitude of the problem. Taking this same population and grouping the data into levels of severity can help identify whether the existing patient population with diabetes is early in its progression of disease, has a normal distribution of severity, or is late in the progression of disease. This information can be used by clinical and business leaders to inform a strategy to address the underlying cause of one or more of the condition categories that is driving the clinical episode, such as avoiding unnecessary emergency department events and hospital admissions. This same analysis can be replicated on the top 5 or 10 clinical episodes driving cost; when coupled with surveillance of cost, utilization, and severity of illness in these populations as cohorts over time, the analysis can be used to develop a multiyear strategy to address the underlying cause of avoidable disease and its associated costs.

Setting Pricing and Payment of Healthcare Services

The cost to provide healthcare services is often described as "rising" and is primarily attributed to both the demand for healthcare services (giving the ability of providers to raise prices of these services) and the significant increase in chronic illness such as cardiovascular disease and diabetes, creating an even higher demand for future services (Peterson–Kaiser Family Foundation, n.d.) As health care moves away from process and procedure-based care to value-based care, alternative financing models have emerged. The models focus on spending less to achieve better health, improving efficiencies and patient satisfaction, reducing patient risk and burden of disease, and aligning spending with patient outcomes. Examples of new value-based financial models include patient-centered medical homes (PCMH), ACOs, hospital value-based purchasing programs, and bundled payment for care improvement initiatives (Centers for Medicare and Medicaid Services [CMS], n.d.-a; NEJM Catalyst, 2017). To be successful in these types of financial models, population health contextualized data can be used to support the following value-based pricing or payment functions (Baird, 2019; Candrilli, Meyers, Boye, & Bae, 2015; Centers for Medicare and Medicaid Services, n.d., Risk Adjustment; Garrett & Martini, 2007; Jeffery et al., 2019; Maltenfort, Chen, & Forrest, 2019; Reschovsky, Hadley, O'Malley, & Landon, 2013; Wasfy & Ferris, 2019).

- Assessing:
  - the risk of the population at a point in time and over time, and
  - the disease burden of the population at a point in time and over time.
- Identifying populations where opportunity exists to:
  - reduce cost,
  - improve health,
  - improve quality of care, and
  - reduce variation in care delivery and pricing.
- Stratifying populations into cohorts that can be targeted for specific:
  - clinical interventions,
  - clinical outcomes,
  - provider behavioral changes, and
  - patient or member behavioral change.
- Directing patient care:
  - clinical decision support,
  - referrals to specialty care, and
  - risk identification and management.
- Adjusting risks by:
  - timely identification of new diagnoses and complications of existing diagnoses, and
  - planning for future risk in the population (underwriting, reinsurance, benefit design).

- Identifying geographic regions where:
  - variation in cost and utilization exists across similar subpopulations,
  - health disparities are concentrated, and
  - poor health outcomes are concentrated.
- Monitoring interventions, cost, clinical outcomes, and behavior change at a point in time and over time.
- Measuring the efficiency, effectiveness, and return on investment of the financial models at a point in time and over time.

Medical Underwriting, Reinsurance, and Stop-Loss Coverage

Medical underwriting is a process used by insurance companies to understand the health status of their memberships, determine risk appetite for new member growth, and anticipate the financial impact of high-cost medical cases (HealthCare.gov, n.d.; Schaudel, Niederman, Kumar, & Reinecke, n.d.). Population health contextualized data can support underwriting activities by assisting the assessment of the health risk of a population, identifying high-cost diseases and the impact of high disease burden, and assisting in understanding the various determinants and behaviors driving the development and progression of disease.

Reinsurance and stop-loss coverage is a financial support method to prevent bankruptcy of organizations from unexpected high costs. According to a 2017 Health Affairs article on this topic, "Some employers and insurers purchase reinsurance, also called stop-loss coverage, to limit their financial risk and prevent extreme cases from bankrupting their funds" (Lambrew & Montz, 2017). In this scenario, it is common to think of financial risk occurring from a few extreme high-cost cases such as severe motor vehicle accident cases or rare genetic diseases in newborn infants. As the population ages and as chronic disease becomes even more prevalent, the future of financial risk can occur from a high number of low- to medium-cost cases such as the progression of disease in patients with diabetes with end-stage renal disease requiring hemodialysis,

patients with congestive heart failure requiring coronary artery bypass surgery, and patients requiring cardiac pacemaker devices. Each case can be a one-time or a multiple-occurrence high-cost procedure, and the financial risk is realized when the majority of the population with these diseases progress to needing these types of services, as is the case with an aging baby boomer population. Population health contextualized data can support the assessment and identification of a population's disease burden and can help inform the financial risk of a high number of low-to medium-cost cases over time.

Health Insurance Plan Types and Subpopulation Analyses

Population health data can support different decisions when applied to specific types of health plans and subpopulations to better understand the unique characteristics, constraints, and behaviors that drive healthcare costs and health outcomes in these populations. Population health analytics is particularly beneficial when analyzing subpopulations, especially when a population health data model is present. Multiple filters can be applied to data that allow for simultaneous and unlimited data combinations to be made in near real time to glean actionable insights quickly and effectively. These insights can be directly applied to enhance the delivery of primary and specialty care, enhance the benefits of specific health plans, engage patients in care-management programs and quality-improvement interventions, and assist provider organizations taking on financial risk to understand and project revenue and spend to ensure profitability.

- Health insurance plan type: Medicare (Advantage and fee for service), Medicaid, commercial or employer, individual (ACA and non-ACA).
- Provider group: primary care medical group, specialty care medical group, and inpatient hospital group.
- Specialty service line: orthopedics, cardiovascular, endocrinology, oncology, neurology,

---

Table 8.5 Adding Context to Data: Best Practices

1. Place data assets into a common staging area as prescribed by the use case.
2. Access data assets from a population health data model.
3. When considering using multiple solutions, include a data-governance process to clearly articulate the established use cases for each market solution and document any overlapping functionality across different market solutions to avoid applying mixed methodologies and results.
4. When considering using multiple market solutions, strive to adopt a single diagnosis grouper, episode grouper, or procedure grouper to avoid confusion and misunderstanding for analysts and end users. Consider "turning off" or "masking" features that are overlapping across different market solutions.
5. Exhaust the use of existing functionality within selected market solutions for optimizing risk adjustment and risk prediction before opting to build custom logic.
6. Display reports and visualize results according to the defined use case, including the category of improvement, intended goal, subpopulation, and action. For example, to lower the total cost of care, reduce the cost associated with avoidable hospital admissions in patients with diabetes at risk of communicable pneumonia through preventive administration of a pneumococcal vaccine.
7. Incorporate benchmark data or comparison populations in all reports and results.

---

pediatrics, obstetrics and gynecology, geriatrics, and so on.

- Accountable care network: group of health systems and hospitals sharing financial and medical responsibility for providing coordinated care to patients to improve quality, reduce costs, and improve patient experience (Gold, 2015).
- Clinically integrated network: collection of health providers such as physicians, hospitals, and postacute specialists join together to improve care and reduce costs (Bires, McMurray, & Coffin, J., n.d.).
- Ancillary care provider group: home care, skilled nursing facility, hemodialysis infusion center, chemotherapy infusion center.
- Disease category: degenerative joint disease, heart failure, diabetes, lung cancer, seizure disorder, infectious disease, and so on.

Best Practices for Population Health Analytic Decision Support

To achieve outstanding results using population health analytics to support clinical and business decision-making, a few best practices are important to consider when planning a population health data and analytics strategy; these are outlined in **Table 8.5**. Many of these are based on the practical experience of multiple authors contributing to this text and are meant to guide the reader when making decisions on tools, methods, and approach as they relate to applying context to data for decision support.

Adding Context to Population Health Data: Pitfalls to Avoid

Caution must be used applying context by grouping population health data and their interpretation because the information from these data can be easily misinterpreted. Many pitfalls of grouping and interpreting population health data exist and can have the following deleterious effects:

- derail an initiative,
- make it difficult to take action or change behavior,
- create unintended harm,
- draw erroneous conclusions,
- validate incorrect assumptions,
- lose credibility with stakeholders, and
- waste time and money.

Poor Calibration of the Magnitude of Opportunity

Poor calibration of the magnitude of opportunity identified to achieve results is a common pitfall. When assigning value to an identified opportunity, it is important to:

1. pair identified opportunities with a relevant prescribed action,
2. understand the relative impact and "doability" of the associated prescribed action relative to the identified opportunity,
3. avoid aggressively assigning estimated savings or improvement that is greater than the magnitude of opportunity and doability, and
4. validate assumptions with stakeholders likely to apply the prescribed action.

When interpreting contextualized population health data, not every patient in the population will be actionable, and not every clinician can or will act on the information. Too often an identified opportunity is calibrated by the analyst to warrant a 10%, 20%, or 30% improvement in a given calendar year despite not having a clearly articulated population definition or a prescribed action or set of actions derived from the evidence-based literature. It is important to review the evidence-based literature to identify possible prescribed actions and to determine the magnitude of the expected outcome to include in the analysis. Simply performing a scenario reduction analysis by applying different percentage savings or improvement is inadequate and can be harmful to patients, frustrating to clinicians, and poorly representative of population health analytics. For example, please see the example highlighted in best practice number 6 from Table 8.5, "Adding Context to Data: Best Practices."

Misrepresentation of the Ability to Lower the Total Cost of Care

Reducing the cost associated with avoidable hospital admissions in patients with diabetes at risk of communicable pneumonia through preventive administration of pneumococcal vaccine demonstrates a desired outcome: *reduced cost* associated with a discreet category of health cost, *avoided hospital admissions* in a defined subpopulation of patients with diabetes at risk of communicable pneumonia with a specific action aimed at mitigating the identified risk *preventive administration of pneumococcal vaccine*. A common pitfall to avoid is calculating a reduction in hospital admissions without pairing the reduction with a clear understanding of the population at risk, the event to be avoided, the clinical appropriateness of the avoided event, and whether an action can be taken to minimize or eliminate the avoidable risk from being realized and the event from taking place. A review of the evidence base must be included in any population health analysis and can produce a relative expected reduction along with the methodologies to track, monitor, and report results.

Pressure for Rapid Results or a Defined Result

Often the desire for quick results can overwhelm a population health and analytics team. The desire for quick results often comes at a time when the financials of an organization are not performing well or there is pressure from the business leaders to achieve results that can be marketed or communicated to create a competitive edge in the marketplace. Caution must always be used when quick results are needed because many population health opportunities and interventions take time because a solution often targets the root cause of a disease, requires behavior change, or warrants clinical transformation. In addition, it takes time to work with multiple stakeholders across various disciplines and to develop analytic solutions that can effectively track and monitor progress over time. It is important to develop and communicate a project timeline that includes forecasting a time period in the future when results will be reported, known as time-to-results before starting the project. This is needed to garner mutual agreement on time-to-results and focuses the population health project team on the expectations of the project sponsor and organization.

Seeking a data-driven solution to justify an already drawn conclusion is an inappropriate use of data and population health methodologies. It is not uncommon for an emerging trend such as an increase in outpatient utilization to be interpreted as actionable and avoidable, particularly to achieve a financial result equal to or exceeding the financial impact of the increased trend. Not all increases in cost or utilization are actionable or preventable. In fact, a population health solution to an increasing trend may be to increase utilization in outpatient care and offset the cost increases by identifying an opportunity to reduce cost in an entirely different area—for example, avoidable hospital readmissions. Another example of pressure for a defined result can occur when an existing program or intervention is no longer demonstrating the intended results. As can happen with any intervention or program, the results may plateau or cease to exist for much of the population at risk when risks are mitigated or the underlying cause is addressed. Not infrequently an existing program or intervention will be brought to a population health team to optimize for improved results. However, caution must be applied in these situations to ensure clear communication such that any opportunity for improved results can be clearly articulated, may require significant changes to the intervention, or may be reduced or no longer exist.

Lack of Transparency, Understanding, or Effectiveness of Analytic Tools

Lack of information in the form of technical documentation, inadequate understanding, and a general lack of effectiveness of an organization's existing analytic toolkit are also common pitfalls to avoid and are explained in more detail here.

Lack of Information in the Form of Technical Documentation

Accurate and detailed technical documentation is paramount to ensure the successful application of population health data. Too often, the documentation fails to include the data sources used as inputs, details of the calculations or data transformations, or the specifications for how the information is meant to be used. In addition, training of end users on analytic tools and contextualized data is often confused with end-user testing, where often the expectation is that the end user will be proficient in the tool's application after one or two user-testing sessions. Organizations might adopt a best practice used in the technology sales industry: hosting dedicated training sessions after each new feature release. This may help increase the data literacy across end users and leaders. Another best practice is to centralize and make available all technical documentation and assign several end users' and information technology (IT) staff as subject matter experts, with dedicated time to train new users on existing tools.

Another challenge in the application of market solutions is the lack of transparency to definitions, calculations, and logic, which are often referred to as *proprietary*. When selecting a market solution, inquire about the ability to validate assumptions and understand calculations and data sources. A common pitfall is learning of the inability to access this information only after the tool is purchased and implemented and being unable to defend or explain any of its insights or assessments. The need to properly validate a market solution's logic and explain findings is imperative to successful population health management and analytics, because the insights gleaned from these tools are often categorized into high or low opportunities to improve quality, reduce cost, and improve the healthcare experience. The inability to accurately explain how a high or low opportunity is calculated renders the tool's use to directional at best. If applied at a patient level, a lack of understanding of the logic can leave providers and operations teams frustrated with and distrustful of the information and can lead to disengagement. A solution to this can be piloting the tool for a period of time to better understand its application and calculations and informing an assessment of the ability to use the tool to change behaviors and transform care in a way that builds trust and confidence.

Inadequate Understanding

A lack of understanding can take multiple forms, including a lack of knowledge of end users, confusion about how the data are intended to be applied, and misinterpretation. Caution must be used when interpreting contextualized data because many business and clinical decisions have already been applied to the data to transform it for one or more specific uses. Inadequate training or a lack of self-motivated learning of the data engineer, data scientist, or analyst can have a detrimental effect on the tool's impact. A lack of understanding on the part of end users also has the potential to incorrectly render judgement on the tool's performance as "ineffective."

Often, there is confusion about how the contextualized data can be used; more times than not, applications go way beyond the intended use cases. For example, it is inappropriate to use data that have been contextualized to predict the likelihood of a future event such as an avoidable hospital admission and apply it to a provider profile that assigns high or low provider performance based on the number of patients in a panel who have predicted future risk of avoidable hospital admissions. Its intended use is to predict future avoidable hospital admissions to assist in the early intervention of these patients to avoid an unnecessary hospitalization. Its misuse is interpreting the number of predicted patients as reflective of provider performance. Improved person-to-person and written materials for training can help reduce the likelihood of misuse. Other options include forming user groups to track and discuss on- and off-label use cases, and written expectations of end users for self-directed learning to improve competence over time.

Lack of Effectiveness

The maturity of data quality, integrity, and accuracy can significantly impact the effectiveness of contextualized data. When developing predictive or prescriptive data models, it is important to perform the appropriate analysis to understand the model's sensitivity, specificity, positive predictive value, negative predictive value (see Chapter 20), and overall robustness. When working with market solutions, look to the evidence base to understand how these tools have been used to achieve results and what methods have been applied to test their validity and reliability. A market solution that has no documented applications in the clinical evidence base and no test results demonstrating robustness of the model will be difficult to determine its applicability or the magnitude of opportunity within which to improve. Request this information when selecting a market solution and be cautious of vendors who cannot produce this information or render it proprietary and not shareable. This caution is not to make a determination that these tools are not effective when used directionally, only that they will likely be ineffective when applied in population health; lacking this information makes it impossible to tailor these models to specific populations to achieve a particular result.

Applied Learning: Use Cases

Use Case 1: Building a Decision Support Tool

You recently graduated with a degree in population health and have been hired into a top-five healthcare clinical decision support system company. You are six months into your new job when you are assigned to work with a team of data scientists and engineers to develop a decision support tool that can support population health strategies and initiatives for health insurance plans across the United States. You are asked that the solution be evidence-based and assist both executives in strategic planning and clinical and business leaders in care delivery at the point of care. What questions need to be asked and answered to focus the team's work? What considerations must be taken to ensure the solution will meet the requirements for being based in the evidence? Used for strategic planning? Used in care delivery? What are some examples of tools in the market that offer this type of decision support? What risks exist in using this solution, and how can they be mitigated?

Use Case 2: Clinical Decision Support

You are the clinical service line director of a small regional hospital with several primary care outpatient clinics in the southwestern United States. You have observed a recent increase in medication-related hospital admissions and would like to develop a plan to assist your colleagues and other clinicians to reduce hospitalizations from adverse drug events (ADEs), including medication errors, toxicity, allergic reactions, and overdoses. During a review of the clinical evidence base, you learn that hospital admissions from ADEs are most common in patients 65 years and older who take multiple medications (Calloway, Akilo, and Bierman, 2013; Rochon, n.d.). During your investigation into how the hospital currently manages medications in this population, you discover that there is little clinical decision support for medication management in patients at your hospital. You consult with the hospital's IT team to propose this be included as a tool to guide clinicians in their clinical decision-making when caring for these patients.

During your consultation, the IT team provides several options to consider, and asks you to answer the following questions to assist it in helping you meet your need for decision support.

1. What is the question or problem to be solved?
2. What market solutions exist that may address your question or problem to be solved?
3. What is the estimated impact, effort, and cost associated with this proposed solution?

Conclusion

Adding context to data can focus analytic efforts, identify actionable opportunities to improve health and reduce avoidable and unnecessary healthcare costs, and support clinical and business decision-making. This chapter reviews methods used to apply context by grouping and trending data into discreet areas of opportunity, optimize strategic planning, and support population health clinical decision-making. When used as intended, data contextualizers not only can speed up the process from insight to action but also provide information on trends and patterns of cost, use, and disease progression. Insights and findings from the use of data contextualizers are important tools to support population health management planning and activities, improve health outcomes, and influence the way care is delivered to improve overall health and well-being.

The chapters that follow provide more detail on how adding context to data can be used to identify and track engagement, the risk of poor health outcomes, and healthcare waste and inefficiency.

Study and Discussion Questions

- What are the differences between decision support and clinical decision support systems? What are examples of each from a basic Internet search?
- If you are on the receiving end of decision support, what are the advantages and disadvantages of building decision support versus buying decision support?
- If you are on the building end of decision support, what are some considerations that can be made to ensure that the decision support will be relevant, accurate, and actionable?

References

3M. (n.d.-a). All patient refined diagnosis related groups (APR DRGs). https://www.3m.com/3M/en_US/health -information-systems-us/drive-value-based-care/patient -classification-methodologies/apr-drgs/

3M (n.d.-b). Clinical risk grouping software. https://www.3m .com/3M/en_US/company-us/all-3m-products/~/3M -Clinical-Risk-Grouping-Software/?N=5002385+32906033 33&preselect=8707795+8709364&rt=rud

3M. (2018). What are the 3M TM clinical risk groups? Health Information Systems. https://www.3m.com/his

American Diabetes Association Primary Care Advisory Group (2020). Standards of medical care in diabetes—2020 abridged for primary care providers. *Clinical Diabetes, 38*(1), 10–38. https://doi.org/10.2337/cd20-as01

Baird, G. S. (2019, March 26). The Choosing Wisely initiative and laboratory test stewardship. *Diagnosis* [Berlin], *6*(1), 15–23. https://pubmed.ncbi.nlm.nih.gov/30205639/

Berwick, D. M., Nolan, T. W., & Whittington, J. (2008, May–June). The triple aim: Care, health, and cost. *Health Affairs, 27*(3), 759–769. https://doi.org/10.1377/hlthaff.27.3.759

Bires, S., McMurray, M., & Coffin, J. (n.d.). Clinically integrated networks: Guidelines and common barriers for establishment. Medical Economics. https://www.medicaleconomics.com/view/clinically-integrated-networks-guidelines-and-common-barriers-establishment

Centers for Medicare and Medicaid. (n.d.-a). Bundled payments for care improvement (BPCI) initiative: General information. https://innovation.cms.gov/innovation-models/bundled-payments

Centers for Medicare and Medicaid. (n.d.-b). Risk adjustment. https://www.cms.gov/Medicare/Health-Plans/MedicareAdvtgSpecRateStats/Risk-Adjustors

Centers for Medicare and Medicaid. (n.d.-c). CY 2020 Medicare hospital outpatient prospective payment system and ambulatory surgical center payment system final rule (CMS-1717-FC). https://www.cms.gov/newsroom/fact-sheets/cy-2020-medicare-hospital-outpatient-prospective-payment-system-and-ambulatory-surgical-center-0

Calloway, S., Akilo, H., & Bierman, K. (2013). Impact of a clinical decision support system on pharmacy clinical interventions, documentation efforts, and costs. *Hospital Pharmacy, 48*(9), 744–752. https://doi.org/10.1310/hpj4809-744

Candrilli, S. D., Meyers, J. L., Boye, K., & Bae, J. P. (2015, May–June). Health care resource utilization and costs during episodes of care for type 2 diabetes mellitus-related comorbidities. *Journal of Diabetes and Its Complications, 29*(4), 529–533. https://doi.org/10.1016/j.jdiacomp.2014.12.009

Cave Consulting Group. (n.d.). Products—home. https://cavegroup.com/#section-554

Centers for Medicare and Medicaid. (2016, November). Medicare program: Hospital outpatient prospective payment and ambulatory surgical center payment systems and quality reporting programs; organ procurement organization reporting and communication; transplant outcome measures and documentation requirements. *Federal Register, 81*(219), 79562–79892. https://pubmed.ncbi.nlm.nih.gov/27906530/

Centers for Medicare and Medicaid. (n.d.). MS-DRG classifications and software. https://www.cms.gov/Medicare/Medicare-Fee-for-Service-Payment/AcuteInpatientPPS/MS-DRG-Classifications-and-Software

Garrett, N., & Martini, E. M. (2007). The boomers are coming: A total cost of care model of the impact of population aging on the cost of chronic conditions in the United States. *Disease Management, 10*(2), 51–60. https://doi.org/10.1089/dis.2006.630

Gold, J. (2015). Accountable care organizations, explained. *Kaiser Health News.* https://khn.org/news/aco-accountable-care-organization-faq/

Han, X., Zhu, S., & Jemal, A. (2016). Characteristics of young adults enrolled through the Affordable Care Act—Dependent coverage expansion. *Journal of Adolescent Health, 59*(6), 648–653. https://doi.org/10.1016/j.jadohealth.2016.07.027

HealthCare.gov. (n.d.). Medical underwriting [Glossary]. https://www.healthcare.gov/glossary/medical-underwriting/

IBM Watson Health. (n.d.). Medical episode grouper: Applications and methodology [White paper]. https://www.ibm.com/downloads/cas/EZALXAMB

Insignia Health. (n.d.). PAM is a predictive powerhouse. https://www.insigniahealth.com/products/pam-survey

Jeffery, A. D., Hewner, S., Pruinelli, L., Lekan, D., Lee, M., Gao, G., Holbrook, L., & Sylvia, M. (2019). Risk prediction and segmentation models used in the United States for assessing risk in whole populations: A critical literature review with implications for nurses' role in population health management. *JAMIA Open, 2*(1), 205–214. https://doi.org/10.1093/jamiaopen/ooy053

Johns Hopkins. (n.d.) ACG system. https://www.hopkinsacg.org/

Kominski, G. F., Nonzee, N. J., & Sorensen, A. (2017, March). The Affordable Care Act's impacts on access to insurance and health care for low-income populations. *Annual Review of Public Health, 38*(1), 489–505. https://doi.org/10.1146/annurev-publhealth-031816-044555

Lambrew, J., & Montz, E. (2017). A different type of public program: National reinsurance. *Health Affairs Blog.* https://www.healthaffairs.org/do/10.1377/hblog20171207.280708/full/

Maltenfort, M. G., Chen, Y., & Forrest, C. B. (2019, August 15). Prediction of 30-day pediatric unplanned hospitalizations using the Johns Hopkins Adjusted Clinical Groups risk adjustment system. *PLoS ONE, 14*(8). https://doi.org/10.1371/journal.pone.0221233

MedInsight. (n.d.). Chronic conditions hierarchical groups (CCHGs). Milliman. https://www.medinsight.milliman.com/-/media/medinsight/pdfs/medinsight-chronic-conditions-cchgs.ashx

Milliman. (n.d.). Ecosystem. MedInsight. https://www.medinsight.milliman.com/en/ecosystem#products

Milliman Grouper. (n.d.). Health cost guidelines (HCG). https://milliman-cdn.azureedge.net/-/media/products/health-cost-guidelines-grouper/hcg_grouper.ashx

Milliman. (n.d.) Health waste calculator. https://mhdo.maine.gov/_boardMtngItems/health%20waste%20calculator_brochure.pdf

naviHealth. (n.d.). Decision support tools. https://www.navihealth.com/decision-support-tools/

NEJM Catalyst. (2017). What is value-based healthcare? https://catalyst.nejm.org/doi/full/10.1056/CAT.17.0558

Optum. (n.d.). Symmetry: Manage clinical resources to assess risk and quality. https://www.optum.com/business/solutions/health-plans/deliver-actionable-clinical-analytics/symmetry.html

Optum. (2011). *Symmetry® Episode Risk Groups® (ERGs®): Health management and population analytics*. https://www.optum.com.br/content/dam/optum/resources/productSheets/Symmetry_Episode_Risk_Groups_ps_06_2012.pdf

Optum. (2012). Symmetry—Episode treatment groups: Measuring health care with meaningful episodes of care. https://www.optum.com/content/dam/optum/resources/whitePapers/symmetry_episode_treatment_groups_wp_06_2012.pdf

Optum. (2018a). Symmetry® Episode Risk Groups® (ERG®): Predict future health care utilization. https://www.optum.com/content/dam/optum3/optum/en/resources/sell-sheet/symmetry-episode-risk-groups-erg-sell-sheet.pdf

Optum. (2018b). *Symmetry Procedure Episode Groups (PEG): Evaluate clinical speciality performance*. https://www.optum.com/content/dam/optum3/optum/en/resources/sell-sheet/symmetry-procedure-episode-groups-peg-sell-sheet.pdf

Optum. (2018c). *Symmetry Procedure Episode Groups: Understanding the cost and qualtity of surgical procedures*. https://www.optum.com/content/dam/optum3/optum/en/resources/white-papers/wf700090-symmetry-peg-whitepaper.pdf

Optum. (2020). *Symmetry® Episode Risk Groups®: A successful approach to health risk assessment*. https://www.optum.com/content/dam/optum3/optum/en/resources/white-papers/Symmetry_ERG_White_Paper_July181.pdf

National Academy for State Health Policy. (n.d.). Population health. https://www.nashp.org/policy/population-health/

Patient Activation Measure. (n.d.). Increasing activation starts with measurement.

Peterson–Kaiser Family Foundation. (n.d.). National health spending explorer. https://www.healthsystemtracker.org/health-spending-explorer/?display=U.S.%2520%2524%2520Billions&service=Hospitals%252CPhysicians%2520%2526%2520Clinics%252CPrescription%2520Drug

Receptiviti. (n.d.) Understand the people who matter to your business. https://www.receptiviti.com

Reinsel, D., Gantz, J., & Rydning, J. (2018, November). *The digitization of the world from edge to core* [IDC White paper]. https://www.seagate.com/files/www-content/our-story/trends/files/idc-seagate-dataage-whitepaper.pdf

Reschovsky, J. D., Hadley, J., O'Malley, A. J., & Landon, B. E. (2013, July 5). Geographic variations in the cost of treating condition-specific episodes of care among Medicare patients. *Health Services Research, 49*(1), 32–51. https://doi.org/10.1111/1475-6773.12087

Rochon, P. A. (2020). Drug prescribing for older adults. In K. E. Schmader (Ed.), *UpToDate*. https://www.uptodate.com/contents/drug-prescribing-for-older-adults

Schaudel, F., Niederman, F., & Kumar, S., & Reinecke, K. R. (n.d.). Underwriting excellence: The foundation for sustainable growth in health insurance. McKinsey on Healthcare. https://healthcare.mckinsey.com/underwriting-excellence-foundation-sustainable-growth-health-insurance

Shafrin, J. (2012, June 19). What is the difference between DRGs, AP-DRGs, and APR-DRGs? Healthcare Economist. https://www.healthcare-economist.com/2012/06/19/what-is-the-difference-between-drgs-ap-drgs-and-apr-drgs/

Simmons, D. (n.d.). *Context is to data what water is to a dolphin*. https://www.goodreads.com/quotes/697053-context-is-to-data-what-water-is-to-a-dolphin

Sokol, E. (n.d.). Data analytic strategies essential for population health management. Health IT Analytics. https://healthitanalytics.com/news/data-analytic-strategies-essential-for-population-health-management

Techopedia. (n.d.). What is garbage in, garbage out (GIGO)? [Definition]. https://www.techopedia.com/definition/3801/garbage-in-garbage-out-gigo

Wasfy, J. H., & Ferris, T. G. (2019, December). The business case for population health management. *Primary Care: Clinics in Office Practice, 46*(4), 623–629. https://doi.org/10.1016/j.pop.2019.07.003

Welltok. (n.d.). How we drive action. https://welltok.com/how-we-drive-action/

CHAPTER 9

Grouping, Trending, and Interpreting Population Health Data for Receptivity, Engagement, and Activation

Ines Maria Vigil, MD, MPH, MBA

Patient engagement is the blockbuster drug of the century.

—Leonard Kish (2012)

EXECUTIVE SUMMARY

Patients' receptivity to care, engagement in their health, and activation level to adopt healthy behaviors that support their well-being are vital components to the success of improving the health of the population. Whereas much is known about how electronic devices, medical records, and health information portals have enabled health care to engage patients in novel ways, much remains to be done to understand what motivates a person to adopt healthier lifestyles, be an active participant in self-care, and care for others. New methods are developing that specifically target the ways in which healthcare organizations and providers can meet people (perhaps not yet patients) where they are in their health journey. Many of these new methods center on the application of nonstandard health data sources in new and different ways, such as the use of self-reported, health determinants data, consumer information, and social media interactions.

Adding context to these novel data sources to drive the improvement of health, reduce total cost, and, most importantly included in this chapter, engage persons to be receptive to changing their behaviors to be more active participants in their health is a new and burgeoning discipline in health care. It will be important for analysts and analytic leaders to think creatively and responsibly when building, applying, and interpreting them in support of population health management planning and activities.

LEARNING OBJECTIVES

At the end of this chapter, the learner will be able to:

1. Define and differentiate patient receptivity, engagement, and activation.
2. Describe the types of data sources that can be used to apply context to improve patient receptivity, engagement, and activation.
3. Understand how predicting and measuring patient receptivity, engagement, and activation in population health can improve health and reduce avoidable and unnecessary healthcare costs.

Introduction

The engagement of patients in their health is an important part of building impactful population health solutions. Patient and caregiver engagement and activation in the fields of healthcare technology and medical informatics has been well studied in the evidence-based literature (Leung et al., 2019; Malhotra et al., 2017; Ricciardi, Mostashari, Murphy, Daniel, & Siminerio, 2013; Risling, Martinez, Young, & Thorp-Froslie, 2017; Schnock et al., 2019). However, combining demographic, consumer behavior, health determinants, and social media information with clinical and financial data is an emerging discipline. The potential impact this information can have on tailoring health interventions to individual preferences in personalized ways is relatively unknown. Several healthcare content and technology companies are embracing the opportunity to enable a deeper understanding of patient engagement through the development of analytic models that predict a patient's willingness and readiness to participate in clinical programs or interventions and encourage a more personalized patient and caregiver experience.

This chapter outlines how adding receptivity, engagement, and activation context to data can enhance patient relationships, promote personal responsibility, detect selection bias, and support planning, prioritization, and triage into the most effective program or intervention that can provide the most benefit. Also discussed in this chapter is the importance of meeting patients where they are along their care journey, with examples of how data and analytics can align a patient's engagement with effective clinical and behavioral health-improvement programs, along with examples of clinically and financially impactful monitoring and evaluation metrics to measure performance.

Defining Receptivity, Engagement, and Activation

Receptivity, engagement, and activation are inextricably linked and are increasingly recommended in the application of population health programs and interventions. A patient must be receptive to adopting a healthier lifestyle, engaging in activities that advance health, and becoming an active participant in his or her health journey to experience sustained success. However, being receptive does not automatically lead to being engaged, and engagement can wax and wane, leading to both active and passive phases of activation over time. It is important to understand how these concepts are defined in the evidence-based literature and their applicability in population health to improve health and quality of care and reduce unnecessary cost and utilization in populations.

Receptivity

Receptivity is defined by the *Oxford Dictionary* as the "willingness to consider or accept new suggestions and ideas" (*Oxford Dictionary*, n.d.-a). Inherent to this willingness is the capacity of a person to listen to and be influenced by the advantages and disadvantages of a specific suggestion or idea. Applying this definition to health care and population health, theory holds that, by increasing receptivity, a healthcare organization or clinician can have the potential to increase people's understanding of the possibility for behavior change and their commitment to transform themselves or others to improve overall health and well-being. Utilizing and measuring receptiveness to reduce risk and engage in healthy behaviors in health care and population health is a relatively new field of study, and more investigation is warranted in the literature (Kim et al., 2017; McDonnell et al., 2020; Shonkoff et al., 2017).

Engagement

Engagement as it relates to health care is well defined in the evidence-based literature within the context of patient engagement in technology, programs, and interventions. This literature leverages the root definition of *engagement* as to participate in or become involved in a named activity (*Oxford Dictionary*, n.d.-b). In a 2013 article in *Health Affairs*, "A National Action Plan to Support Consumer Engagement via E-Health," L. Ricciardi and colleagues outline a plan from the Office of the National Coordinator for Health Information Technology in the Department of Health and Human Services to enhance patient engagement in the use of secure e-mail exchange with providers, mobile health technologies, and electronic information. This plan reviews the evidence to support engagement to monitor and direct health and achieve improved health outcomes (Ricciardi et al., 2013). Additional literature is available that defines engagement in the space of health information and technology (Leung et al., 2019; Malhotra et al., 2017; Milani, Lavie, Bober, Milani, & Ventura, 2017; Prey et al., 2014; Risling et al., 2017; Zhou, Kanter, Wang, & Garrido, 2010). Engagement in health goes beyond participation in technology, with the evidence-based literature providing a wealth of information on patients' engagement in various health programs and clinical interventions. Engaging patients in health programs and clinical interventions is described in a 2019 article by Rahmi, Zomahoun, and Légaré as varying from providing information (passive) to full partnership as equal members of the treatment team (active) (Rahimi et al., 2019). Both aspects of patient engagement will be covered in this chapter.

Activation

Activation stems from the root word *active*, which is defined as participating or engaging in an activity in a positive way that is not passive (*Oxford Dictionary*, n.d.-c). Patient and caregiver activation are well studied in the literature (Hibbard, Stockard, Mahoney, & Tusler, 2004; Prey et al., 2014; Sadak, Korpak, & Borson, 2015; Schnock et al., 2019). Judith Hibbard (Hibbard et al., 2004), the creator of a patient activation measurement (PAM) tool defines patient activation as comprising four elements:

1. acknowledgement that the patient's role in motivating and directing his or her health is important,
2. patients acting to improve their health require both knowledge and confidence,
3. action must be taken by the patient to improve health, and
4. resilience in patients is needed to overcome barriers, setbacks, and stressors.

These definitions assume patients are actively accountable for improving their health and entering a partnership with patients, caregivers, and clinical care teams to achieve improved results. Whereas patient activation has been well studied and a measurement tool exists, there is room to evolve this work and its adoption in population health.

Data Sources to Support the Identification, Prediction, and Measurement of Receptivity, Engagement, and Activation

Many different and emerging data sources can be used to support the identification of the level and type of receptivity of patients, their level of engagement, and their respective degrees of activation. Some data sources have been developed previously and validated in peer-reviewed journals, and some are emerging as having significant influence despite not yet demonstrating results or showing mixed results. Patient self-reported, social determinants of health (SDOHs), consumer, and social media data are identified as data assets that can be leveraged to provide insights into the engagement of individual patients and populations and are defined in the following sections.

Patient Self-Reported Data

Self-reported data is typically provided directly by a patient and includes the patient's accounting of symptoms, health outcomes, behaviors, beliefs, and preferences. These data can be collected in a variety of ways, including during clinical encounters, electronically, or via interviews or surveys. Two types of patient self-reported data commonly used in healthcare research and clinical trial settings are often referred to as *patient reported outcome measures* (PROs) and *patient reported experience measures* (PREMs). These data are used to understand patients' perspectives on their health outcomes and experience and are not meant to reflect any clinical assessment or diagnosis (Ahmed et al., 2017; Arbuckle, Moher, Bartlett, Ahmed, & El Emam, 2017; Bartlett & Ahmed, 2017; Bartlett, Witter, Cella, & Ahmed 2017; Basch, Barbera, Kerrigan, & Velikova, 2018; Bingham et al., 2017; Black, Varaganum, & Hutchings, 2014; Bottomley, Jones, & Claassens, 2009; Groene et al., 2015; Male, Noble, Atkinson, & Marson, 2017; Mamiya et al., 2017; Mayo, Figueiredo, Ahmed, & Bartlett, 2017; Noonan et al., 2017; Sawatzky et al., 2017).

Examples of self-reported health outcomes and experience data include:

- characteristics of health and well-being,
- assessment of health status,
- assessment of health function and disability,
- perceptions and understanding of health conditions and progression of disease,
- quality of life, and
- patient experience with health care, providers, and health plans.

Many instruments exist to capture and track self-reported health outcomes and experience and have undergone significant testing and validation. The instruments in **Table 9.1** represent a selection of tools that can be used effectively to understand and measure receptivity, engagement, and activation in populations as they relate to improving health and reducing avoidable healthcare cost and utilization. This list is a sample and not meant to be exhaustive.

For more measurement tools that contain self-reported data, their methodologies, scales, and their applications in health care, please refer to the "Resources and Websites" section toward the end of this chapter for McDowell (2006).

Social Determinants of Health (SDOH) Data

SDOHs are sets of conditions and environments that have been studied because of their underlying causes, or determinants, of health outcomes. Healthy People.gov's approach to addressing social determinants of health selects five key determinants as impactful to health and include the following (Braveman & Gottlieb, 2014; Centers for Disease Control and Prevention, n.d.-b; Healthy People.gov, n.d.):

- economic stability (employment, poverty, access to food, access to housing),

Table 9.1 Examples of Validated Patient Self-Reported Instruments

Category	Measurement Tool	Description
Health status	Nottingham Health Profile (NHP)	Assesses an individual's perception of his or her health status in the areas of emotional, social, and physical health (Busija et al., 2011; Wiklund, 1990).
	Health Utilities Index (HUI), (HUI-2), (HUI-3)	Measures health status and quality of life. Used to calculate health utility values such as quality-adjusted life years (QALYs) (Furlong, Feeny, Torrance, & Barr, 2001; Grootendorst, Feeny, & Furlong, 2000; Horsman, Furlong, Feeny, & Torrance, 2003; Mo, Choi, Li, & Merrick, 2004; Raat, Bonsel, Essink-Bot, Landgraf, & Gemke, 2002).
Health function and disability	Activities of daily living (ADLs)	Measures fundamental skills for independent living, health function, disability (Edemekong, Bomgaars, Sukumaran, & Levy, 2020; Neo, Fettes, Gao, Higginson, & Maddocks, 2017).
	Disability-adjusted life years (DALYs)	Measures disability, disease burden, and early death from disease (McDowell, 2006; Murray et al., 2012; WHO, 2014).
Quality of life	Short Form 36 (SF-36) and Short Form 12 (SF-12)	Assess the impact of health on an individual's everyday life. The SF-12 is a shortened version of the SF-36 (Gandek et al., 1998; Lacson et al., 2010; Ware, Kosinski, & Keller, 1996).
	Quality of well-being (QWB) scale	Measures overall health status and well-being within the previous three days (Busija et al., 2011; McDowell, 2006).
	Quality-adjusted life years (QALYs)	Measures the quality and quantity of life lived and how treatment improves a patient's quality of life (Health Economics, n.d.; McDowell, 2006; Wani & Blanco-Garcia, 2016).
Patient experience	Consumer Assessment of Healthcare Providers and Systems (CAHPS), Clinician and Group (CG-CAHPS)	Assesses patient experiences with health care, including care from clinicians, hospital staff, outpatient clinic staff, and health plans on experience with communication and access to services (Agency for Health Research and Quality, n.d.; Quigley, Mendel, Predmore, Chen, & Hays, 2015).

- education (early childhood, high school, higher),
- social and community (community, social, discrimination, imprisonment),
- access to health care (access, literacy), and
- neighborhood and built environment (access to healthy foods and exposure to crime, violence, and environmental and housing conditions).

Across health care, determinants of health are increasingly important for understanding and addressing the broader factors affecting health outcomes. It is important to incorporate social determinants of health in the development of population health programs and interventions to understand the contributions of these determinants in influencing health. More investigation is needed to understand the impact of interventions that address the SDOHs on health outcomes, cost, and patient experience. More detailed information on social determinants of health data is available in Chapter 7, "Social and Behavioral Data."

Consumer Data

Consumer data include demographics, lifestyle, and behavioral information on a person or household and are typically collected by marketing and consumer product companies and can also include information from consumers' use of the Internet. These personal and transactional data are primarily collected for the purposes of understanding customer buying behavior and satisfaction and is used to make personalized product recommendations to customers (Collins English Dictionary, n.d.; WhatIs.com, n.d.).

Increased digitization of self-reported consumer information in the form of consumer devices and applications can serve an important role in health care and has been a relatively untapped data source in healthcare analytics and population health. New areas of study are emerging on the applicability and usefulness of consumer data in identifying clinical patterns, improving productivity among frontline staff and analysts, and bringing forward new solutions to existing healthcare challenges (Brown, Kanagasabai, Pant, & Pinto, 2017; Shandrow, n.d.). For additional information on ethical considerations when using consumer data, see Chapter 34.

Examples of consumer data and market solutions for consumer data include those shown in **Table 9.2**.

Social Media Data

Social media data are defined as collections of information from social networks, applications, and Internet content that show how consumers share and use information and engage with others electronically. Social media's data and analytics use in health care is emerging. A few studies in the evidence-based literature have shown significant influence from social media interactions on health, well-being, and self-image. Social media has been used in healthcare settings to create virtual social support networking communities, disseminate education, study behaviors demonstrating decline in mental health status, and track behaviors considered to be high health risks such as substance use and abuse in populations (Bjornestad et al., 2019; Carrotte, Vella, & Lim, 2015; Grajales, Sheps, Ho, Novak-Lauscher, & Eysenbach, 2014; Groth, Longo, & Martin, 2017; Lander, Sanders, Cook, & O'Malley, 2017; Rolls, Hansen, Jackson, & Elliott, 2016).

The link between information obtained through social media and its impact on the health of populations requires more study and research. However, its applicability to population health in understanding the preferences of patients and its use in tailoring clinical programs and interventions is growing. Barnhart (n.d.) summarizes examples of social media data as likes, followers, shares, impressions, hashtag uses, mentions,

Table 9.2 Examples of Market Solutions for Consumer Data

Market Solution	Description
Nielsen Global Connect	Database of consumer-packaged goods (CPGs), demographics, purchasing, electronic point of sale, and consumer behavior (Nielsen Global Connect and Nielsen Global Media Solutions, n.d.).
Numerator OmniPanel	Database of consumer, demographics, purchasing, reasons for purchasing, and consumer purchase panel information (Numerator, n.d.).
Experian ConsumerView	Database of demographics, life events, financial, purchasing, communication preferences, device and social media, political personas (Experian Marketing Services, n.d.).

Table 9.3 Examples of Market Solutions for Social Media Data

Market Solution	Description
Neilson Global Media	Database of consumer use of online social content including audio, television, streaming television, digital advertisements, and social media websites and applications (Nielsen Global Connect and Nielsen Global Media Solutions, n.d.).
Experian ConsumerView	Database of demographics, life events, financial, purchasing, communication preferences, device and social media, political personas (Experian Marketing Services, n.d.).

new followers, URL clicks, keyword analysis, and comments.

Examples of market solutions for social media data are as shown in **Table 9.3**.

Applying Context to Data for Receptivity, Engagement, and Activation

An unlimited number of data combinations exist to combine patient self-reported, SDOHs, consumer, and social media data to better understand the influence of these characteristics on increasing receptivity, engagement,

and activation of patients in their health and well-being. Health care is only scratching the surface of what can be done with these data, and their application in population health management and analytics to improve health, cost, and experience is not well documented in the evidence-based literature. Caution must be applied when making inferences using these data because more work needs to be done to validate findings, insights, and their applicability to generalized populations (Denecke et al., 2015).

The following case studies outline several ways to develop and use contextualized self-reported, health determinants, consumer, and social media data in population health projects to improve patient experience and health outcomes and to reduce avoidable costs.

Case Study 1: Enhancing Patient Experience and Outcomes by Applying Context to Social Media Data

Understanding Norms Related to Health Behaviors Using Data from Social Media

In a 2015 article by Elise Carrotte and colleagues (Carrotte et al., 2015), the authors connected content related to diet and exercise in adolescents and their related activity on social media to determine social norms related to appropriate and inappropriate health behaviors and body image. Using social media—including content, likes, and followers—the team was able to determine the level of positive and negative influence certain content had on adolescent perception of body image. The study also identified the level of accuracy and inaccuracy of information shared and its positive and negative influence on behaviors regarding certain diet and exercise options that claim to improve health and well-being. The authors concluded a need for social media content to include responsible health messages targeted to predominantly teenaged girls to influence positive perceptions of body image and adoption of healthy behaviors.

(continues)

Case Study 1: Enhancing Patient Experience and Outcomes by Applying Context to Social Media Data   *(continued)*

Applying a population health approach and solution to this application, the problem to solve and a proposed intervention can be as follows:

Reversing or avoiding poor body image and adoption of unhealthy habits and behaviors in teenage girls through the development of clinically accurate and positively worded health and fitness-related content in the form of messages, shared content, followers and likes on social media.

An algorithm can then be developed to identify the population of teenage girls, stratify them to receive various combinations of messages using social media, send messages to the participants via social media, and collect responses using social media data types. Insights from an analysis of the data can then be gleaned to identify what type of messages and content receive the most favorable reception from the population receiving the intervention, thereby achieving the improvement of tailoring communications on health and fitness content to improve patient experience and outcomes.

Options exist for applying context to data to determine patient receptivity, engagement, and activation to *enhance the experience and outcomes of the patient or member*. In **Table 9.4**, items have been selected from the content introduced in Chapter 8, "Grouping, Trending, and Interpreting Population Health Data for Decision Support, " to highlight where Case Study 1's use of social media data can be used to generate population health insights, programs, and interventions.

Table 9.4 **Applying Context to Data to Enhance the Experience and Outcomes of the Patient or Member**

Use Case	Description	Example
Receptivity	A person's openness to new ideas, activities, participation	*Likelihood to participate*: Measures a person's likelihood to participate in certain types of events, wellness programs, care-management interventions.
		Mode of communication: Measures a person's preferred method of communication such as face to face or by telephone, e-mail, chat, or text.
		Direct messaging: Measures a person's interaction with automated messaging delivered through chat bots, automated telephonic decision trees, e-mails, and Internet website use.
Clinical decision support	Information used by clinicians at the point of care and business stakeholders in administration to assist in data-driven decision-making	*Appropriateness of care*: Measures whether a given service, encounter, activity, or event follows a standard of care, clinical care guidelines, or the evidence-based medical literature recommendations such as the appropriateness of having standard orders for lab tests that may be unnecessary and costly to the health system and patients.

Case Study 2: Improving Health by Applying Context to Self-Reported Consumer Electronic Device Data

Reducing Burden of Disease in Patients with Diabetes

As of 2016, diabetes has been identified as having the fourth highest number of disability-adjusted life years (DALYs), an increase from the sixth highest since 1990, and it continues to increase in disease burden. Lifestyle risk factors including poor diet, high body mass index, high fasting plasma glucose, low physical activity, and impaired kidney function have all been identified to be significant contributors to disability, morbidity, and death in patients with diabetes (Murray et al., 2012). The National Diabetes Prevention Program (National DPP) is recognized by the Centers for Disease Control and Prevention (CDC) as an evidence-based lifestyle change program, targeting the reduction of risk factors that result in the development of diabetes and prevention of advanced morbidity in patients with early onset type 2 diabetes. According to the CDC, participants of the lifestyle change program reduced their risk of developing type 2 diabetes by as much as 58% by losing weight and increasing exercise.

A 2017 study by Sepah, Jiang, Ellis, McDermott, and Peters investigated the relationship between program engagement via a digital deployment of the National DPP experience and clinical outcomes over a 3-year time frame in patients at risk of type 2 diabetes. The study utilized a 16-week, commercially available digital DPP administered online via health education and tracking of health behaviors. Clinical outcomes, including changes in body weight and average blood glucose levels, were tracked, along with engagement outcomes such as frequency of and depth of access to online patient-education content, group participation, digital tracking of weight, blood glucose, and program website logins. The study concluded that the digital DPP experience showed significant sustained reduction in body weight and average blood glucose levels in study participants over time. In addition, the study identified the number of website logins and level of group participation as statistically significant predictors of weight loss at 16 weeks and 1 year.

Applying a population health approach and solution to this application, the problem to solve and a proposed intervention can be as follows:

Delaying the progression of disease in adult patients with type 2 prediabetes via a digital diabetes prevention program (DPP)

or

Predicting sustained weight loss and reduced average blood glucose in adult patients at risk of type 2 diabetes utilizing an online version of a CDC-recognized evidence-based lifestyle change program, DPP.

A digital population health-improvement program can be developed or adopted and tailored to adult patients at risk of developing type 2 diabetes, focusing analytic monitoring and reporting efforts on the engagement predictors of website logins and group participation and their effect on delaying the progression of type 2 diabetes, along with the costs of avoided health care.

Options exist for applying context to data to determine patient receptivity, engagement, and activation to improve the health of the population. In **Table 9.5**, items have been selected from the content introduced in Chapter 8, " Grouping, Trending, and Interpreting Population Health Data for Decision Support," to highlight where Case Study 2's use of self-reported consumer electronic device data can be used to generate population health insights, programs, and interventions.

(continues)

Case Study 2: Improving Health by Applying Context to Self-Reported Consumer Electronic Device Data *(continued)*

Table 9.5 Applying Context to Data to Improve the Health of the Population

Use Case	Description	Example
Risk or presence of worsened or poor health outcomes	The presence or absence of often clinical or health determinant indicators that categorize a patient as having poor health or an adverse event that has significant impact on day-to-day activities and well-being	*Related diagnoses*: Measures the presence or absence over time of comorbidities, complications, gaps in medications, and health determinants such as patients with diabetes and depression, patients with DJD and morbid obesity, and patients with breast cancer that is invasive. An example of a risk or presence of worsened or poor health outcome use case is the presence of pneumonia in a patient with severe asthma and an inpatient hospitalization to help the patient breathe using supplemental oxygen and inhaled steroid medication.
		Level of severity: Measures the presence or absence over time of comorbidities, complications, gaps in medications, and health determinants within a categorical designation of severity such as patients whose diabetes is unmanaged secondary to untreated depression, patients whose pain associated with DJD is worsened by the wear and tear caused by morbid obesity, and patients with breast cancer that has metastasized to other organs. An example of a risk or presence of worsened or poor health outcome use case is the patient with severe asthma complicated by pneumonia being treated in a hospital who worsens and requires mechanical ventilation to breathe.

Case Study 3: Reduce per Capita Cost of Care by Applying Context to Demographic and Self-Reported Data

Identification of Predictors of Engagement in End-of-Life Care Planning

As defined by the National Hospice and Palliative Care Organization, advanced care planning is the process of stating preferences and making decisions about the care a person would like to receive when facing a medical crisis or near the end of life. Decisions are based primarily on understanding of the severity of illness and likelihood to recover, and they are formed from a combination of preferences, personal values, and input from family (National Hospice and Palliative Care Organization, n.d.). Advance care planning has been shown in the evidence base to improve patient experience and reduce healthcare expenditures to generate a net cost savings in certain populations at or near the end of life (Dixon, Matosevic, & Knapp, 2015; Klingler, Schmitten, & Marckmann 2015). Daniel David and colleagues concluded in the 2018 study *Patient Activation: A Key Component of Successful Advance Care Planning* that increased activation in patients led to both an increased engagement in the advance care planning process and a higher level of confidence in their belief that they can manage their health care. This study utilized patient demographic information and self-reported data to measure patients' knowledge, confidence, and degree of skill required to manage their health using a validated 13-item PAM survey tool (Hibbard et al., 2004; Patient Activation Measure, n.d.).

Applying a population health approach and solution to this application, the problem to solve and a proposed intervention can be as follows:

Predicting patient engagement in advance care planning in populations with high disease morbidity or complex health conditions by measuring patients' level of activation in managing their health care.

Advanced care planning resources can then be prioritized toward those patients demonstrating a high level of activation and are predicted to have a high level of engagement in the planning process. As a result, more patients with a high disease morbidity or complex health conditions will have successfully planned their care in advance, with the potential for net cost savings from avoided unnecessary hospitalizations and procedures. Additional cost savings can be generated from increased productivity of staff administering the advanced care planning resulting from improved completion rates. Evidence-based practice that supports more effective planning, prioritization, and triage of patients to cost-effective and beneficial programs or interventions is the underpinning of population health.

Options exist for applying context to data to determine patient receptivity, engagement, and activation to *reduce per capita cost of care for the benefit of communities*. **Table 9.6** incorporates items that have

Table 9.6 **Applying Context to Data to Reduce per Capita Cost of Care for the Benefit of Communities**

Use Case	Description	Example
Cost and price	The costs and prices associated with the delivery of clinical and administrative healthcare services	*Risk of future high cost*: Measures the predicted costs associated with the delivery of clinical and administrative healthcare services such as the average total predicted cost for caring for patients with congestive heart failure.
Utilization and volume	The utilization and volume of clinical and administrative healthcare services	*Risk of future high volume*: Measures the predicted volume of clinical and administrative healthcare services estimated to be delivered in the future such as the total number of patients with diabetes that involves the kidneys that will likely require dialysis.
Point-of-care events and service types	Information that describes the qualitative aspects of an event or service	*Lower level of care*: Measures the activity of appropriately moving a person from a higher level of care to a lower level of care such as movement from a hospital ICU bed to a medical bed when care needs decrease.
		Appropriateness of care: Refer to Table 9.4, "Clinical Decision Support," in the left column. An example of a point-of-care events or services type use case is the consideration of a surgery in an ambulatory surgical outpatient center for procedures that can be safely performed with less need for high-acuity services such as those provided by a hospital.
		Outcomes-based care: Measures effectiveness or efficiency of an event or service to achieve a specified health or financial outcome such as a technology company receiving payment for use of its medical device only when the patient achieves an improved health outcome as a result of a clinical response to treatment with the medical device.
Procedures	Information that describes a service that is meant to diagnose or treat and can be invasive (an operation) or noninvasive (changing a dressing on a wound)	*Shared decision-making*: Measures the presence of a conversation, event, or service where options for care exist for patients and are used to inform treatment decisions where patient preferences exist. An example of a procedure use case is the different treatment options for male patients with prostate cancer, including an invasive operation and noninvasive radiation-based treatments.

(continues)

Case Study 3: Reduce per Capita Cost of Care by Applying Context to Demographic and Self-Reported Data *(continued)*

been selected from the content introduced in Chapter 8, "Grouping, Trending, and Interpreting Population Health Data for Decision Support," to highlight where Case Study 3's use of demographic and self-reported data combined with administrative claims data can be used to generate population health insights, programs, and interventions.

Many more opportunities exist to personalize and tailor the way health care is delivered to specific populations in addition to the existing use cases documented previously. More detail information on specific data sources can be found in Section 2, "Data Sources." A case study such as what is presented in this chapter that applies context to SDOH data can be found in Chapter 25, "Assessing Populations."

Considerations for Applying Context to Data for Receptivity, Engagement, and Activation

Several considerations must be made when adding context to data to measure or improve receptivity, engagement, and activation in populations. In addition to understanding the problem to solve, the data needed, the state of the data, the audience, and the actions that will be taken outlined in Chapter 8, "Grouping, Trending, and Interpreting Population Health Data for Decision Support," additional discussions are warranted when working on population health projects where self-reported, health determinants, consumer, and social media data are used (Denecke et al., 2015; Kumar et al., 2018).

Understanding the impact to the relationship between patients and their providers and healthcare system requires:

- considering the role and responsibility of the patient in their health,
- meeting patients where they are in their care journey, and
- recognizing when patients may not be ready to act to improve their health and provide the appropriate levels of support along the way.

These discussions are critical to ensuring the right intervention is offered at the right time to optimize patients' engagement and success. An important caveat when working to identify receptivity, engagement, and activation is the potential to select patients for study who may not represent the general population or selection bias. Analytic methods exist to detect selection bias in population health analytics, and more information can be found in Chapter 21, "Risk Adjustment."

Use Case 1

Adding Context to Case Study 1: Understanding Norms Related to Health Behaviors Using Data from Social Media

You work for a healthcare analytics and technology company and have been asked to take Case Study 1 and incorporate it as a product that can be applied to populations across the United States. What is the problem to solve, the data needed, the state of the data, the audience, and the actions that will be taken from interacting with the data? What is the potential impact to the relationship between patients and their providers and healthcare systems?

Use Case 2

Adding Context to Case Study 3: Identification of Predictors of Engagement in End-of-Life Care Planning

You are a student working with Dr. Judith Hibbard, one of the developers of the patient activation measure and have been asked to enhance the existing PAM questionnaire for patients at or near the end of life. You decide to enhance the questionnaire by adding questions that directly address some of the considerations presented in this chapter: What is the role and responsibility of the patient in his or her health? How can the product know where patients are in their healthcare journeys? What are examples of providing support for patients that may not be ready to act to improve their health?

Propose questions that can be included in the PAM or administered alongside that address the considerations posed. Present them in a Likert scale format, with 1 = strongly disagree and 5 = strongly agree (David et al., 2018; Likert Scale Definition and Examples, n.d.).

Conclusion

When building population health solutions, it is important to include analyses that aim to understand a patient's receptivity to new ideas, his or her engagement and participation in tailored evidence-based interventions, his or her level of activation to improve their health, and develop touch points and content to meet patients along the healthcare journey. Combining demographics, health determinants, consumer behavior, and social media data with clinical and financial data can enable a deeper understanding of patient engagement and further the development of analytic models that predict a patient's willingness and readiness to participate in a particular clinical program or intervention. Data and analytics using self-reported and consumer data can also align a patient's engagement with clinical and behavioral health-improvement programs and be clinically and financially impactful to performance. This chapter outlined several ways and examples of how adding receptivity, engagement, and readiness context to data has the potential to go beyond improving patient experience, health outcomes, and cost to be used to enhance patient relationships, promote personal responsibility, detect selection bias, and support planning, prioritization, and triage of the most effective program or intervention that can provide the most benefit.

Study and Discussion Questions

- What additional types of consumer data can be applied to health care to improve health, reduce cost, and improve experience?
- What non-healthcare industries can be partners to develop healthcare solutions that drive a deeper understanding of a patient's motivation and engagement to improve their health?

Resources and Websites

Centers for Disease Control and Prevention. (n.d.). Health-related quality of life (HRQOL).

McDowell, I. (2006). *Measuring health: A guide to rating scales and questionnaires*. New York, NY: Oxford University Press. https://oxford. universitypressscholarship.com/view/10.1093 /acprof:oso/9780195165678.001.0001 /acprof-9780195165678

References

Agency for Health Research and Quality. (n.d.). About CAHPS. https://www.ahrq.gov/cahps/about-cahps/index.html

Ahmed, S., Ware, P., Gardner, W., Witter, J., Bingham, C. O., III, Kairy, D., & Bartlett, S. J. (2017). Montreal Accord on patient-reported outcomes (PROs) use series—Paper 8: Patient-reported outcomes in electronic health records can inform clinical and policy decisions. *Journal of Clinical Epidemiology, 89*, 160–167. https://doi.org/10.1016/j.jclinepi.2017.04.011

Arbuckle, L., Moher, E., Bartlett, S. J., Ahmed, S., & El Emam, K. (2017). Montreal Accord on patient-reported outcomes (PROs) use series—Paper 9: Anonymization and ethics considerations for capturing and sharing patient reported outcomes. *Journal of Clinical Epidemiology, 89*, 168–172. https://doi.org/10.1016/j.jclinepi.2017.04.016

Barnhart, B. (n.d.). How to mine your social media data for a better ROI. Sprout Social. https://sproutsocial.com/insights/social-media-data/

Bartlett, S. J., & Ahmed, S. (2017). Montreal Accord on patient-reported outcomes (PROs) use series—Paper 1: Introduction. *Journal of Clinical Epidemiology, 89*, 114–118. https://doi.org/10.1016/j.jclinepi.2017.04.012

Bartlett, S. J., Witter, J., Cella, D., & Ahmed, S. (2017). Montreal Accord on patient-reported outcomes (PROs) use series—Paper 6: Creating national initiatives to support development and use-the PROMIS example. *Journal of Clinical Epidemiology, 89*, 148–153. https://doi.org/10.1016/j.jclinepi.2017.04.015

Basch, E., Barbera, L., Kerrigan, C. L., & Velikova, G. (2018). Implementation of patient-reported outcomes in routine medical care. *ASCO Educational Book, 38*(38), 122–134. https://doi.org/10.1200/edbk_200383

Bingham, C. O., Noonan, V. K., Auger, C., Feldman, D. E., Ahmed, S., & Bartlett, S. J. (2017). Montreal Accord on patient-reported outcomes (PROs) use series—Paper 4: Patient-reported outcomes can inform clinical decision making in chronic care. *Journal of Clinical Epidemiology, 89*, 136–141. https://doi.org/10.1016/j.jclinepi.2017.04.014

Bjornestad, J., Hegelstad, W. T. V., Berg, H., Davidson, L., Joa, I., Johannessen, J. O., Melle, I., Stain, H. J., & Pallesen, S. (2019). Social media and social functioning in psychosis: A systematic review. *Journal of Medical Internet Research, 21*(6). https://doi.org/10.2196/13957

Black, N., Varaganum, M., & Hutchings, A. (2014). Relationship between patient reported experience (PREMs) and patient reported outcomes (PROMs) in elective surgery. *BMJ Quality and Safety, 23*(7), 534–543. https://doi.org/10.1136/bmjqs-2013-002707

Bottomley, A., Jones, D., & Claassens, L. (2009). Patient-reported outcomes: Assessment and current perspectives of the guidelines of the Food and Drug Administration and the reflection paper of the European Medicines Agency. *European Journal of Cancer, 45*(3), 347–353. https://doi.org/10.1016/j.ejca.2008.09.032

Braveman, P., & Gottlieb, L. (2014, January 1). The social determinants of health: It's time to consider the causes of the causes. *Public Health Reports, 129*(Suppl. 2), 19–31. https://doi.org/10.1177/00333549141291s206

Brown, B., Kanagasabai, K., Pant, P., & Pinto, G. S. (2017, March 15). Capturing value from your customer data. McKinsey & Company. https://www.mckinsey.com/business-functions/mckinsey-analytics/our-insights/capturing-value-from-your-customer-data

Busija, L., Pausenberger, E., Haines, T. P., Haymes, S., Buchbinder, R., & Osborne, R. H. (2011, November). Adult measures of general health and health-related quality of life. *Arthritis Care and Research, 63*(Suppl. 11), S383–S412. https://pubmed.ncbi.nlm.nih.gov/22588759/

Carrotte, E. R., Vella, A. M., & Lim, M. S. C. (2015, August). Predictors of "liking" three types of health and fitness-related content on social media: A cross-sectional study. *Journal of Medical Internet Research, 17*(8). https://doi.org/10.2196/jmir.4803

Centers for Disease Control and Prevention. (n.d.-a). Health-related quality of life (HRQOL). https://www.cdc.gov/hrqol/index.htm

Centers for Disease Control and Prevention. (n.d.-b). Social determinants of health. https://www.cdc.gov/socialdeterminants/

Collins English Dictionary. (n.d.). Customer data definition and meaning. https://www.collinsdictionary.com/us/dictionary/english/customer-data

David, D., Barnes, D. E., McMahan, R. D., Shi, Y., Katen, M. T., & Sudore, R. L. (2018, December 14). Patient activation: A key component of successful advance care planning. *Journal of Palliative Medicine, 21*(12), 1778–1782. https://doi.org/10.1089/jpm.2018.0096

Denecke, K., Bamidis, P., Bond, C., Gabarron, E., Househ, M., Lau, A. Y. S., Mayer, M. A., Merolli, M., & Hansen, M. (2015). Ethical issues of social media usage in Healthcare. *Yearbook of Medical Informatics, 10*(1), 137–147. https://doi.org/10.15265/IY-2015-001

Dixon, J., Matosevic, T., & Knapp, M. (2015). The economic evidence for advance care planning: Systematic review of evidence. *Palliative Medicine, 29*(10), 869–884. https://doi.org/10.1177/0269216315586659

Edemekong, P. F., Bomgaars, D. L., Sukumaran, S., & Levy, S. B. (2020, January). Activities of daily living. *StatPearls*. http://www.ncbi.nlm.nih.gov/pubmed/29261878

Experian Marketing Services. (n.d.). ConsumerView: Marketing data that connects brands with fans. https://www.experian.com/marketing-services/targeting/data-driven-marketing/consumer-view-data

Furlong, W. J., Feeny, D. H., Torrance, G. W., & Barr, R. D. (2001). The health utilities index (HUI) system for assessing health-related quality of life in clinical studies. *Annals of Medicine, 33*(5), 375–384. https://doi.org/10.3109/07853890109002092

Gandek, B., Ware, J. E., Aaronson, N. K., Apolone, G., Bjorner, J. B., Brazier, J. E., Bullinger, M., Kaasa, S., Leplege, A., Prieto, L., & Sullivan, M. (1998). Cross-validation of item selection and scoring for the SF-12 Health Survey in nine countries: Results from the IQOLA Project. *Journal of Clinical Epidemiology, 51*(11), 1171–1178. https://doi.org/10.1016/s0895-4356(98)00109-7

Grajales, F. J., Sheps, S., Ho, K., Novak-Lauscher, H., & Eysenbach, G. (2014, February). Social media: A review and tutorial file. *Journal of Medical Internet Research, 16*(2), 1–68. https://doi.org/10.2196/jmir.2912

Groene, O., Arah, O. A., Klazinga, N. S., Wagner, C., Bartels, P. D., Kristensen, S., Saillour, F., Thompson, A., Thompson, C. A., Pfaff, H., DerSarkissian, M., & Sunol, R. (2015, July 7). Patient experience shows little relationship with hospital quality management strategies. *PloS One, 10*(7), e0131805. https://doi.org/10.1371/journal.pone.0131805

Grootendorst, P., Feeny, D., & Furlong, W. (2000, March). Health utilities index Mark 3: Evidence of construct validity for stroke and arthritis in a population health survey. *Medical Care, 38*(3), 290–299. https://doi.org/10.1097/00005650-200003000-00006

Groth, G. G., Longo, L. M., & Martin, J. L. (2017, February). Social media and college student risk behaviors: A mini-review. *Addictive Behaviors, 65*, 87–91. https://doi.org/10.1016/j.addbeh.2016.10.003

Health Economics. (n.d.). What is a QALY? www.whatisseries.co.uk

Healthy People.gov. (n.d.). Social determinants of health. https://www.healthypeople.gov/2020/topics-objectives/topic/social-determinants-of-health

Hibbard, J. H., Stockard, J., Mahoney, E. R., & Tusler, M. (2004). Development of the Patient Activation Measure (PAM): Conceptualizing and measuring activation in patients and consumers. *Health Services Research, 39*(4, part 1), 1005–1026. https://www.ncbi.nlm.nih.gov/pmc/articles/PMC1361049/

Horsman, J., Furlong, W., Feeny, D., & Torrance, G. (2004, August). The health utilities index (HUI): Concepts, measurement properties and applications. *Health and Quality of Life Outcomes, 1*, 54. https://www.ncbi.nlm.nih.gov/pmc/articles/PMC293474/

Kim, M., Budd, N., Batorsky, B., Krubiner, C., Manchikanti, S., Waldrop, G., Trude, A., & Gittelsohn, J. (2017). Barriers to and facilitators of stocking healthy food options: Viewpoints of Baltimore City small storeowners. *Ecology of Food and Nutrition, 56*(1), 17–30. https://doi.org/10.1080/03670244.2016.1246361

Kish, L. (2012, August 28). The blockbuster drug of the century: An engaged patient [Blog post] https://healthstandards.com/blog/2012/08/28/drug-of-the-century/

Klingler, C., Schmitten, J., & Marckmann, G. (2015, August). Does facilitated advance care planning reduce the costs of care near the end of life? Systematic review and ethical considerations. *Palliative Medicine, 30*(5), 423–433. https://doi.org/10.1177/0269216315601346

Kumar, A., Rahman, M., Trivedi, A. N., Resnik, L., Gozalo, P., & Mor, V. (2018). Comparing post-acute rehabilitation use, length of stay, and outcomes experienced by Medicare fee-for-service and Medicare Advantage beneficiaries with hip fracture in the United States: A secondary analysis of administrative data. *PLoS Medicine, 15*(6). https://doi.org/10.1371/journal.pmed.1002592

Lacson, E., Xu, J., Lin, S. F., Dean, S. G., Lazarus, J. M., & Hakim, R. M. (2010, February). A comparison of SF-36 and SF-12 composite scores and subsequent hospitalization and mortality risks in long-term dialysis patients. *Clinical Journal of the American Society of Nephrology, 5*(2), 252–260. https://doi.org/10.2215/CJN.07231009

Lander, S. T., Sanders, J. O., Cook, P. C., & O'Malley, N. T. (2017, October–November). Social media in pediatric orthopaedics. *Journal of Pediatric Orthopedics, 37*(7), e436–e439. https://doi.org/10.1097/BPO.0000000000001032

Leung, K., Lu-McLean, D., Kuziemsky, C., Booth, R. G., Rossetti, S. C., Borycki, E., & Strudwick, G. (2019). Using patient and family engagement strategies to improve outcomes of health information technology initiatives: Scoping review. *Journal of Medical Internet Research, 21*(10), e436–e439. https://doi.org/10.2196/14683

Likert Scale Definition and Examples. (n.d.). What is the Likert Scale? https://www.statisticshowto.com/likert-scale-definition-and-examples/

Male, L., Noble, A., Atkinson, J., & Marson, T. (2017, June). Measuring patient experience: A systematic review to evaluate psychometric properties of patient reported experience measures (PREMs) for emergency care service provision. *International Journal for Quality in Health Care, 29*(3), 314–326. https://doi.org/10.1093/intqhc/mzx027

Malhotra, A., Crocker, M. E., Willes, L., Kelly, C., Lynch, S., & Benjafield, A. V. (2017, November 15). Patient engagement using new technology to improve adherence to positive airway pressure therapy: A retrospective analysis. *Chest, 153*(4), 843–850. https://doi.org/10.1016/j.chest.2017.11.005

Mamiya, H., Lix, L. M., Gardner, W., Bartlett, S. J., Ahmed, S., & Buckeridge, D. L. (2017, April 20). Montreal Accord on patient-reported outcomes (PROs) use series—Paper 5: Patient-reported outcomes can be linked to epidemiologic measures to monitor populations and inform public health decisions. *Journal of Clinical Epidemiology, 89*, 142–147. https://doi.org/10.1016/j.jclinepi.2017.04.018

Mayo, N. E., Figueiredo, S., Ahmed, S., & Bartlett, S. J. (2017, April 20). Montreal Accord on patient-reported outcomes (PROs) use series—Paper 2: Terminology proposed to measure what matters in health. *Journal of Clinical Epidemiology, 89*, 119–124. https://doi.org/10.1016/j.jclinepi.2017.04.013

McDonnell, K. K., Owens, O. L., Hilfinger Messias, D. K., Friedman, D. B., Newsome, B. R., Campbell Kin, C., Jenerette, C., & Webb, L. A. (2020). After ringing the bell: Receptivity of and preferences for healthy behaviors in African American dyads surviving lung cancer.

Oncology Nursing Forum, 47(3), 281–291. https://doi.org/10.1188/20.ONF.281-291

McDowell, I. (2006). *Measuring health: A guide to rating scales and questionnaires.* New York, NY: Oxford University Press. https://oxford.universitypressscholarship.com/view/10.1093/acprof:oso/9780195165678.001.0001/acprof-9780195165678

Milani, R. V., Lavie, C. J., Bober, R. M., Milani, A. R., & Ventura, H. O. (2017, January 1). Improving hypertension control and patient engagement using digital tools. *American Journal of Medicine, 130*(1), 14–20. https://doi.org/10.1016/j.amjmed.2016.07.029

Mo, F., Choi, B. C. K., Li, F. C. K., & Merrick, J. (2004). Using health utility index (HUI) for measuring the impact on health-related quality of life (HRQL) among individuals with chronic diseases. *The Scientific World Journal, 4,* 746–757. https://doi.org/10.1100/tsw.2004.128

Murray, C. J. L., Vos, T., Lozano, R., Naghavi, M., Flaxman, A. D., Michaud, C., Ezzati, M., Shibuya, K., Saolmon, J. A., Abdalla, S., Aboyans, V., Abraham, J., Ackerman, I., Aggarwal, R., Ahn, S. Y., Ali, M. K., AlMazroa, M. A., Alvarado, M., Anderson, H. R., Lopez, A. D. (2012, December 15). Disability-adjusted life years (DALYs) for 291 diseases and injuries in 21 regions, 1990–2010: A systematic analysis for the Global Burden of Disease Study 2010. *The Lancet, 380*(9859), 2197–2223. https://doi.org/10.1016/S0140-6736(12)61689-4

National Hospice and Palliative Care Organization. (n.d.). Advance care planning. https://www.nhpco.org/patients-and-caregivers/advance-care-planning/

Neo, J., Fettes, L., Gao, W., Higginson, I. J., & Maddocks, M. (2017, December 1). Disability in activities of daily living among adults with cancer: A systematic review and meta-analysis. *Cancer Treatment Reviews, 61,* 94–106. https://doi.org/10.1016/j.ctrv.2017.10.006

Nielsen Global Connect and Nielsen Global Media Solutions. (n.d.). Connect solutions—Media solutions. https://www.nielsen.com/us/en/solutions/

Noonan, V. K., Lyddiatt, A., Ware, P., Jaglal, S. B., Riopelle, R. J., Bingham, C. O., III, Figueiredo, S., Sawatzky, R., Santana, M., Bartlett, S. J., & Ahmed, S. (2017, September 1). Montreal Accord on patient-reported outcomes (PROs) use series—Paper 3: Patient-reported outcomes can facilitate shared decision-making and guide self-management. *Journal of Clinical Epidemiology, 89,* 125–135. https://doi.org/10.1016/j.jclinepi.2017.04.017

Numerator. (n.d.). Consumer panel data. Numerator OmniPanel. https://www.numerator.com/omnipanel-consumer-panel

Oxford Dictionary. (n.d.-a). Receptivity—defined. Lexico.com. https://www.lexico.com/en/definition/receptivity

Oxford Dictionary. (n.d.-b). Engage—defined. Lexico.com. https://www.lexico.com/en/definition/engage

Oxford Dictionary. (n.d.-c). Active—defined. Lexico.com. https://www.lexico.com/en/definition/active

Patient Activation Measure. (n.d.). Increasing activation starts with measurement.

Prey, J. E., Woollen, J., Wilcox, L., Sackeim, A. D., Hripcsak, G., Bakken, S., Restaino, S., Feiner, S., & Vawdrey, D. K. (2014, July). Patient engagement in the inpatient setting: A systematic review. *Journal of the American Medical Informatics Association, 21*(4), 742–750. https://doi.org/10.1136/amiajnl-2013-002141

Quigley, D. D., Mendel, P. J., Predmore, Z. S., Chen, A. Y., & Hays, R. D. (2015, July 7). Use of CAHPS patient experience survey data as part of a patient-centered medical home quality improvement initiative. *Journal of Healthcare Leadership, 7.* https://doi.org/10.2147/JHL.S69963

Raat, H., Bonsel, G. J., Essink-Bot, M. L., Landgraf, J. M., & Gemke, R. J. B. J. (2002). Reliability and validity of comprehensive health status measures in children: The child health questionnaire in relation to the health utilities index. *Journal of Clinical Epidemiology, 55*(1), 67–76. https://doi.org/10.1016/S0895-4356(01)00411-5

Rahimi, S. A., Zomahoun, H. T. V., & Légaré, F. (2019). Patient engagement and its evaluation tools—Current challenges and future directions. *International Journal of Health Policy and Management, 8*(6), 378–380. https://doi.org/10.15171/ijhpm.2019.16

Ricciardi, L., Mostashari, F., Murphy, J., Daniel, J. G., & Siminerio, E. P. (2013, February). A national action plan to support consumer engagement via E-health. *Health Affairs, 32*(2), 376–384. https://doi.org/10.1377/hlthaff.2012.1216

Risling, T., Martinez, J., Young, J., & Thorp-Froslie, N. (2017, September). Evaluating patient empowerment in association with eHealth technology: Scoping review. *Journal of Medical Internet Research, 19*(9). https://doi.org/10.2196/jmir.7809

Rolls, K., Hansen, M., Jackson, D., & Elliott, D. (2016, June). How health care professionals use social media to create virtual communities: An integrative review. *Journal of Medical Internet Research, 18*(6). https://doi.org/10.2196/jmir.5312

Sadak, T., Korpak, A., & Borson, S. (2015). Measuring caregiver activation for health care: Validation of PBH-LCI: D. *Geriatric Nursing, 36*(4), 284–292. https://doi.org/10.1016/j.gerinurse.2015.03.003

Sawatzky, R., Chan, E. K. H., Zumbo, B. D., Ahmed, S., Bartlett, S. J., Bingham, C. O., III, Gardner, W., Jutai, J., Kuspinar, A., Sajobi, T., & Lix, L. M. (2017, September 1). Montreal Accord on patient-reported outcomes (PROs) use series—Paper 7: Modern perspectives of measurement validation emphasize justification of inferences based on patient reported outcome scores. *Journal of Clinical Epidemiology, 89,* 154–159. https://doi.org/10.1016/j.jclinepi.2016.12.002

Schnock, K. O., Snyder, J. E., Fuller, T. E., Duckworth, M., Grant, M., Yoon, C., Lipsitz, S., Dalal, A. K., Bates, D. W., & Dykes, P. C. (2019, July). Acute care patient portal intervention: Portal use and patient activation. *Journal of Medical Internet Research, 21*(7). https://doi.org/10.2196/13336

Sepah, C. S., Jiang, L., Ellis, R. J., McDermott, K., & Peters, A. L. (2017). Engagement and outcomes in a digital diabetes prevention program: 3-year update. *BMJ Open Diabetes Research and Care, 5*(1), e000422. https://doi.org/10.1136/bmjdrc-2017-000422

Shandrow, K. L. (n.d.). 10 questions to ask when collecting customer data. Entrepreneur. https://www.entrepreneur.com/article/231513

Shonkoff, E. T., Anzman-Frasca, S., Lynskey, V. M., Chan, G., Glenn, M. E., & Economos, C. D. (2017, July 25). Child and parent perspectives on healthier side dishes and beverages in restaurant kids' meals: Results from a national survey in the United States. *BMC Public Health, 18*(1). https://doi.org/10.1186/s12889-017-4610-3

Wani, P., & Blanco-Garcia, C. (2016, February 3). A round-up on cost-effectiveness of hypertension therapy based on the 2014 guidelines. *Current Cardiology Reports, 18*(3), 1–5. https://doi.org/10.1007/s11886-016-0703-3

Ware, J. E., Kosinski, M., & Keller, S. D. (1996). A 12-item short-form health survey: construction of scales and preliminary tests of reliability and validity. *Medical Care, 34*(3), 220–233. https://doi.org/10.1097/00005650-199603000-00003

WhatIs.com. (n.d.). What is consumer data? https://searchcio.techtarget.com/definition/consumer-data

Wiklund, I. (1990). The Nottingham Health Profile—A measure of health-related quality of life. *Scandinavian Journal of Primary Health Care, 1*(Supplement), 15–18.

World Health Organization. (2014). Metrics: Disability-adjusted life year (DALY). Author.

Zhou, Y. Y., Kanter, M. H., Wang, J. J., & Garrido, T. (2010). Improved quality at Kaiser Permanente through e-mail between physicians and patients. *Health Affairs, 29*(7), 1370–1375. https://doi.org/10.1377/hlthaff.2010.0048

CHAPTER 10

Grouping, Trending, and Interpreting Population Health Data for Assessing Risk and Disease Burden

Ines Maria Vigil, MD, MPH, MBA

Everything in life has some risk. What you have to actually learn to do is how to navigate it.

—Reid Hoffman (Medhi, 2020)

EXECUTIVE SUMMARY

A fundamental element of any population health analyses is a robust identification and stratification of the population of interest regarding its realized (historical), existing (concurrent), and rising (predicted) risk. Categorization of data into subsets of clinically informed and relevant condition sets is a core method of assigning various levels of risk to patients in population health management and analytics. Several technology and analytic companies exist with market solutions in this space, and new products and solutions are introduced every year that establish new methodologies and use cases. Identification of risk in population health primarily utilizes a combination of demographic; health plan claims; electronic medical records (EMRs); pharmacy, lab, imaging, and ancillary data; and supplemental data such as social and behavioral data. Various risk categories can exist simultaneously for a patient and is dependent on the combination of various risk factors and their respective likelihood to negatively impact health. When developing population health programs and interventions, it is important to consider the root cause of the risks identified, the ways in which these risks can be mitigated, the required time frame to truly reduce or eliminate a risk, and the relative cost savings and avoidance that may occur as a result of delaying the progression of a health risk into a disease, comorbidity, complication, or death.

The *data contextualizers* outlined in this chapter can be used in combination with one another or in isolation, and it will be important for analysts and analytic leaders to apply and interpret them appropriately in support of population health management planning and activities.

LEARNING OBJECTIVES

At the end of this chapter, the learner will be able to:

1. Describe the ways in which data can be placed into context to assess realized, concurrent, and predicted risk.
2. Identify the data assets required to develop a risk assessment or risk predictor.
3. Demonstrate knowledge in several existing applications and use cases of risk identification and stratification used commonly in population health analytics.

Introduction

Grouping, trending, and interpreting population health data into discreet categories of realized (historical), existing (concurrent), and rising (future or predicted) risk requires an equal amount of artistry as it does science. The introduction of new analytic techniques such as the use of artificial intelligence, machine learning, and natural language processing (NLP) are bringing forward new opportunities to assess and assign risk to populations with greater accuracy and timeliness than ever before. The exponential growth of healthcare data available since 2010 is outpacing any one clinician's ability to absorb and synthesize the data and their applicability to patient populations, let alone tailor them to the unique needs of individual patients (Reinsel, Gantz, & Rydning, 2018; Shah, Steyerberg, & Kent, 2018).

Parsing out vast amounts of healthcare data into usable bits of actionable population health insights is rooted in the identification of risk in populations and the ability to turn these risks into opportunities to improve the health of populations, reduce the cost while maintaining or improving quality of care delivered, and improve the healthcare experience for patients. An unlimited number of combinations exist when bringing together clinical, financial, and supplementary data, and success is gained when a clear path of context can be applied and the logic of the algorithms developed can be clearly articulated and followed by both clinicians and business leaders.

This chapter outlines definitions for realized, existing, and rising risk data categorizations and case studies where healthcare data has been contextualized to produce population health data insights that can be translated into action to improve patient experience, health outcomes, and reduce the total cost of care. Also covered in this chapter are the challenges associated with assigning understated or suspected risk, uncertainty when identifying patients for participation in population health clinical programs and interventions, and uncertainty when reporting outcomes.

Defining Health Risk and Disease Burden

A *health risk* is defined as an adverse event or the likelihood that one's health will be affected in a negative way by a specific event, disease, or condition (Stoppler, n.d.). Risk is not a guarantee; it is a possibility based on statistical probabilities from studies conducted in the clinical evidence base. Health risks are often called *risk factors* and are typically reported as being low, moderate, or high. Health risks can originate from genetics, environmental exposures, and lifestyle behaviors. Some risks are inherent and cannot be changed, and some are within a person's control to change. For example, certain types of breast cancers can have a genetic risk component, and certain types of lung cancers are caused by the risk of prolonged exposure to cigarette smoke. Examples of health risks that are within a person's control to change are listed in **Table 10.1**, "Examples of Health Risks."

Table 10.1 Selected Health Conditions and Risk Factors, by Age: United States, Selected Years 1988–1994 Through 2015–2016

Health condition	1988–1994	1999–2000	2001–2002	2003–2004	2005–2006	2007–2008	2009–2010	2011–2012	2013–2014	2015–2016
Diabetes	Percent of adults aged 20 and over									
Total, age-adjusted	8.8	9.0	10.6	10.9	10.4	11.4	11.5	11.9	11.9	—
Total, crude	8.3	8.6	10.3	10.9	10.9	11.9	12.1	12.5	12.7	—
Hypercholesterolemia										
Total, age-adjusted	22.8	25.5	24.6	27.9	27.4	27.6	27.2	28.2	27.4	26.9
Total, crude	21.5	24.5	24.2	27.9	28.1	28.8	28.6	30.4	29.3	29.6
High total cholesterol										
Total, age-adjusted	20.8	18.3	16.5	16.9	15.6	14.2	13.2	12.7	11.1	12.2
Total, crude	19.6	17.7	16.4	17.0	15.9	14.6	13.6	13.1	11.1	12.5
Hypertension										
Total, age-adjusted	25.5	30.0	29.7	32.1	30.5	31.2	30.0	30.0	30.8	30.2
Total, crude	24.1	28.9	28.9	32.5	31.7	32.6	31.9	32.5	33.5	33.2
Uncontrolled high blood pressure among persons with hypertension										
Total, age-adjusted	77.2	71.9	68.3	63.8	63.0	56.2	55.7	54.6	51.3	59.7
Total, crude	73.9	69.1	65.4	60.8	56.6	51.8	46.7	48.0	46.1	51.5
Overweight or obesity										
Total, age-adjusted	56.0	64.5	65.6	66.4	66.9	68.1	68.8	68.6	70.4	71.3
Total, crude	54.9	64.1	65.6	66.5	67.3	68.3	69.2	69.0	70.7	71.6
Obesity										
Total, age-adjusted	22.9	30.5	30.5	32.3	34.4	33.7	35.7	34.9	37.8	39.7
Total, crude	22.3	30.3	30.6	32.3	34.7	33.9	35.9	35.1	37.9	39.8
Untreated dental caries										
Total, age-adjusted	27.7	24.4	21.3	29.8	24.4	21.7	—	25.5	31.5	—
Total, crude	28.2	25.0	21.7	30.2	24.5	21.8	—	25.5	31.3	—

(continues)

Table 10.1 Selected Health Conditions and Risk Factors, by Age: United States, Selected Years 1988–1994 Through 2015–2016   *(continued)*

Health condition	1988–1994	1999–2000	2001–2002	2003–2004	2005–2006	2007–2008	2009–2010	2011–2012	2013–2014	2015–2016
Obesity	Percent of persons under age 20									
2–5 years	7.2	10.3	10.6	14.0	11.0	10.1	12.1	8.4	9.4	13.9
6–11 years	11.3	15.1	16.3	18.8	15.1	19.6	18.0	17.7	17.4	18.4
12–19 years	10.5	14.8	16.7	17.4	17.8	18.1	18.4	20.5	20.6	20.6
Untreated dental caries										
5–19 years	24.3	23.6	21.2	25.6	16.2	16.9	14.6	17.5	19.6	—

Data from Centers for Disease Control and Prevention. (2017). Selected health conditions and risk factors, by age: United States, selected years 1988–1994 through 2015–2016. https://www.cdc.gov/nchs/data/hus/2017/053.pdf

Health risk can also be categorized into realized (historical) risk, existing (concurrent) risk, and rising (predicted) risk based on the temporal understanding of the risk and the relative probability that the risk will result in a worsened health outcome. Identifying health risks and effective interventions to mitigate health risks is the foundation of population health, and it is important to understand and differentiate different types of risks when performing analytics to support population health.

Disease burden was first described in 1990 by a collaboration between the World Health Organization, the Harvard School of Public Health, and the World Bank as "death and loss of health due to diseases, injuries, and risk factors for all regions of the world" (World Health Organization, n.d.). Disease burden can be calculated in the form of disability-adjusted life years (DALYs) and quality-adjusted life years (QALYs) as the impact of a health condition, injury, or risk factors as measured by morbidity, financial cost, and mortality, and it is regularly studied in the United States and around the world (Murray et al., 2012, 2018).

Realized Risk and Disease Burden (Historical)

Historical or realized risk is the most common form of analytics and reporting on risk. A realized risk model uses data from the base period prior to the risk score being calculated, and they typically have the best predictive power when compared to existing or rising risk models. Descriptive in nature, the identification and stratification of realized risk is a vital component of syndromic surveillance, population health trending, and tracking the overall prevalence, incidence, and burden of disease in populations. Analyzing and reporting on realized risk allows for population health insights and learnings to become known and for the nuances of how health is impacted by various interventions in diverse subpopulations to be understood. In addition, understanding the realized risk of populations is a foundational analytic element needed for the timely identification of existing risk and prediction of risk that more advanced analytics provides. The historical trending of population health data is what has identified the health risks that are commonly reported on in health care today and where interventions to address risk are continuously being developed, studied, and translated into standard clinical practice in the form of clinical care pathways and standards of care. Numerous examples exist across the evidence-based literature and include the identification of comorbid conditions that serve as risk factors to the use and abuse of opioid prescription medications, cumulative environmental risk factors for the development of lung cancer in smoking and nonsmoking adults, and a multi-decade review of burden of illness, injuries, and risk factors in the U.S. population (Canizares, Power, Rampersaud, & Badley, 2019; Lipfert & Wyzga, 2020; Livingston et al., 2020; Murray et al., 2018).

Existing Risk and Disease Burden (Concurrent)

Existing or *concurrent risk* is defined as the estimation of risk in the current period. A concurrent model uses data from the same period as the risk score being calculated. For example, if calculating a calendar year concurrent risk score, all data for that calendar year are included in the model. Typically, existing risk models have a better predictive power as compared to rising risk models and less predictive power than realized risk models. Diagnostic in nature, the identification and stratification of existing risk is foundational to confirming diagnoses across populations, proactively assessing and managing the health of patients, improving the quality of care delivery, affording timely intervention to avoid unnecessary cost and utilization, and in health insurance or for those healthcare organizations that are financially accountable, the accurate capture and protection of revenue. Analyzing and reporting on existing risk requires the continuous review of medical record and medical encounter data, and these are often reported with a time lag of 1 to 3 months to allow for any test results, billing, and payment adjustments in the data to complete. Abstraction

of data directly from the EMR can provide more timely assessment of existing risk and allow for timely patient outreach, education, and intervention. Abstraction of data from administrative medical claims allows for more accurate assessment of cost and utilization associated with the existing risk, are auditable in nature, and are typically used in health care to confirm diagnoses relative to risk-adjusted revenue payments from Centers for Medicare and Medicaid Services (CMS) (Dudley et al., 2003; Haas et al., 2013; Hileman, Mehmud, & Rosenberg, 2016; Hill et al., 2011; Mark, Ozminkowski, Kirk, Ettner, & Drabek, 2003).

Rising Risk and Disease Burden (Predicted or Prospective)

An established definition of rising risk does not yet exist in the evidence-based literature (Cantor, Haller, & Greenberg, 2018). However, many examples exist in that literature of populations with risk factors that can contribute to the development of risk models to identify rising risk of worsened health outcomes in populations (Canizares et al., 2019; Chang & Weiner, 2010; Irvin et al., 2020; Lipfert & Wyzga, 2020). These clinical and financial risk models are also referred to as *predicted* or *prospective risk* in many studies. In 2016, the Society of Actuaries (Hileman et al., 2016) defined prospective risk as models that are developed for the purpose of prediction and use data from a baseline period of time to predict a risk score in the future.

For the purposes of this textbook, *rising risk* refers to individuals whose modifiable health risks and morbidity is projected to result in higher healthcare utilization and costs. In this situation, timely capture of health data allows for the identification and stratification of individuals with the intent of intervening to reduce or eliminate their rising risk trend. It is important to recognize that the risk in these models is predicted to occur according to a probability and within a defined time frame in the future and is not a guarantee. Uncertainty exists and, as a result, rising risk models have less predictive power than both historical and existing risk models. However, the benefit of using these models is to allow for the most lead time to intervene to mitigate risk factors and disease burden. Identifying rising risk in populations and intervening early and effectively has been demonstrated to reduce healthcare costs and improve health outcomes in populations across subsets of risk factors and diverse populations (Cantor et al., 2018; Goetzel et al., 2012; Ozminkowski et al., 2006; Seow & Sibley, 2014; Yen, McDonald, Hirschland, & Edington, 2003).

Assessing and Addressing Health Risk and Disease Burden

Assessing health risks and disease burden can occur in many ways. Self-reported questionnaires called *health risk assessments* (HRAs) are a common way of identifying health risks and disease burden associated with lifestyle behaviors such as diet, exercise, smoking, alcohol intake, stress, and sleep. Assessing and addressing health risks and disease burden using HRAs has been demonstrated to have significant cost savings potential, delay progression of chronic disease, and improve health outcomes (Anderson et al., 2000; Mills, Kessler, Cooper, & Sullivan, 2007; Ozminkowski et al., 2006; Yen et al., 2003). Assessment of risks and health outcomes can also be calculated using combinations of administrative claims and EMR data (Gavrielov-Yusim & Friger, 2014; Riley, 2009; Wanken et al., 2020). Using administrative claims data has been identified to be particularly useful in assessing cost and utilization information, whereas use of clinical registry and EMR data have been identified to be best when

assessing clinical risk and health outcomes (Lawson et al., 2016). Linking these different data assets is critical in population health and preferably done through a population health data model as highlighted in Chapter 13, "The Population Health Data Model." Additional supplemental data can inform risk models, including but not limited to data on demographics, social and behavioral determinants of health, consumer-reported, device, and social media. Refer to Chapter 7, "Social and Behavioral Data," and Chapter 9, "Grouping, Trending, and Interpreting Population Health Data for Receptivity, Engagement, and Activation," for more detailed information on these data sources.

The key to addressing health risks and disease burden in populations is understanding the natural progression of disease, the standard of care, the clinical care pathway, and the time frames by which health declines and disease advances in populations. Understanding each item as it relates to conditions of interest guides the identification of the data assets needed to develop the algorithms for identification, stratification, and interventions in population health. In addition, timely identification and intervention enables clinicians the ability to intervene and avoid an unnecessary procedure, therapy, or emergency department or hospital admission. It is important to understand the timeliness, completeness, and accuracy of each data asset when linking them together to determine health risk and disease burden, particularly when developing more advanced analytic risk models that predict rising risk and future disease burden.

More detailed information on analytics to support the targeting, development, and monitoring of interventions to address health risks and disease burden can be found in Chapter 26, "Targeting Individuals for Interventions," Chapter 27, "Analytics Supporting Population Health Analytics," and Chapter 28, "Monitoring and Optimizing Interventions."

Data Sources to Support the Identification, Prediction, and Measurement of Health Risk and Disease Burden

A variety of data sources can be used to identify and determine risk. The most common sources for data come from administrative medical claims, laboratory, pharmacy, electronic medical records, social and behavioral determinants of health, and self-reported, consumer, and social media. Additional methods can be added to these data combinations to enhance the predictability and accuracy of risk models, such as machine learning, artificial intelligence, and NLP (Irvin et al., 2020; Jeffery et al., 2019; Liang et al., 2020; Shah et al., 2018; Yen et al., 2003).

Section 2, "Data Sources," and Chapter 9, "Grouping, Trending, and Interpreting Population Health Data for Receptivity, Engagement, and Activation," provide detailed information on all data sources that can be used to identify and determine risk.

Applying Context to Data for Health Risk and Disease Burden

As with self-reported and consumer data, an unlimited number of data combinations exist to combine data assets in ways that enable the identification and prediction of risk. Utilizing a population health data model—where the data assets have been linked together to provide a comprehensive view of the patient and his or her health—enables rapid prototyping of identification and prediction models to be developed to confirm, identify, and predict risk in an unlimited number of patient populations.

A review of the clinical evidence base in databases such as the National Institute of Health's National Library of Medicine's PubMed provides a plethora of modifiable risk factors, stratification of subpopulations based on morbidity of disease, and interventions targeted to reduce or remove risk and harm to patients from a variety of diseases such as chronic conditions, cancers, and environmental hazards. Many of the established findings, insights, and learnings from peer-reviewed clinical publications have not yet been translated into clinical practice. A 2011 study by Morris, Wooding, and Grant (2011) found that the time lag from clinical evidence-based research to clinical practice is 17 years and identified the need to speed up the time from research to clinical practice.

> The study concludes that understanding lags first requires agreeing models, definitions and measures, which can be applied in practice. A second task would be to develop a process by which to gather these data.

The opportunity to improve the speed of translation of research to practice in medicine is enormous and can be achieved through the development of codifiable data and algorithms to support decision-making. The data are available. The mechanism by which these data can be translated into information that can be applied at the point of care is the current gap, particularly as it relates to tailoring the existing evidence to clinical and business outcomes and individual patient preferences (Curtis, Fry, Shaban, & Considine, 2017; Morris et al., 2011; Shah et al., 2018).

The following case studies outline several ways to develop and use contextualized medical claims, laboratory, pharmacy, EMR, and social and behavioral health data in population health projects to improve patient experience, health outcomes, and reduce avoidable costs.

Case Study 1: Enhancing Patient Experience and Outcomes

Applying Context to Social Determinants of Health Data
Including Health Determinants in Predictive Models to Reduce Health Disparities

Social and behavioral determinants of health are increasingly gaining traction as important data to include in population health analyses to understand and reduce healthcare disparities at both the individual patient and community levels. Social and behavioral determinants of health are factors that have been demonstrated to affect the health and well-being of communities and include poverty, access to food and housing, education, literacy, crime, violence, and environmental conditions (Braveman & Gottlieb, 2014; Healthy People.gov, n.d.). More detailed information on social and behavioral data and application can be found in Chapter 7, "Social and Behavioral Data," and Chapter 9, "Grouping, Trending, and Interpreting Population Health Data for Receptivity, Engagement, and Activation."

A 2020 study by Dr. Marissa Tan and colleagues outlines the advantages and challenges associated with including select social and behavioral determinants of health in analytic models to predict risk and health outcomes and to reduce health disparities whose underlying causes are social or economic in nature. Although including health determinants in predictive models has been shown to have similar predictive power as clinical factors alone, Tan and her colleagues advocate for inclusion of these factors in predictive models to promote health equity, address the role of poverty and lack of education or literacy in clinical and population health interventions, and to connect health care to social care resources that address social needs as a way to improve the quality of care delivery and experience.

Applying a population health approach and solution to this application, the problem to solve and a proposed intervention can be practiced as presented in the following section:

Using Predictive Risk Models That Incorporate Social and Behavioral Data to Improve Community Engagement in Health Programs

The use of social and behavioral data in predictive analytics can assist in tailoring any program or intervention to the unique needs of the population of interest and can be used to inform decisions for the allocation of funding, resources, and the geographic locations best suited to where the challenges may be the greatest. **Table 10.2** provides recommendations from the article to advance the use of health determinants in predictive and population health analytics.

Options exist for applying context to data to determine health risk and disease burden to enhance the experience and outcomes of the patient/member. **Table 10.3** includes items that have been selected from the content introduced in Chapter 8, "Grouping, Trending, and Interpreting Population Health Data for Decision Support," to highlight where Case Study 1's use of social and behavioral determinants of health data can be used to generate population health insights, programs, and interventions.

Table 10.2 Recommendations to Effectively Include SDOH and SBDH in Predictive Analytics

Privacy Standards, Patient Consent, and Ethical Use of SBDH Data
Develop consensus on transparency, privacy protections, and ethical uses of SBDH data in predictive models
Create guidelines to reduce inherent bias in predictive models
Technical Challenges Associated with SBDH Data Sources and Analytics
Determine best practice guidelines for SBDH data sources and predictive model design as well as open-source access
Expand standardized coding and taxonomies of SBDH risk factors that enhance interoperability

Expanding the Knowledge Base to Inform 'Best-Practice' Guidelines for SBDH Analytics
Support national shared research and development to advance the SBDH predictive model development and application
Establish a national agenda to create a shared evidence base regarding the importance of SBDH factors and the best approach for including SBDH in analytics

SBDH: social and behavioral determinants of health.
Tan, M., Hatef, E., Taghipour, D., Vyas, K., Kharrazi, H., Gottlieb, L., & Weiner, J. (2020). Including social and behavioral determinants in predictive models: Trends, challenges, and opportunities. *JMIR Medical Informatics, 8*(9), e18084. https://doi.org/10.2196/18084

Table 10.3 Applying Context to Data to Enhance the Experience and Outcomes of the Patient or Member

Use Case	Description	Example
Receptivity	A person's openness to new ideas, activities, participation	*Likelihood to participate*: Measures a person's likelihood to participate in certain types of events, wellness programs, and care-management interventions.
		Mode of communication: Measures a person's preferred method of communication such as face to face or by telephone, e-mail, chat, or text.
		Direct messaging: Measures a person's interaction with automated messaging delivered through chat bots, automated telephonic decision trees, e-mails, and Internet website use.
Engagement	A person's participation in ideas, activities, programs, interventions	*Meaningful encounter*: Measures a person's participation in certain activities, programs, and interventions such as the number of visits, activities, or goals set and completed.
		Touchpoints: Measures the number and type of interactions with patients across an activity, intervention, program, organization, or system such as the number of health outreach communications made each year.
Activation	A person's level self-confidence, motivation, and ability to set and accomplish tasks and goals to get results	*Readiness to take action*: Measures the self-confidence, motivation, comprehension, and ability to set and accomplish tasks and goals such as the self-assessment results of a person who is motivated to lose weight to reduce the risk of diabetes, including the person's perceived ability to exercise.
		Level of activation: Measures the change in the level of self-confidence, motivation, comprehension, and ability to set and accomplish tasks and goals such as the self-assessment results over time of a person who initially was motivated to lose weight and then participated in weight-loss activities to lose a total of 30 lbs.

Case Study 2: Improving Health

Applying Context to Demographic and Medical Record Retrospective Data
Predicting Risk of Severity of Disease in Patients with COVID-19

The 2019 outbreak of coronavirus disease placed a significant number of people at risk of developing severe disease morbidity and death. The severity of illness associated with infection with COVID-19 in certain populations resulted in the need for advanced life support and recovery services. Identified as a novel disease in late 2019 and lacking proven treatment or prevention protocols, several clinician researchers and public health officials focused efforts early in 2020 on identifying subsets of populations that were at increased risk of requiring critical care support in an inpatient setting to initiate early treatment and avoid the need for advanced life support resulting in disability or death.

An article in the *Journal of the American Medical Association* (JAMA) by Dr. Wenhua Liang and colleagues (2020) reviewed retrospective demographic and medical record data of close to 1,600 patients admitted to a hospital with both a confirmed laboratory and clinical presentation of COVID-19. This information was used to generate a list of more than eight demographic variables, including age, smoking status, and recent travel to areas where COVID-19 was present in high concentrations. Another 65 medical history, clinical signs and symptoms, imaging results, and laboratory findings were selected to identify the epidemiologic and clinical characteristics that most closely correlates with severe illness requiring critical care, advanced life support such as mechanical ventilation, or death. The findings of a retrospective data analysis identified 10 independent risk factors of patients with laboratory and clinically confirmed COVID-19 infection that reliably predicts increased severity of disease. The predictors were a combination of the following indicators (Liang et al., 2020; Taber's Online, n.d.):

- Demographics
  - age
- Medical history
  - number of comorbidities
  - cancer history
- Clinical signs and symptoms
  - hemoptysis (coughing up blood)
  - dyspnea (difficulty breathing)
  - unconsciousness
- Imaging results
  - chest X-ray abnormality
- Laboratory findings
  - neutrophil to lymphocyte ratio (indicator of systemic inflammation)
  - lactate dehydrogenase (energy production enzyme, indicator of tissue damage, or cellular destruction)
  - direct bilirubin (indicator of increased red blood cell destruction)

Applying a population health approach and solution to this application, the problem to solve and a proposed intervention can be as follows:

Early detection and prevention of critical illness requiring advanced life support in patients with confirmed COVID-19

or

Predicting burden of disease and impact on critical and advanced care teams to support resource and facility planning in response to Coronavirus disease.

As part of the study results, Dr. Liang and colleagues developed and validated a calculation algorithm to predict COVID severity in the form of a risk score that can be applied to patients admitted to the hospital with COVID-19 to score the risk associated with the need for critical and advanced care services.

This calculation tool and the findings from the published journal article can be applied to quickly and effectively identify the risk of severity of disease and the potential burden the disease may have on frontline responders, hospital staff, resource planning, supply chain, and overall patient and staff safety. This information can be used to estimate the projected percentage of patients who may require critical or advanced care and the number of patients expected to die from the infection. In addition, this information also assists in focusing triage and testing to the imaging studies and laboratory tests that are most predictive of increased severity and avoid unnecessary and potentially harmful testing.

Options exist for applying context to data to determine health risk and disease burden to *improve the health of the population*. **Table 10.4** contains items that have been selected from the content introduced in Chapter 8, "Grouping, Trending, and Interpreting Population Health Data for Decision Support," to highlight where Case Study 2's use of demographic and medical record data can be used to generate population health insights, programs, and interventions.

Table 10.4 Applying Context to Data to Improve the Health of the Population

Use Case	Description	Example
Presence of diagnosis or disease	Presence or absence of a specified health condition or disease	*Diagnoses*: Measures the presence or absence of a specified health condition, set of conditions, or disease such as diabetes, degenerative joint disease (DJD), and breast cancer.
Progression of diagnoses or disease	Worsening or advancement of a specified health condition or disease over time	*Related diagnoses*: Measures the presence or absence over time of comorbidities, complications, gaps in medications, and health determinants such as patients with diabetes and depression, patients with DJD and morbid obesity, and patients with breast cancer that is invasive.
		Level of severity: Measures the presence or absence over time of comorbidities, complications, gaps in medications, and health determinants within a categorical designation of severity such as patients whose diabetes is unmanaged secondary to untreated depression, patients whose pain associated with DJD is worsened by the wear and tear caused by the morbid obesity, and patients with breast cancer that has metastasized to other organs.
Care and treatment pathways	A documented set of standards of care, care guidelines, and care pathways that indicates a disease's life cycle from risk factors to symptoms, diagnosis, morbidity, treatments, and death	*Related diagnoses*: An example of a care or treatment pathway's use case is the translation and incorporation of the 2020 American Diabetes Association's (Johnson et al., 2020) set of clinical guidelines to treat patients with diabetes in a health system's EMR.
		Level of severity: An example of a care or treatment pathway's use case is the identification of patients where they are along the care pathway or the time and way in which a patient deviates from a care pathway or care guideline to alert clinicians to make adjustments to their care or treatment plan.

(continues)

Table 10.4 Applying Context to Data to Improve the Health of the Population

Use Case	Description	Example
Risk or presence of worsened or poor health outcomes	The presence or absence of often clinical or health determinant indicators that categorize a patient as having poor health or an adverse event that has significant impact on his or her day-to-day activities and well-being	*Related adverse outcomes*: Measures the presence or absence over time of comorbidities, complications, gaps in medications, health determinants, and harm of patients within a categorical designation of outcomes such as patients with diabetes that have been unmanaged over time that resulted in kidney failure requiring dialysis.
		Related procedures: Measures utilization of specified surgical and pharmacy procedures such as patients with diabetes that have been unmanaged over time that resulted in multiple leg amputations because of poor wound healing and blood circulation complicated by multiple wound infections.
		Related events: Measures utilization of specified hospital-based emergency department, admission, and readmission events such as recurring admissions of patients with congestive heart failure with volume or fluid overload.
		Quality of care: Measures the level of value assigned to care provided in an encounter, service, or treatment according to a clinical evidence base, clinical pathways, care guidelines such as measuring the presence of retinal eye exams in patients with diabetes to screen for and prevent advanced severity of disease. An example of a risk or presence of worsened or poor health outcome use case is the harm caused to a patient who had an allergic reaction to a medication that resulted in a loss of hearing.
		Related diagnoses: An example of a risk or presence of worsened or poor health outcome use case is the presence of pneumonia in a patient with severe asthma and an inpatient hospitalization to assist the patient to breathe using supplemental oxygen and inhaled steroid medication.
		Level of severity: An example of a risk or presence of worsened or poor-health outcome use case is the patient with severe asthma complicated by pneumonia being treated in a hospital who worsens and requires mechanical ventilation to breathe.
		Adherence: Measures a patient's actions in following a given care plan, medication regimen, or treatment such as a patient with hypertension who suffers a heart attack from years of not following heart-healthy lifestyle and not consistently taking blood pressure medication.

Case Study 3: Reduce per Capita Cost of Care

Applying Context to Demographic, Health Determinants, Administrative Claims, and Medical Record Data

Applying Risk-Adjusted Methods to Calculate Health Services Payments

Adjusting for realized, existing, and rising risk can be applied in many ways, including the use of risk-adjusted data to determine healthcare payments and understand mortality across populations. One of the most common examples of healthcare data being adjusted for risk to set healthcare payments and understand mortality is the development and use of the All Patient Refined Diagnosis Related Group, an inpatient classification system that assigns a diagnostic related group, a Risk of Mortality subclass and a Severity of Illness subclass and is primarily used to adjust payments to hospitals for the provision of hospital-based care (Baram et al., 2008; De Marco, Lorenzoni, Addari, & Nante, 2002; McCormick, Lin, Deiner, & Levin, 2018; Vertrees, Averill, Eisenhandler, Quain, & Switalski,2013; Yee et al., 2019). As health risk and complexity increases, so does the need for more treatment services. As the number and complexity of services to treat the health conditions and severity increases, so does the cost. Payments to cover the cost of these services can therefore be adjusted prospectively or concurrently based on the historical costs. The payment amounts are set or weighted by both the disease category and complexity of services required. Risk-adjustment methodologies are also used in determining payments for patients with chronic conditions in insurance health plans and to predict healthcare expenditures (Chang & Weiner, 2010; Lawson et al., 2016; Mark et al., 2003). Refer to Chapter 21, "Risk Adjustment," for more detailed information.

CMS's Comprehensive Care for Joint Replacement Model (CMS, n.d.) is a bundled payment and quality-measurement reimbursement innovation model for hip and knee replacements with more than 450 participating hospitals across the United States. The goals of the innovation model are to reduce Medicare healthcare spending by providing a set payment to participating hospitals for hip and knee surgeries to incentivize improved quality and reduced variation of care based on historical spending analyses showing variation in cost more than two times, depending on geographic region. The model holds hospitals financially accountable for the total cost of an episode of care and incentivizes care coordination to improve quality and decrease the rate of complications associated with these types of procedures.

A 2016 study by Clement and colleagues (Clement et al., 2016) and later validated by two additional 2018 studies by Courtney and colleagues and Cairns and colleagues (Cairns, Ostrum, & Carter Clement, 2018; Courtney et al., 2018) of the accuracy and validity of Medicare's bundled payment reimbursement model demonstrated the need for more robust methods to adjust reimbursements to account for risk and disease burden in patients receiving hip or knee surgeries as part of the bundle. All three proposed including risk-adjustment methods in the payment methodology using historical data from demographic, administrative claims, and medical record data. The proposed risk-adjustment methodology provides a solution to the potential adverse selection of healthier patients to maximize hospital profitability and avoids the creation of barriers to accessing care for patients with more health risks and morbidity.

Across the studies, the following risk factors were identified to contribute to increased risk and cost associated with a hip- or knee-replacement procedure (Cairns et al., 2018; Clement et al., 2016; Courtney et al., 2018).

- Demographics:
  - age
  - male gender
  - geographic location
- Surgical risk:
  - risk of complications resulting from anesthesia or surgery
- Social determinants of health:
  - lower socioeconomic status
- Clinical morbidity:
  - malnutrition
  - depression

(continues)

Case Study 3: Reduce per Capita Cost of Care *(continued)*

- lung disease
- rheumatoid arthritis
- neurologic disease

Applying a population health approach and solution to this application, the problem to solve and a proposed intervention can be as follows:

Applying clinical, social, and demographic data to properly adjust for risk in populations with significant orthopedic joint disease as a method to calculate payments and improve health outcomes.

All three studies concluded that a methodology incorporating the adjustment of risk based on demographic, health determinants, and specific comorbid conditions would improve the accuracy of the bundled payment reimbursement for hospitals and reduce the risks of adverse selection of healthier patients and barriers to accessing care. In addition, understanding the risk of a patient developing a costly complication before a surgery can be used to develop pre- and postsurgical optimization programs and identify select populations that may benefit from more robust postsurgical services such as home health care.

Options exist for applying context to data to determine health risk and disease burden to *reduce per capita cost of care for the benefit of communities*. **Table 10.5** contains items selected from the content introduced in Chapter 8, "Grouping, Trending, and Interpreting Population Health Data for Decision Support," to highlight where Case Study 3's use of demographic, social, and behavioral health determinants; and administrative and medical records data can be used to generate population health insights, programs, and interventions.

Table 10.5 Applying Context to Data to Reduce per Capita Cost of Care for the Benefit of Communities

Use Case	Description	Example
Cost and price	The costs and prices associated with the delivery of clinical and administrative healthcare services	*High cost*: Measures the costs associated the delivery of clinical and administrative healthcare services such as the total cost of care of a patient with lung cancer or the per member per month cost of a patient with hepatitis C. *Risk of future high cost*: Measures the predicted costs associated with the delivery of clinical and administrative healthcare services such as the average total predicted cost for caring for patients with congestive heart failure.
Utilization and volume	The utilization and volume of clinical and administrative healthcare services	*High volume*: Measures the volume of clinical and administrative healthcare services delivered such as the average number of chemotherapy medication infusions for a patient with lung cancer. *Risk of future high volume*: Measures the predicted volume of clinical and administrative healthcare services estimated to be delivered in the future such as the total number of patients with diabetes that involves the kidneys that will likely require dialysis.
Point-of-care events and service types	Information that describes the qualitative aspects of an event or service	*Lower level of care*: Measures the activity of appropriately moving a person from a higher level of care to a lower level of care such as movement from a hospital ICU bed type to a medical bed type when their care needs decrease.

		Outcomes-based care: Measures effectiveness or efficiency of an event or service to achieve a specified health or financial outcome such as a technology company receiving payment for use of its medical device only when the patient achieves an improved health outcome as a result of a clinical response to treatment with the medical device.
Procedures	Information that describes a service that is meant to diagnose or treat and can be invasive (an operation) or noninvasive (changing a dressing on a wound).	*High cost*: Refer to "Cost and price" in the left column. An example of an invasive procedure use case that is high cost and invasive is the placement of a pacemaker device in a patient with a heartbeat irregularity, also called an arrhythmia. *High volume*: Refer to "Utilization and volume" in the left column. An example of a noninvasive procedure use case that is high volume is the use of electrocardiography to monitor heart rate, rhythm, and function in patients with cardiovascular disease or symptoms of disease.
Variation in care	Differences in cost and volume of services across providers, facilities, geographic regions, services, ancillary services or DMEs, imaging, laboratory, pharmacy, and so on	*High cost*: Refer to "Cost and price" in the left column. An example of a variation in care cost use case is the differences in cost across provider networks of the delivery of medication regimens to treat a specified type of lung cancer.

Considerations for Applying Context to Data for Health Risk and Disease Burden

Additional applications of risk include context that can be applied to data to identify coding patterns for suspected clinical conditions or to verify clinical indicators for illness in the form of risk-adjusted reporting to more accurately adjust reimbursements for care delivered concurrently and prospectively (Dudley et al., 2003). Of note, using data when the presence of a health

condition is suspected must be done with caution because identifying a patient with a health condition that may not be confirmed or not yet communicated can create confusion, fear, and distrust in both patients and providers (Johnson, 2003; Lawson et al., 2016; Mark et al., 2003).

A 2018 quote by Jeremy Cantor in "Rising Risk: An Overview of Identification and Intervention Approaches" highlights the challenges that may occur when communicating suspected and rising risk to patients:

Focusing on "rising-risk" populations is also a bridge between after-the-fact treatment and broad public health prevention efforts aimed at the majority of the population, who make up the bottom of the utilization pyramid. This variation is understandable given this is a new field in the early stages of development, innovation, and evidence generation. There is also a warranted concern that the concept of rising risk be developed with an awareness of potential adverse effects (such as stigma, anxiety, and criticism) that can result from labeling individuals and communities with labels such as "high risk" and "potentially high cost." (Cantor et al., 2018)

Identification of risk, severity of illness, and disease burden can also be applied to verify patients' existing health conditions for participation in population health programs and interventions, and this is best achieved when administrative claims and medical record data are combined with self-reported data such as would be found in HRAs. Each type of data asset contributes differently to the accuracy of determining that a health condition exists, the comorbidities and complications that indicate severity of the health condition, incidence, prevalence, and associated comorbidities

(Bagley & Altman, 2016; Glassberg, Trygstad, Wei, Robinson, & Farley, J. 2019; Haas et al., 2013; Ho et al., 2018). For detailed information on each of these data assets, refer to Section 2, "Data Sources," and Chapter 21, "Risk Adjustment."

Another consideration in determining risk in populations occurs when soliciting vendor or market solutions. It is important to understand the respective tools' methodologies for calculating risk; analysts and data scientists must understand data sources and linkages and the product's existing use cases along with related clinical evidence. Often an organization can become enticed by the idea of having multiple ways of determining the risk to intervene. If multiple solutions are available for use, then it is important for analytic leaders and staff to understand the gaps that exist in a given solution, the full suite of functionality that a given solution provides, and the dangers of overlapping functionality that derives meaning from different and potentially conflicting methods. As always, the presence of benchmarks and analytic methods such as calculating observed to expected ratios can assist in understanding the magnitude of the problem and the opportunity interventions can realize across diverse solutions. Refer to Chapter 21, "Risk Adjustment," for more information on calculating observed to expected ratios.

Applied Learning: Use Case

Use Case 1: Predicting Cardiovascular Risk

You manage a team of web application developers and healthcare analysts in the health division at a software technology company named—HealthPredictors–that has recently partnered with the Cleveland Clinic. You have been asked to work with the clinical advisor team from the Cleveland Clinic to develop a smartphone application of their existing Heart Risk Factor Calculator for Men and Women, a tool that predicts the risk of developing a heart attack or death from cardiovascular disease within a 10 year period. You are provided the following link (https://my.clevelandclinic.org/health/diagnostics/17085-heart-risk-factor-calculators) to two risk factor calculators (Reynolds Risk Score & ACC/AHA Cardiovascular Risk Score) for review and are scheduled to meet with the clinical advisor team in two weeks.

In preparation for your meeting and following your company's process of applying a population health approach to health product designs, you come across several additional risk factors and data assets that have been identified in the evidence-based literature to improve upon the accuracy of the risk prediction model and relevancy to certain subpopulations (Flueckiger et al., 2018; Tzoulaki et al., 2009; Zhou et al., 2017). You would like to incorporate these new risk factors into the product's design to improve upon Cleveland Clinic's existing use of these tools. What are the steps you can propose to guide the meeting in two weeks and the work to develop the electronic application of the improved risk prediction model?

Conclusion

It is important to add context to healthcare data to render it useful from both a population analytic perspective and to drive decision-making at the point of care. Contextualizing risk by linking various data sources to develop categorizations of clinical conditions that predict future utilization, cost, and disease burden are a staple of population health management and analytics. Understanding the methods to develop and apply analytic models to identify realized, existing, and rising risk are key skills for analysts, data scientists, and analytic leaders to master. All the examples and case studies presented in this chapter demonstrate the importance of identifying risk with early intervention to understand and prevent the development of health conditions and their associated utilization and cost. Multiple examples and case studies were provided in this chapter on how a variety of healthcare data sources can be linked to identify clinical indicators for illness, monitor morbidity and mortality trends, and predict future cost, utilization, and worsening health outcomes.

Study and Discussion Questions

- What additional types of data can be applied to assess, stratify, and intervene to prevent or reduce health risk and disease burden?
- What are examples of ways machine learning, artificial intelligence, and natural language processing methods and techniques can identify and stratify health risk and disease burden?
- What are some existing technologies and tools that demonstrate the capability of predicting health risks and disease burden? That demonstrate results that improve patient experience? Improve health outcomes? Reduce the total cost of care?

Resources and Websites

Cochrane Library. (n.d.). Database of systematic reviews. https://www.cochranelibrary.com/

National Institute of Health. (n.d.). National Library of Medicine's PubMed. https://pubmed.ncbi.nlm.nih.gov/

Taber's Online. (n.d.). Medical dictionary. https://www.tabers.com/tabersonline/

UpToDate Clinical Decision Support Resource Library. (n.d.). *Evidence-based clinical decision support at the point of care.* Riverwoods, IL: Wolters Kluwer. https://www.uptodate.com/home

References

Anderson, D. R., Whitmer, R. W., Goetzel, R. Z., Ozminkowski, R. J., Wasserman, J., & Serxner, S. (2000, September 1). The relationship between modifiable health risks and group-level health care expenditures. *American Journal of Health Promotion, 15*(1), 45–52. https://doi.org/10.4278/0890-1171-15.1.45

Bagley, S. C., & Altman, R. B. (2016, October). Computing disease incidence, prevalence and comorbidity from electronic medical records. *Journal of Biomedical Informatics, 63*, 108–111. https://doi.org/10.1016/j.jbi.2016.08.005

Baram, D., Daroowalla, F., Garcia, R., Zhang, G., Chen, J. J., Healy, E., Riza, S. A., & Richman, P. (2008, April 18). Use of the All Patient Refined-Diagnosis Related Group (APR-DRG) risk of mortality score as a severity adjustor in the medical ICU. *Clinical Medicine: Circulatory, Respiratory and Pulmonary Medicine, 2.* https://doi.org/10.4137/ccrpm.s544

Braveman, P., & Gottlieb, L. (2014, January 1). The social determinants of health: It's time to consider the causes of the causes. *Public Health Reports, 129*(Suppl. 2), 19–31. https://doi.org/10.1177/00333549141291s206

Cairns, M. A., Ostrum, R. F., & Carter Clement, R. (2018). Refining risk adjustment for the proposed CMS surgical hip and femur fracture treatment bundled payment program. *Journal of Bone and Joint Surgery, 100*(4), 269–277. https://doi.org/10.2106/JBJS.17.00327

Canizares, M., Power, J. D., Rampersaud, Y. R., & Badley, E. M. (2019). Patterns of opioid use (codeine, morphine or meperidine) in the Canadian population over time: Analysis of the Longitudinal National Population Health Survey 1994–2011. *BMJ Open, 9*(7), e029613. https://doi .org/10.1136/bmjopen-2019-029613

Cantor, J., E., Haller, R., & Greenberg, E. (2018, January). Rising risk: An overview of identification and intervention approaches. JSI Research & Training Institute. https:// publications.jsi.com/JSIInternet/Inc/Common/_download _pub.cfm?id=19182&lid=3

Centers for Medicare and Medicaid Services. (n.d.). Comprehensive care for joint replacement model. Baltimore, MD: CMS Innovation Center. https://innovation .cms.gov/innovation-models/cjr

Chang, H. Y., & Weiner, J. P. (2010). An in-depth assessment of a diagnosis-based risk adjustment model based on national health insurance claims: The application of the Johns Hopkins Adjusted Clinical Group case-mix system in Taiwan. *BMC Medicine, 8.* https://doi.org/10.1186/1741 -7015-8-7

Clement, R. C., Derman, P. B., Kheir, M. M., Soo, A. E., Flynn, D. N., Levin, L. S., & Fleisher, L. (2016). Risk adjustment for Medicare total knee arthroplasty bundled payments. *Orthopedics, 39*(5), e911–e916. https://doi.org /10.3928/01477447-20160623-04

Cleveland Clinic. (n.d.). What's your risk of developing a heart attack of coronary disease? https://my.clevelandclinic.org /ccf/media/files/heart/Framingham.pdf

Courtney, P. M., Bohl, D. D., Lau, E. C., Ong, K. L., Jacobs, J. J., & Della Valle, C. J. (2018). Risk adjustment is necessary in Medicare bundled payment models for total hip and knee arthroplasty. *Journal of Arthroplasty*, 33(8), 2368–2375. https://www.arthroplastyjournal.org/article /S0883-5403(18)30258-4/abstract

Curtis, K., Fry, M., Shaban, R. Z., & Considine, J. (2017). Translating research findings to clinical nursing practice. *Journal of Clinical Nursing, 26*(5–6), 862–872. https:// onlinelibrary.wiley.com/doi/full/10.1111/jocn.13586

De Marco, M. F., Lorenzoni, L., Addari, P., & Nante, N. (2002). Evaluation of the capacity of the APR-DRG classification system to predict hospital mortality [English translation from Italian]. *Epidemiologia e Prevenzione, 26*(4), 183–190. https://pubmed.ncbi.nlm.nih.gov/12408005/

Dudley, R. A., Medlin, C. A., Hammann, L. B., Cisternas, M. G., Brand, R., Rennie, D. J., & Luft, H. S. (2003). The best of both worlds? Potential of hybrid prospective/concurrent risk adjustment. *Medical Care, 41*(1), 56–69. https://doi .org/10.1097/00005650-200301000-00009

Edington, D. W. (2001, May 1). Emerging research: A view from one research center. *American Journal of Health Promotion, 15*(5), 341–349. https://journals.sagepub.com /doi/10.4278/0890-1171-15.5.341

Flueckiger, P., Longstreth, W., Herrington, D., & Yeboah, J. (2018, January 8). Revised Framingham stroke risk score, nontraditional risk markers, and incident stroke in a multiethnic cohort. *Stroke, 49*(2), 363–369. https://doi .org/10.1161/STROKEAHA.117.018928

Gavrielov-Yusim, N., & Friger, M. (2014). Use of administrative medical databases in population-based research. *Journal of Epidemiology and Community Health, 68*(3), 283–287. https://doi.org/10.1136/jech-2013-202744

Glassberg, M. B., Trygstad, T., Wei, D., Robinson, T., & Farley, J. F. (2019, December). Accuracy of prescription claims data in identifying truly nonadherent patients. *Journal of Managed Care and Specialty Pharmacy, 25*(12), 1349–1356. https://doi.org/10.18553/jmcp.2019.25.12.1349

Goetzel, R. Z., Pei, X., Tabrizi, M. J., Henke, R. M., Kowlessar, N., Nelson, C. F., & Metz, R. D. (2012). Ten modifiable health risk factors are linked to more than one-fifth of employer-employee health care spending. *Health Affairs, 31*(11), 2474–2484. https://doi.org/10.1377 /hlthaff.2011.0819

Haas, L. R., Takahashi, P. Y., Shah, N. D., Stroebel, R. J., Bernard, M. E., Finnie, D. W., & Naessens, J. M. (2013, September). Risk-stratification methods for identifying patients for care coordination. *American Journal of Managed Care, 19*(9), 725–732. https://pubmed.ncbi .nlm.nih.gov/24304255/

Healthy People.gov. (n.d.). Social determinants of health. https://www.healthypeople.gov/2020/topics-objectives /topic/social-determinants-of-health

Hileman, G., Mehmud, S., & Rosenberg, M. (2016, July). *Risk scoring in health insurance: A primer.* Schaumburg, IL: Society of Actuaries. https://www.soa.org/globalassets /assets/Files/Research/research-2016-risk-scoring -health-insurance.pdf

Hill, J. C., Whitehurst, D. G. T., Lewis, M., Bryan, S., Dunn, K. M., Foster, N. E., Konstantinou, K., Main, C. J., Mason, E., Somerville, S., Sowden, G., Vohora, K., & Hay, E. M. (2011). Comparison of stratified primary care management for low back pain with current best practice (STarT Back): A randomised controlled trial. *The Lancet, 378*(9802), 1560–1571. https://doi.org/10.1016/S0140-6736(11)60937-9

Ho, T. W., Ruan, S. Y., Huang, C. T., Tsai, Y. J., Lai, F., & Yu, C. J. (2018, October 2). Validity of ICD9-CM codes to diagnose chronic obstructive pulmonary disease from National Health Insurance claim data in Taiwan. *International Journal of COPD, 13*, 3055–3063. https://doi .org/10.2147/COPD.S174265

Irvin, J. A., Kondrich, A. A., Ko, M., Rajpurkar, P., Haghgoo, B., Landon, B. E., Phillips, R. L., Petterson, S., Ng, A. Y., & Basu, S. (2020, May 1). Incorporating machine learning and social determinants of health indicators into prospective risk adjustment for health plan payments. *BMC Public Health, 20*(1). https://doi .org/10.1186/s12889-020-08735-0

Jeffery, A. D., Hewner, S., Pruinelli, L., Lekan, D., Lee, M., Gao, G., Holbrook, L., & Sylvia, M. (2019, April). Risk prediction and segmentation models used in the United States for assessing risk in whole populations: A critical literature review with implications for nurses' role in population health management. *JAMIA Open, 2*(1), 205–214. https://doi.org/10.1093/jamiaopen/ooy053

Johnson, M. L. (2003, January). Risk assessment and adjustment: Adjusting for sick patients or a sick system? *Medical Care, 41*(1), 4–7. https://doi.org/10.1097/00005650-200301000-00002

Lawson, E. H., Louie, R., Zingmond, D. S., Sacks, G. D., Brook, R. H., Hall, B. L., & Ko, C. Y. (2016, January). Using both clinical registry and administrative claims data to measure risk-adjusted Surgical outcomes. *Annals of Surgery, 263*(1), 50–57. https://doi.org/10.1097/SLA.0000000000001031

Liang, W., Liang, H., Ou, L., Chen, B., Chen, A., Li, C., Li, Y., Guan, W., Sang, L., Lu, J., Xu, Y., Chen, G., Guo, H., Guo, J., Chen, Z., Zhao, Y., Li, S., Zhang, N., Zhong, N., & He, J. (2020, May 12). Development and validation of a clinical risk score to predict the occurrence of critical illness in hospitalized patients with COVID-19. *JAMA Internal Medicine, 180*(8), 1081–1089. https://doi.org/10.1001/jamainternmed.2020.2033

Lipfert, F. W., & Wyzga, R. E. (2020, January). Longitudinal relationships between lung cancer mortality rates, smoking, and ambient air quality: A comprehensive review and analysis. *Critical Reviews in Toxicology, 49*(9), 790–818. https://doi.org/10.1080/10408444.2019.1700210

Livingston, G., Huntley, J., Sommerlad, A., Ames, D., Ballard, C., Banerjee, S., Brayne, C., Burns, A., Cohen-Mansfield, J., Cooper, C., Costafreda, S. G., Dias, A., Fox, N., Gitlin, L. N., Howard, R., Kales, H. C., Kivimaki, M., Larson, E. B., Ogunniyi, A., . . . , Mukadam, N. (2020). The Lancet Commissions Dementia prevention, intervention, and care: 2020 report of the Lancet Commission. *The Lancet, 396*, 413–446. https://doi.org/10.1016/S0140-6736(20)30367-6

Mark, T. L., Ozminkowski, R. J., Kirk, A., Ettner, S. L., & Drabek, J. (2003, September 1). Risk adjustment for people with chronic conditions in private sector health plans. *Medical Decision Making, 23*(5), 397–405. https://doi.org/10.1177/0272989x03257264

McCormick, P. J., Lin, H.-m., Deiner, S. G., & Levin, M. A. (2018, March 22). Validation of the All Patient Refined Diagnosis Related Group (APR-DRG) risk of mortality and severity of illness modifiers as a measure of perioperative risk. *Journal of Medical Systems, 42*(5). https://doi.org/10.1007/s10916-018-0936-3

Medhi, T. (2020, March 23). 20 powerful quotes by Reid Hoffman, the former COO of PayPal and the man behind LinkedIn. Your Story. https://yourstory.com/2020/03/20-powerful-quotes-reid-hoffman-paypal-linkedin?utm_pageloadtype=scroll

Mills, P. R., Kessler, R. C., Cooper, J., & Sullivan, S. (2007). Impact of a health promotion program on employee health risks and work productivity. *American Journal of Health Promotion, 22*(1), 45–53. https://doi.org/10.4278/0890-1171-22.1.45

Morris, Z. S., Wooding, S., & Grant, J. (2011, December 16). The answer is 17 years, what is the question: Understanding time lags in translational research. *Journal of the Royal Society of Medicine, 104*(12), 510–520. https://doi.org/10.1258/jrsm.2011.110180

Murray, C. J. L., Mokdad, A. H., Ballestros, K., Echko, M., Glenn, S., . . . , Troeger, C. (2018). The state of US health, 1990–2016: Burden of diseases, injuries, and risk factors among US states. *Journal of the American Medical Association, 319*(14), 1444–1472. https://doi.org/10.1001/jama.2018.0158

Murray, C. J. L., Vos, T., Lozano, R., Naghavi, M., Flaxman, A. D., Michaud, C., Ezzati, M., Shibuya, K., Salomon, J. A., Abdalla, S., Aboyans, V., Abraham, J., Ackerman, I., Aggarwal, R., Ahn, S. Y., Ali, M. K., AlMazroa, M. A., Alvarado, M., Anderson, H. R., Lopez, A. D. (2012, December 15). Disability-adjusted life years (DALYs) for 291 diseases and injuries in 21 regions, 1990–2010: A systematic analysis for the Global Burden of Disease Study 2010. *The Lancet, 380*(9859), 2197–2223. https://doi.org/10.1016/S0140-6736(12)61689-4

Ozminkowski, R. J., Goetzel, R. Z., Wang, F., Gibson, T. B., Shechter, D., Musich, S., Bender, J., & Edington, D. W. (2006, November). The savings gained from participation in health promotion programs for Medicare beneficiaries. *Journal of Occupational and Environmental Medicine, 48*(11), 1125–1132. https://doi.org/10.1097/01.jom.0000240709.01860.8a

Reinsel, D., Gantz, J., & Rydning, J. (2018). *The digitization of the world from edge to core* [IDC white paper]. Cupertino, CA: Seagate. https://www.seagate.com/files/www-content/our-story/trends/files/idc-seagate-dataage-whitepaper.pdf

Riley, G. F. (2009). Administrative and claims records as sources of health care cost data. *Medical Care, 47*(7), Suppl 1. https://doi.org/10.1097/MLR.0b013e31819c95aa

Seow, H. Y., & Sibley, L. M. (2014, August 30). Developing a dashboard to help measure and achieve the triple aim: A population-based cohort study. *BMC Health Services Research, 14*(1). https://doi.org/10.1186/1472-6963-14-363

Shah, N. D., Steyerberg, E. W., & Kent, D. M. (2018, July 3). Big data and predictive analytics: Recalibrating expectations. *Journal of the American Medical Association, 320*(1), 27–28. https://doi.org/10.1001/jama.2018.5602

Stoppler, M. C. (n.d.). Medic al definition of health risk. MedicineNet. https://www.medicinenet.com/script/main/art.asp?articlekey=205099

Taber's Online. (n.d.). Medical dictionary. https://www.tabers.com/tabersonline/

Tan, M., Hatef, E., Taghipour, D., Vyas, K., Kharrazi, H., Gottlieb, L., & Weiner, J. (2020, September). Including social and behavioral determinants in predictive models: Trends, challenges, and opportunities. JMIR Medical Informatics, 8(9). https://doi.org/10.2196/18084

Tzoulaki, I., Liberopoulos, G., & Ioannidis, J. P. A. (2009, December 2). Assessment of claims of improved prediction beyond the Framingham risk score. *Journal of the American Medical Association, 302*(21), 2345–2352. https://doi.org/10.1001/jama.2009.1757

Vertrees, J. C., Averill, R. F., Eisenhandler, J., Quain, A., & Switalski, J. (2013). Bundling post-acute care services into MS-DRG payments. *Medicare & Medicaid Research Review, 3*(3). https://www.cms.gov/mmrr/Downloads/MMRR2013_003_03_a03.pdf

Wanken, Z. J., Anderson, P. B., Bessen, S. Y., Rode, J. B., Columbo, J. A., Trooboff, S. W., Moore, K. O., & Goodney, P. P. (2020, February 18). Translating coding lists in administrative claims-based research for cardiovascular procedures. *Journal of Vascular Surgery, 72*(1). https://doi.org/10.1016/j.jvs.2019.09.040

World Health Organization. (n.d.). Publications. https://www.who.int/healthinfo/global_burden_disease/publications/en/

Yee, P., Tanenbaum, J. E., Pelle, D. W., Moore, D., Benzel, E. C., Steinmetz, M. P., & Mroz, T. E. (2019). DRG-based bundled reimbursement for lumbar fusion: implications for patient selection. *Journal of Neurosurgery, 31*(4), 1–6. https://doi.org/10.3171/2019.3.SPINE18875

Yen, L., McDonald, T., Hirschland, D., & Edington, D. W. (2003, October). Association between wellness score from a health risk appraisal and prospective medical claims costs. *Journal of Occupational and Environmental Medicine, 45*(10), 1049–1057. https://doi.org/10.1097/01.jom.0000088875.85321.b9

Zhou, X. H., Wang, X., Duncan, A., Hu, G., & Zheng, J. (2017). Statistical evaluation of adding multiple risk factors improves Framingham stroke risk score. *BMC Medical Research Methodology, 17*(1). https://doi.org/10.1186/s12874-017-0330-8

CHAPTER 11

Grouping, Trending, and Interpreting Population Health Data for Waste and Inefficiency

Ines Maria Vigil, MD, MPH, MBA

Healthcare waste and inefficiency account for 25 cents of every healthcare dollar spent in the United States. Population health programs that integrate across stakeholders throughout the continuum of care, and deliver targeted actionable insights at the point of care are invaluable in reducing waste and inefficiency to deliver better outcomes.

—Raj Lakhanpal, MD, FACEP, Founder and CEO, SpectraMedix

EXECUTIVE SUMMARY

Waste and inefficiency in health care has been identified as an area that greatly needs analytics to support decision-making (Ardoin & Malone, 2019). Waste and inefficiency in health care is typically categorized into areas of unnecessary care, administrative inefficiency, inaccurate diagnosis, diagnostic errors, clinical variation, medical overuse, pricing variation, and fraud and abuse (Berwick, 2019; Klein, 2012; Shrank, Rogstad, & Parekh, 2019; Yong et al., 2017). Population health analytics can assist in determining clinical practice pattern variation, support decision-making, define the magnitude of variation in cost and utilization, and promote appropriate care to reduce inefficiency and waste. Identifying, trending, and reporting variation allows clinicians to compare their practice patterns to their peers, drives improvement efforts to reduce variation, and promotes the use of evidence-based protocols and interventions that reduce unnecessary laboratory, imaging, procedures, and medications where effective alternatives exist.

Contextualizing data allows analysts to decide which data assets to link to define variation, what the data points represent, and how to interpret them to best support the development and implementation of population health programs and interventions.

LEARNING OBJECTIVES

At the end of this chapter, the learner will be able to:

1. Differentiate the categories that define healthcare waste and inefficiency.
2. Describe the types of data sources that can be used to apply context to identify healthcare waste and inefficiency opportunities to improve experience, health outcomes, and reduce cost.
3. Understand the ways that healthcare waste and inefficiency are contributing to the rise in the total cost of care.

Introduction

Variation in the provision of medical services can be significant, and clinical and administrative reduction in variation is a strong focus of many healthcare organizations seeking to reduce unnecessary services and waste in health care to achieve financial success and optimize health outcomes. A 2019 study in the *Journal of the American Medical Association* (JAMA) estimated current levels of healthcare waste to be approximately 25% of total annual healthcare spending, or a range of between $760 billion and $935 billion (Shrank et al., 2019). Various studies categorize healthcare waste and inefficiency in different ways, although the most commonly reported areas are unnecessary care, administrative inefficiency, inaccurate diagnosis, diagnostic errors, clinical variation, and medical overuse, pricing variation, and fraud and abuse (Klein, 2012; National Academy of Medicine, n.d.; Shrank et al., 2019). Reducing waste and inefficiency in health care is believed to be a significant contributor to lowering the total cost of health care in the United States, and many analytic and technology market solutions are focused on identifying areas of opportunity to reduce variation and inefficiency in health care (Cave Consulting Group, n.d.; naviHealth, n.d.; Milliman, n.d.).

This chapter looks at the ways data can be grouped into clinical episodes of care, practical applications of evidence-based practice of medicine, and clinical and administrative care pathways to identify diagnostic and clinical errors, lower administrative and transactional waste, and promote cost-effective and cost-efficient programs and interventions.

Defining Healthcare Waste and Inefficiency

Waste is defined by *Oxford Dictionary* as "the use or [to] expend carelessly, extravagantly, or to no purpose" (*Oxford Dictionary*, n.d.-a, Waste). Inefficiency is defined by the same source as "the failure to make the best use of time or resources" (*Oxford Dictionary*, n.d.-b, Inefficiency). Together, these two concepts applied to health care represent a significant spend and result in potential harm to patients, both financially and clinically. Included in **Table 11.1** are commonly referred to categories of healthcare waste and inefficiency and their definitions.

Waste and inefficiency are well defined in a 2019 JAMA article by Dr. William Shrank, Teresa Rogstad, and Dr. Natasha Parekh, and it is defined into categories, costs associated with each category, and suggested interventions to reduce variation, healthcare failures, and inefficiency (Shrank et al., 2019).

The different categories of waste span many areas of health care, and solutions can be derived at the clinical level of patient care (micro), management level of the provision of care (meso), and policy and government (macro) levels. There is a significant opportunity to improve in any one or more of these categories to improve health and reduce the total

Table 11.1 Areas of Healthcare Waste and Inefficiency

Provision of Unnecessary Care	The overuse, overutilization, or overtreatment of healthcare services
Administrative Inefficiency	The failure to maximize productivity, resources, and time
Inaccurate Diagnosis	The failure to diagnose, delay diagnosis, or incorrectly diagnose
Diagnostic Errors	The failure to identify or communicate a diagnosis in an accurate and timely manner
Clinical Variation	The overuse, underuse, different use of healthcare services with varying health outcomes
Medical Overuse	The overdiagnosis, overtreatment, and overuse of healthcare services
Pricing Variation	The difference between the actual and standard price of a product or service multiplied by how much input was used
Fraud and Abuse	The deliberate and dishonest act committed with the knowledge that the deception could result in some unauthorized benefit

Data from Fuchs, V. R. (2018). Is US medical care inefficient? *Journal of the American Medical Association, 320*(10), 971–972). https://doi.org/10.1001/jama.2018.10779; Morgan, D. J., Dhruva, S. S., Coon, E. R., Wright, S. M., & Korenstein, D. (2019). 2019 update on medical overuse: A review. *JAMA Internal Medicine, 179*(11), 1568–1574. https://doi.org/10.1001/jamainternmed.2019.3842; Shrank, W. H., Rogstad, T. L., & Parekh, N. (2019). Waste in the US health care system: Estimated costs and potential for savings. *Journal of the American Medical Association, 322*(15), 1501–1509. https://doi.org/10.1001/jama.2019.13978

cost of care and population health methods and analytics can be an effective way of supporting decision-making in this area.

Assessing and Addressing Healthcare Waste and Inefficiency

Several strategies have been proposed for how to identify and reduce healthcare waste and inefficiency, and several market solutions are available that target specific areas of health care such as reducing variation in utilization and cost in home health and skilled nursing (naviHealth, n.d.). Note that opportunity can be identified at the micro, meso, and macro levels of healthcare delivery and developing population health teams to identify and address healthcare waste and inefficiency is an effective way to assess and address identified challenges. For more detailed information on the process of developing a high-performing population health team, see Chapter 31, "Building a Team Culture for Population Health."

Dr. Douglas Ardoin and John Malone published two thought pieces in 2019 for the Healthcare Financial Management Association on "Reducing Clinical Variation to Drive Success in Value-Based Care (Parts 1 and 2)" (Ardoin & Malone, 2019a, 2019b), highlighting four key components and several tactics to assess and address clinical variation. **Figure 11.1**, "Components of Clinical Variation," summarizes the information in a graphic.

The four key components highlighted in both thought pieces help connect clinician leaders to apply evidence-based best practices to populations, utilizing risk-adjusted analytics to identify opportunity and stratify populations to appropriate interventions, and measuring performance through the development of scorecards. All these components are foundational elements within population health management and analytics.

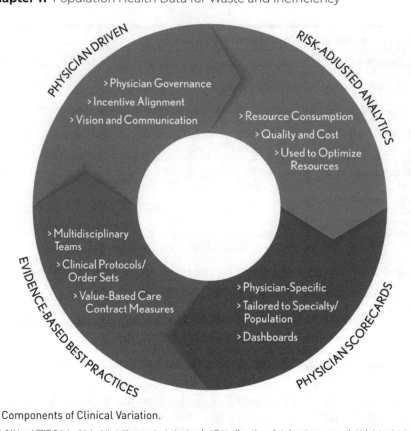

Figure 11.1 Components of Clinical Variation.

Data Sources to Support the Identification and Measurement of Healthcare Waste and Inefficiency

Many data sources can be used to identify and measure healthcare waste and inefficiency. Data from medical claims, lab, pharmacy, and electronic medical records (EMRs) are primarily used to identify opportunities to reduce waste and inefficiency. New work is being done in this field to understand how machine learning and artificial intelligence can assist in identifying clinician practice patterns that vary from standard practice or evidence-based care (Ardoin & Malone, 2019a, 2019b; Morgan, Dhruva, Coon,

Wright, & Korenstein, 2019; Oren, Kebebew, & Ioannidis, 2019; Sanders, n.d.). Section 2, "Data Sources," provides detailed information on data sources that can be used to identify and measure healthcare waste and inefficiency.

Applying Context to Data to Identify and Monitor Healthcare Waste and Inefficiency

When using data to identify healthcare waste and inefficiency, it is important to follow the process outlined in Chapter 8, Figure 8.1, "Process to Apply Context to Population Health Data Process," by asking the following questions:

- What is the question or problem to be solved?
- What data are needed?
- What is the state of the data?
- Who is the audience for the data?
- What action will be taken as a result of interacting with the data?

In addition, it is important to align the problem identified to solve to an area of healthcare waste and inefficiency to target, outlined in Table 11.1 and Figure 11.1. The process can occur in any order such that if an area of waste is known to be a challenge, then the population health process questions can be applied to the known challenge. If a challenge is unknown, the population health questions can be applied to assist in identifying opportunities.

Engaging clinicians at the point of care is vital to the success of identifying, verifying, and addressing variation. Often and when working at the patient level, it is a practice or behavior that is the cause of the variation and requires clinician participation to understand the drivers of the behavior and correct for them. For example, overutilizing laboratory testing as is the case of standing laboratory orders, can result in incidental findings that can cause the patient to undergo unnecessary additional testing and potentially harmful treatments. These are often referred to as "incidentalomas" and can cause significant mental and physical harm to patients and their families, waste needed resources, and create unnecessary cost for health systems (Bejjanki et al., 2018; Morgan et al., 2019).

The following case studies outline several ways to develop and add context to administrative medical claims, laboratory, pharmacy, and EMR data in population health projects to improve patient experience, health outcomes, and reduce avoidable costs.

Case Study 1: Enhancing Patient Experience and Outcomes

Applying Context to Radiographic Imaging Medical Record Data
Using Artificial Intelligence to Differentiate Non-small Cell Lung Cancer

Wrong diagnoses, incorrect diagnoses, and errors in the diagnostic process (such as lab testing errors) are all examples healthcare waste and inefficiency and can have a harmful effect on patients' quality of care and their care experience. Dr. Mark Jarett, the chief quality officer of Northwell Health, stated it best:

> "The wrong diagnosis leads to delays in treatment and increased cost of care. It puts a burden on the healthcare system as a whole." (Castellucci, 2019)

Castellucci (2019) identified six barriers to the ability to make accurate and effective diagnoses, including:

- poor communication when patients' care is transferred,
- lack of monitoring metrics and outcomes measures,
- lack of timely and efficient access to information and resources to support clinical reasoning,
- lack of appropriate time with patients,
- lack of workflows to ensure proper follow-up of test results and referrals and communication to patients, and
- lack of research funding to improve diagnostic testing accuracy and treatment effectiveness.

A 2018 review by Hosny, Parmar, Quackenbush, Schwartz, and Aerts of the use of deep learning analytic techniques in medicine summarized the use of artificial intelligence to support clinical reasoning and improve diagnostic testing accuracy in non-small cell lung cancer (NSCLC). The study outlines how *radiomics*—radiographic images paired with data on clinical outcomes—can assist in clinical decision-making to predict distant metastases, differentiate tumor subtypes, predict disease recurrence, identify

(continues)

Case Study 1: Enhancing Patient Experience and Outcomes   *(continued)*

mutations and gene-expression profiles for treatment, and predict overall survival with greater accuracy than human review alone. Additional artificial intelligence methods have been applied to other cancer types such as breast cancers to assist radiologists in diagnosing disease, improving the quality of radiographic imaging, and monitoring performance and health outcomes (Fazal, Patel, Tye, & Gupta, 2018; Hosny et al., 2018).

Applying a population health approach and solution to this application, the problem to solve and a proposed intervention can be summarized as:

Combining advanced analytic techniques with clinical discretion to enhance diagnosis and treatment accuracy of [NSCLC] for the purpose of tailoring treatment to patients' unique characteristics and healthcare needs.

The combination of clinical discretion and artificial intelligence techniques such as neural networks and variational autoencoders has only begun to be explored and applied to areas of health care to improve on existing processes to diagnose and stratify disease. Population health and quality-improvement projects aim to reduce diagnostic errors and increase diagnostic accuracy to reduce overall failures in the diagnostic process that can harm patients. Population health techniques can help scale many of these learnings using big data to identify optimal treatments and tailor treatments to the unique needs of individual patients.

Options exist for applying context to data to identify healthcare waste and inefficiency to reduce diagnostic errors to *enhance the experience and outcomes of the patient or member*. In **Table 11.2**, items have been selected from the content introduced in Chapter 8, "Grouping, Trending, and Interpreting Population Health Data for Decision Support," to highlight where Case Study 1's use of radiographic imaging from medical records data can be used to generate population health insights, programs, and interventions.

Table 11.2 Applying Context to Data to Enhance the Experience and Outcomes of the Patient or Member

Use Case	Description	Example
Clinical decision support	Information used by clinicians at the point of care and business stakeholders in administration to assist in data-driven decision-making	*Appropriateness of care*: Measures whether a given service, encounter, activity, or event follows a standard of care, clinical care guidelines, or evidence-based medical literature recommendations such as the appropriateness of having standard orders for lab tests that may be unnecessary and costly to the health system and patients.
Patient decision support	Information used by patients to assist in data-driven decision-making for point-of-care services and treatments	*Quality of care*: Measures the level of value assigned to care provided in an encounter, service, or treatment according to clinical evidence-based pathways, care guidelines such as measuring the presence of retinal eye exams in patients with diabetes to screen for and prevent advanced severity of disease. Uses administrative medical claims data, EMR, pharmacy, laboratory, imaging, and safety types of data.

Case Study 2: Improving Health

Applying Context to Administrative Medical Claims and Pharmacy Data

Identifying Medical Overuse of Antibiotics in Patients

The widespread medical overuse of antibiotics has been deemed a public health crisis and has resulted in significant medical harm, avoidable cost, and low-value care (Daniel, Keller, Mozafarihashjin, Pahwa, & Soong, 2018; Pulia, Redwood, & May, 2018). Overtreatment with wide-spectrum antibiotics when not clinically indicated has resulted in the global emergence of antibiotic-resistant strains of bacteria and increased severity of disease in patients who formerly could have been adequately treated (Segura-Egea et al., 2017). In addition, use of antibiotics can cause adverse health outcomes in patients with an incidence as high as 20%, including allergic reactions, gastrointestinal, kidney, and blood abnormalities requiring additional treatments (Pulia et al., 2018; Tamma, Avdic, Li, Dzintars, & Cosgrove, 2017).

Several studies have demonstrated the medical overuse and overtreatment of patients with antibiotics, including a study that identified almost 40% of patients treated in urgent care and emergency department settings were prescribed antibiotics (Morgan et al., 2019; Pulia et al., 2018). There remains a significant global opportunity to decrease the medical overuse of antibiotics to treat non-bacterial infections and simultaneously improve the health of the population. Using a population health approach to identify prescribing patterns indicating overuse of broad-spectrum antibiotics can help focus the allocation of resources to address the challenge and prevent the occurrence of adverse events and associated illness.

Applying a population health approach and solution to this application, the problem to solve and a proposed intervention can be as follows:

Preventing antibiotic resistance in populations via the identification of the medical overuse of broad-spectrum antibiotics in outpatient care settings.

Profiling clinician prescribing patterns of broad-spectrum antibiotics in outpatient care settings help identify practices that may be overprescribing treatment of nonbacterial infections such as sinusitis, upper respiratory infections, and allergic rhinitis.

Options exist for applying context to data to identify and address healthcare waste and inefficiency to *improve the health of the population*. In **Table 11.3**, items have been selected from the content introduced in

Table 11.3 Applying Context to Data to Improve the Health of the Population

Use Case	Description	Example
Presence of diagnosis or disease	Presence or absence of a specified health condition or disease	*Diagnoses*: Measures the presence or absence of a specified health condition, set of conditions, or disease such as diabetes, degenerative joint disease (DJD), and breast cancer.
Progression of diagnoses or disease	Worsening or advancement of a specified health condition or disease over time	*Related diagnoses*: Measures the presence or absence over time of comorbidities, complications, gaps in medications, and health determinants such as patients with diabetes and depression, patients with DJD and morbid obesity, and patients with breast cancer that is invasive.
		Level of severity: Measures the presence or absence over time of comorbidities, complications, gaps in medications, and health determinants within a categorical designation of severity such as patients whose diabetes is unmanaged secondary to untreated depression, patients whose pain associated with DJD is worsened by the wear and tear caused by morbid obesity, and patients with breast cancer that has metastasized to other organs.

(continues)

Table 11.3 **Applying Context to Data to Improve the Health of the Population**   *(continued)*

Use Case	Description	Example
Care and treatment pathways	A documented set of standards of care, care guidelines, or care pathway that indicate a disease's life cycle from risk factors to symptoms, diagnosis, morbidity, treatments, and death	*Related diagnoses*: Refer to "Progression of diagnoses or disease" in the left column of this table. An example of a care or treatment pathway's use case is the translation and incorporation of the 2020 American Diabetes Association's (Johnson et al., 2020) set of clinical guidelines to treat patients with diabetes in a health system's EMR. *Level of severity*: Refer to "Progression of diagnoses or disease" in the left column of this table. An example of a care or treatment pathway's use case is identifying where patients are along the care pathway or the time and way in which a patient deviates from a care pathway or care guideline to alert clinicians to make adjustments to his or her care or treatment plan.
Risk or presence of worsened or poor health outcomes	The presence or absence of often clinical or health determinant indicators that categorize a patient as having poor health or an adverse event that has significant impact on their day-to-day activities and well-being	*Related adverse outcomes*: Measures the presence or absence over time of comorbidities, complications, gaps in medications, health determinants, and harm of patients within a categorical designation of outcomes such as patients with diabetes that have been unmanaged over time and resulted in kidney failure requiring dialysis. *Related procedures*: Measures utilization of specified surgical and pharmacy procedures such as patients with diabetes that have been unmanaged over time that resulted in multiple leg amputations because of poor wound healing and blood circulation complicated by multiple wound infections. *Related events*: Measures utilization of specified hospital-based emergency department, admission, and readmission events such as recurring admissions of patients with congestive heart failure with volume or fluid overload. *Quality of care*: Refer to Table 11.2, "Patient decision support," in the left-hand column. An example of a risk or the presence of a worsened or poor health outcome use case is the harm caused to a patient who had an allergic reaction to a medication that resulted in a loss of hearing. *Related diagnoses*: Refer to "Progression of diagnoses or disease" in the left-hand column. An example of a risk or presence of worsened or poor health outcome use case is the presence of pneumonia in a patient with severe asthma and an inpatient hospitalization to help the patient breathe using supplemental oxygen and inhaled steroid medication. *Level of severity*: Refer to "Progression of diagnoses or disease" in the left-hand column. An example of a risk or the presence of worsened or poor health outcome use case is the patient with severe asthma complicated by pneumonia being treated in a hospital who worsens and requires mechanical ventilation to breathe.

| | | *Adherence*: Measures a patient's actions in following a given care plan, medication regimen, or treatment such as a patient with hypertension who suffers a heart attack from years of not following a heart-healthy lifestyle and not consistently taking blood pressure medication. |
| | | *Factors influencing health status*: Measures a patient's social and behavioral factors that influence health such as a patient with severe asthma who lives in a geographic region with significant air pollution who requires a hospital admission to treat an asthma attack. |

Chapter 8 "Grouping, Trending, and Interpreting Population Health Data for Decision Support," to highlight where Case Study 2's use of administrative medical claims and pharmacy data can be used to generate population health insights, programs, and interventions.

Case Study 3: Reduce per Capita Cost of Care

Applying Context to Administrative Medical Claims, Laboratory Data, and Pharmacy Data

Identifying Laboratory Testing Patterns Not Indicated by the Clinical Standard of Care

Laboratory accuracy testing has identified both underuse of certain drug-testing methodologies and overuse of others. The worsening epidemic of prescription drug abuse over recent years has placed a spotlight on drug addiction and addiction medicine. Specifically, the accuracy and appropriate use of blood and urine drug screening as a test for screening versus treatment has undergone scrutiny (Jarvis et al., 2017; Krasowski et al., 2020). Widespread use of urine drug screening to monitor active use of prescription pain medication has increased in the United States dramatically following the rise in prescription drug abuse.

A Kaiser Health News and Mayo Clinic (Schulte & Lucas, 2017) analysis of administrative medical claims from 2011 to 2014 demonstrated a fourfold increase in urine drug screens and related genetic tests, representing $8.5 billion a year. In addition, the study found that national standards were lacking on criteria indicated for testing, frequency of testing, and which drugs to test when. Further troubled by the practice of for-profit physician-owned drug-testing laboratories, the area of drug testing was identified to be an area of concern for waste and abuse.

Applying a population health approach and solution to this application, the problem to solve and a proposed intervention can be as follows:

Profiling clinician laboratory ordering patterns to identify excessive testing of drug use, dependency, and abuse in addiction medicine.

or

Profiling clinician prescription pain medication patterns to identify excessive or inappropriate prescribing of opioids that contribute to drug use, dependency, and abuse.

Clinical pathways are being developed to guide clinicians on the appropriate indications, frequency, and type of laboratory testing for testing and treatment for users of prescription pain medications. Population health interventions have been developed to monitor opioid prescribing across the United States to identify and focus resources to educate providers of the health dangers and downstream negative financial impact of overprescribing addictive pain medications. Research is currently underway to identify alternatives to manage pain effectively to avoid the need for treatment of pain with opioids (Jarvis et al., 2017; Trasolini, McKnight, & Dorr, 2018). Profiling clinician prescribing and ordering patterns can also be performed on other medications, imaging studies, laboratory tests, emerging technology, and unproven treatments.

(continues)

Case Study 3: Reduce per Capita Cost of Care   *(continued)*

Options exist for applying context to data to determine healthcare waste and inefficiency to *reduce per capita cost of care for the benefit of communities*. In **Table 11.4**, items have been selected from the content introduced in Chapter 8, "Grouping, Trending, and Interpreting Population Health Data for Decision Support," to highlight where Case Study 3's use of administrative claims, laboratory, and pharmacy data can be used to generate population health insights, programs, and interventions.

More detail on specific data sources can be found in Section 2, "Data Sources."

Table 11.4 Applying Context to Data to Reduce per Capita Cost of Care for the Benefit of Communities (Excerpt from Chapter 8)

Use Case	Description	Example
Utilization and volume	The utilization and volume of clinical and administrative healthcare services.	*High volume*: Measures the volume of clinical and administrative healthcare services delivered such as the average number of chemotherapy medication infusions for a patient with lung cancer.
		Risk of future high volume: Measures the predicted volume of clinical and administrative healthcare services estimated to be delivered in the future such as the total number of patients with diabetes involving the kidneys that will likely require dialysis.
Point-of-care events and service types	Information that describes the qualitative aspects of an event or service.	*Appropriateness of care*: Refer to Table 11.2, "Clinical decision support," in the left-hand column. An example of a point-of-care event or service type use case is the consideration of a surgery in an ambulatory surgical outpatient center for procedures that can be safely performed with less need for high-acuity services such as would be provided by a hospital.
Variations in care	Differences in cost and volume of services across providers, facilities, geographic regions, services, ancillary services or DMEs, imaging, laboratory, pharmacy, etc.	*High volume*: Refer to "Utilization and volume" in the left-hand column. An example of a variation in care volume use case is the differences in volume across provider networks of the use of CT scan imaging studies in the management of a specified type of lung cancer.
Inefficient or unnecessary care (waste or harm)	Avoidable encounters, events, services, procedures, tests, treatments that are not needed to diagnose, treat, or manage health.	*Appropriateness of Care*: Refer to Table 11.2, "Clinical decision support," in the left-hand column. An example of an inefficient or unnecessary care use case is a laboratory test for vitamin D deficiency when it is suspected as the treatment with supplements or sunlight with recovery is appropriate and low harm.
		Fraud and abuse: Measures the overutilization and inappropriate utilization of services for financial gain or some other personal reward such as the billing to CMS for home healthcare visits to patients that were never performed for financial gain.

Use Case 1

Equitable Distribution of Philanthropic Funding

You are the director at a foundation with a mission to improve the health of populations across the United States and have received a generous donation of $3 million targeted for improving equitable access to high-quality, low-cost healthcare services through the reduction in variation of cost and utilization of care. You are charged with overseeing the allocation of the funding to areas of need defined as high variability in cost or utilization. Your goal is to reduce variation to standardize costs to provide more affordable access to services for populations in need. Where do you start? What information do you need to understand to most effectively allocate the funding?

Use Case 2

Improving Quality of Care Delivery

You are a recent graduate from a master's program in biostatistics and have been working at a national health insurance plan in its clinical analytics and improvement team. You love your team, and you are learning so much about how health care is administered. You are asked to review a set of evidence-based guidelines from Choosing Wisely, an initiative of the ABIM Foundation (Baird, 2019; Choosing Wisely, n.d.; Colla, Morden, Sequist, Schpero, & Rosenthal, 2014). After a review of its website at www.choosingwisely. org, you select one guideline that you believe has the potential to be programmed into a dashboard that profiles performance across the different regions of the United States.

Which one do you choose? Why? What about it interests you? What value does it appear to bring (improve experience, health, or reduce cost)?

Conclusion

Multiple domains of healthcare waste and inefficiency were defined by Dr. William Shrank and colleagues in a JAMA Special Communication (Shrank et al., 2019) and represented approximately 25% of total annual healthcare spending. In addition, healthcare waste and inefficiency have significant negative downstream impacts of worsened health outcomes and poor care quality. Unnecessary care, administrative inefficiency, inaccurate diagnosis, diagnostic errors, clinical variation, medical overuse, pricing variation, and fraud and abuse are all areas of opportunity for population health analytics to play a critical role in identifying opportunity and measuring performance. Several market solutions exist in this space and have only scratched the surface of what can be realized in the near future. Adding context to data to define variation and selecting data that can assist in identification, stratification, and monitoring performance can effectively support clinical and business decision-making and drive results.

Study and Discussion Questions

- What are examples of healthcare waste and inefficiency within the domains of failure of care coordination, pricing failure, and administrative complexity mentioned in Shrank et al. (2019) and not specifically detailed in this chapter?

- What market solutions exist that identify healthcare waste and inefficiency in the form of opportunity to improve patient experience? Improve health? Reduce cost?

Resources and Websites

Choosing Wisely. (n.d.). Promoting conversations between providers and patients; https://www.choosingwisely.org/

Shrank, W. H., Rogstad, T. L., & Parekh, N. (2019, October 7). Waste in the US health care system: Estimated costs and potential for savings. *Journal of the American Medical Association, 322*(15), 1501–1509. https://doi.org/10.1001/jama.2019.13978

References

Ardoin, D., & Malone, J. (2019a). Reducing clinical variation to drive success in value-based care (Part 1). (March 26). Healthcare Financial Management Association. https://www.hfma.org/topics/operations-management/article/reducing-clinical-variation-to-drive-success-in-value-based-care0.html

Ardoin, D., & Malone, J. (2019b). Reducing clinical variation to drive success in value-based care (Part 2). (April 20). Healthcare Financial Management Association. https://www.hfma.org/topics/operations-management/article/reducing-clinical-variation-to-drive-success-in-value-based-care.html

Baird, G. S. (2019). The Choosing Wisely initiative and laboratory test stewardship. *Diagnosis, 6*(1), 15–23. https://www.unboundmedicine.com/medline/citation/30205639/The_Choosing_Wisely_initiative_and_laboratory_test_stewardship_

Bejjanki, H., Mramba, L. K., Beal, S. G., Radhakrishnan, N., Bishnoi, R., Shah, C., Agrawal, N., Harris, N., Leverence, R., & Rand, K. (2018). The role of a best practice alert in the electronic medical record in reducing repetitive lab tests. *ClinicoEconomics and Outcomes Research, 10*, 611–618. https://doi.org/10.2147/CEOR.S167499

Berwick, D. M. (2019, October 7). Elusive waste: The Fermi paradox in US health care. *Journal of the American Medical Association, 322*(15), 1458–1459. https://doi.org/10.1001/jama.2019.14610

Castellucci, M. (2019, January 26). Coalition tackling diagnostic errors gains some traction. Modern Healthcare. https://www.modernhealthcare.com/article/20190126/NEWS/190129972/coalition-tackling-diagnostic-errors-gains-some-traction

Cave Consulting Group. (n.d.). Products—Home. https://cavegroup.com/#section-554

Choosing Wisely. (n.d.). Promoting conversations between providers and patients. https://www.choosingwisely.org/

Colla, C. H., Morden, N. E., Sequist, T. D., Schpero, W. L., & Rosenthal, M. B. (2014, November 6). Choosing Wisely: Prevalence and correlates of low-value health care services in the United States. *Journal of General Internal Medicine, 30*(2), 221–228. https://link.springer.com/article/10.1007%2Fs11606-014-3070-z

Daniel, M., Keller, S., Mozafarihashjin, M., Pahwa, A., & Soong, C. (2018). An implementation guide to reducing overtreatment of asymptomatic bacteriuria. *JAMA Internal Medicine, 178*(2), 271–276). https://doi.org/10.1001/jamainternmed.2017.7290

Fazal, M. I., Patel, M. E., Tye, J., & Gupta, Y. (2018). The past, present and future role of artificial intelligence in imaging. *European Journal of Radiology, 105*, 246–250. https://doi.org/10.1016/j.ejrad.2018.06.020

Fuchs, V. R. (2018, September 11). Is US medical care inefficient? *Journal of the American Medical Association, 320*(10), 971–972. https://doi.org/10.1001/jama.2018.10779

Bill Gates. (n.d.). The first rule of any technology used. . . . Brainy quote. https://www.brainyquote.com/quotes/bill_gates_104353

Hosny, A., Parmar, C., Quackenbush, J., Schwartz, L. H., & Aerts, H. J. W. L. (2018, May 17). Artificial intelligence in radiology. *Nature Reviews Cancer, 18*(8), 500–510. https://doi.org/10.1038/s41568-018-0016-5

Jarvis, M., Williams, J., Hurford, M., Lindsay, D., Lincoln, P., Giles, L., Luongo, P., & Safarian, T. (2017, May–June). Appropriate use of drug testing in clinical addiction medicine. *Journal of Addiction Medicine, 11*(3), 163–173. https://doi.org/10.1097/ADM.0000000000000323

Klein, I. (2012). Eliminating low-value health care: Where pathways approaches have succeeded. *Journal of Clinical Pathways, 5*(2). https://www.journalofclinicalpathways.com/article/eliminating-low-value-health-care-where-pathways-approaches-have-succeeded

Krasowski, M. D., McMillin, G. A., Melanson, S. E. F., Dizon, A., Magnani, B., & Snozek, C. L. H. (2020, February 1). Interpretation and utility of drug abuse screening immunoassays: Insights from laboratory drug testing proficiency surveys. *Archives of Pathology and Laboratory Medicine, 144*(2), 177–184. https://doi.org/10.5858/arpa.2018-0562-CP

Lumina Health Partners. (n.d.). Trusted experts, proven strategies, leaders in healthcare consulting. https://www.luminahp.com/about-lumina-health-partners/

Milliman. (n.d.). MedInsight. https://www.medinsight.milliman.com/en/ecosystem#products

Morgan, D. J., Dhruva, S. S., Coon, E. R., Wright, S. M., & Korenstein, D. (2019, September 9). 2019 Update on medical overuse: A review. *JAMA Internal Medicine, 179*(11), 1568–1574. https://doi.org/10.1001/jamainternmed.2019.3842

National Academy of Medicine. (n.d.). Home. https://nam.edu/naviHealth. (n.d.). Decision support tools. https://www.navihealth.com/decision-support-tools/

Oren, O., Kebebew, E., & Ioannidis, J. P. A. (2019). Curbing unnecessary and wasted diagnostic imaging. *Journal of the American Medical Association, 321*(3), 245–246. https://doi.org/10.1001/jama.2018.20295

Oxford Dictionary. (n.d.-a) Waste—Definition. Lexico.com. https://www.lexico.com/definition/waste

Oxford Dictionary. (n.d.-b) Inefficiency—Definition. Lexico.com. https://www.lexico.com/definition/inefficiency

Pulia, M., Redwood, R., & May, L. (2018, November). Antimicrobial stewardship in the emergency department. *Emergency Medicine Clinics of North America, 36*(4), 853–872. https://doi.org/10.1016/j.emc.2018.06.012

Sanders, M. (n.d.). Using AI to reduce clinical variation: An idea whose time has come. Becker's Health IT. https://www.beckershospitalreview.com/healthcare-information-technology/using-ai-to-reduce-clinical-variation-an-idea-whose-time-has-come.html

Schulte, F., & Lucas, E. (2017). Liquid gold: Pain doctors soak up profits by screening urine for drugs. *Kaiser Health News*. https://khn.org/news/liquid-gold-pain-doctors-soak-up-profits-by-screening-urine-for-drugs/

Segura-Egea, J. J., Gould, K., Şen, B. H., Jonasson, P., Cotti, E., Mazzoni, A., Sunay, H., Tjäderhane, L., & Dummer, P. M. H. (2017, December). Antibiotics in endodontics: A review. *International Endodontic Journal, 50*(12), 1169–1184. https://doi.org/10.1111/iej.12741

Shrank, W. H., Rogstad, T. L., & Parekh, N. (2019, October 7). Waste in the US health care system: Estimated costs and potential for savings. *Journal of the American Medical Association, 322*(15), 1501–1509. https://doi.org/10.1001/jama.2019.13978

Tamma, P. D., Avdic, E., Li, D. X., Dzintars, K., & Cosgrove, S. E. (2017). Association of adverse events with antibiotic use in hospitalized patients. *JAMA Internal Medicine, 177*(9), 1308–1315. https://doi.org/10.1001/jamainternmed.2017.1938

Trasolini, N. A., McKnight, B. M., & Dorr, L. D. (2018). The opioid crisis and the orthopedic surgeon. *Journal of Arthroplasty, 33*(11), 3379–3382. https://doi.org/10.1016/j.arth.2018.07.002

Yong, P. L., Saunders, R. S., & Olsen, L. (Eds.). (2010). The healthcare imperative: Lowering costs and improving outcomes [Workshop series summary]. Washington, DC: National Academies Press. https://www.nap.edu/catalog/12750/the-healthcare-imperative-lowering-costs-and-improving-outcomes-workshop-series

SECTION IV

Creating the Population Health Data Model

CHAPTER 12

Development of a Data Model

Martha Sylvia, PhD, MBA, RN

The bitterness of poor quality remains long after the sweetness of low price is forgotten.

—Benjamin Franklin

EXECUTIVE SUMMARY

Readily available data infrastructure for population health analytics requires that a data model be developed that brings together data from multiple data sources in a cohesive way and on which the tools used for analytics can be placed. A population health data model allows users to easily combine and contrast multiple data variables to describe events, examine relationships, identify patterns, derive insights, and support the operations of population health management. Data modeling is the part of data architecture that defines the structures in which data reside and evolve. It is a powerful technique to define, create, and maintain data structures and enable data integrity, gather business requirements, and communicate the scope of population health data along with its organization, levels of aggregation, and constraints (Berson & Dubov, 2011).

LEARNING OBJECTIVES

At the end of this chapter, the learner will be able to:

1. Define the process for developing prototypes and moving them into production.
2. Define levels of abstraction in data modeling.
3. Distinguish between conceptual, logical, and physical data models.
4. Define the roles required for each level of data abstraction.

Introduction

When done well, a strong data-modeling architecture is flexible in that it can accommodate changes when business rules and clinical logic changes.

A data model can be as large as the entire model for data across an organization, which is referred to as the *master data model,* or can be sized to meet the needs of critical business functions like population health management. The goal of data

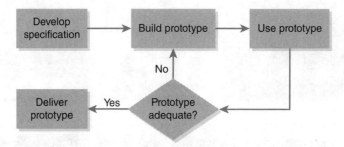

Figure 12.1 Prototyping Process.

Data from Sommerville, I. (2016). *Software engineering* (10th ed., p. 63). Pearson Education.

modeling in population health is to optimize the ability to perform the analytic functions in support of the population health process. Refer to Chapter 2, "Guiding Frameworks for Population Health Analytics," for more information on the population health process.

This chapter describes key components of the approach to use when developing data models for population health management. Agile project management supports the use of prototypes in developing population health data models. Conceptual, physical, and logical data models are used in this chapter to support the development of a population health data model. The process of moving from conceptual to physical to logical data models allows all stakeholders in the model the ability to actively participate with each and understand the important role they play in developing a high-functioning data model.

Prototyping

Data modeling is considered a highly technical endeavor with considerable uncertainty in the process. For this reason, data models are best developed through a prototyping process. In prototyping, an executable model of the desired end product is created to facilitate early feedback in support of the development process (Kordon & Luqi, 2002). The first iteration of a protype meets the needs set out in the use case. A use case is a data request with a description from a stakeholder of how they will use the information provided by the prototype to accomplish a goal. Multiple use cases may be requested

simultaneously and must be clearly articulated individually and shown how they will be used together if appropriate. Note that a final prototype may not take into consideration all aspects of requirements for production or scalability. The main goal of a prototype is to quickly demonstrate a proof of concept to drive value. In model development, an *evolutionary approach* to prototype development is taken where a series of prototypes are developed based on techniques that allow rapid iterations (Sommerville, 2016). The final version is what will go into production and requires:

- precise specifications,
- clear documentation, and
- optimization in the transfer-to-production process.

When prototyping, *validation* is defined as demonstrating the adequacy of the system (Sommerville, 2016). **Figure 12.1** depicts a process of prototyping in which specifications are developed, a prototype is built, and the prototype is used, tested for adequacy, and delivered for use once deemed adequate.

Agile Project Management

Projects that are highly technical, complex, and with a high degree of uncertainty about the final result require a project management approach, which can be thought of as a spiral approach in which only core requirements are met in the first prototype followed by further development in sequential cycles of definition, design, building, and testing. This spiral approach is considered to take on a spiral-like shape of ever-enlarging circles of development (Flahiff & Liker, 2014). *Agile* is a method of development that takes a spiral approach. Agile development uses an iterative approach to deliver as much functioning within a data model as early as possible to maximize value and return on investment and identify issues, miscommunications, and misunderstandings early in the development process (Agile Manifesto, 2001). Agile methods are advantageous in that:

- "value is achieved through quicker releases to the end user,
- frequent releases expose flaws faster and reduce waste,
- iterative processes are better able to adopt to inevitable changes and evolving business needs, and
- earlier customer feedback and development team collaboration leads to user-centered solutions." (van der Lans, 2015)

Agile methods are guided by a manifesto developed by a group of 17 software developers as follows:

We are uncovering better ways of developing software by doing it and helping others do it. Through this work we have come to value:

- "individuals and interactions over process and tools
- working software over comprehensive documentation
- customer collaboration over contract negotiation
- responding to change over following a plan"

That is, while we value the items on the right, we value the items on the left more. (Agile Manifesto, 2001)

The manifesto is achieved through a set of 12 guiding principles within three domains of execution:

Regular Delivery of Software

- "Our highest priority is to satisfy the customer through early and continuous delivery of valuable software.
- Deliver working software frequently, from a couple of weeks to a couple of months, with a preference to the shorter timescale.
- Working software is the primary measure of progress.
- Agile processes promote sustainable development. The sponsors, developers, and users should be able to maintain a constant pace indefinitely." (Agile Manifesto, 2001)

Team Communication

- "Business leaders and developers must work together daily throughout the project.
- The most efficient and effective method of conveying information to and within a development team is face-to-face conversation.
- The best architectures, requirements, and designs emerge from self-organizing teams.
- Build projects around motivated individuals. Give them the environment and support they need and trust them to get the job done.
- At regular intervals, the team reflects on how to become more effective and then tunes and adjusts its behavior accordingly." (Agile Manifesto, 2001)

Design Excellence

- "Continuous attention to technical excellence and good design enhances agility.
- Simplicity—the art of maximizing the amount of work not done—is essential.
- Welcome changing requirements, even late in development. Agile processes harness change for the customer's competitive advantage." (Agile Manifesto, 2001)

Multiple resources exist for learning about the Agile methodology and processes as well as certification opportunities that are not included in the scope of this textbook. Resources are provided at the end of this chapter.

Data Models

For the purposes of this book, a data model is a description of the structure for data. This description includes data elements to be stored and the way in which they will be stored. This description also includes the relationships between data elements and any limitations or constraints that need to be considered.

The data model specifies the following:

- *Data types*—for example date, integer, character, string, and more.
- *Constraints*—rules that are applied to the data. These rules help ensure accuracy and reliability of the data within a data model. For example, a constraint may prevent null values from being entered into a data field.
- *Relationships*—or how the rows in one table of data can be related to the rows in another table of data. For instance, one data table may have one row per person whereas a related table can have multiple rows per person.
- *Metadata*—"data about the data" describe the intended meaning and use of each data element.

Levels of Abstraction

When building a data model, it is highly beneficial to gain multiple perspectives and input from each stakeholder. This ensures that all interested parties and end users actively participate in development of the model, understand the end product, and know how to use it. These perspectives are referred to as *levels of abstraction* and are defined by three levels: conceptual, logical, and physical.

Producing three perspectives of the data model allows for better communication and mutual understanding. This ensures that business and clinical needs for information are met and that the design helps develop insights. Technical developers have line of sight from the technical physical model to the concepts connecting them to the purpose of the model. The process of developing the three perspectives facilitates collaboration among all stakeholders. Data governance objectives are supported and enhanced through multiple perspectives of the model.

Conceptual Models

Conceptual models represent concepts or domains and the relationships between them and are depicted and described in a way that business and clinical stakeholders can understand. The conceptual model uses common language to explain a domain such as *enrollment* or *outreach*. The conceptual model explains entities within the domain such as *contact attempts* that evolve into data tables in a logical model. The conceptual model also explains the relationships between entity classes. A conceptual model is independent of the method that will be used to ultimately design or implement the data model. The aim of the conceptual model is to express the meaning of terms and is used by domain experts to discuss the concept and find the correct relationships (Beshears, 2019).

A conceptual model is usually developed by a team of analysts with a business or clinical owner of the model. An *owner* is the person who has decision-making authority over the business or clinical rules applied in the model (data definitions and constraints) and the ways in which the model will be used to answer questions of interest in population health.

Figure 12.2 displays an example of a portion of a conceptual data model that explains the concept or domain of patient outreach. Two entities are described. The first entity is the list of eligible members that is used for outreach to people who are eligible for the intervention. The second entity is outreach attempts and provides information about the attempts to contact the patient for outreach.

Logical Models

A logical model uses the conceptual model to structure the data in terms of tables and variables and the relationship between them; it is depicted as a diagram. The logical model is expressed independently of a particular database management product or storage technology (Beshears, 2018). The primary key identifies a unique record in the table, and the foreign key, a

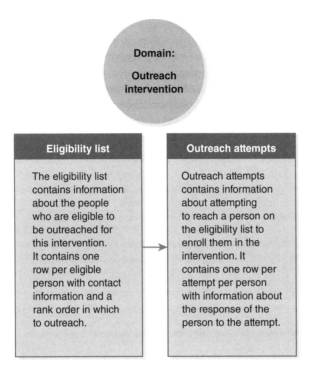

Figure 12.2 Conceptual Model.

field in the table that is a primary key in another table, is also identified in a logical model. The analyst or data scientist from the team that developed the conceptual model works with a data architect to make this transition from the conceptual to the logical model.

Figure 12.3 is an example of a logical model that was developed from the conceptual model in Figure 12.2. The text descriptions are replaced with the names of variables or columns that will be in the table. In addition, the primary and foreign keys are noted.

Physical Models

The physical data model is the most technical of all of the data model perspectives, representing the structure as it exists in its environment or database system. It is usually derived from a logical data model but can also be reverse engineered from a given database structure. It describes all of the table structures, indexes, relationships,

constraints, and primary and foreign keys and also contains storage-allocation details (Beshears, 2018). The structure of the physical model depends on the type of database model used, which is often dictated by data warehouse specifications (see Chapters 14 and 15).

Figure 12.4 depicts an example of a physical model that was developed from the logical model and uses the technical terminology in the structure of the database. In addition, variables representing primary and foreign keys are directly associated according to their relationships. In this example, ID number is a primary key in the eligibility table that links to the foreign key in the attempt table. This is called a *one-to-many relationship*. The physical model would be accompanied by a data dictionary that provides the metadata to support the model and would include a detailed description of the use case in easy-to-understand plain business or clinical language, the variable names, a brief description, the data formats, and example values.

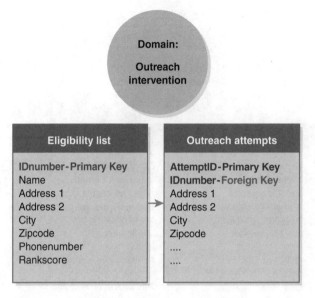

Figure 12.3 Logical Model.

Metadata

The final data model contains information about the data itself, which is called *metadata*. A data dictionary is a common way to communicate and document metadata and contains a complete set of data points that explain the use cases, data types, tables and variables, formatting, constraints, relationships, and other important information. Metadata also include other documentation about the data model like the annotated code used to

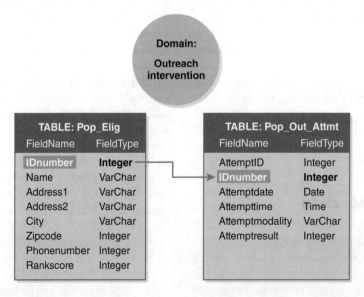

Figure 12.4 Physical Model.

Data Table	Variable Name	Description	Format	Data Type	Ln	Example Values
Pop_Out_Attmt	attemptID	The ID number assigned at the time the attempt is documented by the outreach worker	XXXXXXX	INT	10	111324739
Pop_Out_Attmt	Idnumber	The unique person ID number assigned as of initial eligibility. Any number above 99999 will not be inputted. Leading zeros are acceptable	XXXXXX	INT	6	000101
Pop_Out_Attmt	attempdate	The date at the time the attempt is documented by the outreach worker.	XX/YY/ZZZZ	DATE	10	02/15/2021
Pop_Out_Attmt	attemptime	The time at the time the attempt is documented by the outreach worker in military time	XX:YY	TIME	5	13:15
Pop_Out_Attmt	attemptmodality	The modality used for the outreach attempt selected from a drop-down list at the time the attempt is documented by the outreach worker	XXXXXXX	VARCHAR	12	Phone/ Email/ Text/Postal
Pop_Out_Attmt	attemptresult	The result of the outreach attempt selected from a drop-down list at the time the attempt is documented by the outreach worker. The result is documented as a number representing different result types	XX	INT	2	1-25

Figure 12.5 Data Dictionary.

Reproduced from Sylvia, M. (2020). *The population health data model.* Population Health Management Learning Series. ForestVue Healthcare Solutions.

create the tables and relationships, data lineage, and business rules.

Figure 12.5 shows a data dictionary from the data model created in Figure 12.4 and provides detailed information about the outreach attempt data table. A complete set of information would contain all metadata about the intervention outreach domain.

Conclusion

Data models in population health are complex and highly technical, requiring a prototyping approach to development where incremental executable portions of the model are delivered for use and acceptance. Agile project management supports prototyping goals and ensures that sequential cycles of valuable functionality are provided frequently and within reasonable time frames.

When building a data model, the analyst, clinical, and business leaders must work together to clearly articulate and document in plain language the various use cases so they can develop a conceptual model that serves as a mechanism for mutual understanding for the clinical and business needs from the model and the technical translation of those needs. In addition, it serves as a way to communicate the structure of the model to various stakeholders. The analyst works with the data architect to develop a logical model to ensure that high-level concepts are accurately translated into technical requirements. The architect then works with developers to create the physical model, which completes the technical development and complete set of information and specifications for the model.

Study and Discussion Questions

- Why is prototyping the best way to develop a data model?
- Discuss aspects the Agile manifesto and principles and the way in which they support prototyping.
- Working as a team, select a use case from the literature or from another chapter in this textbook and design a conceptual model which will ultimately be used to measure results for a population health intervention.

Resources and Websites

Agile Methodology: https://agilemethodology.org/

ScrumAlliance: https://www.scrumalliance.org/

Project Management Institute: www.pmi.org

References

Agile Manifesto. (2001) Manifesto for agile software development. https://agilemanifesto.org/

Berson, A., & Dubov, L. (2011). Master data modeling. Pp. 167–194 in A. Berson & L. Dubov (Eds.), *Master data management and data governance* (2nd ed.). McGraw-Hill.

Beshears, F. (2018). Levels of abstraction in data modelling. Innovation Memes. https://innovationmemes.blogspot.com/2018/06/levels-of-abstraction-in-data-modelling.html

Flahiff, J., & Liker, J. (2014). *Being agile in a waterfall world: a practical guide for complex organizations.* CreateSpace Corporation.

Kordon, F., & Luqi. (2002). An introduction to rapid system prototyping. *IEEE Transactions on Software Engineering, 28*(9), 817–821. https://doi.org/10.1109/TSE.2002.1033222

Sommerville, I. (2016). Coping with change. In I. Sommerville (Ed.), *Software engineering* (10th ed.). Pearson.

Sylvia, M. (2020). The population health data model. Population Health Management Learning Series. ForestVue Healthcare Solutions.

CHAPTER 13

The Population Health Data Model

Martha Sylvia, PhD, MBA, RN

Current healthcare data models are designed to analyze utilization events and financial impacts . . . it's time to organize our data in terms of the person and their health determinants.

—Anonymous

EXECUTIVE SUMMARY

Data in health care are not naturally structured to understand health determinants and outcomes for individuals and populations. Ask a question of an analyst in an organization that does not have a population health data model (PHDM) about morbidity burden; clinical, behavioral, and health system drivers of poor quality; healthcare costs and utilization; or any other population health question that seems on the surface easy to answer and you may get a puzzled look. Absent a population health data model, an analyst may approach the question by going to one siloed data source like medical claims data and, if more advanced, try to integrate this data with another source like pharmacy claims data. The process would require a great deal of querying, cleansing, transforming, and integrating of data by writing reams of code; making assumptions about the meaning of data; and using multiple tools to analyze the data and make it presentable. The analyst has every desire to provide high-quality results that address the question in a timely manner but is not set up to successfully do so without a population health data model.

LEARNING OBJECTIVES

At the end of this chapter, the learner will be able to:

1. Describe the core features of a population health data model.
2. Distinguish the population health data architecture from event-based architecture.
3. Design a conceptual model for population health data.
4. Describe the advantages of a population health data model.

Introduction

Population health management is made possible by translating data into information. Aggregated data are used to carry out clinical processes of care in a population in the same way that the tools of the clinician are used in the clinical process of care for individual patients. Individual data collected at multiple points of contact within the care system are aggregated to understand the health of an entire population. For instance, where an individual blood pressure value is used to determine the treatment and prescription for one patient, the range and mean of blood pressure in a population is used to determine evidence-based programs for masses of patients with hypertension. Population health management seeks to obtain person-level data from multiple data sources on an ongoing basis to develop evidence-based strategies directed at reversing negative trends in the health status of a defined population that have been shown in the health literature to lead to overall increased costs, inappropriate utilization of health care services, and overall decline in the health of the population.

The population health data model (PHDM) is designed to support population health management strategy. In its fully functioning state, the analytic infrastructure consists of a team of analysts using various software tools applied to multiple sources of patient-centric data that are organized within an enterprise data warehouse with the overarching goal of driving innovation in population health management. The PHDM supports care delivery based on population indicators and outcomes, supports organizational processes for intervention, and facilitates care that meets the goals of the Triple Aim.

This chapter describes the core components and functionality of a PHDM, proposes a process for developing the model, and provides an example conceptual model. With these basic principles in mind, stakeholders and resources can be organized to develop a population health data model that is uniquely tailored to unique organizational strategy, data availability, and technical capabilities.

The Core Population Health Data Model

Although a population health data model is developed with specific organizational goals in mind, all population health data models share certain basic features. These features make up the core of the data model. At its core, the model has person-level observations from multiple data sources at equally distant points in time that can be aggregated to an entire population and segmented by smaller subgroupings.

The Person-Centric View

Although it may sound simple, the person-centric view of data is subtly complex. Healthcare organizations—whether they are payers, providers, large health systems, small community hospitals, or other types—are often at the lower end of data maturity where the data systems are built to support healthcare transactions. These data structures support billing and payment in fee-for-service models of care. The data about a patient are derived from and stored as information about the transaction. For instance, an electronic medical record assigns diagnoses and procedures based on a patient visit with a provider; a bill to the patient and payer is then produced based on that visit. Some electronic medical records (EMR) have more advanced person-level transactional functionality to indicate when a patient may have a gap in care services provided such as being due for a vaccination or screening test. However, this is not driven by a person-level data model. Some EMRs are even more advanced in that they house patient registries in their associated data warehouse; although these registries are person centric and can populate aspects of a data model, they are not population health data models in and of themselves.

Payers or health insurers have some of the most sophisticated data warehouses for healthcare data but are still new to the concept of structuring a person-centric data model. Payers have developed sophisticated data infrastructures and data models around the elements of a claim for healthcare services in performing functions like integrating medical, pharmacy, and enrollment data; aggregating claims data to events such as hospitalizations, readmissions, emergency department visits, and primary and specialty care visits; measuring volume and cost by providers and health systems; becoming efficient at diagnosis coding for risk adjustment; and more. However, these functions have not required or resulted in the robust development of person-centric data models in healthcare organizations.

The population health data model has people at its center. The model is designed to organize observations about people and provide the ability to aggregate person-level observations to both larger subgroups and the entire population (Hennessy et al., 2015). All observations are from the viewpoint of a person. For example, a demographic indicator like Zip Code is linked to a person and defined as the Zip Code where the person lives. An indicator like hospital admissions is attached to a person and can indicate if a person had a hospitalization during a period of time or indicate the number of admissions a person had over a certain period of time. All variables in a population health data model are defined in the context of a person within a period of time. Individuals represent the denominator for measures and metrics in population health analytics, and the population health data model supports this context (Sylvia, 2020).

Multiple Data Sources

Identifying opportunities to improve the health of a defined population requires data inputs from multiple sources including but not limited to administrative medical and pharmacy claims, self-reported health-risk assessment, lab and radiology results, EMRs, and data contextualizing software outputs. The ability to concisely and consistently match patients by ID numbers and the accuracy and reliability of the various types of data and information gathered throughout the analytic process are the most crucial steps required to fully understand the health risks of the defined population (see Chapter 18).

Data sources used in the population health data model should reflect the experiences people have in their encounters not only with the healthcare system but also in their lives as a whole. These experiences are captured in multiple and varied data sources. Data sources include those that usually exist within a healthcare system or health plan related to the delivery of healthcare services and clinical evaluation of patients. Sources also include those that are available outside the healthcare system and are reflective of how individuals live their lives and their interactions with family, communities, digital monitoring tools, and environment. There is some overlap between data sources available inside and outside the healthcare system.

Table 13.1 provides more information about the data sources that are commonly used for a population health data model. Some of these sources are described in greater detail in Section 2 of this textbook. Depending on data availability, the core population health data model usually is initiated with one or two of these data sources; as iterative prototypes are developed, more data sources are added.

Whole Populations

The core PHDM includes all individuals, broadly defined. A health insurer would define the population as anyone who is or ever has been enrolled in one of its health plans, and a provider would include any past or present patient who has been under its care. Geographic terms can also be used to define a population as in the people of an entire county, state, or country, which are also referred to as *macro populations*. The PHDM can be defined by a geographic community or region, members of a health plan, employees, or a provider's catchment area. The health of the population included in the PHDM spans the full spectrum from wellness to illness (Jeffery et al., 2019).

The data model contains a wide variety of indicators about people that allow for subgroupings and comparisons within a population, including important health determinants. For example, subgroupings can be created by age, Zip Code, chronic condition, and other morbidity

Table 13.1 Data Sources Commonly Used in the Population Health Data Model

Category	Description	Key Data Points	Examples of Uses for Population Health Analytics
Enrollment data	Any data used to track enrollment of individuals in health insurance plans or in risk-bearing care-delivery entities like accountable care organizations and clinically integrated networks	Age, gender, race, ethnicity, address, dependent family members, start and stop dates of enrollment	Geomapping Linking information about social determinants of health to census track, Zip Code, county, state Determining impact of length of enrollment on outcomes
Administrative medical claims data (see Chapter 3)	Data points that are submitted on a bill to a payer of healthcare benefits for medical services	Medical diagnoses, date, place, provider, and type of service; procedure performed; type of provider performing the service; billed amount by the provider; paid amount by the payer; and any copayment by the patient	Presence of disease conditions, comorbidities, complications, and sequelae Treatment and clinical pathways Access to care and health disparities Care coordination Value-based care and bundled healthcare services Utilization and cost outcomes
Administrative pharmacy claims data (see Chapter 5)	Data points that are submitted on a bill to a payer of healthcare benefits for medication prescriptions obtained by patients	Fill date, prescribing physician, pharmacy, National Drug Code, drug manufacturer, drug strength, drug form, route of delivery, and packaging; days of supply of the medication; and cost to the payer and patient	Presence and treatment of disease conditions, comorbidities, complications, and sequelae Medication adherence Clinical and quality outcomes
Electronic medical record data (see Chapter 6)	Data points generated in the delivery of healthcare services to patients	Demographics, progress notes, diagnoses, medication prescriptions, vital signs, past and family medical histories, social determinants of health, clinician assessment of health status, care plans, immunizations, laboratory data, and radiology reports	Presence, actual and prescribed treatment of disease conditions, comorbidities, complications, and sequelae Clinical assessment, care planning, and goal setting Applying clinical indictors, family history, social determinants of health and otherwise unobtainable information in population health analytics Clinical and quality outcomes

Laboratory data (see Chapter 6)	Data points representing the collection, testing, and results of laboratory services	Includes any combination of date and type of laboratory test, payer, ordering physician, diagnosis for laboratory test, result, normal range for result, and any special notes	Monitoring of disease condition severity Surveillance of new onset of disease, comorbidities, and complications Clinical and quality outcomes
Health information exchange	Contains data derived through the electronic transfer of health data across stakeholders in a healthcare system for the purpose of improving overall quality of care and health outcomes in a specific region of the United States	Commonly admissions, discharge, and transfer data between inpatient settings of care Less common and widely varying data from administrative claims and enrollment and electronic medical records	Real-time data for inpatient admissions and emergency department visits allow for more accurate risk prediction, monitoring metrics, and ability to intervene during events Integration of clinical data with cost and utilization data
Health-risk assessments	Data derived from tools that are used to assess the health status of individuals through self-reported responses to health-related questions	Common areas of assessment within a health risk assessment include chronic condition and cancer disease risk, family history, nutritional status, fitness level, stress level, mental health status, substance use, safety risks, follow-up of medical conditions, use of preventive health examinations, self-perception of health status, readiness to change risky health behaviors, and absenteeism or lost productivity at work or at school	Assessing and surveilling the health status of populations Gain patient's perspective about his or her own health Disclosure of risky behaviors Developing population health interventions
Personal device monitoring data	Include data from hospital monitoring systems such as cardiac and vital sign devices, remote chronic condition monitoring, and personal devices such as weight scales and blood pressure cuffs, and health-monitoring applications	Large volumes of data representing biological, behavioral, and other self-reported indicators, such as nutritional intake, exercise routines, vital signs, symptom reporting, and chronic condition indicators like blood glucose levels	Assessing and surveilling health status Understanding health behaviors Developing population health interventions and treatment plans Measuring health outcomes
Publicly available data sources	Includes any publicly available data (by both public and private organizations) or reporting on health indictors or outcomes	Data sources contain a variety of information depending on the organization reporting such as incidence and prevalence of disease conditions, cost and utilization impact of health determinants, and quality indicator rates	Support problem identification for population health analytics Comparison of internal population health findings to other sources Setting targets and benchmarks

Reproduced from Sylvia, M. (2020). *The population health data model.* Population Health Management Learning Series. ForestVue Healthcare Solutions.

indicators; health system indicators such as where a person receives care and the types of treatment provided for certain conditions; behavioral indicators like smoking and illicit drug use; and much more. Individuals within whole populations can be segmented according to their risk for adverse events, need for healthcare services, level of illness burden, health disparities, access to healthcare services, care gaps, and more (Lynn, Straube, Bell, Jencks, & Kambic, 2007).

Longitudinal

The core PHDM is longitudinal, facilitating multiple data points over evenly distributed time intervals. The determination of the right time interval depends on the type of healthcare organization, the organization's population health management strategy, the timeliness in which the data sources feeding the PHDM are refreshed with new data, and data warehousing and storage capabilities. Indicators used in population health do not change as frequently as they do for people who are in acute care situations, so it is not as important to have real-time data for the PHDM. At its core, unique observations in the PHDM are usually defined by a unique member in a unique week, month, or quarter.

Determinations are made about the time component for each person-level observational data point placed in the model. Most observations represent the last known value such as the last assigned primary care provider or the most recent. Some observations may be a count over a time period like the number of hospitalizations in the month or in the last year. Other indicators could be selected as the "best" value or the average value like weight (Sylvia, 2020).

Assembling the Core Population Health Data Model

The best way to develop a population health data model is to use *prototyping techniques*. Prototyping techniques using Agile project methods are described in detail in Chapter 12. In addition, the core is built using a use-case–based approach where the interactions between the users of the PHDM and the PHDM structure are defined and the functionality is built incrementally to achieve prescribed goals (see Chapter 12). The PopHealth Troika team triad in combination with information technology staff (see Chapter 31) work together to build the population health data model.

Structure

Table 13.2 is a simplified example of the core structure for a population health data model. In this example, a unique year, month, and patient ID makes up each row of the structure. Each

Table 13.2 Simplified Example of the Core PHDM Structure

Year Month	Person ID	Age	PCP	Weight in lbs	Hospital Admit	#Hospital Admits
202001	0001	34	Dr. B	175	No	0
202001	0002	65	Dr. X	129	Yes	2
202002	0001	35	Dr. B	175	No	0
202002	0002	65	Dr. Y	129	No	0
202003	0001	35	Dr. B	175	No	0

202003	0003	72	Dr. X	156	No	0
202004	0001	35	Dr. B	165	No	0
202004	0003	72	Dr. X	156	Yes	1
202004	0004	47	Dr. C	142	No	0

variable is defined in terms of the person and the time dimension. Age is calculated as of the last day of the month. Patient 0001 became a year older in February 2020. The primary care physician is the last known. The weight is also the last documented weight, which could be from six or more observations before the current month. The weight value changes in a month when a new weight is entered. Hospitalizations are measured in two ways, one in terms of having a hospitalization in the month, and the other in terms of the number of hospitalizations in the month. Each variable in the core structure of the population health data model is defined in terms of the person and the time relationship to the month in which it is measured.

The core data structure for the PHDM is made up of multiple types of data tables all linking at the person level. These connections are made technically through one-to-one and one-to-many person-level connections in data structures. These connections can be made to provide more granular data points about observations in the core structure such as linking the person to a data structure that details individual hospitalizations to find out more data points about each hospitalization or the connections can be made to link completely different information such as associating a person's Zip Code with census data to make a person-level estimate about an economic indicator like salary. **Figure 13.1** displays this example using a simplified structure.

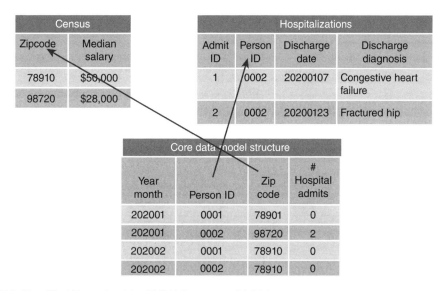

Figure 13.1 Simplified Example of the PHDM Structure with Linkages.

The OMOP Common Data Model

An existing example of a population health data model in practice was developed and maintained by the Observational Health Data Sciences and Informatics (OHDSI) organization. The Observations Medical Outcomes Partnership (OMOP) Common Data Model (CDM) is an open source solution that allows for systematic analysis of observational data and provides a view of what happens to a patient while receiving care. The model exists to collect and organize research data in the form of surveys and registries, electronic healthcare data, and data used to manage payment for healthcare services. For more than a decade, the OMOP community has and continues to develop this model to ensure that research methods can be systematically applied to produce meaningfully comparable and reproduceable results (Blaketer, 2020).

The OMOP CDM is under continuous development with the tools and principles described in this section of use-case–based development, with multiple stakeholder prototype development, using agile project methods. As prototypes are used, tested, and accepted, they are moved into use for research and other purposes. Although the OMOP CDM has a community of users mainly in research, the model could potentially be used as a core beginning structure for developing a population health data model within healthcare organizations.

Figure 13.2 shows a conceptual model of the OMOP CDM. At its core, the model is person centric, housing a vast variety of meaningful data points for unique individuals over discrete time periods of observation. The model identifies patient populations and outcomes and characterizes patients using such parameters

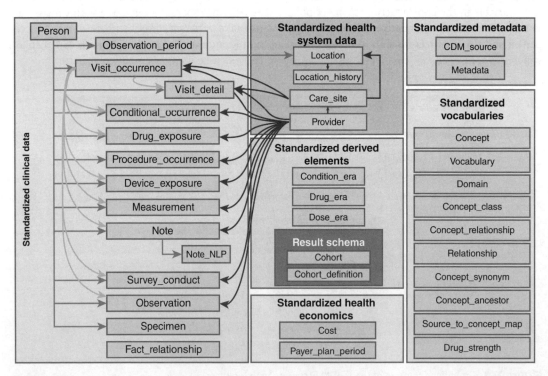

Figure 13.2 The Conceptual Model of the OMOP Common Data Model.

Reich, C., Van Zandt, M., Voss, E. A., Abedtash, H., Dymshyts, D., Philofsky, M., & Torok, D. (2019). *OMOP common data model and standardized vocabularies.* https://www.ohdsi.org/wp-content/uploads/2019/09/OHDSI-Vocabulary-CDM-Tutorial.pdf

as demographics, disease history, healthcare delivery, morbidities, treatments and sequence of treatment, utilization and cost, and more. The model is also used to predict outcome occurrence over time and estimate the effects of intervention (Blaketer, 2020).

To achieve its goals, the OMOP CDM community follows these principles for development:

- Suitability for purpose: The CDM aims to provide data organized in a way optimal for analysis, rather than for the purpose of addressing the operational needs of health care providers or payers.
- Data protection: All data that might jeopardize the identity and protection of patients, such as names, precise birthdays, etc., are limited. Exceptions are possible when the research expressly requires more detailed information, such as precise birth dates for the study of infants.
- Design of domains: The domains are modeled in a person-centric relational data model, where for each record the identity of the person and a date is captured as a minimum. Here, a relational data model is one where the data is represented as a collection of tables linked by primary and foreign keys.
- Rationale for domains: Domains are identified and separately defined in an entity-relationship model if they have an analysis use case (conditions, for example) and the domain has specific attributes that are not otherwise applicable. All other data can be preserved as an observation in the observation table in an entity-attribute-value structure.
- Standardized vocabularies: To standardize the content of those records, the CDM relies on the standardized vocabularies containing all necessary and appropriate corresponding standard healthcare concepts.
- Reuse of existing vocabularies: If possible, these concepts are leveraged from national or industry standardization or vocabulary definition organizations or initiatives, such as the National Library of Medicine, the Department of Veterans Affairs, the Center of Disease Control and Prevention, etc.
- Maintaining source codes: Even though all codes are mapped to the standardized vocabularies, the model also stores the original source code to ensure no information is lost.
- Technology neutrality: The CDM does not require a specific technology. It can be realized in any relational database, such as Oracle, SQL Server, etc., or as SAS analytical datasets.
- Scalability: The CDM is optimized for data processing and computational analysis to accommodate data sources that vary in size, including databases with up to hundreds of millions of persons and billions of clinical observations.
- Backwards compatibility: All changes from previous CDMs are clearly delineated in the github repository (https://github.com/OHDSI/Common DataModel). Older versions of the CDM can be easily created from the current version, and no information is lost that was present previously. (Blaketer, 2020)

Advantages of a Population Health Data Model

There are a multitude of advantages to having a fully operational and automated population health data model that is updated at regular time intervals. Although not exhaustive, this list highlights some of the most important advantages. The population health data model:

- represents all stakeholder input in the business and clinical rules applied to data and the technical execution of the model,
- collects and integrates core data content (internal and external) into a pertinent model within an enterprise data warehouse where it can be linked to other important data models and datamarts, and
- provides ease and efficiency by facilitating:
  - the assembly of sets of patients into populations at will;
  - informative and actionable financial risk analyses;
  - measurement of key clinical, quality, and financial performance metrics in populations;

- automated (on-demand and self-service) internal and external reporting;
- risk prediction and prescription techniques;
- segmentation and targeting algorithms to stratify populations into varying levels of intervention intensity;
- advanced statistical and risk adjustment techniques to key metrics;
- tailored patient care based on population outcomes and metrics;
- analytic techniques to reward healthcare outcomes that meet the Triple Aim of improved healthcare experience, quality, and costs; and
- strategic contractual decisions with affiliates and payers.

Conclusion

A well-designed population health data model using a use-case–based approach, prototyping, and an Agile project-management approach facilitates ease and efficiency for analytic support in all phases of the population health process.

When building a population health data model, it is important for the analyst, clinical, and business leaders to work together to develop a conceptual model that serves as a mechanism for mutual understanding for the clinical and business needs from the model and the technical translation of those needs. In addition, it serves as a way to communicate the structure of the model to various stakeholders.

At its core the population health data model is person centric. It is longitudinal, facilitating multiple person-level data points over evenly distributed time intervals. Observations about people are defined in terms of the time frame used. The population health data model links to other data sources that provide granular details and expanded data points about people.

Study and Discussion Questions

- Compare and contrast the core structure of a population health data model from the perspective of a health insurer, accountable care organization, provider organization, and hospital.

- What are some of the basic data elements required to build a first phase of a population health data model?
- Why is it important to use a prototyping and use-case–based approach to building a population health data model?

Resources and Websites

Observational Health Data Sciences and Informatics (OHDSI): https://www.ohdsi.org/

Patient-Centered Outcomes Research Institute (PCORI) Research network data: https://www .pcori.org/research-results/pcornet%C2%AE -national-patient-centered-clinical-research -network

References

Blaketer, C. (2020). The common data model. The Book of OHDSI. https://ohdsi.github.io/TheBookOfOhdsi/Common DataModel.html#fn20

Hennessy, D. A., Flanagan, W. M., Tanuseputro, P., Bennett, C., Tuna, M., Kopec, J., Wolfson, M. C., &, Manuel, D. G. (2015). The Population Health Model (POHEM): An overview of rationale, methods and applications. *Population Health Metrics*, *13*(24). https://doi.org/10.1186 /s12963-015-0057-x

Jeffery, A. D., Hewner, S., Pruinelli, L., Lekan, D., Lee, M., . . . , Sylvia, M. (2019, April). Risk prediction and segmentation models used in the United States for assessing risk in whole populations: A critical literature review with implications for nurses' role in population health management. *JAMIA Open*, *2*(1), 205–214. https://doi .org/10.1093/jamiaopen/ooy053

Lynn, J., Straube, B. M., Bell, K. M., Jencks, S. F., & Kambic, R. T. (2007, June). Using population segmentation to provide better health care for all: The "bridges to health" model. *Milbank Quarterly*, *85*, 185–208. https://pubmed.ncbi.nlm.nih.gov/17517112/

Reich, C., Van Zandt, M., Voss, E. A., Abedtash, H., Dymshyts, D., Philofsky, M., & Torok, D. (2019, September 15). OMOP common data model and standardized vocabularies. OHDSI. https://www.ohdsi .org/wp-content/uploads/2019/09/OHDSI-Vocabulary -CDM-Tutorial.pdf

Sylvia, M. (2020). The population health data model. Population Health Management Learning Series. ForestVue Healthcare Solutions.

SECTION V

Data Infrastructure

CHAPTER 14

Options for Warehousing Data for Population Health Analytics

Timothy C. Zeddies, MHSA, PhD
Ines Maria Vigil, MD, MPH, MBA

In the world of population health analytics, data is oxygen. Ready access to clean data is critical for success. Yet, it's only the beginning. Any robust population health program transforms that data using a sophisticated data warehousing framework that affords ready access at the member or patient level across all available data stores. Only this type of system can offer the promise of sustainable clinical and financial improvement across a population.

—Raj Lakhanpal, MD, FACEP, Founder and CEO, SpectraMedix

EXECUTIVE SUMMARY

Data warehouses come in many shapes and sizes. Many are developed and readily available in the marketplace. Some are even specifically targeted to store, query, and analyze healthcare data. Because several options exist, the choices are primarily driven by the goals of the analytic effort *and* the constraints of the organization. The goals of the analytic effort can range from simple queries to complex modeling, and each requires a unique database system for support. The constraints of the organization can include a general lack of understanding of the need for and complexity of a database system, budget, availability of resources, and skill set of technical staff. It is important to understand the current and future needs of the organization to select an option for warehousing data that can effectively support population health analytics.

LEARNING OBJECTIVES

At the end of this chapter, the learner will be able to:

1. Describe the ways in which a data warehouse supports population health analytics.
2. Identify the components of a comprehensive data warehouse.
3. Explain alternatives to a comprehensive data warehouse.
4. Identify factors that affect the choice of a data warehouse (or alternative) and its components.
5. Analyze the implications of the choice of data warehouse factors in supporting population health analytics.

Introduction

A data warehouse is a relational database system used to store, query, and analyze the data and to report functions.
                    —Panneerselvam, Liu, & Hill, 2015

A data warehouse environment is built to hold historical data integrated from several source systems, often operational, in an organized manner. Operational systems are built for specific functions and traditionally are not built to serve the purpose of data analytics or data mining. To support the activities of population health analytics, new environments must be created to merge the population health data from these systems and other more traditional data sources into one central area called a *population health data warehouse system* for overall enterprise use. This is best performed using a population health data model.

Various types of data are required for the population health data model. Population health data can be analyzed to help to make decisions on how better to manage the health and well-being of populations. Examples include identifying opportunities to prevent illness, slowing the progression of disease, understanding what interventions work and how well, predicting outcomes, and ultimately informing actions to prevent, mitigate, or reverse disease. How does one manage all the data needed to do this? The solution to support population health data outlined in this chapter is a type of organized data repository—usually a data warehouse in combination with a population health data model. Refer to Chapter 12, "Creating the Population Health Data Model," for information on how a data model can work together with a data warehouse to comprehensively support population health analytics.

To optimize population health analytic performance, data and data contextualizers from many data sources are needed, including but not limited to clinical interaction data (such as from an electronic medical record (EMR)), administrative claims, financial, social, behavioral, and other supplemental or reference data. A common pitfall of many organizations is to gather the population data needed each time a data request is made. Rather than attempting to pull together data from many sources each time a report is needed, it is best practice to bring these data together into some centralized data repository (CDR). When this best practice is followed, analysts can easily and quickly choose and combine needed data to support reporting, analysis, and decision-making. Analysts and organizational leaders can then use the CDR to identify trends, compare data from various reports, or analyze the data in search of correlates or predictors of desired outcomes.

This chapter outlines options for storing the data used for population health analytics. Understanding and storing these data are best supported by the organization's overall data strategy. If no strategy exists, data needs—including those required for population health analysis—tend to get parceled out into several small, noncoherent, and sometimes contradictory data siloes. In addition, knowing and working within the overall data strategy will assist the organization in selecting an option for warehousing population health analytics data that best suits their needs.

Note that in every organization, data already exist in some form, model, and structure. Larger, more established organizations are likely to have established data models and data structures that may resemble an enterprise data warehouse, with (usually) predetermined data integration. Smaller or newer organizations are likely to have multiple data models and structures holding data with little or no data integration. In both cases, it is likely that these models and structures will not fully support population health management and analytics. The goal of this chapter is to outline a roadmap to a more robust, useful, population-oriented data warehouse that can be used to inform healthcare decisions and drive results.

Terminology

Before describing aspects of data warehousing, it is important to understand commonly used terms and their definitions. **Table 14.1** defines commonly used terms in data warehousing.

Table 14.1 Terms and Acronyms Used in Data Warehousing

Source Data	Data contained in transaction and operational systems representing information about patients, clinicians, and encounters, extracted into the data repository
Unstructured Data	Data that do not have a predefined data model or are not organized in a predefined manner
Extraction, Transformation, and Load (ETL)	The process for creating data repositories used in analytics. Data are extracted from the source system and transformed (e.g., normalized, organized, redefined) to conform to reference standards (e.g., all date information are reformatted to a single predefined format for date fields) and loaded into the target data repository for use by analysts.
Metadata	Information about data. For example, for a given instance of data, the data source, date and time of creation, location in the data architecture, and the reference standards used in transformation
Central Data Repository (CDR)	Where the data are kept for use by analysts—for example, a data warehouse
Operational Data Store (ODS)	Used for operational reporting and decision support; designed to integrate data from multiple data sources and one or more production systems
Staging Area	The area in the data warehouse in which the source data are readied for transformation
Interface Layer	Where the data are loaded for users: graphic interfaces, visualization tools, reports

Snowflake. (2020). Data warehousing glossary. https://www.snowflake.com/data-warehousing-glossary/data-warehousing/

Central Data Repositories (CDRs)

Population health analytics requires the use of many types of data—clinical, demographic, financial, and transactional. Data may exist in several different storage types from spreadsheets to operational transaction system databases and existing enterprise data warehouses. These data storage entities are referred to as *data repositories* (commonly *centralized*, which are referred to as CDRs). Typical terms used for data repositories include the following and are listed from least to most complex or comprehensive, with a strong positive correlation to the amount of time and cost to develop:

- data marts,
- relational databases,
- operational data stores,
- enterprise data warehouses,
- early-binding data warehouses,
- late-binding data warehouses, NS
- data lakes.

A comprehensive functional population health analytics program will ultimately require one of the more complex types of CDRs and extensive involvement from information technology (IT) experts. A recent article on big data states, "A data warehouse has both a business and an IT symbiotic relationship: one cannot survive without the other" (Laberge, 2011). IT is needed to implement the CDR project, maintain the data warehouse system, and make needed improvements. IT must not drive the CDR, however, because CDR requirements must be driven by the business to be successful and meet the needs of the organization, particularly as they relate to supporting a population health data infrastructure.

Data Marts, Relational Databases, and Operational Data Stores

Data marts are referred to as independent business and operations-oriented data structures and include simple relational databases and operational data stores. Typically built for a specific department or other subcategory of an organization, data marts aggregate data from multiple existing data sources—for example, clinical, financial, or demographic—that focus on domain-specific information related to a specific department, category, or business function. They are primarily structured and built to support existing business operations or transactions in the form of static reports. For example, an operating room data mart is used in a hospital setting to understand all transactions taking place before, during, and after a surgical procedure. For population health analytic purposes, such aggregated and domain-specific data do not provide the required detail for fully understanding information regarding what happened, what might happen, or how an undesired event or outcome could be prevented.

Because a data mart is usually built for the needs of a specific department, an analysis requiring information from *all* departments cannot be accomplished using this type of warehousing option. Combining information from multiple data marts is cumbersome, time-consuming, and often impossible because of different marts' definitions and values for same or similar data elements (Bresnick, 2013). Data marts, although an effective way of getting to a specific set of information quickly, can often impede a population health approach to assessing a population and developing predictive and prescriptive information to improve health. For instance, a patient may be assigned an identifier in the hospital setting and be assigned a different identifier in an outpatient provider setting. A population health analysis requires the information about a given person to be aggregated across all clinicians and settings, which requires a unique identifier for that person. The effort to create unique patient

identifiers is best performed in a data warehouse in partnership with IT.

Data marts have an advantage in that they meet the needs of individual departments or functional areas. Reporting and analysis of existing operations can be quickly and easily done from a departmental data mart. An advantage of warehousing data in data marts is that the tools are typically easy to use and understood by many analysts. Whether in the presence or absence of an enterprise data warehouse, many departments within an organization choose to elect one or more computer and data-savvy data analysts and data engineers to build one or more data marts, often using a tool such as Microsoft Excel, and extracting data from the operational system. However, it is vital that the data mart be derived from the data warehouse data—or uses the same rules, governed definitions, and source systems used by the data warehouse system. Otherwise, analyses and reports from each system will soon diverge from each other, resulting in useless arguments and even misleading information because of disagreements about definitions or even underlying data. This can also lead to unnecessary costs from significant rework, time, and frustration among analysts and IT staff as the work to bring together already existing but divergent data marts is time-consuming, expensive, and at times impossible.

> The data warehouse architecture may include a data mart, which is an additional layer used to access the data warehouse. Data marts are important for many data warehouses because they customize various groups within an organization. The data within the data mart is generally tailored according to the specific requirements of an organization. (Panneerselvam et al., 2015)

When the needs for analysis are on this smaller scale, a data mart will suffice because it is easier to contain and produces more immediate results. However, because data marts are based on requirements from one department or other smaller business unit, data silos may unintentionally be created that cannot be translated to other business units. In addition, individually built data marts may have interoperability issues with other organizational data and transactional systems (Bresnick, 2013). For these reasons, bringing together many varying data marts can require many more IT, analytic and data engineer resources than is cost-effective and thus is not recommended to support a population health analytics strategy.

Enterprise Data Warehouses

A data warehouse is the entire system for collecting, organizing, holding, and sharing historical data in order to facilitate managing the business beyond the data needed for its day-to-day operations (Inmon, 1999). The data warehouse is a central storehouse of current and historical data, a description of the data, and a system for retrieving that data. A comprehensive data warehouse system will extract, transform, and load (ETL) data from multiple and disparate operational and historical data sources. *Extraction* is the process of reading data from a database and is where the data are collected from multiple sources. *Transformation* is the process of converting the extracted data so that they conform to the data warehouse structure. *Load* is the process of writing the data to the final destination in the data warehouse (Beal, 2020). During this process, the data warehouse system ensures data quality and data security, manages the data dictionary, and provides tools for managing metadata, business intelligence, decision support, and analytics (Inmon, 2005; Ponniah, 2010). A structure and process of data governance should oversee the creation and maintenance of the data warehouse. Refer to Chapter 17, "Assessing Data Quality," for more details on data quality for population health analytics. Data governance, data security, and managing a data dictionary are all important topics and are beyond the scope of this book. Additional resources for these topics, however, have been included in the "Resources and Websites" section at the end of this chapter.

The core function of any data warehouse is storing the information that most closely represents the fundamental operations comprising key business processes of an organization. For example, in most commercial organizations, the key business process and fundamental operation to represent is when a customer purchases a product. Information about the customer, the location of the purchase, the price of the product, and the product itself are used in conducting a full analysis of these processes and would be key data elements when storing the information in a data warehouse. In health care, the key business process and fundamental operation to represent are the transaction of services and interactions between the community, provider, health system, payer, and patient.

A data warehouse that supports population health analytics provides an in-depth, comprehensive view of the key unit of analysis: the interaction of a person with the healthcare system, including the characteristics of each person, each provider and the community in which they receive and access care.

Various types of data are needed from multiple sources: patient (person) information, community information, provider information, and information about transactions. No one source contains *all* this information. An electronic health record or electronic medical record will contain much of the data, but not, for example, costs or many of the characteristics of the patient, community, or provider. Information from other sources is also needed to provide comparisons such as administrative claims data. To facilitate combining and comparing, data from these multiple sources is stored in one data repository—ideally, a fully comprehensive population health data warehouse combined with a population health data model.

Data Warehouse System

As with any system, the main components of a data warehouse system are input, process, output, and feedback (Laberge, 2011).

- *Input* is the capture, collection, or acquisition of all needed data from all source systems.

- *Processing* refers to the conversion, collation, analysis, or storage of input data into a meaningful or useful format in a way that facilitates delivering information needed by the business. The central environment is typically one large database (the CDR). Processing occurs within this environment, transforming and holding the data in a structured and organized manner conforming to the population data model.
- *Output* is the delivery or presentation of processed information to end users, including analysts. The output part of the system transfers data to the end users. Typically, many of the requirements are satisfied by reports or visualizations of outcomes, trends, predictions, and prescriptions.
- *Feedback* refers to the information used to communicate interesting or useful information to the input and processing activities.

The data input step requires high levels of data quality. Data quality can be an issue in any system. When merging disparate systems, it is especially important at the input step to account for and improve the quality of the data. Refer to Chapter 17, "Assessing Data Quality," for more details on data quality for population health analytics.

When merging multiple systems, a data warehouse must pay attention to modeling (also known as *structuring* or *organizing*) the data to

ensure a common vocabulary and flexible design. Often, needed data can be created only in the processing step of the system—from simple calculations such as length of stay to complicated categorizations of people into relative risk categories of short-term or long-term morbidity. These calculations and definitions occur during the initial processing phase. Data from the results of these calculations create facts about clinicians or people and are then fed back into the input stage to be processed and stored in the CDR. Refer to Chapter 12, "Development of a Data Model," and Chapter 13, "The Population Health Data Model," for more details specific to supporting population health analytics.

One chief value of a data warehouse is in having a central common business-wide area for *all* business users to access the same underlying data with common vocabulary and definitions. Furthermore, the process of building the data warehouse often generates a better understanding of what information is needed to support the enterprise purpose (population health management), determine the key questions needing answers, and provide a deep understanding of the data itself.

Figure 14.1 shows a modern healthcare enterprise data warehouse system—encompassing the source data which is made available in the staging environment, also known as a central data repository, along with information about

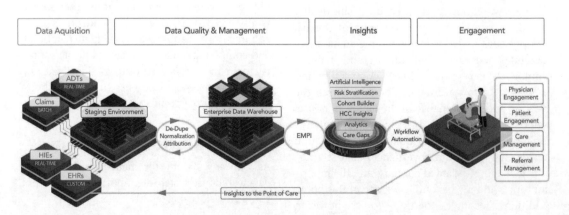

Figure 14.1 Data Warehouse System to Support Population Health Analytics.
Lightbeam Health Solutions. (2021). World class data. https://lightbeamhealth.com/world-class-data

the data used for presentation purposes such as analytics and reporting. Of note, many visual representations of data warehouses are not publicly available or are proprietary. This represents a challenge for learners in this space because many different data warehouse systems exist in the industry but were not available for inclusion in this chapter.

Early- and Late-Binding Data Warehousing

To fit into a traditional enterprise data model, data must undergo massive transformations. Binding is the process of mapping the data in an enterprise data warehouse from source systems to standardized vocabularies. Examples of standardized vocabularies include:

- Logical Observation Identifiers Names and Codes (LOINC), a common terminology for laboratory and clinical observations (LOINC, n.d.);
- Systemized Nomenclature of Medicine (SNOMED), a standardized clinical healthcare terminology (SNOMED, n.d.); and
- RxNorm, a set of normalized names for clinical drugs and drug vocabularies (National Library of Medicine, n.d.).

Binding also maps data to business rules such as length of stay, admissions, transfers, and discharge rules and definitions so it can be brought together for analysis (Sanders, 2018). Because of the rapidly changing environment of population health management, challenges exist when connecting all data elements to predefined rules, as is the case when a database is created or compiled.

Enterprise data warehouses are typically designed from a set of requirements that are inclusive of all known specifications and are modeled into the data warehouse at its onset. Once the design is determined, multiple data sources representing the required elements are extracted, transformed, and loaded into a central space where users can access them. More established data warehouses are often built to support extensive business reporting across a large organization. Business and clinical stakeholders determine the necessary reports, drill downs, and aggregations needed to support key business functions. Ideally, these specifications are known, and the data warehouse is built to support these specifications.

Transformations are key to a usable data warehouse; this is where the binding or connecting happens. Data fields that describe the same thing (such as a patient's name) but are different in content or format across different systems must be brought into conformity with each other. Values must be linked to definitions and calculations must be linked to rules. This is also the stage at which data are governed and new data elements are added to an existing data dictionary.

In a traditional enterprise data warehouse model, the data extractions, transformations, and linkages are designed into a main data repository and remain the same at every refresh of the data. This promotes ease of integration, maintenance, troubleshooting, definitions, and so on, and it promotes speed and ease of reporting.

Traditional or Early Binding

The early-binding method of data warehousing is an option that binds elements to definitions, terms, and rules that rarely change or are unlikely to change—for example, making patient names all conform. In this method, elements that do change are bound only when reports and analyses are created. This option is similar to the traditional data warehouse but attempts to optimize the virtues of that type of option (building the binding for some elements into the basic structure at the initial stages of programming compilation) *when those elements have low volatility*, and delaying binding for those elements, or types of elements, which are more likely to change. The advantage of using the early-binding method is the ease of development and strong technical performance.

An example of an element with low volatility is provider identification, often considered to be the provider's National Provider Identifier, or NPI. The NPI is a 10-digit number code used by the Centers for Medicare and Medicaid Services (CMS) as an administrative simplification standard to identify clinicians who are authorized to provide healthcare services on behalf of CMS (CMS, 2019). This variable is conducive to using an early-binding method because the identifier rarely if ever changes over time.

The promise of the traditional early-binding enterprise data warehouse includes:

- access to all needed data,
- quick access to data, and
- one source of truth.

The reality of the traditional early-binding enterprise data warehouse includes:

- no complete agreement on the "source of truth"—reports continue to differ;
- new data, computations, and reports are constantly being desired;
- adding new data, computations, and reports is hard to do and takes a long time; and
- access to the original data is fast but access to new data is slow.

Data warehouses are not new in the world of computing and information management, but traditional data warehouses tend to be built to optimize transaction data and support operational systems and basic reporting by using structures and processes that are not optimal as the only option when supporting population health analytics. Conflicting requirements between the infrastructure needed to support population health analytics and more traditional uses of data can lead to disagreements within an organization on data architecture, especially if the organization has an older or dated IT infrastructure built to support primarily operations functions of an enterprise, including transactional reporting.

Enterprise data warehouses are typically designed from the top down, with all existing use cases and functionality modeled as part of the original architecture design, usually in one big program. The advantage of this approach is primarily so the data extractions, transformations, and linkages are designed cohesively and remain the same at every refresh of the data. This approach also promotes ease of integration, maintenance, troubleshooting, uniformity across definitions, and much more. This type of design

works best when all the desired data elements, calculations, and transformation are known at the onset of the build.

The disadvantage of this approach and design when used to support population health analytics is that the data required for a given analysis are constantly evolving in that tomorrow may bring a request for a new data element, outcome, transformation, or linkage. If this need to constantly add new data sources has not already been accounted for in the design of the data warehouse, it must be completed as a new requirement and the data warehouse must be recoded and tested repeatedly. This can take an exceptionally long time, limiting the agility of the analysis, often impeding the ability to provide analytics quickly, and ultimately limiting its use for data-driven business decision-making.

Late Binding

Late binding, or delaying the linkages, is best used when the data are unknown and variables and properties of the data are addressed at the run time because the data are considered highly volatile. Note that early binding is used by most compiled programming languages, and late binding is used by most script programming languages (Net-informations.com, 2020).

An example of an element with high volatility is the presence or absence of an acute illness such as influenza and COVID-19. The data element may or may not apply to any given patient; changes in subtype can bring forward a different strain and severity as the disease evolves and can result in acute illness with short duration or complications that can impact chronic illness with a longer duration. This variable is conducive to using a late-binding method because the identifier is subject to constant change over time.

Binding or coupling the data to uniform definitions, formats, and calculations is a necessary step to create a useful CDR. As the goals, rules, and calculations needed for population health management change, the approach to binding data also needs to change. Using a combination of early- and late-binding techniques when constructing the data warehouse can create the advantage of a more flexible and adaptable data infrastructure to support population health analytics. This flexibility can be achieved by applying early-binding techniques to data that is unlikely to change much over time (e.g., date of birth, NPI) and applying late-binding techniques to data that is expected to change over time (e.g., health risk score, social determinants). Building into a workflow the review of new data on a use-by-use basis and determining the approach used to build the data warehouse will provide for a much more flexible and adaptable data infrastructure. On a technical note, this approach involves using object-oriented programming and binding at run time rather than at compilation time.

However, such architecture and processes are quite different from the traditional (early-binding) data warehouse approach that is commonly used in many large organizations. In the instance where a traditional data warehouse exists, one of the first steps to adopting population health management and analytics within an organization will be building an overall data strategy to accommodate responsive solutions to new data, redefining terms or calculations, and perhaps even reviewing the marketplace for more modern warehousing solutions (Sanders, 2018).

Both types of data warehouses require a substantial commitment in time and resources from IT and business leaders and subject matter experts from across the organization. Constructing and testing a traditional data warehouse can take as few as 2 years and as many as 5 years before it can be used to support population health analytics. Although traditional early-binding data warehouse technology is readily available, late-binding data warehouse technology for health care is relatively new. HealthCatalyst (n.d.), SAS (SAS), AWS (n.d.), Microsoft Azure-Apache Hadoop (Azure, n.d.), Snowflake (2020), and Google Cloud (Cloud Healthcare API, n.d.) are the most frequently mentioned organizations in this space. Despite IT resources existing in an organization, it is likely additional expertise will be needed in building data warehouses specifically structured to support population health analytics.

Data Lakes (Unstructured and Unbound)

Data lakes can also be considered repositories of data compiled from multiple source systems and are stored in a lightly or unstructured format. Data transformations, calculations, and connections are performed by the data scientist or analyst at the time of analysis. To compare, in a traditional data warehouse, some source system data may not be loaded into the repository if it appears to have no use in the goals of the warehouse. In a data lake, *all* data are kept, including data not used at all now but that *might* have some use in the future.

In addition, almost any data type can be stored in a data lake. In a data warehouse, the data are usually alphanumeric—letters and numbers. It is difficult to find a way to bind, for example, weblogs, social media output, images, and other nontraditional forms of data. Such instances can be kept in the data lake. This option of data warehousing also requires a different type of architecture. Data warehouses and data marts use typical relational databases at their core; data lakes generally distribute unstructured data across multiple clusters of storage. Apache™ Hadoop® is an example of this type of warehousing (Campbell, 2015).

Data lakes have traditionally been used as storage containers to hold raw data until they are incorporated into the data warehouse. The lack of required binding or connection, early or late, rapidly speeds the ability to use the data housed in data lakes, while at the same time requires special expertise. However, data lakes are growing in their popularity among data scientists for their use in developing machine-learning algorithms and can be used as one of many data sources for more sophisticated and computationally advanced analysis, such as that needed in population health analytics. In addition, the growing interest of health care in using large volume, variety, and velocity of data ("big data") has renewed interest in using data lakes to house these data. The market has responded with several companies offering support in this area, including Apache Hadoop and Microsoft Azure.

Note that when using a data lake approach to warehousing data, the need for expertise in the source systems' data and the ability to transform data as needed, grow and require more specialized technical and business resources than either a data mart or data warehouse. Primarily, data lakes require more and different IT resources than may traditionally exist in an organization. The technologies used in this space are new, and expertise is scarce. Second, the types of analysts required to use these unstructured data are also uncommon; typically, highly skilled data scientists are needed to monitor the output to ensure data quality. Data security, data quality, and access to data are all handled differently than in a traditional data warehouse.

The needs and characteristics of the organization drive needed data and the data warehousing options. Any data can be fitted into a traditional data warehouse structure; any data can be left unstructured in a data lake. However, the poorer the quality and the less knowledge there is about the data, the more time and resources are needed to corral it into a data warehouse. Data already of a high quality and well understood are best suited for a data warehouse; data of dubious quality and poorly understood (assuming they seem useful someday) should perhaps be stored in a data lake for the time being. Refer to Chapter 17, "Assessing Data Quality," for more details on data quality for population health analytics.

Approaches to Data Storage

Traditionally, there are two approaches to store the data in data warehouses: dimensional and normalized. A *dimension* is a category of data, such as people, locations, dates, or diagnoses that are needed to fully describe the unit of analysis. A dimensional data warehouse has the various categories used in health care and needed to support population health analytic functions, along with the facts or values about each category.

The dimensional approach provides an understanding of the data warehouse and

facilitates retrieval of the information. Note that many traditional enterprise data warehouses are built using a dimensional approach. Challenges associated with a dimensional approach lie in properly loading data from different data sources into the data warehouse and in properly modifying the stored data to represent the business context accurately.

In the normalized approach, the tables are grouped together by subject areas under defined data categories. This structure divides the data into entities and creates several tables in the form of relational databases. The process of loading information into the data warehouse is straightforward, although merging of data from different sources is not easy because of the high number of tables involved. Also, users may experience difficulties in accessing information in the tables if they lack precise understanding of the data structure and the data elements housed within.

Structured and Standardized Data

Data management requires an understanding of the differences between structured and standardized data. *Structured data* means that there is a discrete data field or data element for a concept, whereas *standardization* means that there is a commonly used code set or *controlled vocabulary* for expressing the data in each field. Standardized data are structured, but the opposite is not necessarily true. Structured data may or may not be standardized. **Figure 14.2**, "Example of Structured and Standardized Data," shows an example of pharmacy data. Each field or variable in this data set is a structured field in that they are all discrete data elements. The National Drug Code (NDC) field is the only one that is standardized because it uses a standardized code set developed and maintained by the U.S. Food and Drug Administration. Each number in the NDC value has meaning related to the labeler, product, packaging, and manufacturer. This standardization allows the ability

Patient_ID	Prescription_ID	Service_Date	National_Drug_Code	Quantity_Dispensed	Days_Supply	Patient_Paid	Total_Paid
00001C24EE7B06AC	376274477280599	1/23/2020	67544027594	240	30	$10	$10
00001C24EE7B06AC	376444478082254	2/3/2020	51129391601	360	10	$0	$0
00001C24EE7B06AC	376404478575218	3/1/2020	68788062509	30	90	$0	$10
00001C24EE7B06AC	376734479470427	3/12/2020	54868581601	90	90	$0	$50
00001C24EE7B06AC	376604482751046	5/5/2020	62584099190	90	30	$0	$10
00001C24EE7B06AC	376864479453649	5/14/2020	68624000114	60	30	$0	$190

Figure 14.2 Example of Structured and Standardized Data.

Reproduced from Sylvia, M. (2020). Data sources and context. In Population Health Management Learning Series. ForestVue Healthcare Solutions.

to perform tasks like recalling bad medications but also allows a way to uniquely identify medications in population health analytics (Sylvia, 2020).

Advantages and Disadvantages of Various Options for Warehousing Data

Several advantages and disadvantages exist for applying the various options for warehousing population health data. It is important to become familiar with the flexibility and limitations of each to fully understand how to translate the data into insights, trends, and findings used for business and clinical decision-making.

Timing of the Data

Source systems such as EMRs must provide real-time information for clinicians. Thus, their databases are refreshed on a real-time basis, nearly immediately. Other data sources, such as revenue cycle or cost information, may not be updated more frequently than weekly or monthly. Population health analytics is a retrospective, concurrent, and prospective predictive and prescriptive analysis using all source systems. New information

is provided to the CDR whenever the source data are extracted and loaded. Typically, this is no more frequent than daily and may be weekly, monthly, quarterly, or even yearly, depending on the data. However, ingesting new information and performing the necessary transformations or calculations must occur in a timely fashion to be usable by analysts working in population health. This means that the ETL process will start after the end of the business day of the latest performing source system and must finish before the start of the next business day when analysts can then utilize the updated information. Note the various ETL dates for each data source and time any analysis so that the information is the most timely and relevant to the decision it is driving.

Performance of the CDR

Performance can be described as the responsiveness of the CDR to analytic queries calling data. Frequently, utilities such as dashboards or other statistics will use the same CDR as their data source. Utilities that are frequently refreshed can overwhelm the system and cause delays in processing time. Best practice states that analysis should be refreshed at times other than during normal analytic business hours to avoid overloading the system and slowing its responsiveness—although clearly not until the ETL process is completed.

Speed and Cost of Setting up the Data

One of the most fundamental and oppositional forces in warehousing data are speed to data insight and cost to deliver a sustainable data product. In any organization, the speed to insight that data has to offer always appears to take the lead to setting up the data such that it is stable, secure, governed, and flexible. In most organizations, there is a constant trade-off between the following technology and analytic needs:

- data model design,
- need for descriptive reporting,
- need for predictive reporting,
- ease of transactions and maintenance, and
- flexibility and preparation for an unknown future.

All users of data want excellent, high-quality analysis quickly and inexpensively. Among the three desires of good, fast, and cheap, an organization may have any two, but not all three. It is vital to the success of population health analytics to understand the implications of the choices made by requestors when bringing in various data sources, the compelling influence analysts and health care data leaders can have in helping to make these decisions (when and how to ask for forgiveness rather than permission), and communicating the limitations of how and when the insights and conclusions can be used to drive decisions.

To fully support population health analytics, multiple data types are needed, often coming from disparate sources, and usually without common data elements to link them. These data sources, then, must be cleaned, ensured of data quality, transformed to ensure a common data key with another relevant data source, transformed to common data definitions, and placed into categories to allow for ease of analysis. The more complex the data model, the greater the number of sources; the greater the number of transformations needed, the more necessary it is to have a powerful data repository like a data warehouse. Building a data warehouse can be expensive and time-consuming. However, the requirements of today will not be the requirements of tomorrow. Many data and analytics companies are working to solve for this challenge, and the future promises to bring solutions that are less expensive and more timely and have improved data models and governance, thereby avoiding the challenge of having to make trade-offs within an organization. Refer to Chapter 17, "Assessing Data Quality," for more details on data quality for population health analytics.

Considerations for Applying Options to Support Population Health Analytics

All options for warehousing data outlined previously will support some level of population health analytics. In fact, more than one option will likely be required, depending on the data type, their use, whether they are used internally in the organization or shared externally to the organization, and the risk associated with their use to make business or clinical decisions. When choosing one option over another, it is important to consider the type and amount of IT and analytic resources available, the overall organizational data strategy, and the advantages and disadvantages of the various options.

The design of the data warehouse sounds simple—take source data, centralize into a nicely structured database, and run some reports—but it is actually a complicated system. As such, building a data warehouse requires a strong partnership between the business and IT (Schmarzo, 2013). A best practice is to approach building a data warehouse with the goals of both stakeholders in mind, remembering the business purpose while communicating any limitations of the data and their efficient structure and organization.

Contributing to the complexity of this system is the atomic level of the data needed to support population health analytics—typically the lowest possible level and the finest level of data able to be captured from each source system. This is best represented in the example of encounters between patients and their clinicians. A patient can see more than one provider a day, and a provider will care for more than one patient a day. To adequately support population health analytics, each encounter must be captured individually in the data warehouse, even though much of the reporting and analysis occurs at a higher level of aggregation.

Types and Sources of Data Needed

When considering types and sources of data needed to warehouse population health data, consider the question, "What is the fundamental unit of analysis needed to understand a population?" The fundamental unit of health care can be described as a patient possessing various personal characteristics and lifestyle behaviors, living in a community that possesses certain characteristics, having an interaction that possesses several characteristics with a provider who possesses certain characteristics, for a diagnosis (or set of diagnoses) with a said interaction ultimately rendering a cost for a certain amount. The need for clearly identifiable data is also a major differentiator of population health analytics and healthcare research or education. Often in healthcare research or education, data are de-identified as a standard practice. This is not feasible and is contradictory to the goal of population health analytics in its practical use because opportunities are identified to intervene at a patient level. Refer to Chapter 18, "Person Identity Management," for more information on developing analytics at a patient level of detail.

Understanding a population using population health analytics often includes posing questions to the data that combine these fundamental units in various ways and often compare the results over time to some standard or goal, whether it be past, present, or future performance. The world of health care

is one in which a person can interact with their community, a provider (or payer), or a health system at any time on any given day. All information about that interaction and all the ancillary data about that person, provider, payer, or community must be captured and made available to any question about the person, the provider, the payer, the community, or the type of interaction. Section 2, "Data Sources," and Section 3, "Data Contextualizers," indicate the variety of data sources and contextualizers used in population health analytics.

Data must be mapped to a standard data model. Although the population, provider, and interactions data models will differ (because they have different characteristics), each model must contain at least one field that can be universally linked to the others. For example, the transaction data model will have a unique person identifier (which will always link to the same person in any population-centered data set) and a unique provider identifier, which will always link to the same provider in any provider-centric data set.

Thus, population health analytics requires clean, standardized, and often encrypted clinical, financial, demographic, and transaction data about:

- individuals in the population being analyzed (e.g., everyone in the organization, every patient seen by every provider, or every person insured by a financial entity);
- the community in which the population resides (e.g., census tract information, social determinants, places and types of employment, and places and types of access to health care);
- every healthcare provider, personal and institutional (e.g., labs, physicians, hospitals, pharmacies, registries, health plans), in which individuals may interact;
- each encounter between an individual and a healthcare provider (e.g., annual health exam, acute care visit, preventive care visit); and
- each financial transaction and its amount by individual for each encounter (e.g., cost of a

prescribed medication, lab, imaging study, annual health exam, or acute care visit).

These data must be processed to use them simply, accurately, quickly, efficiently, and easily for analytic purposes. More detailed information on each data element is available in Section 2, "Data Sources," and Chapter 18, "Person Identity Management."

Data Infrastructure in Support of Population Health Analytics

Different healthcare sectors have unique data needs—for example:

- IT departments need data to support various business transactions, meet the demand for reports, and exchange data across organizations.
- Clinicians need access to clinical information on their patients and real-time insights in their clinical scheduling and workflows.
- Population health leaders, as the number and type of populations served grow, need data to identify trends and areas of opportunity to improve in a way that is scaled up from population sizes previously managed at the individual level.
- Financial leaders need data to develop new methodologies of financial accounting and effectiveness in an environment of decreasing revenue and increasing healthcare cost.
- Health system leaders undergoing mergers and acquisitions need data to integrate EMRs to a single system to understand the health needs of the communities they serve.
- Managed care companies and other insurers need data to design and test programs to measure the quality and effectiveness of care and optimize best practices for managing care.
- Independent software vendors need access to clinical data to integrate into clinical workflows.

Basic descriptive reporting and analytics that report individual-level indicators, means, proportions, and distributions using historical data is common across all types of industries. Analyzing historical data can be useful in making comparisons and drawing conclusions on what has already occurred in the past. This type of analysis is particularly useful to help form the hypotheses used to develop predictive analytics. For example, basic descriptive reporting and analytics can be applied in a population health analysis when describing the prevalence or the total number of individuals with one or more health conditions in the population of interest during a specific period of time, typically conveyed as a percentage of the population (Chapter 20, "Epidemiologic Methods," provides more information). Most data warehouse architecture can support basic descriptive reporting and analytics because this type of analysis is considered a preliminary stage of data processing using historical data to summarize information.

Depending on the type of data warehouse and the level of detail provided in each data asset, diagnostic analytics can also be supported to perform a more complex analysis in an attempt not only to summarize but also to understand the causes of events and behaviors in the population selected. This type of analytics provides the ability to understand what percentage of the population identified as having one or more diseases also have significant risk factors for the disease, along with any social determinants of health that may have an effect on the health of the selected population. An additional level of detail of data is required to perform diagnostic analytics, and it is important to request that the most granular level of detail of data be provided to support analytics in the data warehouse. See Chapter 2, "Guiding Frameworks for Population Health Analytics," and Chapter 27, "Analytics Supporting Population Health Interventions," for detailed examples of the analytics derived from data from a data warehouse.

Supporting Advanced Population Health Analytic Needs

Additional considerations must be applied when selecting a data warehouse option to support population health analytics, predictive and prescriptive modeling, and machine learning. Refer to Chapter 22, "Predictive and Prescriptive Analytics," and Chapter 23, "Advanced Analytic Methods."

Some level of data standardization must be present to support the development and operationalization of predictive analytic methods used in population health. This is a fundamental shortfall of most traditional data warehouse options, particularly if each data asset is governed differently. It can be an expensive and time-consuming venture to rearchitect all existing data assets to support the ability to perform predictive analytics. The development of a population health data model in conjunction with a flexible data warehouse is the key to supporting predictive and prescriptive analytic capabilities.

Prescriptive analytics require a data warehouse that both normalizes different data assets similarly and is flexible enough to combine, compare, and contrast different data assets and data elements in an unlimited number of ways. This is key to identifying in the data what is effective in achieving a positive health outcome or result. Population health analytics, and specifically prescriptive analytics, requires multivariate analysis of more than one dependent variable, or in the case of prescriptive analytics, more than one outcome variable at a time (see Chapter 19, "Overview of Analytic Methods Used in Population Health"). An unlimited number of queries may be necessary to identify behaviors, treatments, or the timeliness of action taken that help mitigate risk to avoid the undesired event or health outcome. The accuracy and relevance of the prescription primarily depends on the completeness, timeliness, and accuracy of the data in the data warehouse.

A considerable number of decisions must be made when selecting the right data warehouse options to meet the organization's current and future needs. To specifically support population health analytics and the analytic capabilities of descriptive, diagnostic, and predictive and prescriptive analytics, specific questions will need to be asked and addressed, important capabilities will need to be assessed, and a review of existing or planned processes will be required. **Table 14.2** describes the questions to ask, the capabilities to assess, and the processes to review.

Summarizing Designs and Considerations

Table 14.3 summarizes key characteristics and considerations for decision-making around central data repositories.

Table 14.2 Considerations When Choosing A Data Warehouse Option to Support Population Health Analytics

(a)

Questions to Ask and Address	Considerations to Selecting a Data Warehouse Option
Who is the patient population?	■ Accommodate for populations changing over time, with persons entering and exiting the population constantly. ■ Incorporate historical data capture over a period of time historically (typically 5–7 years). ■ Include capabilities to prospectively follow cohorts or subsets of populations over time. ■ Include a group to compare data and results.

(continues)

Table 14.2 **Considerations When Choosing A Data Warehouse Option to Support Population Health Analytics**   *(continued)*

What are all the filters that will be applied or ways that this population will need to be described?	■ Understand from the business all required and optional elements of data that are commonly used to support business decision-making and operations. ■ Decide whether an early-binding or late-binding or combination is the best method to apply for each data element.
What types of data will need to be connected? ■ Clinical, laboratory, pharmacy, administrative claims data, etc. ■ Financial: allowed, paid, incurred but not reported, inpatient, outpatient, emergency department, pharmacy, etc. ■ Self-reported: patient experience, surveys, electronic communications, etc.	■ As the number and types of data increase, the complexity also increases to transform, integrate, and standardize the data, likely requiring a hybrid approach to data warehousing. ■ When a hybrid approach is used, consider the staff and skill sets needed to implement and maintain complete, accurate, and timely data.
What is the most granular level of detail that is needed?	■ Not every data set will need to be structured and governed at the most granular level of detail. ■ If the data are being used to support descriptive or diagnostic types of analytics, then high-level data are sufficient. ■ If the data are being used or are anticipated being used to support predictive or prescriptive analytics, then detail-level data are required.
What are the goals or desired results and how will they be measured?	■ Financial and clinical performance measures source from different data assets and require various data elements to be linked or bound in combinations specific to each goal or desired result. The data warehouse needs to be agile enough to allow for an unlimited number of data element combinations to be made.
What are the time frames within which the stated goals are expected to be achieved?	■ The time frames within which goals are needed to be achieved often drive the data warehouse option selected. ■ Note that often the business need to get to results quickly can often drive the development of a data mart warehouse solution at the risk of not being able to support more advanced analytics in the future. ■ Assess the number of data marts that exist in the organization and compare to other types of warehousing options to understand the current state and to inform the future state. ■ Constructing IT infrastructure to support population health analytics is a marathon, not a race. It is important to set expectations with business leaders on the complexity inherent in warehousing data and the trade-offs between speed and agility when selecting a data warehouse option informed by the business time lines to achieve results. ■ Consider vendor solutions if time lines are aggressive.

What types of reimbursements are expected to cover the costs of the services provided? ■ Fee for service ■ Capitated payment ■ Shared savings risk contract ■ Bundled payments	■ Various payment methods require the tracking and reporting of financial and clinical performance within a specified time. ■ This performance is then tied to a payment; the method of payment can be quite complex and unique to a single provider or provider group. ■ Include the ability to audit the data for completeness, accuracy, and timeliness. ■ Include the ability to produce audit scripts for business analysts to resolve any discrepancies in the data.
Will the information and data be shared internal to the organization? External?	■ Consider the level of role-based access and data security, particularly as it relates to access to and sharing of protected health information (PHI) and the sharing of competitive or antitrust information with competing provider networks. ■ Consider the requirements necessary for data sharing, legal agreements, and the technology needed to house and store data (hosted vs. cloud-based). ■ Consider how the data will be accessed by analysts, business, and clinical leaders.
What clinicians will be included in managing this population? ■ Primary care (MD, NP, RN, PA, CM, UM, social work, etc.) ■ Specialty care (pulmonology, cardiology, infectious disease, etc.) ■ Ancillary care (home health, skilled nursing facility, durable medical equipment, etc.) ■ Vendor-provided care (care management, utilization management, telemonitoring, etc.)	■ Accommodate the multiple ways clinicians can be identified (NPI, facility ID, employee ID, DEA pharmacy identifier). ■ Accommodate the multiple board certifications and specialty certifications that differentiate clinicians from one another. ■ Account for the multiple methods used to group clinicians together to support business use cases (single provider, independent physician association, preferred provider organization, employed, accountable care organization, accountable care network, clinically integrated network) and decide whether these definitions should be standardized and available from the data warehouse to ensure consistency in analytics and reporting across various teams that use these elements. ■ Understand and incorporate standardization across the different code sets that are typically used to designate various clinicians (administrative claims data).

(b)

Capabilities to Assess	Considerations to Selecting a Data Warehouse Option(s)
What technology will best help manage these populations?	■ A patient-centered data model is required to support population health analytics. ■ Methods to structure data ■ Methods to standardize data ■ Methods to integrate data ■ Integration and standardization of multiple data assets
What technology will best help manage the financial payment associated with services provided?	■ Billing and transaction payment system ■ Value-based care and value-based payment system ■ Methods to attribute patients and members to and assign care team members ■ Custom contract payment, incentive payment, and administrative payment system

(continues)

Table 14.2 **Considerations When Choosing A Data Warehouse Option to Support Population Health Analytics** *(continued)*

What technology is needed to integrate the various data sets?	■ Data marts ■ Early binding data warehouse ■ Late binding data warehouse ■ Data lakes ■ Hybrid data warehouse ■ Support of multiple programming languages: C++ (C++, n.d.), Python (Python, n.d.), R Studio (R Studio, n.d.), SAS (SAS, n.d.), SQL (International Organization for Standardization, n.d.-a, n.d.-b), etc. ■ Support of multiple data visualization tools: Alteryx (n.d.), Tableau (n.d.), etc.
What data privacy or security technology is needed to ensure protected health information is secure and that competitive information does not violate antitrust laws?	■ Role-based access to data ■ Security operations systems 1 or 2 (SOC 1 or SOC 2) (Joshi, Thorpe, & Waldron, 2020) ■ Data security, integrity, availability, privacy, and confidentiality (Joshi et al., 2020) ■ Deidentification of patient data and all PHI.
What technology is needed to standardize data elements across various types of patient, provider, community, and payer data as they relate to the provision of healthcare services?	■ Conduct a data source audit ■ Standardize the data sources ■ Standardize the database ■ Interoperability (foundational, structural, semantic) (Joshi et al., 2020). ■ Explore gold standards (HL7, C-CDA, FHIR, etc.) (Joshi et al., 2020).
What are the key data sets that will be utilized across multiple teams, departments, or divisions that work with data?	■ Conduct a data asset audit ■ Conduct a data owner audit (business owner, technical owner) ■ Rank data assets (general use, frequency of use, importance to the business, regulatory, compliance, level of effort to maintain, level of data governance, etc.) ■ Develop a plan for how to work with business and technical data owners to layer these assets into the enterprise data warehouse options
What are the supplemental data sets that will be utilized by specific teams, departments, or divisions that work with specific data?	■ From the list of data assets within the audit, identify the data sets that are infrequently used or are used by only one department. ■ Conduct a data owner audit (business owner, technical owner, governance owner). ■ Develop a plan for how to work with business, technical, and governance data owners to house data, apply data-governance standards, privacy, and security to these assets.
For each key and supplemental data set, what is the optimal structure, content, frequency, and quality needed to support both existing and future use cases?	■ Develop criteria for if and when a supplemental data asset is eligible to be layered into enterprise data warehouse options.

(c)

Processes to Review	Considerations to Selecting a Data Warehouse Option(s)
What are the workflows for and structure of care teams and staff when implementing new technologies?	■ Mobile or tablet enabled ■ Cloud-based storage and processing speed
What are the workflows for and structure of care teams and staff when implementing new data and information?	■ Data visualization, access, sharing ■ Understand how the data processing speed and refresh frequency will affect the results and use of the data. ■ Complete, accurate, and timely data delivery
What are the time frames for when the technology is needed by the business to begin implementing population health analytics and activities? The time frame for when the business needs to achieve results?	■ 1-, 3-, and 5-year strategy ■ 1-, 3-, and 5-year time frame for results ■ Daily, weekly, monthly, quarterly, and annual monitoring and performance reporting ■ Consider vendor solutions if time lines are aggressive
What are the data assets, elements, and data-refresh time frames that are required to effectively report clinical and financial results that are complete, accurate, and timely?	■ Understand how the cadence and sequence of data refreshes affect the performance of the data and their use. ■ Financial and clinical performance measures source from different data assets and require various data elements to be linked or bound in combinations specific to each goal or desired result. The data warehouse needs to be agile enough to allow for an unlimited number of data element combinations to be made. ■ Include the ability to audit the data for completeness, accuracy, and timeliness. ■ Include the ability to produce audit scripts for business analysts to resolve any discrepancies in the data.

Data from Bresnick, J. (2018). Top 5 questions for payers about population health initiatives. https://healthitanalytics.com/news/top-5-questions-for-payers-about-population-health-initiatives; Castilla, F. (2020). What is SOC 1 and SOC 2 compliance? [Blog post]. Nerds Support. https://nerdssupport.com/soc-1-soc-2-compliance; Chick, S. (2017). Defining the components of a modern data warehouse. SQL Chick. https://www.sqlchick.com/entries/2017/1/9/defining-the-components-of-a-modern-data-warehouse-a-glossary; Coombs, B. (2017). 4 steps to standardize your data and get better insights. Oracle Marketing Cloud. https://blogs.oracle.com/marketingcloud/4-steps-to-standardize-your-data-and-get-better-insights; Kuo, M.-H., Sahama, T., Kushniruk, A. W., Borycki, E. M., & Grunwell, D. K. (2014). Health big data analytics: Current perspectives, challenges and potential solutions. *International Journal of Big Data Intelligence, 1*(1/2), 114. https://doi.org/10.1504/ijbdi.2014.063835; Monica, K. (2018). How health data standards support healthcare interoperability. https://ehrintelligence.com/features/how-health-data-standards-support-healthcare-interoperability; Narra, L., Sahama, T., & Stapleton, P. (2015). Clinical data warehousing: A business analytics approach for managing health data. In A. Maeder & J. Warren (Eds.), *Proceedings of the 8th Australian Workshop on Health Informatics and Knowledge Management* (pp. 101–104). https://50years.acs.org.au/content/dam/acs/50-years/journals/crpit/Vol164.pdf

Table 14.3 Summary of Key Characteristics and Considerations for Central Data Repositories

Attribute	Relational Databases	Data Marts	Traditional Data Warehouse	Late-Binding Data Warehouse	Data Lakes
Data	Structured, numerical data, text, and dates organized in a relational model, usually captured from a single source such as a transactional system	Usually one data source	Transactional systems, operational databases, and line of business applications	Transactional systems, operational databases, and line of business applications	Nonrelational and relational from transactional systems, operational databases, and line of business applications, websites, mobile apps, social media, and corporate applications
Schema	Simple relational database	Simple relational database	Designed prior to the data warehouse implementation; difficult to change	In part, designed before implementation; amenable to future changes	Written at the time of analysis
Price and performance	Inexpensive, fast, easy to build, easy to use, hard to change	Inexpensive, easy to use, fast, hard to change	Costliest and slowest to build; fastest query results using higher-cost storage	Faster to build than traditional data warehouses, ability to add new data quickly, fast query results usually using similar storage	Query results getting faster using low-cost storage; dependent on skill of users

Data quality	Solely dependent on the quality of the data source and the database builder—but is organized and consistent	Often unexamined data, depending on skill of builder	Highly curated data that serves as the central version of the truth	Highly curated data that serves as the central version of the truth	Any data that may or may not be curated (e.g., raw data); data curated as needed
Users	Staff, business analysts	Business analysts, regular staff	Business analysts	Business analysts	Data scientists, Data developers, and Business analysts (using curated data)
Analytics	Can be used for analytics, but is not intended for that purpose	Simple business reporting, trends, visualizations	Batch reporting, business intelligence, and visualizations	Batch reporting, Business Intelligence, and visualizations	Machine Learning, Predictive analytics, data discovery, and profiling
Benefits	Provides consistent business data for critical applications	Provides quick and easy-to-use data, lower cost; holds detailed information	Keeps data analysis separate from production systems; brings consistency to disparate data sources	Do not have to make lasting decisions about a data model up front; quickly adapt to new use cases	Ability to store multiple types of data, increased flexibility; supports structured and unstructured data.

Applied Learning: Use Cases

Use Cases for Selecting Various Data Warehouse Options to Support Population Health

Use Case 1: Clinician Group Needing to Connect Data from Multiple Applications

You are the leader of a small organization supporting more than 50 healthcare clinicians. These clinicians reach out to patients having difficulty getting into clinical offices or in complying with postdischarge care and provide home health, transportation, and other personalized services to ensure proper care and follow-up. Over the course of many years, your organization has built or bought various applications to communicate with and provide services to patients, clinicians, and other service organizations such as telehealth visits, online monitoring of vital signs, and direct secure messaging to patients. To support a population health approach using these technologies and workflows, the organization chooses to focus your staff on connecting data across the technologies used. What information do you need? What type of data repository system and architecture will you need to support the effort?

Use Case 2: Care Management Team Needing to Implement Improved Identification of High-Risk Members

You are the leader of an outpatient care management team at a regional insurance company who is finding that the patients identified for care management interventions have either already accessed the care they need or the opportunity to intervene has passed and the patients have readmitted and are in an inpatient care setting. Your company produces many typical financial and operations reports. To succeed at identifying new methods of patient identification and stratification appropriate for outpatient care management services, you would like to implement population health analytics and management. What type of data repository system and architecture will you need to support this new type of analysis to identify the most appropriate patients for outpatient care management? What type of questions would be beneficial to ask to best support the ongoing financial and health outcomes of the patients engaged in the interventions?

Conclusion

Strong analytics are needed to support any type of population health management initiative. Multiple sources of information about patients, clinicians, patient–provider interactions, and patient–provider–payer interactions all need to come together to answer questions of the data, measure results, and report performance over time that is common to population health management activities. The essence of data warehousing is collating the data from multiple data sources, transforming the data so that they are high quality, and ensuring ease of access for use in analytics.

Connecting the data to achieve uniform definitions, linking data elements to all the possible connections for each element, and locating them where analysts can use them in an efficient, less-expensive, and maintainable and improvable way is the hard work of data warehousing. All options—data marts, enterprise data warehouses, and data lakes—have advantages and

disadvantages; there is no one right answer suitable for every organization. Each organization must thoroughly understand its goals and objectives, resources and limitations, and its strategic future to choose a good option—once undertaken, it will be difficult to stop and start over down a different pathway.

When supporting a population health analytics strategy, note that the IT or data analyst or data engineer relies on resources that currently exist within a given organization but that may not be sufficient to build or implement population health analytics. Additional resources of varying skills and expertise will likely be needed to create a data infrastructure to support population health analytics. Chapter 15, "Process for Warehousing Data for Population Health Analytics," will review the steps needed to achieve some of the common processes chosen for data warehousing.

Study and Discussion Questions

- What are the elements needed for any comprehensive data warehouse?
- What are some reasons for choosing or not choosing a comprehensive data warehouse?
- What are some figures and examples in the industry of visual representations of data warehouse architecture?

Resources and Websites

Some useful resources for further details about data warehouses:

Chelico, J. D., Wilcox, A. B., Vawdrey, D. K., & Kuperman, G. J. (2016). Designing a clinical data warehouse architecture to support quality improvement initiatives. AMIA Annual Symposium Proceedings, 381–390. https://www.ncbi.nlm.nih.gov/pmc/articles/PMC5333328/

Inmon, W. (1992). *Building the data warehouse*. Hoboken, NJ: Wiley & Sons.

Inmon, W. (2008). *DW 2.0: The architecture for the next generation of data warehousing*. Amsterdam, Netherlands: Elsevier Press. Inmon wrote the first book, held the first conference (with Arnie Barnett), wrote the first column in a magazine, and was the first to offer classes in data warehousing.

Joshi, A., Thorpe, L., & Waldron, L. (2020). *Population health informatics: Driving evidence-based solutions into practice*. Burlington, MA: Jones & Bartlett Learning. https://www.jblearning.com/catalog/productdetails/9781284103960

Kimball, R. (2014). *Kimball's data warehouse toolkit classics* (3-volume set) (2nd ed.). New York, NY: Wiley & Sons. Ralph Kimball has been a leading visionary in the data warehouse industry since 1982 and is one of today's most internationally well-known speakers, consultants, and teachers on data warehousing. He is regarded as one of the founders of the enterprise data warehouse.

Laberge, R. (2011). *The data warehouse mentor: Practical data warehouse and business intelligence insights*. New York, NY: McGraw-Hill.

Some useful websites for information about data warehouses and options:

Data warehouse vs. data lake vs. data mart: Beyond the RDBMS. (2019, August 28). https://searchdatamanagement.techtarget.com/feature/Beyond-the-RDBMS-Data-warehouse-vs-data-lake-vs-data-mart

Defining the basics of the healthcare big data warehouse. https://hitinfrastructure.com/news/defining-the-basics-of-the-healthcare-big-data-warehouse

healthcatalyst.com: Provides a wealth of essays and white papers about many aspects of data warehousing. Note that the company is a provider of a solution—the late-binding comprehensive data warehouse—so it is not entirely impartial.

Hersh, W. R. (2014). Healthcare data analytics. Chapter 3 in R. E. Hoyt & A. Yoshihashi (Eds.), Health informatics: Practical guide for healthcare and information technology professionals (6th ed.). Pensacola, FL: Lulu.com. https://dmice.ohsu.edu/hersh/hoyt-14-analytics.pdf

What is a data lake? https://aws.amazon.com/big-data/datalakes-and-analytics/what-is-a-data-lake/

References

Alteryx. (n.d.). Free trial. Alteryx. https://www.alteryx.com/designer-trial/free-trial-alteryx?utm_medium=cpc&utm_source=google&utm_campaign=NA_Search_Demgen_Mixed_Brand_New_AO&gclid=CjwKCAiAnvj9BRA4EiwAuUMDf5c7Tl-pDLMwNqJPTWYBy94iEBa3npOrd4G8elq6y6M9PR-xHIKLvBoCCT0QAvD_BwE

AWS. (n.d.). AWS free tier. Amazon. https://aws.amazon.com/free/?all-free-tier.sort-by=item.additionalFields.SortRank&all-free-tier.sort-order=asc

Azure. (n.d.). Run open source analytics with Azure. Microsoft. https://azure.microsoft.com/en-us/free/hdinsight/search/?&ef_id=Cj0KCQjw1qL6BRCmARIsADV9JtbD9Yc5t8lB

w6NrHQKtBwSCBlxHMOjNA2Y2hXpsQmIu0Pvjm
DOXVGkaAsntEALw_wcB:G:s&OCID=AID2100131
_SEM_Cj0KCQjw1qL6BRCmARIsADV9JtbD9Yc5t8lB
w6NrHQKtBwSCBlxHMOjNA2Y2hXpsQmIu0PvjmD

Barlow, S. (2014). 3 approaches to healthcare data warehousing: A comparison. Health Catalyst. https://www.healthcatalyst .com/whitepaper/3-approaches-healthcare-data -warehousing

Barlow, S. (2017). What is the best healthcare data warehouse model? Comparing enterprise data models, independent data marts, and late-binding solutions. https://www .healthcatalyst.com/wp-content/uploads/2014/07/Best -Healthcare-Data-Warehouse-Model.pdf

Beal, V. (2020). Extract, transform, load. Webopedia Definition. https://www.webopedia.com/TERM/E/ETL.html

Bresnick, J. (2013). Understanding the data warehouse model for healthcare analytics. https://healthitanalytics.com/news /understanding-the-data-warehouse-for-healthcare -analytics

Bresnick, J. (2016). Defining the basics of the healthcare big data warehouse. HIT Infrastructure. https://hitinfrastructure .com/news/defining-the-basics-of-the-healthcare-big-data -warehouse

Bresnick, J. (2018). Top 5 questions for payers about population health initiatives. Health IT Analytics. https:// healthitanalytics.com/news/top-5-questions-for-payers -about-population-health-initiatives

C++. (n.d.). ISO–ISO/IEC 14882:2017—Programming languages—C. ISO. https://www.iso.org/standard/68564 .html

Campbell, C. (2015, January 26). Top five differences between data lakes and data warehouses. Blue Granite. https://www.blue-granite.com/blog/bid/402596/top-five -differences-between-data-lakes-and-data-warehouses

Castilla, F. (2020, August 11). What are SOC 1 & SOC 2 reports? Nerds Support. https://nerdssupport.com/soc-1 -soc-2-compliance/

Cloud Healthcare API. (n.d.). Google Cloud. https://cloud .google.com/healthcare

Centers for Medicare and Medicaid Services. (2019). National Provider Identifier standard (NPI). https://www.cms.gov /Regulations-and-Guidance/Administrative-Simplification /NationalProvIdentStand

Coombs, B. (2017). 4 steps to standardize your data and get better insights. Oracle Modern Marketing Blog. https:// blogs.oracle.com/marketingcloud/4-steps-to-standardize -your-data-and-get-better-insights

Data Warehouse Terms. (n.d.). blink. https://blink.ucsd.edu /technology/help-desk/queries/warehouse/terms.html

Data Warehousing Glossary. (n.d.). https://www.1keydata.com /datawarehousing/glossary.html

HealthCatalyst. (n.d.). Healthcare analytics and data warehousing. https://www.healthcatalyst.com/?_bt=3426 56051985&_bk=%2Bhealth%2Bcatalyst&_bm=b&_ bn=g&_bg=71664853151&gclid=Cj0KCQjw1qL6BRC mARIsADV9JtZN5Np2MLSSpVNA2jYR3Z-ERU8cIzm NY5Z5LHZ0bSllcv8_c3a8-hMaAgNmEALw_wcB

LOINC. (n.d.). The international standard for identifying health measurements, observations, and documents. https://loinc.org/

Inmon, W. H. (1999). *Building the operational data store* (2nd ed.). John Wiley & Sons.

Inmon, W. H. (2005, October). *Building the data warehouse* (4th ed.). John Wiley & Sons.

International Organization for Standardization. (n.d.-a). ISO/ IEC 9075-1:2016—Information technology—Database languages—SQL—Part 1: Framework (SQL/Framework). https://www.iso.org/standard/63555.html

International Organization for Standardization. (n.d.-b). ISO—ISO/IEC 9075-2:2016—Information technology— Database languages—SQL—Part 2: Foundation (SQL /Foundation). https://www.iso.org/standard/63556.html

Joshi, A., Thorpe, L., & Waldron, L. (2020). *Population health Informatics: Driving evidence-based solutions into practice.* Jones & Bartlett Learning. https://www .jblearning.com/catalog/productdetails/9781284103960

Kuo, M. H., Sahama, T., Kushniruk, A. W., Borycki, E. M., & Grunwell, D. K. (2014). Health big data analytics: Current perspectives, challenges and potential solutions. International *Journal of Big Data Intelligence, 1*(1–2), 114. https://www.inderscience.com/info/inarticle.php?artid =63835

Laberge, R. (2011). *The data warehouse mentor: Practical data warehouse and business intelligence insights.* McGraw-Hill.

Lightbeam Health Solutions. (2021). World class data. https:// lightbeamhealth.com/world-class-data/

Monica, K. (2018). How health data standards support healthcare interoperability. EHR Intelligence. https:// ehrintelligence.com/features/how-health-data-standards -support-healthcare-interoperability

Narra, L., Sahama, T., & Stapleton, P. (2015). Clinical data warehousing: A business analytics approach for managing health data. Pp. 101–104 in A. Maeder & J. Warren (Eds.), *Proceedings of the 8th Australian Workshop on Health Informatics and Knowledge Management.* https://50years .acs.org.au/content/dam/acs/50-years/journals/crpit /Vol164.pdf

National Library of Medicine. (n.d.). RxNorm. https://www .nlm.nih.gov/research/umls/rxnorm/index.html

Net-informations.com. (2020). Difference between early binding and late binding. http://net-informations.com /faq/oops/binding.htm

Panneerselvam, J., Liu, L., & Hill, R. (2015). Requirements and Challenges for Big Data Architectures. In B. Akhgar, G. B. Saathoff, H. R. Arabnia, R. Hill, A. Staniforth, & P. S. Bayerl (Eds.), *Application of big data for national security* (pp. 131–139). Elsevier. https://doi.org/10.1016/b978-0 -12-801967-2.00009-4

Ponniah, P. (2010). *Data warehousing fundamentals for IT professionals.* John Wiley & Sons. http://business .baylor.edu/gina_green/teaching/dw/spr16/Ponniah_data -warehousing-fundamentals-for-it-professionalsSecond Edition.pdf

Python. (n.d.). Compound data types. https://www.python .org/

R Studio. (n.d.). We think serious data science should be done in code. https://rstudio.com/

Rainer, R. K., Prince, B., & Cegielski, C. (2014). Data and knowledge management. In *Introduction to information systems* (5th ed.). John Wiley & Sons.

Sanders, D. (2018). The late binding data warehouse technical overview. HealthCatalyst. https://www.healthcatalyst.com /late-binding-data-warehouse-explained/

SAS. (n.d.). SAS: Analytics, artificial intelligence and data management. https://www.sas.com/en_us/home.html

Schmarzo, B. (2013). Data warehousing 101. Dell Technologies. https://infocus.delltechnologies.com/william_schmarzo /data-warehousing-101/

SNOMED. (n.d.). SNOMED International. http://www.snomed .org/

Snowflake. (2020). Data warehousing glossary. https:// www.snowflake.com/data-warehousing-glossary/data -warehousing/

SQL Chick. (2017). Defining the components of a modern data warehouse. https://www.sqlchick.com/entries/2017/1/9 /defining-the-components-of-a-modern-data-warehouse -a-glossary

Sylvia, M. (2020). Data sources and context. In Population Health Management Learning Series. ForestVue Healthcare Solutions.

Tableau Software. (n.d.). Changing the way you think about data. The Silicon Review. https://thesiliconreview.com /magazine/profile/tableau-software-changing-the-way -you-think-about-data

CHAPTER 15

Process for Warehousing Data for Population Health Analytics

Ines Maria Vigil, MD, MPH, MBA

A basic principle of data processing teaches the folly of trying to maintain independent files in synchronism.

—Frederick P. Brooks Jr.

EXECUTIVE SUMMARY

To build a data warehouse, several existing processes ensure the data received are complete, accurate, timely, and usable for transactions, reporting, and analytics. Many of these processes center around the ETL: *extraction* (copying of raw data), *transformation* (cleansing and optimizing the data), and *loading* (getting data into the warehouse) process of making data available for use by the organization (GeeksforGeeks, n.d.). Best practices are available to optimize these processes to support a majority of healthcare reporting, analytics, and management. In addition, commercially available products are available that automate several processes involved in building a data warehouse and should be considered.

To build a data warehouse that supports population health analytics and management requires additional processes to ensure the data can be used to identify opportunities to achieve the goals of the Triple Aim (Institute for Healthcare Improvement, n.d.). These processes include the development of a population health data model, a population health framework, and an understanding of the business needs to effectively support end users of population health analytics.

This chapter describes the basic processes associated with building an effective data warehouse and the additional processes that are required to effectively support population health analytics and management. Resolving data inconsistencies, denormalizing or normalizing data, and inserting frequently used calculations and definitions are critical aspects of the process for warehousing data to support population health analytics. This chapter also includes best practices to incorporate and pitfalls to avoid when optimizing the data to support a population health data model, framework, and the maturation of analytics over time.

LEARNING OBJECTIVES

At the end of this chapter, the learner will be able to:

1. Identify the basic processes involved in warehousing data.
2. Define the processes and techniques used to develop and maintain a data warehouse that are specific to supporting population health analytics.
3. Demonstrate awareness of the best practices and pitfalls of not preparing the data to support population health analytics.
4. Apply the knowledge of processes used to warehouse population health data using multiple case studies.

Introduction

Processes to warehouse data for use in population health analytics requires the collection and management of data from various sources, is often large in volume, requires electronic storage and updating, and is most often used by analysts to query and analyze data to identify meaningful insight for clinicians and business leaders. The processes used to support population health data differ in both the basic elements and techniques from those that support more traditional healthcare transaction processing and reporting. These differences are important to understand because the use cases for processing and reporting on transactions, such as claims paid to providers rendering healthcare services to patients, are much different than providing a targeted list of patients to a provider to mitigate a health risk factor or prevent the occurrence of a complication of an existing disease, such as a heart attack in a patient with cardiovascular disease.

Incorporating the basic elements and techniques to support population health analytics and management into an existing or new data warehouse brings forward the opportunity to make data accessible to providers, payers, and business leaders who can use the insights gleaned from analyzing population and patient-level data to inform clinical care, operational, and business decisions. Population health data analytics identifies trends and patterns to assist clinicians and business leaders to reduce unnecessary care and improve both the quality of care delivered and the patient's experience in seeking healthcare services. The potential for value that this work brings forward is exponential and can often serve to differentiate effective from ineffective healthcare organizations.

This chapter outlines the basic elements and techniques used to develop and support population health analytics, how these compare to more traditional processes for warehousing data, and best practices for storing and managing population health data.

Traditional and Population Health Processes to Warehousing Data

As discussed in previous chapters, a data warehouse is a database system used to store, query, analyze, and report current and historical data (Panneerselvam, Liu, & Hill, 2015), and it can include the entire system of data to facilitate not only day-to-day operations of the business but also population health analytics (Inmon, 1999).

A few key best practice processes underscore the development of a data warehouse and are described in the following section.

Understanding What the Data Will Be Used to Achieve

Warehousing data to support day-to-day transaction reporting and analysis is quite different from using data to support outcomes improvement and population health analytics (Johnson, n.d.). Different decisions are made regarding data warehouse architecture; types of data sources; *extract*, *transfer*, and *load* (ETL) versus *extract*, *load*, and *transfer* (ELT); and requirements for what is included in the metadata. Understanding the organization's needs and uses will drive many of these decisions and must be carefully considered before embarking on the process to build a data warehouse (Sarad, n.d.).

An example of an organizational need for a population health supported data warehouse includes outcomes-based reporting and analytics. Applying this example, a population health outcome can be an improvement in hemoglobin A1c (HbA1c) test results over time in patients with diabetes undergoing treatment with a new brand medication. Tests for this population may be performed as many as four times a year, and each test result may be the same or different from the one before. To determine an improvement in the HbA1c lab test result of patients with diabetes over time as a result of taking the new brand medication, the following must occur:

1. Patients receiving the new brand medication must be identified and tracked prospectively over time to identify those patients in the treatment group.
2. Patient-level detail data, such as age, gender, type of diabetes, other medications must be linked to each patient to support a cohort analysis.
3. The presence or absence of one or more lab test results—in this case, the HbA1c—is needed to establish a link to the desired outcome (an improved test result over time).
4. Test results must be linked in sequence of earliest to most recent date of service to establish an accurate time line of results.
5. Patients who would otherwise have qualified to receive the new brand medication but did not or patients who currently receive another medication such as a generic substitute are also needed to establish an adequate comparison group, along with their respective 1 through 4 data.

Other outcomes of interest may include:

6. Diabetes severity of illness such as comorbidities and complications.

7. Social determinants of health such as lack of transportation, unsafe conditions at home, and lack of caregiver support.

Many of the data elements required to produce the use case just described are replicated in population health analytics, meaning that much of the data in the example above can be loaded into the data warehouse using the same process and applied repeatedly across several different disease states and patient health outcomes.

Building on the previous example, a financial outcome in population health can be the comparison of cost between a brand versus generic medication to treat patients with diabetes. When comparing costs to derive financial impact, it is important to ensure there is no difference between the two medications' efficacy or intended use. All the same tracking of information and level of detail is needed as previously, with the addition of the total cost of each medication over time. The cost comparison of two seemingly similar medications may appear to be straightforward, however, many elements of data must be considered when applying a population health approach. Additional information to connect to the patients include the following:

1. the cost of medications to the health plan, including manufacture rebates and pharmacy benefit manager discounts;
2. the cost of the medications to patients, including all copays, cost shares, deductibles, and discounts associated with mail order or 90-day bulk supply; and
3. the amortized cost of any devices or supplies associated with administration of the medications such as insulin pumps, glucometers, syringes, and blood glucose test strips.

Other costs of interest may include:

4. the cost of the lab tests, accounting for frequency of testing; and
5. the costs associated with clinical services needed to treat diabetes by level of severity, including use of emergency department services, hospital admission, hospital readmission, and elective procedures.

Again, many of the data elements required for reporting financial outcomes are reproducible across different medications and lab tests and can be connected to one or more common health conditions. The availability of care pathways that outline an organization's standards of clinical care and progression of common diseases is critical to providing the clinical and business acumen needed to effectively build a data warehouse flexible enough to support a variety of population health analytic capabilities and functions. Ultimately, an understanding of the patients and their outcomes of interest, whether outcomes are health or financial, will guide the architectural design differently than if outcomes are not of interest.

Building a Data Warehouse Model That Fits the Needs of the Organization

The traditional process of building a data warehouse uses a dimensional or normalized model. A dimensional model is a structured database that allows for the querying and analysis of various data. It typically comprises *dimensions*, or information of interest to the business, and *facts*, or numeric values to count (Kimball, 2013). In a normalized or relational model, columns of data or *attributes* and tables of data or *relations* are organized to ensure that the relationship between the attributes and relations are understood and prescribed in the model. The goal of normalization is to minimize any redesign in the data warehouse structure when adding new or updated data and to make the data more usable for analysts, clinicians, and business leaders (Date, 1999, 2015). Supporting population health analytics requires further advancement of these fundamental processes. Dimensional models tend to be more denormalized and optimized for data querying, and normalized models are optimized for de-duplicating and updating varying types of data. The need for both processes to support population health analytics has brought forward a new process for modeling data called *dimension normalization* or *snowflaking*. Snowflaking can also be referred to as a starlike schema and primarily comprise dimensions surrounding a fact table (Golfarelli & Rizzi, 2009). The primary challenge associated with adoption of this best practice process for warehousing data is best summarized by the Kimball Group:

> [Teams] often struggle on the first step. They struggle to articulate the business process, [defined as] an event or activity [that] generates or collects metrics. . . .
>
> Determining your organization's core business processes is critical to establishing your overall framework of dimensional models. The easiest way to determine these processes is by listening to the business users. (Kimball & Ross, 2013)

Population health analytics requires a warehousing process that allows for a variety of data assets to be related to one another; whose results of interest by the business can be easily queried, analyzed and filtered; where inputs and outputs require monitoring; and where data can be compared and contrasted by drilling into it across several business processes. In combination with an expectation for data that are complete, accurate, and timely, this is an unlimited number of simultaneous queries and a processing speed to match make for a challenge that many organizations may not be able to deliver on. It is important to evaluate the organization's commitment, information technology capabilities, skill sets, and availability of subject matter experts before embarking on a build solution. However, many companies exist that can provide these processes and capabilities, including the Snowflake cloud data platform (Snowflake, n.d.; Qlik, n.d.; and Actian, n.d.).

Applying a Standard Set of Tools and Techniques

Several tools and techniques are available to warehouse data. Applying a standard set of tools and techniques is important to ensure process consistency, standardization, and maximized interoperability. Organizational commitment to the tools and techniques that follow is critical to successfully developing capabilities to deploy population health analytics and are described in greater detail in other chapters in this book as indicated:

- ETL versus ELT,
- data asset management (DAM) framework and ownership,
- data asset maturity model,
- population health data model (refer to Chapter 13, "The Population Health Data Model"),
- analytics maturity model (refer to Chapter 2, "Guiding Frameworks for Population Health Analytics"), and
- a team and use-case approach (refer to Chapter 31, "Building a Team Culture for Population Health," and Chapter 12, "Creating the Population Health Data Model," respectively).

ETL versus ELT

This technology is an important element of a data warehouse and is defined across the industry as an easy-to-use graphical interface to quickly map data between the source data and target applications and databases (GeeksforGeeks, n.d.). This enables the data to be processed or converted into a format meaningful for analytic use. **Figure 15.1** illustrates a common structure for the ETL process.

Alternatively, another process is emerging and is popular among data scientists working in population health analytics that utilizes the same ETL process and reverses the process steps of loading and transformation (ELT). The ELT process is also gaining more use among companies that offer cloud-based database services featuring high-speed data processing. The following advantages of ELT are summarized best by Sarad (n.d.) and make this process ideal for supporting population health analytics when data scientists are leading the process to transform the data for business use.

- The business acumen and transformation logic are not needed before being loaded into

the data warehouse (however, these data may be unstructured or semistructured).

- The data made available in the data warehouse are only that needed (all other data in the data warehouse may be unstructured or semistructured).
- The ELT method is best for handling unstructured data and for data warehouses with high data-processing speed (see **Figure 15.2**).

Some of the challenges associated with data moving into the data warehouse before being transformed include poor data quality, large volumes that exceed capacity, data that appear similar but are different, data that are undefined, or data that are invalid. These challenges render the data inappropriate for immediate use. The potential advantages and disadvantages of using an ETL versus ELT approach requires a deep understanding of how each data warehousing process works, the use of data lakes versus more traditional data warehouse options, and a commitment to a standard process to which the organization must adhere.

Data Asset Management (DAM) Framework and Ownership

Data asset management refers to the processes associated with the following (Inmon, 2005; Ponniah, 2010):

- inventory and assessment of the various data sources;
- mapping of the data from the trusted source of truth to the various applications and end-user analytic tools and technologies;
- documentation of all program code required to meet the business objectives;
- development of testing and audit code scripts to ensure the data are complete, accurate, and timely;
- documentation of the metadata, including business use cases, data variable title, source data, and data assets; and
- explanations of the rationale behind any calculations, including length of stay, admit, discharge, and transfer rules, average length of stay, and 30-day all-cause readmissions.

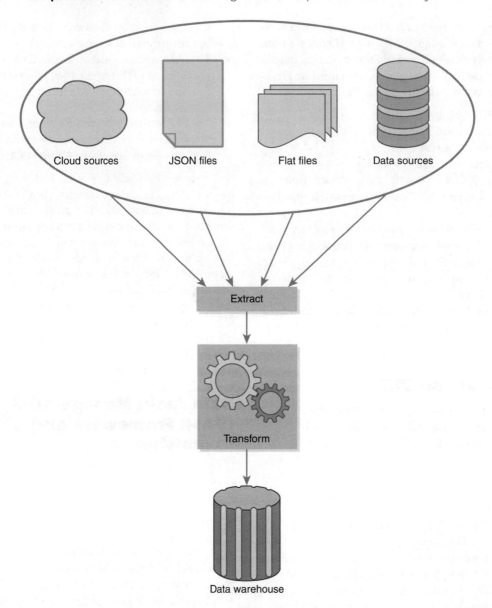

Figure 15.1 ETL Process in a Data Warehouse.

It is important for the organization to select both an owner for and process of data asset management. Presence of a single data asset management owner allows for the development of a data-management strategy with a focus on optimizing data to drive clinical and business value. In addition, having a data asset management strategy and framework is critical to the success of population health analytics, accuracy of predictive and prescriptive modeling, and the robustness of a population health data model. Where population health initiatives are combined with incentive payments or risk-share payments, having a data asset management process can be

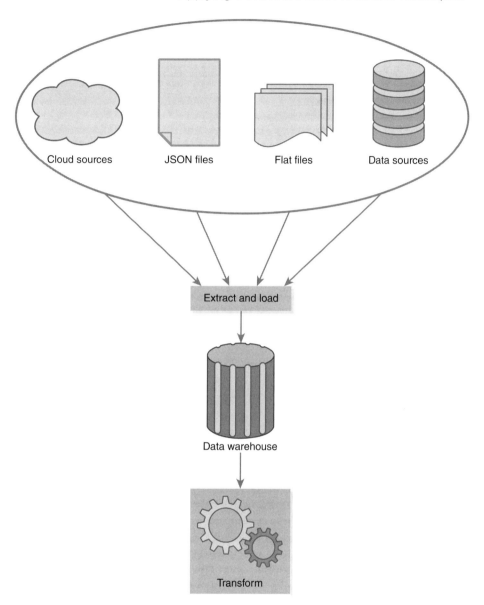

Figure 15.2 ELT Process in a Data Warehouse.

the difference between profit gain or loss. The following quote summarizes the importance of managing the maturity of data assets over time for organizations:

> In every industry sector, companies are in a race to accumulate unique data assets and develop data exploitation methods. Those companies [that] do not see data as a core enterprise asset or are unable to develop a Data Asset Management Strategy are in danger of decline—and ultimately risk business failure. (Tebbutt, 2017)

Presence of a data asset management strategy and framework and a single organizational owner of the strategy enables data governance, data quality, data architecture, and the data operations process to be linked to one or more of the organization's overall value streams. **Figure 15.3** shows an example of a framework to manage data assets.

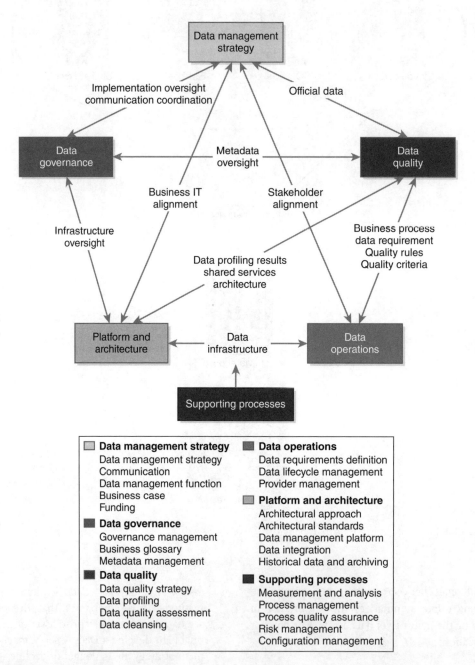

Figure 15.3 Example of a Data Asset Management Framework.

Data from Tebbutt, N. (2017). Data Asset Management (DAM). *The Digital Transformation People.* https://www.thedigitaltransformationpeople.com/channels/delivery/data-asset-management-dam/

Without a framework, applying the information the organization needs to drive decision-making and strategy development cannot be successful. The volume of healthcare data alone will quickly overwhelm an organization and has the potential to consistently introduce fragmented and inconsistent data with no inherent value.

Data Asset Maturity Model

Over time, data can be perceived to lose its applicable value to the organization. It is common practice that once the inherent known value of a data asset is captured by the clinical and business teams in an organization, it is deemed no longer useful. However, this view can create limitations for the organization over time and, when combined with a never-ending pursuit of new and unique data assets, can be an expensive and time-consuming venture. The introduction of a data asset maturity model, specifically one aimed at supporting population health initiatives and analytics, can leverage existing data assets to continue to drive value over time and be used as building blocks for a population health data model. In addition, as the volume and complexity of healthcare data grow, the need for a model to update, refresh, and mature data over time becomes increasingly important to a healthcare organization's overall success and budget.

Absence of a data asset maturity model can increase risk of making decisions on bad or inaccurate data and can increase this risk over time—to the point that data can quickly become untrustworthy and harmful to patient care. Note that it takes only one or two bad experiences with data for a clinical or business leader to reject all data within an organization. To avoid this scenario, introduce a process to govern data to ensure a high level of quality before maturing it for use by the organization.

Regarding the maturity of data assets over time, there is a significant difference between data that are made available for ad hoc queries and data that are optimized for population health analytics. **Figure 15.4** illustrates a

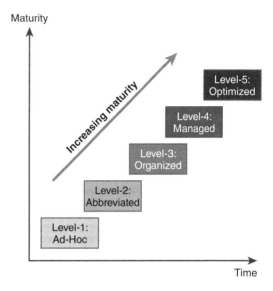

Figure 15.4 Data Asset Maturity Model.

Data from Tebbutt, N. (2017). Data Asset Management (DAM). *The Digital Transformation People.* https://www.thedigitaltransformationpeople.com/channels/delivery/data-asset-management-dam/

stepwise approach to increasing the maturity of data assets over time and the categories of maturity that are applicable to healthcare data and considered to be a best practice when applying these data to a population health data model to support analytics (Tebbutt, 2017).

Population Health Data Model

Whether an ETL or an ELT process of warehousing data is selected, it is critical to have a population health data model in place to support population health analytics. A population health data model forms a 360-degree view of the patient by connecting multiple varying data sets to create a wealth of information that can be used to describe a patient's unique characteristics, and addresses the following (Sylvia, 2020):

- includes data elements to be stored,
- defines the way in which data elements will be stored,
- describes the relationships between data elements,

- outlines any limitations or constraints, and
- describes the intended meaning and use of each data element in the metadata.

During the transformation process, often occurring in the area where data are staged, a population health data model can be layered onto multiple data assets (transformed or loaded) to collate and analyze and to be stored in a way that closely follows clinical and business healthcare workflows. In 2011, Laberge referred to the need to process, transform, and hold data that are structured and organized to conform to a population data model (Laberge, 2011). Best practices in population health analytics require a population health data model, along with the development of analytic prototypes, be present to ensure accuracy of information, be consistent in results over time, and be able to track small and large populations prospectively in time and compare the information to historical results. More detailed information on the population health data model and the development of analytic prototypes can be found in Section IV, "Creating the Population Health Data Model."

Analytics Maturity Model

To effectively support both advanced analytics and population health analytics, the data warehouse must include an assessment of the maturity of the current analytics model and a commitment to or a defined path toward maturing analytics over time (HIMSS, n.d.-a, HIMSS, n.d.-b). Analytics can only advance as quickly as the process to warehouse data, the degree to which data assets are managed and matured, and the robustness of a population health data model will allow. Any inefficiencies in any of the tools, techniques, and processes discussed in this chapter can negatively impact an organization's ability to perform more advanced levels of analytics, such as predictive and prescriptive analytics and personalized medicine.

Chapter 2 of this textbook describes the healthcare analytics adoption mode, which is a well-known way to quantify and measure maturity of analytic capabilities within healthcare organizations. Another similar maturity model is the HIMSS Analytics Maturity Model (HIMSS Analytics, n.d.-b), which recommends an eight-stage analytics maturity model that allows organizations to measure their internal process and technology capabilities and is designed to provide a stepwise approach to maturing analytics, enabling increasingly advanced levels of analysis to be performed over time. Following the steps in either model provides a way for any organization to move from fragmented point solutions to enabling predictive and prescriptive analysis. Including a process for data analytics maturity is an important aspect of any organization's data analytics strategy and road map.

A Team and Use-Case Approach

Significant input from clinical and business leaders is required to model and mature data and is typically performed in collaboration with a team of data scientists, engineers, and analysts using a use-case–based approach. Use-case modeling is typically used to document requirements for clinical, business, and technical leaders. In this method, use cases are structured to clearly articulate the way in which data will be used and the value inherent to the organization. The process of maturing data to develop use-case models for population health requires a multidisciplinary team of clinical and business subject matter experts, data stewards, analysts, data engineers, data architects, business intelligence developers, and the data warehousing team. A multidisciplinary team is needed to ensure leadership commitment to a data warehouse architecture and process focused on achieving outcomes improvement using a population health and data-driven method. Of note, not every resource previously listed will be required to be dedicated to the process for warehousing data. Whereas certain information technology and data architecture team members may be 100% dedicated, other members of the team will need to allocate time in sprints where and when their expertise is a critical function to ensure success. This requires significant planning and scheduling, and it is best achieved with the presence of a data strategy and road map, thus the need for a centralized data strategy and strategy owner. Building the right team, providing ongoing training and educational support, and having a commitment of the organization to outcomes and data-driven decision-making are all requirements to building a successful population health analytics capability (Johnson, 2017).

For more information on the benefits of team collaboration to support population health analytics, refer to Chapter 31, "Building a Team Culture for Population Health." For more information on the applying a use-case based approach, refer to Chapter 12, "Development of a Data Model" (Yue, Briand, & Labiche, 2009).

Best Practices and Pitfalls to Avoid with Processes Used to Warehouse Data

Warehousing data can be a daunting and expensive venture if not organized through a set of standardized processes. In addition, warehousing data to support advanced and population health analytics is a relatively new field with lots of room for interpretation and therefore misinterpretation. The following paragraphs highlight some best practices and pitfalls to avoid when selecting the process to warehouse data.

Best practices and pitfalls to avoid for selecting processes to support population health analytics can be summarized by an organization's *three C's: capabilities, commitment,* and *cause.* Understanding the organization's capabilities, commitment, and cause before embarking on building or buying what can be expensive tools and processes can be the difference between success and failure. Knowing an organization's capabilities can help build a path toward a strong foundation to support both

operations and analytic functions by acknowledging and closing technical and operational process gaps. This is an important step; if skipped, it can lead to an inability to produce complete, accurate, and timely data that are understood by users and trusted for use in clinical and business decision-making.

Having an organization's commitment is also a best practice; if the commitment is unknown or not present, then this lack can create barriers along the way. Nothing prevents a population health analytics strategy from moving forward faster than a change in leadership direction or commitment. This is often represented when needed clinical, business, and technical resources are pulled away to other, higher priority work. Planning and working with the business to ensure the availability and skill sets of critical team members can ensure the right people are included in the process when needed. It is also important to continuously educate leaders about the value population health analytics can create for an organization, the need to build capabilities and mature those capabilities over time, and what may be needed from them and others to succeed.

Cause is likely the most important element to understand, defined as the reasons an organization has selected to pursue population health analytics. What problem or problems is the organization is trying to solve? How would population health analytics help it solve these problems? What does success look like for the leaders asking for this capability to exist? Who is needed or available to participate, and what is needed to achieve success? Knowing the answers to these questions up-front can save time and expense and prevent significant frustration along the way.

Developing a data warehouse and the processes to support one does not happen overnight. It is a multiyear project that requires the development of a road map and continuous funding to ensure the right capabilities are made available and that the map is trusted, understood, and used by the organization to drive results. Wherever the start, do not underestimate the impact the processes selected can have on results.

Special Considerations When Selecting Processes for Warehousing Data

Table 15.1 provides a checklist to ensure a successful data warehousing process.

It is important to conduct the assessment that follows before building a data warehouse to support population health analytics. If completion of this assessment shows the organization has more "No" than "Yes" responses, it is highly recommended to pursue a vendor option. If, on the other hand, the organization discovers more "Yes" than "No" responses, the next step would be to perform an assessment of the quality of each of the preceding processes to identify and close any gaps. Consider running three small example projects through this process to test each one and understand the strengths and weaknesses of each step in each process. This will prepare your organization to tackle any challenges that may arise in one or more steps along the journey toward effectively supporting population health analytics.

Table 15.1 Considerations When Choosing a Process to Warehouse Data to Support Population Health Analytics

YES	NO	Data Warehouse—Process Assessment
		Does the organization understand how the data will be used? Use Case 1.
		Does the organization understand how the data will be used? Use Case 2.
		Does the organization understand how the data will be used? Use Case 3.
		Does a process exist to copy raw data (extract)?
		Does a process exist to cleanse and optimize data (transform)?
		Does a process exist to load raw or cleansed or optimized data (load)?
		Does a data warehouse model exist (dimensional or relational)?
		Does the organization understand the core business processes and workflows it uses—as they relate to Use Case 1?
		Does the organization document its core business processes and workflows—as they relate to Use Case 1?
		Does the organization understand its core business processes and workflows—as they relate to Use Case 2?
		Does the organization document its core business processes and workflows—as they relate to Use Case 2?
		Does the organization understand its core business processes and workflows—as they relate to Use Case 3?
		Does the organization document its core business processes and workflows—as they relate to Use Case 3?
		Does a process to manage data assets exist (DAM framework)?
		Does an owner of data asset and management exist?
		Does a process exist to mature data assets over time (DAM model)?

		Does a population health data model exist?
		Does a process exist to mature data analytics over time (analytics maturity model)?
		Does a process exist to develop a prototype for one or more of the preceding use cases?
		Does a process exist to advance a prototype into production for one or more of the preceding use cases?
		Does a process exist to identify and secure the technical resources needed?
		Do the technical resources have the skill sets to be successful?
		Are the technical resources available to participate?
		Does a process exist to identify and secure the clinical resources needed?
		Do the clinical resources have the skill sets to be successful?
		Are the clinical resources available to participate?
		Does a process exist to identify and secure the business resources needed?
		Do the business resources have the skill sets to be successful?
		Are the business resources available to participate?
		Overall, does the organization have the processes needed to build a data warehouse to support population health analytics (capabilities)?
		Overall, does the organization understand the need for and value of a data warehouse to support population health analytics (commitment)?
		Overall, is the organization committed to building a data warehouse that supports population health analytics (cause)?

Applied Learning: Use Cases

Use Case 1: A Disease Registry for Heart Failure

You are the chief information officer at a regional hospital. Your hospital is pursuing a strategy to improve the health outcomes of patients with advanced heart failure and is asking for technology that would support both the monitoring of patients over time and support advanced analytics using population health methods. What are some foundational process elements needed to successfully support this effort with technology?

Use Case 2: A Target List of Patients Identified to Benefit from One or More Clinical Programs or Interventions

You are part of a team of enterprise data architects who have been asked to assist the medical team at a large national health plan to standardize the process to identify health plan members for one or more of the clinical programs or interventions offered by their network of providers across the country. Luckily, you discover that many of the clinical programs and interventions can be categorized into a handful of similar or like programs. If the goal is to be able to provide clinicians a monthly list of their patients who qualify to participate and would benefit from a given program or intervention, then what would be the data warehouse process needed to achieve this goal?

Conclusion

Critical elements to the process of warehousing data successfully include the need to understand the initiatives and goals of the business, develop processes to support outcomes-based population health analytics and reporting, seek out existing care pathways for common health conditions or seek out clinical and business subject matter experts who can assist in the warehouse design process, select a data model and warehouse that meets the needs of the organization, and ensure universal commitment to a standard set of tools and techniques. Tackling just one element can be daunting for any organization, and a data analytics strategy is needed to ensure progress and realize value along the way.

For those organizations that currently have parts and pieces of the needed elements, the strategy can include identifying and removing any process gaps to optimize existing solutions. For organizations that have not yet embarked on this journey, several options exist where these processes are included in the cost of purchasing a vendor data warehouse solution and should be considered, particularly when the preceding elements cannot be implemented with confidence. Regardless of the organization's current state, specific processes must be in place before embarking on performing population health analytics. When available, the value that population health analytics can bring to an organization can be exponential.

Study and Discussion Questions

- How does the process for warehousing healthcare data to support population health analytics compare to other industries such as banking or retail?

- What advances in data warehousing tools and techniques can be applied to health care in the future?
- What are some of the pitfalls of not having a data process strategy, framework, or model?

Resources and Websites

Barlow, S. (2014). Comparing the three major approaches to healthcare data warehousing: A deep dive review [White paper]. https://www.healthcatalyst.com/whitepaper/3-approaches-healthcare-data-warehousing

Rizi, S. A. M., & Roudsari, A. (2013). Development of a public health reporting data warehouse: Lessons learned. PubMed.gov. https://pubmed.ncbi.nlm.nih.gov/23920680/

References

Actian. (n.d.). Hybrid data management, integration & analytics. https://www.actian.com/

Barlow, S. (2014, November 19). Comparing the three major approaches to healthcare data warehousing: A deep dive review [White paper]. HealthCatalyst. https://www.health catalyst.com/whitepaper/3-approaches-healthcare-data -warehousing

Das, A. (2020). An overview of ETL and ELT architecture. SQLShack.

Date, C. J. (1999). *An introduction to database systems*. Addison-Wesley.

Date, C. J. (2015, Deccember 21). The new relational database dictionary: Terms, concepts, and examples [Online]. O'Reilly Media, Inc. https://www.oreilly.com/library/view /the-new-relational/9781491951729

GeeksforGeeks. (n.d.). ETL process in data warehouse. https:// www.geeksforgeeks.org/etl-process-in-data-warehouse/

Golfarelli, M., & Rizzi, S. (2009). Data warehouse design, modern principles and methodologies. (pp. 1–42, 420–423). McGraw-Hill.

HIMSS Analytics. (n.d.-a). Adoption model for analytics maturity. https://www.himssanalytics.org/amam

HIMSS Analytics. (n.d.-b). *Data content instruction Grow your data content to improve operational, clinical and financial performance*. (n.d.). www.himssanalytics.org /amam

Inmon, W. H. (1999). *Building the operational data store* (2nd ed.). John Wiley & Sons.

Inmon, W. H. (2005, October). *Building the data warehouse* (4th ed.). Hoboken, NJ: John Wiley & Sons.

Institute for Healthcare Improvement. (n.d.). The IHI Triple Aim Initiative. http://www.ihi.org/Engage/Initiatives/Triple Aim/Pages/default.aspx

Johnson, P. (n.d.). A 5-step guide for successful healthcare data warehouse operations. Healthcare Enterprise Data Warehouse (EDW).

Johnson, P. (2017, April 11). A 5-step guide for successful healthcare data warehouse operations. HealthCatalyst. https://www.healthcatalyst.com/a-five-step-guide-to -healthcare-data-warehouse-operations

Kimball, R., & Ross, M. (2013). The data warehouse toolkit: The definitive guide to dimensional modeling (3rd ed.). John Wiley & Sons.

Laberge, R. (2011). *The data warehouse mentor: Practical data warehouse and business intelligence insights*. McGraw-Hill.

Panneerselvam, J., Liu, L., & Hill, R. (2015). Requirements and challenges for big data architectures. Chapter 9, pp. 131–139, in *Application of big data for national security*. Elsevier Press. https://doi.org/10.1016/b978-0-12-801967 -2.00009-4

Ponniah, P. (2010). *Data warehousing fundamentals for IT professionals*. John Wiley & Sons. http://business .baylor.edu/gina_green/teaching/dw/spr16/Ponniah_data -warehousing-fundamentals-for-it-professionalsSecond Edition.pdf

Qlik. (n.d.). Qlik business intelligence: Data analytics & data integration. https://www.qlik.com/us/

Sarad. (n.d.). Data warehouse best practices: 6 factors to consider in 2020. https://hevodata.com/blog/data -warehouse-best-practices/

Snowflake. (n.d.). Try the cloud data platform. https:// www.snowflake.com/try-the-cloud-data-platform/?_bt =335521178155&_bk=snowflake&_bm=e&_bn=g&_bg =64805047909&utm_medium=search&utm_source =adwords&utm_campaign=NA-Branded&utm_adgroup =NA-Branded Snowflake-Computing-Exact RSA&utm _term=snowflake&utm_region=NA&gclid=CjwKCAjwh 472BRAGEiwAvHVfGlkwFZVvDBeMTe6Qpiem3 -E76gvjA_qGHNAXmt5G8z91naQ1fvif9RoCp2MQAvD _BwE

Sylvia, M. (2020). The population health data model. Population Health Management Learning Series. ForestVue Healthcare Solutions.

Tebbutt, N. (2017). Data asset management (DAM). *The Digital Transformation People*. https://www.thedigital transformationpeople.com/channels/delivery/data-asset -management-dam/

Yue, T., Briand, L. C., & Labiche, Y. (2009). A use case modeling approach to facilitate the transition towards analysis models: Concepts and empirical evaluation. In A. Schürr & B. Selic. (Eds.), *Model driven engineering languages and systems* (MODELS 2009). *Lecture notes in computer science*, *5795*. Springer. https://doi.org/10.1007/978-3 -642-04425-0_37

CHAPTER 16

Data Management and Preparation

Martha Sylvia, PhD, MBA, RN

Give me six hours to chop down a tree and I will spend the first four sharpening the axe.

—Abraham Lincoln

EXECUTIVE SUMMARY

The majority of data used for population health analytics is secondary data, meaning that the data were collected for a purpose other than understanding the health determinants and outcomes for populations and subgroupings. As such, these data are rarely, if ever, in a state to answer questions of interest or identify opportunities for improving population experience, health, and cost. The lack of data management is detrimental to a successful population health process and can result in the following challenges:

- poor data quality,
- data-management processes maintained differently across multiple systems,
- missed opportunities to understand populations and intervene,
- lost opportunities to improve quality and health outcomes,
- added inefficiency and waste in delivering healthcare interventions, and
- higher costs and utilization.

It is important to ensure data are readied for population health analytics, and this requirement is upstream of many of the processes outlined in this textbook. The adage "garbage in, garbage out" defines the challenge of poor data management and preparation and must not be ignored or underestimated when performing population health analytics (Quinion, 2005).

LEARNING OBJECTIVES

At the end of this chapter, the learner will be able to:

1. Describe the advantages of an organizational master data management strategy.
2. Determine a repeatable process for approaching data preparation.
3. Identify methods for managing commonly identified issues in data preparation.

Introduction

Creating reports, data visualizations, and running sophisticated statistical and machine-learning data models are often considered the fun part of performing population health analytics. However, considerable time is necessary to prepare data for these types of analyses. For any question in population health analytics answered with data, it is common to spend 60% to 70% of the time preparing data, 10% of the time running the analysis, and the remaining time interpreting the results. The process becomes less cumbersome when data-preparation techniques are automated and a part of data operational processes.

Ideally, healthcare organizations have a *master data management* (MDM) program in place that ensures data integrity from all source systems with data fed from these manicured source systems to a population health data model. In this ideal world, analysts and all stakeholders need not worry about data-integrity issues impacting population health analyses. However, this is not usually the case for population health analytics.

This chapter provides a broad overview of the ideal state of data preparation in which robust MDM processes are in place to manage person-level identification, linking of data files, and scouring of data fields for acceptable levels of data error. Absent MDM, the chapter describes a process to handle some of the most commonly found errors in data when performing population health analyses, offers methods for managing these issues, and encourages placing these methods into automated processes.

Master Data Management

Master data encompasses all of the data within a healthcare organization that are at the core of business operations and interactions with patients and affects its ability to achieve success in patient outcomes and costs. Master data are those that are crucial to the ability of healthcare organizations to remain financially viable in the delivery of healthcare services. A health insurer needs to understand the volume and cost of healthcare services to understand how to contract with providers, hospitals, and pharmacies to obtain cost-efficient rates when paying for healthcare services. Hospitals need to understand the costs of delivering medical, surgical, laboratory, radiological, and other services in order to charge competitive rates for their services. In value-based arrangements, providers need to understand whether individual patients have received required services and whether goals for quality and outcomes are met.

An MDM program for population health goes beyond the ability to manage organizational data for transactional purposes in healthcare organizations. It means managing data for the purposes of robust analytics at the person level, culminating in the population health data model (see Chapter 13, "The Population Health Data Model"). Because MDM in population health requires higher aspirations than MDM for organizational transactions, most healthcare organizations have not reached this level of analytic maturity for population health. Nonetheless, it is important to understand MDM and this ideal method of handling data preparation.

Master data management is a

> technology-enabled discipline in which business and IT work together to ensure the uniformity, accuracy, stewardship, semantic consistency, and accountability of the enterprise's official shared master data assets. Master data [are] the consistent and uniform set of identifiers and extended attributes that describe the core entities of the enterprise, including customers, prospects, citizens, suppliers, sites, hierarchies, and chart of accounts. (Gartner, 2020)

In health care, the patient-centric variant of MDM is considered to be the combination of the Enterprise Master Patient Index (see Chapter 18, "Person Identity Management"), along with interoperability certification standards such as Health Level Seven (see Chapter 14, "Options for Warehousing Data for Population Health Analytics," and Chapter 15, "Process for Warehousing Data for Population Health Analytics"); both are imperative to accomplishing goals of interoperability for the electronic medical record (EMR) (Berson & Dubov, 2011).

In health care, master data are divided into two types: *identity data* (e.g., patients, providers, location, sites of care) and *reference data*, which includes common linkable vocabulary like *International Classification of Diseases, 10th Revision, Clinical Management* (ICD-10-CM); diagnosis-related groups; the Systemized Nomenclature of Medicine; Logical Observation Identifiers Names and Codes; and RxNorm) (see Chapter 14, "Options for Warehousing Data for Population Health Analytics"). The crux of MDM is the ability to link identifying data and reference data across multiple systems (Eliason, Burke, & Hess, 2014).

The approach and definitions of master data management in health care are intricately linked to the transactions in health care and are focused on meeting the standards of interoperability and ensuring safe and efficient healthcare delivery.

This is a first step in ensuring well-prepared data for population health analytics, but it is not enough. Preparation of data for population health analytics requires a data-management strategy executed in a repeatable way in a production environment within the data warehouse. Absent this ability, the analyst will need to deploy strategies for preparing data that combine manual processes with varying levels of automation. The next section lays out a process for preparing data absent an MDM strategy for population health purposes.

An Analytic Approach to Data Preparation

Preparing data requires a methodical and repeatable approach that, once put into place, can be used as a way to approach any analysis used to answer questions of interest for population health. **Figure 16.1** is used to frame the process

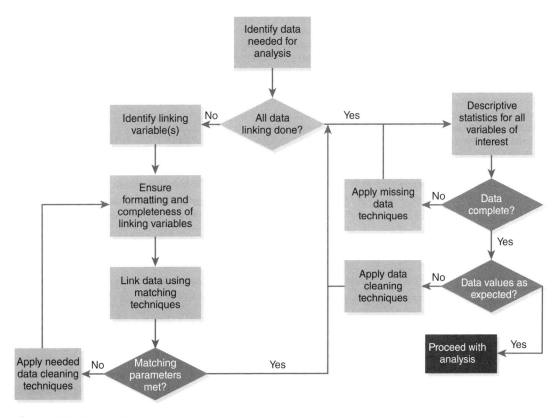

Figure 16.1 Process for Preparing Data for Analysis.

that will be laid out in this chapter. The process begins with identifying the data files and variables that will be required for the analysis. This step requires thought about how the question is posed and ensuring that there is clarity among all stakeholders surrounding the details of the posed question and data needed. For instance, the question of "What is the readmission rate for hospital X?" requires a different data set and structure than "What is the readmission rate for the population of people with congestive heart failure?" The first question has hospital admissions as a denominator, and the second question has people as a denominator. It is helpful at this point to write out the numerators and denominators for the final desired answer as well as envision with stakeholders how the final reported results will be presented.

Data Linking

In the next step of the process it is necessary to determine whether it is necessary to link data files. If that is necessary, then analyses must be undertaken to ensure optimal data linking. Data in population health are most often and best linked at the person level. First, an assessment must be made to ensure that the person-level identifiers have the same definition and format. If the data files are determined to be linked using the same person-level identifiers, then the files must be checked to ensure that the same formatting is used, that identification numbers are not missing for any individuals, and that there are not unexpected duplicate identification numbers in any of the files. Methods for accomplishing data checks using exploratory techniques are described in the next section, and the setting of tolerance parameters is discussed in a subsequent section of this chapter.

Identification numbers are often not the same if the data files do not come from the same source system. For instance, people are identified with a different set of identification numbers in the EMR than they are in payer claims data. If the identifiers are not the same, then the first step is to determine whether there is a file structure in either source system that links the two types of identification numbers. For instance, the EMR usually collects the health insurance identification number for payment services. This number would have to be included in the person-level data set from the EMR in order to link to the health insurer's data file.

Unfortunately, identifiers to exact match two data sources are not always available. In one example, accountable care organizations (ACOs) receive Medicare administrative claims data from the Centers for Medicare and Medicaid Services (CMS) that contain a Medicare Beneficiary Identifier (MBI). In one ACO, the EMR of one of the provider organizations did not collect the MBI and therefore the administrative claims data from CMS could not be directly linked to the EMR data. This linkage is critical to be able to relate aspects of clinical care and outcomes to cost and utilization. In this case, patient-matching techniques such as deterministic and probabilistic matching must be undertaken. Chapter 18, "Person Identity Management," provides more detail about these methods.

Files for data linking may not always be connected at the person level. Occasionally, files must be linked at the event level or they are linked to understand descriptions for certain coding. For instance, a person-level file may contain a date for the most recent hospitalization in a time period, but to find out more information about the hospitalization, the file may have to be linked to another file that contains detailed information about the hospitalization such as diagnoses, procedures, and length of stay. In the latter case, codes are often provided for indicators like an ICD-10-CM code for a diagnosis or a hierarchical condition category code for a grouper assignment. These code sets need to be linked to descriptions of the codes so that clinical meaning can be gleaned. Ideally, each healthcare organization maintains up-to-date descriptions for all used code sets and updates them regularly in the data warehouse.

Preparing Variables of Interest

Data preparation focuses on the variables of interest once the data-linking procedures are executed, files are linked as expected, and the population contains the anticipated number of people. Variables of interest are examined using exploratory and descriptive analysis techniques. These techniques are explored in more detail in Chapter 19, "Overview of Analytic Methods Used in Population Health Management." Here we provide an example of data examination using graphical displays and measures of dispersion. Percentages will be reviewed and suggestions for managing commonly identified issues will be provided.

Assessing for Missing Data

The first round of exploration focuses on understanding the amount of data missing for each field. This can be accomplished for continuous variables by looking at the distribution of the values or by looking at the percentage occurrence for each value of the variables of interest. Categorical and dichotomous variables are examined by looking at the percentage occurrence for each value. Although a simple sorting of the data can reveal the amount of missing values, using exploratory techniques can determine the impact of missing values in relationship to other values for each variable, and voluminous data are better examined.

Table 16.1 shows an example of reviewing a categorical variable for missing data. In this figure, the categorical race data collected within an EMR was examined for 65,677 unique patients with 7.6% of the values missing. **Figure 16.2** displays a histogram of the distribution of values for the continuous variable of *age* for a population of 15,100 people. There are 14,337 values in the data, with values missing for 763 people.

Addressing Missing Data

The first step in addressing missing data is to determine whether the percentage of missing values are worth the resources to investigate further.

Table 16.1 Determining Missing Values for Categorical Variable

Race	Count
American Indian or Alaska Native	140
Asian	1,409
Black or African American	13,672
Caucasian	43,623
Multiracial	80
Other	1,753
Pacific Islander	13
Missing	4,986

It is helpful to set a threshold of tolerance for missing data. The thresholds may depend on the importance of the variable to the question being asked of the data and the source of the data. For instance, when the purpose of the analysis is to determine risk-adjusted payment, variables used for risk adjustment are critical to the analysis and come from the organization's source systems. Because the organization's financial viability is dependent on accurate risk adjustment and source systems are within its control, it is often worth the effort to further address missing data. Alternatively, if the data are used to deliver information to patients that is not tailored or specific to a need, then it may not be worth the effort to address the missing data.

The first step to address missing data is to ensure that the data actually are missing or whether some glitch in the way the data were retrieved missed some values. If access to the source system is available, then a few randomly selected missing values can be checked against the user interface of the system to see if the data exist from that viewpoint. If the data are not in the source system, then a decision can be made to seek the data from another system. For instance, date of birth and age usually exist in more than one source system.

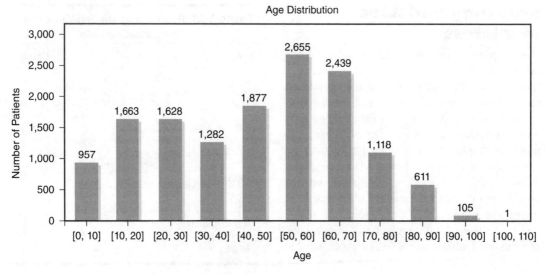

Figure 16.2 Determining Missing Values for Continuous Variable.

If the data are missing and cannot be supplemented, two commonly used options remain. The first is to perform the analysis with the limited number of people for whom the values on the variable are complete. This often happens with laboratory results; for instance, it is common to have missing hemoglobin A1c (HbA1c) values for an entire population of patients with diabetes. Many quality measures use two-part measurements for this reason. Using this example, the first part of a quality measurement for diabetes measures the percentage of people who have an HbA1c test during the measurement period and the second part of the measure determines the percent of people with a value for HbA1c within a desirable range.

Depending on the type of analysis, missing data may be supplemented with the mean or median for the distribution of values of the missing variable. This is necessary when performing advanced multivariate statistical techniques that require complete data for all fields used in the analysis, otherwise the analysis will remove entire rows (rows represent people in most population health analyses) of data from the analysis where any value is missing. When the desire is to keep all rows of data in the analysis, missing values may be imputed by using the mean or median. In the case of a categorical variable,

a decision can be made as to the most suitable way to impute values based on the meaning of the variable to the analysis. For instance, the case of the missing race data in Figure 16.2, the missing data may be given a value of "other," which in the case of exploring health disparities is the best way to ensure that inaccurate conclusions are minimized.

Assessing for Erroneous Data

Erroneous, unexpected data values come in multiple varieties. They are seen more often with manually entered clinical and electronic medical record data but can occur in any source data. Common types are described as follow:

- *Values outside of an expected range* occur when a value is more than an outlier. Outliers represent valid values for a variable and occur within an expected range. However, when values fall outside of the entire expected range, including outliers, they are considered erroneous. For example, the low end of a measure of body mass index (BMI) even considering outliers should not be below 14. Any values below this level are considered out of an expected range.

- *Invalid values* are those that should not occur. This often happens when values for measures are entered in a different unit of measurement than what should be entered. For example, weight in pounds is entered in kilograms and lab data obtained for urine is entered in the unit of measure in which it would be expressed if it were obtained from blood and vice versa.

- *Unexpected value combinations* occur when the value for one variable is not congruent with the value on another variable. For example, a male cannot be pregnant, an infant cannot weigh 100 pounds, and a person with no

hospitalizations should not have a value of greater than zero for the length of hospital stay (Sylvia, 2018).

Addressing Erroneous Data

The best way to assess for these types of errors is similar to that used for understanding missing data. Ranges, distributions, percentages, and measures of dispersion are calculated for each variable and combinations of variables of interest. **Table 16.2** shows an example of the

Table 16.2 Determining Erroneous Data

Blood Pressure Variables	Number of Occurrences	Unique People	Smallest Value	Largest Value	Example of Value
BP systolic (SYS)	295,444	28,679	0	986	
BP diastolic (DIA)	295,327	28,543	0	852	
BP SYS 2	37,689	10,060	0	410	
BP DIA 2	37,603	9,987	0	700	
BP SRC ELEC	32,961	6,578	—	—	Electronic
BP SITE 1	7,433	1,335	—	—	Left arm
BP SYS 3	7,213	1,897	0	454	
BP DIA 3	7,167	1,786	0	146	
BP SITE 2	1,525	876	—	—	Left arm
BP SYS L ARM	407	356	82	220	
BP DIA L ARM	405	354	0	770	
BP SYS R ARM	396	275	88	218	
BP DIA R ARM	396	289	0	130	
BP SYS STAND	359	276	68	200	
BP DIA STAND	358	257	0	114	
BP SITE 3	286	178	—	—	Left arm
BP SYS SUP R	277	168	30	213	
BP DIA SUP R	276	178	38	821	
BP DIA SIT	198	126	0	141	
BP SYS SIT	198	135	72	210	

complexity involved in creating a quality measure for blood pressure. All data fields in an EMR representing any type of blood pressure were queried from the EMR database. Table 16.2 shows all of the variables that indicated some type of blood pressure measurement, the number of occurrences for that variable, the number of unique people with a value, and the smallest and largest values for the variable. Diastolic blood pressure is an important measure of the heart's health between beating and measures below 40 or above 200 are incompatible with life. The known diastolic blood pressure variables are highlighted in gray in Table 16.2, and it is clear that most have erroneous values based on the smallest and highest values.

Addressing erroneous errors in data requires reviewing data and decision-making with the entire population health team that includes the clinical lead, business lead, and analyst lead (Chapter 31, "Building a Team Culture for Population Health"). Indicators derived from clinical data such as blood pressure, diagnoses, assessment results, and more require the expertise of the clinician for interpretation. In Table 16.2, a clinician who worked at the site where the EMR data was generated needed to work with the analyst to determine which variables were appropriate to use for the diastolic reading and the appropriate range for removing erroneous values. Decisions regarding administrative data such as provider and network attribution, price differentials for services, and benefit structure require the expertise of the business leader.

Figure 16.3 shows the distribution of the diastolic blood pressure readings after the decision was made to use only the variable with the most amount of readings for diastolic blood pressure and set the acceptable range between 25 and 145.

Automating Data-Preparation Techniques

Once data files are analyzed in a manual way for a population health analysis, if there are any plans to repeat the analysis, the data-preparation techniques should be automated for future use. Given that indicators of interest change over time and that a core function of population health analytics is to measure trends over time, the majority

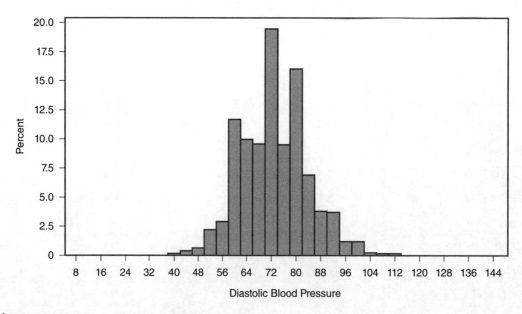

Figure 16.3 Addressing Erroneous Data.

of analytics undertaken are usually repeated. In the blood pressure example in Table 16.2 and Figure 16.3, once the decisions are made about using EMR data for population-level blood pressure assessment, the plan will be to intervene to improve blood pressure and subsequently monitor the impact of the intervention on blood pressure results. This requires monthly monitoring of blood pressure measures. The rules and parameters applied to the data at the onset of data preparation need to be automated into a code set that can be applied every month.

Automation rules and parameters are determined by the population health team and documented and maintained through the organization's data governance structure. **Table 16.3** is an example of automated parameters applied to EMR and lab data for clinical indicators.

Table 16.3 Example of Parameters used for Acceptance of Data Points

Variable Name	Parameters for Acceptance
BP systolic	>= 50 or < 380 mmHg
BP diastolic	>= 25 or < 200 mmHg (cannot be > associated systolic value)
Weight	> 70 or < 1,000 pounds
Height	> 5.6 or < 97.6 inches
BMI	> 13 or < 100 kg/m^2
Triglyceride	> 5.4 mmol/L
LDL	> 30 or < 170 mg/dL
HbA1c	> 3.5 or < 25 %

Conclusion

This chapter sought to highlight major considerations in preparing data for population health analyses. The information presented here represents only a portion of that which is encountered in reality when working with multiple, varied, and disjointed data sets collected for healthcare operational purposes and transformed secondarily for use in population health analytics. Master data management is the recommended solution for sustainably managing population health data and is a requirement for performing successful population health analytics.

Absent an organizational MDM strategy, procedures must be put into place to prepare data for analysis. A methodical analytic approach to preparing data involves first designing the analysis required to answer the population health question and then acquiring the necessary data sources. After the data sources have been identified, a determination is made whether data linking is necessary and, if so, whether this is completed first. After a final data set is created, each variable used for the analysis is analyzed to determine the extent to which there is missing or erroneous data present. Methods are applied to address these data issues before executing an analysis. Ideally these methods are then coded, placed into production, and managed through a data governance process, allowing for a repeatable process of data preparation. It is important to understand and ensure these processes are in place at your organization and, if absent or inconsistent, there is a strategy to reconcile. Any inconsistencies are important to address before or in alignment with a population health analytics strategy.

Study and Discussion Questions

- Discuss the advantages and disadvantages of a MDM strategy.
- Why is it important to spend time preparing data before interpreting analytic results?
- Map out a data-preparation strategy for an analytic project undertaking.

Resources and Websites

DAMA International, Global Data Management Community: https://dama.org/

Data Quality Pro: https://www.dataqualitypro.com/about

References

Berson, A., & Dubov, L. (2011). MDM applications by industry. Pp. 55–78 in A. Berson & L. Dubov (Eds.), *Master data management and data governance* (2nd ed.). McGraw-Hill.

Eliason, B., Burke, J., & Hess, P. (2014). *Master data management in healthcare: 3 approaches*. HealthCatalyst. https://www.healthcatalyst.com/master-data-management-in-healthcare-3-approaches

Gartner. (2020, June 27). Gartner glossary: Master data management. https://www.gartner.com/en/information-technology/glossary/master-data-management-mdm

Quinion, M. (2005). Garbage in, garbage out. World Wide Words. http://www.worldwidewords.org/qa/qa-gar1.htm

Sylvia, M. L. (2018). Creating the analysis data set. In M. L. Sylvia & M. F. Terhaar (Eds.), *Clinical analytics and data management for the DNP* (2nd ed., pp. 157–196). Springer Publishing.

CHAPTER 17

Assessing Data Quality

Martha Sylvia, PhD, MBA, RN

The only thing worse than no data is bad data.

—Michael Hansen, ForestVue Healthcare Solutions

EXECUTIVE SUMMARY

Building sustainable data infrastructure for population health requires an understanding and monitoring of the quality of data assets. The measurement of health determinants, health outcomes, and the financial viability of healthcare organizations are all critically dependent on having and using high-quality data. Across all industries, only 45% of analytic leaders report using some type of metric to measure data quality at the organizational level, and 8% report tying a financial value to key analytic assets. It is not surprising that the small number of organizations who do measure financial value of data are also more likely to be ahead of their peers and competitors in annual revenue growth and their ability to attract top talent (Logan, Duncan, Logan, & Jones, 2019).

In health care and as it applies to population health analytics, the extent to which data quality is assessed is in the context of interoperability, focusing on the ability to match patient records and transfer important health indicators about patients between care settings and providers. At this very basic level of healthcare data quality assessment, it's estimated that patient matching rates within healthcare organizations can be as low as 80% and as low as 50% between organizations using the same electronic medical record vendor (Pew Charitable Trusts, 2018).

Attainment of population health objectives is not possible without data. Data are transformed to insights throughout the population health process to improve care delivery and patient outcomes and to gain efficiency in healthcare delivery. There is a difference between having data and having data of high enough quality to optimize population health strategies. Multidimensional components of data quality must be understood, assessed, and maximized within healthcare organizations as part of an ongoing program of data quality management.

LEARNING OBJECTIVES

At the end of this chapter, the learner will be able to:

1. Describe approaches to data quality assessment.
2. Interpret a process for assessing data quality.
3. Compare and contrast the domains of data quality.
4. Identify metrics used to measure data quality domains.

Introduction

Data used for population health analyses include that generated within the healthcare organization and that obtained by the healthcare organization because it is deemed necessary to provide care to its patients. Assessment of data quality encompasses the integration of data that is internal to the healthcare organization, data received from partner organizations, and data received directly from patients or health plan members. A strong program of data quality assessment and improvement ensures that these data sources are providing value for population health management.

This chapter defines the domains of data quality and their ability to assess the value of data in their entirety so that data points can represent their intended meaning completely and accurately in a timely manner. Emphasis is placed on a data-profiling approach to data quality evaluation where proactive measures are put into place and regularly monitored and where results are used to improve data quality.

Defining Data Quality

Data quality is best defined in terms of the multiple domains in which the quality can be measured. Data quality is quantified through an analysis of the data itself and the metadata, or the data about the data. Data points are examined through the lens of data quality domains. Metadata in the form of documentation of the origins of data, processes for transferring and managing data, and data dictionaries are also evaluated. Multiple domains of data quality exist. This chapter explains the data domains in the context of data used for population health analytics.

Domains of Data Quality

Data quality domains are criteria against which data quality is measured. Depending on the purpose of the data, a combination of domains are chosen for a program of data profiling. **Table 17.1** lists domains commonly used to measure data quality, a description, and an example of metrics.

Not all domains of data quality are applied to the data but take the perspective of measuring overall aspects of the data as an asset. For instance, the "accessibility" domain addresses the question of whether data are overall easily retrieved and analyzed for population health purposes. Table 17.1 distinguishes domains as being measured "about the data" when they measure overall infrastructure and "within the data" when they measure attributes within the data itself. Note that some metrics, especially those about the data, can be obtained through surveying analysts, clinicians, and business stakeholders.

Data Quality Assessment

Data quality assessment represents the activities that assist healthcare organizations evaluate critical data assets against defined quality objectives (Office of the National Coordinator, n.d.). Ideally, this assessment results in a quantifiable measure of data quality, an understanding of issues that goes deep enough to design and plan measures to address them, and a repeatable process for removing data issues such that high-quality data are all that remains.

There are two main approaches to quantifying data quality. The first approach is use-case–driven and referred to as *fit for purpose*. Often while performing population health analyses, data are not returning expected results and deeper examination reveals issues with the data related to the purpose at hand. This discovery that the data are not fit for purpose is one way in which data quality is evaluated. This is aligned with the use-case–based approach where business and clinical use cases are used to frame the data quality assessment (see Chapter 12, "Development of a Data Model"). The fit-for-purpose methodology is advantageous by aligning with population health analytic needs in real time, although it is a reactionary approach dependent on a business request, observation, or perhaps a complaint. Therefore, this type of approach may lead to an inability to understand

Table 17.1 Domains of Data Quality

About or Within Data	Data Quality Domain	Description for Population Health Analytics	Population Health Analytics Example	Example Domain Metric
About	Accessibility	Data are quickly retrievable and analyzable without cumbersome code writing and linking of data tables.	Data are modeled in a way that supports ease of population health analyses.	Average number of tables needed to join for a population health analysis % of total analysis time spent preparing data
About	Appropriate amount	The volume of data is appropriate for the analysis. Data are available for the entirety of a population or subgroup of interest and the measures of interest.	An analysis requires measurement of asthma medication adherence in children with asthma uses data that have the complete population of children and their complete set of asthma medication procured over the time period.	Ratio of number of data units needed to number of units available % of people falling within population definition (assessed for adequacy) % of people in population definition with observations of interest (assessed for adequacy)
About	Believability	Data are regarded as true and believable.	When reporting population health analytic results, one data point may be identified as inaccurate, which can lead to a disregard for all of the reported results.	Survey: % of stakeholders reporting data are believable, credible, or trustworthy
About	Credibility or reputation	Data are highly regarded in terms of their source and content.	Diagnoses on the problem list in an electronic medical record have been designated as having a poor reputation when the problem list is not regularly maintained or when multiple providers are entering diagnoses on the problem list.	Survey: % of stakeholders reporting data have a good reputation for quality Survey: % of stakeholders reporting data have a good reputation for quality
About	Ease of manipulation	Data are easy to manipulate and apply at a person level and aggregate to populations.	A person-level, longitudinal data model is available to analysts, updated and refreshed regularly, and maintained through a program of data governance.	% of population health analyses that are able to be derived from a person-level data model

(continues)

Table 17.1 Domains of Data Quality *(continued)*

About or Within Data	Data Quality Domain	Description for Population Health Analytics	Population Health Analytics Example	Example Domain Metric
About	Relevancy	Data are applicable and helpful for the given population health analytics use case.	When performing population health analyses, the data are relevant when organized at the person level over time and contain the observations needed to perform the analysis at hand.	Survey: % of stakeholders reporting data are relevant, useful, or applicable to their work
About	Timeliness	Data are sufficiently up to date.	In a longitudinal person-level data model with monthly observations, data are updated on a schedule such that observations are never lagging by more than one month.	Average lag time of entire data model Average lag time for each data source
About	Traceability	Data can be tracked back to their creation, and updates to data are tracked.	Demographic and other person-level characteristics can be traced back to their source from the population health data model.	Metadata contain tracking mechanisms to origins of data and their updates.
About	Understandability	Data are easily comprehended.	Data are supported with documentation about their content, origin, and processing. This includes a data dictionary.	% of data fields represented in comprehensive documentation, including a data dictionary Survey: % of stakeholders reporting data are understandable
About	Value added	Data are beneficial and provide advantages from their use.	The data available for population health analytics provide value to the organization for accomplishing the goals of the Triple Aim.	Survey: % of stakeholders reporting data are valuable for achieving population health strategic objectives

Within	Accuracy	Data are correct and free of errors.	Text in a data field; for instance, a value of 5'6" for height when 66 is expected to be entered as a numerical value for height in inches. See Chapter 17 for more erroneous error types.	% of data fields with erroneous errors Average number of erroneous errors Percentage of data in each field with erroneous errors
Within	Completeness	Data are not missing.	When integrating hemoglobin A1C lab values for a population of people with diabetes, many of the people may be missing a value over a time period.	% of data fields with missing data % of missing values for each data field
Within	Consistent representation or conformity	Data are presented in the same format in the same fields across data tables and sources and over time.	ICD-10 CM diagnosis codes use the same leading digits and a decimal point in the appropriate position across multiple sources like billing data from the electronic medical record and medical claims data.	% of data fields across data sources with alternating formats for the same variable % of data within the same data field with alternating formats
Within	Integrity	Accuracy of representing of relationships in data.	Mother linked to correct baby. Systolic and diastolic blood pressure readings linkable for the same person at the same date and time of measurement.	% of data fields across data sources with alternating formats for the same variable % of data within the same data field with alternating formats
Within	Uniqueness	People can be unambiguously and mutually exclusively identified. There is no data redundancy.	A process is in place for person identity management (see Chapter 20).	% false negatives when matching multiple data sources at a person level % false positives when matching multiple data sources at a person level

Data from Feder, S. L. (2018). Data quality in electronic health records research: Quality domains and assessment methods. *Western Journal of Nursing Research, 40*(5), 753–766. https://doi.org/10.1177/0193945916689084; Lee, Y. W., Strong, D. M., Kahn, B. K., & Wang, R. Y. (2002). AIMQ: A methodology for information quality assessment. *Information & Management, 40*(2). 133–146. http://web.mit.edu/TDQM; Pipino, L. L., Lee, Y. W., & Wang, R. Y. (2002). Data quality assessment. *Communications of the ACM, 45*(4), 211–218. https://doi.org/10.1145/505248.506010; Terry, A. L. Stewart, M., Cejic, S., Marshall, J. N., de Lusignan, S., Chesworth, B. M., Maddocks, H., Shadd, J., Burge, F., & Thind, A. (2019). A basic model for assessing primary health care electronic medical record data quality. *BMC Medical Informatics and Decision Making, 19*(1), 30. https://doi.org/10.1186/s12911-019-0740-0; Vaziri, R., & Mohsenzadeh, M. (2012). A questionnaire-based data quality methodology. *International Journal of Database Management Systems, 4*(2), 55–68. https://doi.org/10.5121/ijdms.2012.4204; Vetrò, A., Canova, L., Torchiano, M., Minotas, C. O., Iemma, R., & Morando, F. (2016). Open data quality measurement framework: Definition and application to Open Government Data. *Government Information Quarterly, 33*(2), 325–337. https://doi.org/10.1016/j.giq.2016.02.001

and solve data issues, a lack of organizational trust in the data, and a haphazard understanding of the extent to which data issues exist (Berson & Dubov, 2011).

Data profiling is a proactive and measurable approach to evaluating data quality. In this method, a set of data quality profiling metrics is generated to find and measure data issues such as missing data, invalid attributes, duplicate records, acceptable values, violations of referential integrity, and more (Berson & Dubov, 2011). Data profiling requires that the organization define data quality before taking on population health analytics, define measures and thresholds for acceptable data quality, and follow through in addressing identified data issues. This requires more organizational resources in terms of technical staff and tools and an organizational culture of treating data as a valuable asset. Data profiling can be executed through ad hoc queries and business intelligence tools, but more organizations are starting to use packaged data-profiling tools that calculate metrics of data quality and run in a production environment (Chien, Judah, & Jain, 2020). The remainder of this chapter focuses on a data-profiling approach to evaluating and managing organizational data quality.

Process for Monitoring Data Quality

An organized and repeatable process for data quality monitoring is required to ensure a proactive data-profiling approach. The process involves making decisions about data and acting on those decisions with those who are involved in creating, modifying, and deleting data across every phase of the data lifecycle. Decisions include defining the best metrics to track improvements, determining whether the data are sufficiently complete and accurate, establishing the desired state of specific attributes (or targets), and determining the minimum acceptable level of quality (or thresholds) (Office of the National Coordinator, n.d.). Steps in this

process include defining data quality, defining metrics, profiling data, setting benchmarks, and making adjustments (Chien et al., 2020).

The process begins with *defining data quality* from the healthcare organization's perspective. The domains of data quality are examined to determine if and how each applies to organization-specific data. For instance, the domain of accuracy when applied to laboratory data may include an assessment of whether laboratory results are associated with the right person and that laboratory results are within expected ranges. There are multiple domains of quality, with any combination or all being applicable, depending on the data source and use of the data.

Once the domains of data quality are identified, the process moves to *defining metrics* for data quality. Metrics are specific to the domain and the way that the domain is used to assess the specific data. Example metrics are provided for each data domain in Table 17.1. When initiating a program of data quality monitoring, the next step in this process is to *profile the data* by deriving the values for the quality metrics. This initial data profiling is assessed by the analytic and stakeholder team to determine reasonableness of the results given contextual understanding. For instance, if the team knows that a laboratory vendor only sends laboratory results for a subset of an entire population, then it may be acceptable to have a high rate of missing data; however, if the data are expected to be complete across an entire population, a low tolerance for missing data is expected.

This initial process of profiling the data leads to *setting benchmarks* for each quality metric based on multiple factors. One factor for determining the benchmark is based on an understanding of the unique characteristics of the data within the healthcare organization. For instance, an organization may understand where problems with data quality exist (such as workflow and documentation issues in the clinical setting) and can set benchmarks with this understanding. In one organization, the electronic medical record was known to be configured incorrectly for drop-down selections when care managers were indicating the type

All items are measured on a 0 to 10 scale where 0 is not at all and 10 is completely											
Relevancy											
The data is useful to our work	0	1	2	3	4	5	6	7	8	9	10
The data is relevant to our work	0	1	2	3	4	5	6	7	8	9	10
The data is appropriate for our work	0	1	2	3	4	5	6	7	8	9	10
The data is applicable to our work	0	1	2	3	4	5	6	7	8	9	10

Figure 17.1 Example of Stakeholder Survey Questions for Data Domains About the Data.

Data from Pipino, L. L., Lee, Y. W., Wang, R. Y., & Yang, R. Y. (2002). Data quality assessment. *Communications of the ACM, 45*(4), 211–218. https://doi.org/10.1145/505248.506010; Vaziri, R., & Mohsenzadeh, M. (2012). A questionnaire-based data quality methodology. *International Journal of Database Management Systems, 4*(2), 55–68. https://doi.org/10.5121/ijdms.2012.4204

of contact with patients. Therefore, the benchmark for accuracy on this field was set liberally with a high tolerance for error. Other considerations for setting benchmarks are the timeliness of data file imports, the percentage of the population covered by each data source, and the level of structured and standardized data used. Benchmarks may change as time goes on and data issues are addressed.

Once data quality elements and metrics are defined, the data are initially profiled, and benchmarks are set, the data quality process should move from initiation to operations. When in operations, the data quality monitoring program follows quality-improvement methodologies where data are profiled on a regular basis, reporting of the data quality metrics are produced with results compared to benchmarks, and a process is in place to *adjust the data or process* if results are not within benchmarks.

The process of monitoring data quality is twofold. Metrics about the data, which require input from data stakeholders, can be measured using survey techniques on an annual or semiannual basis. One way to accomplish this is to use a five-point Likert scale ("strongly disagree," "disagree," "neutral," "agree," "strongly agree") or a 10-point scale of "no agreement" to "full agreement" on statements about each domain. An example of one domain is shown in **Figure 17.1**. A full set of evaluative questions is available in published literature (Lee, Strong, Kahn, & Wang, 2002; Vaziri & Mohsenzadeh, 2012).

Metrics measured within the data use a structured process for data profiling. **Figure 17.2** shows an example of a portion of this process in one accountable care organization contracted with the Centers for Medicare and Medicaid Services to manage a population of Medicare beneficiaries. This example shows part of the quality-monitoring process where the patient-linking process and medical claims data are assessed for linkages and completeness, respectively. Notice that adjustments can be made to the data file or to the benchmarks based on the results of diagnostic analytics performed to understand the issue.

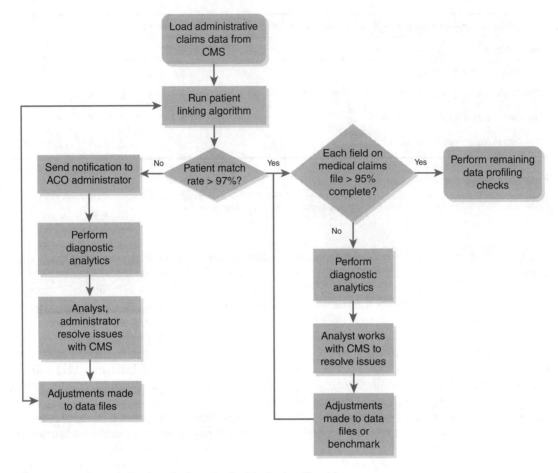

Figure 17.2 Example Portion of a Data Quality Monitoring Algorithm.

Conclusion

Data quality assessment is an important component of population health analytics. A selection of data quality domains is used to define data quality in a way that is meaningful to individual healthcare organizations and their population health management objectives. Data domains are defined from the perspective of data as a whole and measure aspects about the data by surveying and questioning data stakeholders and from the perspective of the data points and values, measuring aspects of completeness, accuracy, conformity, integrity, and uniqueness. Ideally, an automatic system is designed to perform data profiling where data are continuously improved over time. Data quality assessment is a strategic investment for any organization considering or implementing population health analytics. Failing to adequately ensure data quality or assuming the data are ready for analytic use when they are not can create significant downstream inconsistency, inaccuracy, and distrust among frontline staff expected to use the data to support population health initiatives.

Study and Discussion Questions

- What are the considerations when planning a program of data quality evaluation?
- Compare and contrast fit for purpose versus a data-profiling approach to evaluating data quality.

- In thinking about a healthcare organization with which you are familiar, what domains of data quality would be important to measure?

Resources and Websites

Office of the National Coordinator for Health Information (ONC): https://www.healthit.gov/

American Health Information Management Association (AHIMA): http://www.ahima.org

References

Berson, A., & Dubov, L. (2011). Master data governance. Pp. 399–428 in A. Berson & L. Dubov (Eds.), *Master data management and data governance* (2nd ed.). McGraw-Hill.

Chien, M., Judah, S., & Jain, A. (2020, January 29). Build a data quality operating model to drive data quality assurance. Gartner Research. https://www.gartner.com /en/documents/3980235/build-a-data-quality-operating -model-to-drive-data-quali

Feder, S. L. (2018). Data quality in electronic health records research: Quality domains and assessment methods. *Western Journal of Nursing Research, 40*(5), 753–766. https://doi.org/10.1177/0193945916689084

Lee, Y. W., Strong, D. M., Kahn, B. K., & Wang, R. Y. (2002). AIMQ: A methodology for information quality assessment. *Information & Management, 40*(2), 133–146. http://web .mit.edu/TDQM/

Logan, D., Duncan, A. D., Logan, V., & Jones, L. J. (2019). Survey analysis: Gartner's fourth annual CDO survey— Key capabilities that enable business success. https://www .gartner.com/en/documents/3942023/survey-analysis -gartner-s-fourth-annual-cdo-survey-key-c

Office of the National Coordinator for Health Information Technology. (n.d.). Data quality. https://www.healthit.gov /playbook/pddq-framework/data-quality/data-cleansing -and-improvement/

Pew Charitable Trusts. (2018). Enhanced patient matching is critical to achieving full promise of digital health records contents: Accurately linking individuals with their records essential to improving care. https://www.pewtrusts.org /en/research-and-analysis/reports/2018/10/02/enhanced -patient-matching-critical-to-achieving-full-promise-of -digital-health-records

Terry, A. L., Stewart, M., Cejic, S., Marshall, J. N., de Lusignan, S., Chesworth, B. M., Chevendra, V., Maddocks, H., Shadd, J., Burge, F., & Thind, A. (2019). A basic model for assessing primary health care electronic medical record data quality. *BMC Medical Informatics and Decision Making, 19*(1), 30. https://doi.org/10.1186/s12911-019-0740-0

Vaziri, R., & Mohsenzadeh, M. (2012, April). A questionnaire-based data quality methodology. *International Journal of Database Management Systems, 4*(2), 55–68. https://doi .org/10.5121/ijdms.2012.4204

Vetrò, A., Canova, L., Torchiano, M., Minotas, C. O., Iemma, R., & Morando, F. (2016, April). Open data quality measurement framework: Definition and application to Open Government Data. *Government Information Quarterly, 33*(2), 325–337. https://doi.org/10.1016/j.giq .2016.02.001

CHAPTER 18

Person Identity Management

Martha Sylvia, PhD, MBA, RN

Always remember that you are absolutely unique. Just like everyone else.

—Margaret Mead

EXECUTIVE SUMMARY

Achieving the Triple Aim requires a comprehensive view of a population to identify opportunities to reduce waste and inefficiencies in the healthcare system and improve health. Patient identity management is a critical element of population health analytics and is foundational to establishing a comprehensive view of a person and population. When patient identity management is poorly performed, healthcare dollars are needlessly spent on duplicate testing; multiple submissions, and rejections by payers to providers; the wrong results given to the wrong person; and, much worse, wrong treatments provided to patients. On average, 18% of an organization's patient records are duplicates, contributing to an average cost per person per inpatient stay of $1,950 and per emergency department visit of $800 because of issues with duplicate records. In addition, it is estimated that 33% of all denied health insurance claims are a result of inaccurate patient identification, causing the U.S. healthcare system to waste more than $6 billion annually (Black Book Research, 2018).

Healthcare executives agree on the following as they relate to person identity management:

- Match rates are far below the desired level for effective data exchange.
- The increased demand for exchange of data among different systems is pushing the need for improvements.
- Match rates are difficult to measure.
- The methods in which records are received can affect match results.
- Different healthcare providers vary in their perspective on the extent of the problem.
- And, most important, opportunities do exist to more accurately link individuals' health records (Pew Charitable Trusts, 2019).

The differences are astonishing between being able to identify unique patients when a program of unique patient identity management is in place and not having one in place. Hospitals with master patient-index programs in place experience an overall correct patient identification rate of 93% for internal records and 85% for external records compared to 24% with no program in place (Black Book Research, 2018).

LEARNING OBJECTIVES

At the end of this chapter, the learner will be able to:

1. Articulate the importance of the ability of healthcare organizations to identify unique individuals for population health analytics.
2. Describe the challenges and solutions for identifying unique individuals within and across organizations.
3. Compare and contrast deterministic and probabilistic matching techniques.
4. Determine the trade-offs for achieving differing levels of match rates when identifying unique individuals in multiple data sets.

Introduction

The population health data model at its core is person centric. This is absolutely critical in being able to understand health determinants, their relationship to health outcomes, and their trajectory over time. The World Health Organization describes health determinants as the conditions in which a person is born, grows, lives, works, learns, worships, and plays (World Health Organization, 2017). Combining the data representing these life experiences with data from the multiple interactions with the healthcare system for unique individuals requires the ability to organize data at the unique person level.

We cannot overstate the importance of matching data at the person level for population health analytics and the enormity of the challenges in doing so. Every day providers and care management teams receive hundreds and even thousands of admissions, transfer, and discharge data as alerts for targeted interventions for people who are hospitalized. These at-risk entities for population health outcomes must be able to readily respond to patient's needs and prevent worse outcomes, but the identification of the patient with internal organizational records needs to be first reconciled. The same is true with laboratory data in which tens of thousands of records are shared with health plans and providers on a regular basis so that important indicators of chronic illness trajectory can be combined with clinical care data to provide action and reduce poor sequelae.

The term *person level* is used purposely to describe the level at which the unique observation needs to occur. As will be pointed out in this chapter, a unique person can be identified by many terms, depending on the perspective. However, it is at the person level that the uniqueness must be maintained. Although this may sound simple, it can be quite challenging. At one healthcare organization, 2,488 unique health records with the same name were identified, and 231 of them had the same birthdate (Pew Charitable Trusts, 2016). The methods of patient identity management and master data management are used in this chapter to solidify the tenets by which unique person identification can be optimized and maintained for population health analytics.

All the Ways a Person Can Be Identified in Data

A person can be identified in data multiple ways, depending on the perspective of the defining healthcare organization. **Figure 18.1** displays some of the ways a person can be assigned an identifier. When it comes to health insurance, a person can be a subscriber, a member, or a dependent at the same time and in more than one health insurance policy. When 65 and older, a person can be a Medicare beneficiary and dependent or an employee in a self-funded employer health plan. It becomes even more complex when the person is identified as a patient because each organization providing healthcare services usually has its own way of assigning patient identifiers; a laboratory, a primary care physician, a skilled nursing facility,

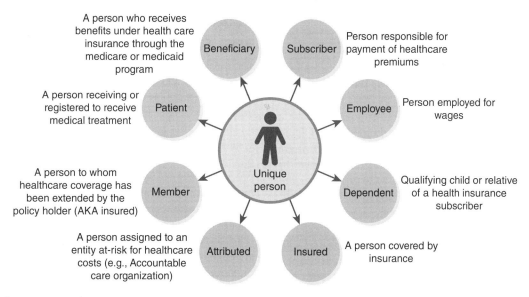

Figure 18.1 Terms Used to Reference a Person.

a hospital, and an outpatient surgical clinic might all assign the same person a separate and unique identifier.

Ideally, a person is uniquely identified for the purposes of population health analytics, with the population health data model assigning one unique identification number per person. This identification number follows the person over time and across settings where health determinants are identified and applied. However, this ideal state of person identification is not possible in the way that health care is delivered in the United States. Multiple entities are usually at risk financially for the same individual with all of the entities requiring a person-centric view. This results in multiple unique person identifiers assigned. For example, a person insured by a Medicare Advantage (MA) plan that is contracted with a Clinically Integrated [Provider] Network (CIN) would be assigned a Medicare Beneficiary Number, a member number in the MA plan, and perhaps an attribution number in the CIN. Each entity has a vested interest in understanding person-level information over time and the ability to uniquely identify people over time. When exchanging healthcare information, it is easy to see why it is difficult to uniquely identify a person with one identifier.

Unique Patient versus Unique Person Identifier

Ideally, every person in the country would be assigned a unique identifier that could be used for any type of personal or healthcare-related transaction, whether it be signing up for health insurance, seeing a provider, making purchases at a drug store, receiving dental care, and more. Social Security numbers are not able to serve this purpose because they are tied to too many other financial aspects of people's lives and are not required to be shared in patient transactions (Umansky, 2019). In addition, federal restrictions in the United States on using funds to establish a national identifier leave the onus on private organizations for such a solution. Other proposed solutions include the use of smartphones by patients to provide identity information when seeking care, agreement on data standardization by provider organizations for patient demographic information, and referential matching using third-party data such as credit bureaus and the postal service (Pew Charitable Trusts, 2019).

Absent an assigned unique person identifier for this purpose, healthcare organizations are left to create their own unique patient identifier.

The distinction between a patient and a person is important because each healthcare organization can create an identifier only for those patients of which it is aware. A patient of a provider organization is either one who is registered to receive or has received medical treatment or one who has been attributed to them through a risk-bearing contract. From the perspective of an insurer, however, the interest is in identifying a unique "member" who is defined as one who is either primarily insured or who is a dependent of the insured. From the perspective of a self-insured employer, unique employees and their dependents are the unit for unique identification. Great strides have been made in creating universal patient identifiers (UPIs) through the use of sophisticated matching techniques, with one company boasting that 100% of the U.S. population now has a UPI (Rivera, 2020).

Person Identity Management

For organizations to achieve success in uniquely identifying people, they must decide on the methods that will be used to match persons between systems. Considerations for the chosen method include the complexity and multitude of the systems in which person-level data is housed, the quality of the data in terms of ability to be confident in matching people between systems, and the level of tolerance for errors in matching. Once these decisions are made, the organization first develops a method for creating and maintaining a unique person identifier for all persons for whom it pays for or provides healthcare services. This method is applied to systems data and stored in the organizations data warehouse for use in population health analytics and other operational purposes. Second, the organization must be able to apply this method when managing linkages to external sources of data (usually received as file imports from external vendors, healthcare providers, and other relevant organizations sharing person-level data) used in population health management.

Level of Granularity and Tolerance for Error

The first step in person identification is the ability to identify an entity—in this case, a person—in the most granular way that makes sense for the organization. This level of granularity depends on the way that source data are stored in legacy systems and the reconciliation among the multiple systems that an organization has to identify people (Berson, 2011). For example, a health insurer may have outdated claims payment systems and current operational systems as well as member data generated in enrollment systems, claims payment systems, utilization management systems, care management systems, and more. A provider organization may have similar complexity with paper charts, legacy, and current electronic medical record systems; files indicating attributed patients from a risk-bearing contract; files indicating attributed patients for value-based quality measures from insurers; and more. The organization must spend time defining the person entity in the way that best ensures that the people it needs to include within the scope of its population over time are actually included.

The assessment of the level of granularity includes an inventory of the amount of information available to identify each person uniquely and to carry out the linkage. Variables chosen must be considered in terms of their *stability*, or the expected amount of change over time; *universality*, or the extent to which everyone in the population will have the attribute; *availability*; and *ease of validation* (Berson, 2011). Variables commonly used to match are:

- ID numbers from the source system;
- name;
- gender;
- birthdate;
- other ID numbers such as Social Security number, driver's license numbers, and employee or student ID numbers;
- address;
- phone; and
- other dates of interest such as enrollment dates or dates of healthcare services.

Table 18.1 Challenges to Identifying Unique People

Subscriber Number	Name	Address	Phone Number
1109892234	Bruce Smith	22 Plains Way, Plaintown, GA 23456	555-678-9023
1109892234	Bruce A. Smith	22 Plains Way, Plaintown, GA 23456	555-678-9023

Note that time must be spent ensuring the data used for matching are clean and high quality (see Chapter 17, "Assessing Data Quality"). This chapter assumes that these concepts are applied before attempting unique person identification techniques.

Once this level of granularity is determined, the granular-level information about the people must be assembled from all relevant records across the organization, which is referred to as getting a "360-degree view of the person" (Berson, 2011). This may seem simple, but there are challenges to achieving this milestone because it is not always clear that one person is the same person across multiple and varied records. **Table 18.1** shows two records for Bruce Smith; all of the information is the same except for the difference in the names. Even though all of the other information is the same, they could be different people living in the same household and covered under the same subscriber number for their insurance—for instance, if one is the son and one is the father. Even if the addresses or phone numbers were different, they could be the same person who had a change in address or phone number.

Considerations for Applying Matching Techniques

Although great pains can be taken to identify unique individuals, we must consider the feasibility of the matching methodology in terms of computing power and resources needed to develop and maintain the methodology. When linking records to identify unique people, three major difficulties must be addressed:

1. Using personal identifiers to discriminate between the person to whom a record refers and all other people in the population.

2. Deciding whether discrepancies in identifiers are the result of mistakes in reporting for a single individual or whether they represent the presence of additional individuals.
3. Processing large volumes of data necessary for the record linkage while using a reasonable amount of computer time. (Roos, Wajda, & Nicol, 1986)

The methods for undertaking matching must take these difficulties into consideration within the context of what amount of effort is reasonable to address them. For example, a considerable amount of time and resources could be spent in obtaining extra identifiers for matching data and only produce a minimally incremental increase in the match rate.

Deterministic and Probabilistic Matching

Two commonly used methods of computerized record linkage are deterministic and probabilistic matching. *Deterministic matching* links unique people based on the complete agreement between two records on the values of a defined set of variables. For example, in Table 18.1, if the variable *subscriber number* was the only variable used for matching, the two people in Table 18.1 would match as the same unique person based on this deterministic method. Deterministic matching is a simplified method that can be applied easily and without a great deal of computing power. Deterministic methods are advantageous when the data are of high quality, the matching must be carried out quickly, and when this method produces minimal duplicates and nonmatches. However, when this is not the case and data are not of high quality and deterministic matching produces an intolerable match rate, then probabilistic matching is considered (Roos & Wajda, 1991). Deterministic methods also include manual techniques used to match people—for instance, when a person laboriously compares records and uses reference information to make the determination of matches.

Probabilistic matching is a more complex approach to matching where agreement is along a spectrum ranging from full agreement to partial agreement to no agreement. In this methodology, numerical weights are used to quantify values for linking variables such as names and addresses with rarer values carrying more discriminating power when they agree than common values. For instance, and depending on your population, the last name of "Afify" would carry more weight on agreement than the last name "Smith." Logarithms are used for the weights so they can be added with the sum of the weights indicating the probability that the two records match (Smith, 1984). A threshold is then applied to this probability; based on that cutoff, a match is or is not made. Probabilistic matching is typically performed by specialized electronic master patient indexing (EMPI) systems that are available commercially.

Often the best methodology uses a combination of deterministic and probabilistic matching to achieve an optimal match rate using a manageable amount of resources. In one study that sought to match a nationwide death registry with a health services database, a combined method of deterministic and probabilistic methods was carried out in five stages. Applying deterministic methods in the first stage, a proportion of the data sets were linked by person, requiring an exact match on a set of nine variables, including sex, death year, death month, death day, birth year, birth month, initials of name, and locality of residence. Stages 2 through 4 parameterized the values on these nine variables so that the discriminating power was still high enough to be confident in matches. By stage 5, probabilistic matching was used with weighting applied based on tolerance for agreement and disagreement for the values on a smaller set of variables. In the end, this strategy resulted in a 96% match rate of individuals in the death

data being linked to the health services data and an understanding that it was not feasible to try to link the remaining 4% (Roos et al., 1986).

In another study, a technique called *naturalistic matching* is used to describe a hybrid method of deterministic and probabilistic methodologies, allowing for manual adjudication of matches when needed. The algorithm compares the values of a given data element across two records and determines whether there is strong evidence that the two records are associated with the same patient, whether there is strong evidence that the two records are not associated with the same patient, or whether there is weak evidence that the two records are or are not associated with each other. The algorithm is based on the selection of various rule sets applied to the data elements with override logic that restrict certain relationships between data sets. Records are also marked for manual review according to the rule sets. This method resulted in a less than 1% false positive and false negative rate (Lee, Clymer, & Peters, 2016).

Tolerance for Error in Patient Matching in Population Health Analytics

Regardless of the methods used to match records, they will not be matched with 100% accuracy. These matching scenarios lead to concerns of *overmatching* in which the records of two or more individuals are mistakenly assigned to a single individual (known as *false positives*) or *undermatching* where the records are assigned to two individuals in error (known as *false negatives*) (Berson, 2011). When determining methods to match records, an important decision is the level of tolerance for false positives and false negatives. See Chapter 20, "Epidemiologic Methods," for a detailed definition of false positives and negatives.

False positives result in the records for two different people being linked to one individual. This means that the individual to whom the information is linked may falsely be assigned health determinants such as chronic conditions, lab results, clinical indicators, costs, and utilization.

Depending on the population health intervention, this could have little impact with interventions such as patient education but could have broader impact when the interventions are invasive or resource intensive such as the diversion of chronic illness care to specialty clinics or tailored medication-management initiatives.

False negatives lead to incomplete individual records, with a limited set of all of the existing records for an individual actually being linked to that individual. The records that are not assigned are either lost because they are never matched or are misassigned to another individual. This may be a bigger problem in population health initiatives where the goal is to prevent adverse outcomes from occurring. If information is incomplete, individuals may not get targeted for interventions in which they are eligible. This means that they may miss out on necessary care and are more likely to be identified when worse outcomes are realized.

Managing Person-Level Identity Intraorganizationally

Internally, organizations with strong capabilities in person identity management have created a unique person identifier for everyone within their purview. Ideally, the organization sets up an EMPI (commonly called the *enterprise master patient index*). The EMPI maintains consistent and accurate information about each person within the organization, linking several different identifiers for the same person together and aggregating data contained in separate systems within the organization.

The EMPI is accomplished through the use of algorithms that constantly scour electronic records looking for duplicates and determining whether records belong to the same person or if more investigation is needed. The EMPI uses deterministic methods to look for exact match records on certain data elements like the patient's first and last name and address. Where deterministic methods do not result in a match, probabilistic matching assigns a rank to different data elements based on a preset acceptable level of certainty (Rouse, 2017).

Managing Interorganizational Identity Management

Healthcare organizations do not solely rely on their own internal operational data to understand populations, they need to import data from other organizations in which their patient populations receive healthcare services or payment for healthcare services. For example, a provider at risk financially for its patient panel needs data from the payer to understand cost and utilization, and a payer needs clinical information to measure quality and healthcare outcomes in its population. Lab and hospital data are shared across healthcare delivery and payer organizations; in states where robust health information exchange exists, data are shared between the majority of healthcare organizations.

Matching data across organizations to identify unique individuals is vastly different than matching within organizations. The following data characteristics can facilitate or hinder the ability to match data (Sequoia Project, 2016):

- quality, completeness, consistency, default values, and vocabulary versioning;
- scope of data in terms of whether the external organization uses a system to manage its own unique identifiers and legal requirements;
- organizational culture around sharing data exhibited in the way that organizations approach sharing data and managing data transfer; and
- application of policies for consent, security, and sensitive data sharing.

Data transfer and management with vendors provides additional challenges related to the company's software limitations and versioning, change management, internal enterprise software architecture, service levels and response times, and data-exchange latency (Sequoia Project, 2016).

Table 18.2 The Patient-Matching Maturity Model

Level	Description
0	People are disorganized, processes are not well understood or defined, and the overall view of cross-organizational patient identity management is that of a chaotic system because of the lack of replicable results. Success often depends on individual heroic efforts. The organization is often in reactive mode instead of being proactive.
1	There is a growing awareness of the critical role of cross-organizational patient matching and a corresponding recognition of the need to apply basic management controls by lower and midlevel management staff. At this level, some processes are repeatable, but not all. Success is more predictable.
2	All key processes related to cross-organizational patient matching are understood and documented. They may be enforced inconsistently. The organization is normally not in a reactive mode, and unexpected events become relatively rare where they were the norm in levels 0 and 1.
3	Organizations monitor, analyze, and systematically improve their ability to manage patients across organizational boundaries. Most if not all processes are defined and documented. The processes are somewhat rigid. However, at level 3, the processes are largely documenting the system behaviors "as is" as opposed to level 4 where the processes are innovative. At level 3, the organization achieves consistency, but it is not optimal.
4	Innovation becomes a standard component of patient matching. Management uses data accumulated to the model; as is deemed viable, implement sometimes significant improvements. Key staff members are considered leaders in this domain and contribute to the community.

Reproduced from Heflin, E. (2018). A framework for cross-organizational identity management. https://sequoiaproject.org/wp-content/uploads/2018/06/The-Sequoia-Project-Framework-for-Patient-Identity-Management-v31.pdf

When linking records, two key considerations are understanding the best way to achieve a high linkage rate in a cost-effective manner and determining the correct linkage rate among the records that are linked (Li, Quan, Fong, & Lu, 2006). The Sequoia Project in collaboration with the Care Connectivity Consortium has developed a set of minimal acceptable cross-organizational patient-matching rules, suggested matching traits, a framework for improving matching methods, and a maturity model as a road map for improved patient matching. The maturity model is laid out in five levels, with each level providing minimal acceptable criteria for achieving more advanced patient identity matching processes (**Table 18.2**) (Heflin, 2018).

The Sequoia Project documentation is freely available, and organizations are welcome to contribute to the evolution of this work. The documentation also provides a detailed example in the form of a case study of these principles applied at Intermountain™ Healthcare (Heflin, 2018).

Conclusion

Person identity management is a foundational capability that healthcare organizations must master to mature their program of population health analytics. The person is at the center of the population health data model, and all data points are linked back to that person at a point in time and longitudinally over multiple time periods. Without this foundational element, the persons identified for intervention and the opportunities identified for improvement risk not being trusted or actionable. This chapter described the methods and provided resources for healthcare organizations to develop their ability to identify unique people in their population and to evolve those capabilities into automated, on-demand processes. Time spent developing these capabilities lead to organizational success in the population health management process.

Study and Discussion Questions

- Discuss the importance of false positives and false negatives in identifying unique people for population health analytics.
- Discuss the feasibility trade-offs when aspiring to achieve a 100% match rate for person level identity. Is this a reasonable goal?

- How is the strategy for identifying unique persons different within healthcare organizations compared to across organizations?

Resources and Websites

The Sequoia Project: https://sequoiaproject.org/

RAND Corporation Evaluation of Record Matching Approaches: https://www.rand.org/pubs/research_reports/RR2275.html

G2 Software Review: https://www.g2.com/categories/patient-identity-resolution

References

Berson, A. (2011). Entity resolution: Identification, matching, aggregation, and holistic view of the master objects. In A. Berson & L. Dubov (Eds.), *Master data management and data governance* (2nd ed., pp. 329–350). McGraw-Hill.

Black Book Research. (2018). Improving provider interoperability congruently increasing patient record error rates. Cision. https://www.prnewswire.com/news-releases/improving-provider-interoperability-congruently-increasing-patient-record-error-rates-black-book-survey-300626596.html

Heflin, E. (2018). *A framework for cross-organizational identity management.* https://sequoiaproject.org/wp-content/uploads/2018/06/The-Sequoia-Project-Framework-for-Patient-Identity-Management-v31.pdf

Lee, M. L., Clymer, R., & Peters, K. (2016). A naturalistic patient matching algorithm: Derivation and validation. *Health Informatics Journal, 22*(4), 1030–1044. https://doi.org/10.1177/1460458215607080

Li, B., Quan, H., Fong, A., & Lu, M. (2006, April 5). Assessing record linkage between health care and vital statistics databases using deterministic methods. *BMC Health Services Research, 6,* article 48. https://doi.org/10.1186/1472-6963-6-48

Pew Charitable Trusts. (2016, November). Electronic health records: Patient matching and data standardization remain top challenges. https://www.pewtrusts.org/-/media/assets/2016/11/ehr_inoperability_v3.pdf

Pew Charitable Trusts. (2019). Hospital and clinic executives see rising demand for accurate exchange of patient records: Health care administrators share perspectives on current experiences and needed improvements. https://www.pewtrusts.org/en/research-and-analysis/issue-briefs/2019/05/hospital-and-clinic-executives-see-rising-demand-for-accurate-exchange-of-patient-records

Rivera, K. (2020). 100% of the U.S. population now has a Universal Patient Identifier: Q&A with Experian Health leader on why this matters. https://www.experian.com/blogs/healthcare/2020/01/100-of-the-u-s-population-now-has-a-universal-patient-identifier-qa-with-experian-health-leader-on-why-this-matters/

Roos, L. L., & Wajda, A. (1991). Record linking strategies. Part I: Estimating information and evaluating approaches. *Methods of Information in Medicine, 30,* 117–123.

Roos, L. L., Wajda, A., & Nicol, J. P. (1986). The art and science of record linkage: Methods that work with few identifiers. *Computers in Biology and Medicine, 16*(1), 45–57. https://doi.org/10.1016/0010-4825(86)90061-2

Rouse, M. (2017). What is enterprise master patient index (EMPI)? TechTarget. https://searchhealthit.techtarget.com/definition/master-patient-index-MPI

Smith, M. E. (1984). Record linkage: Present status and methodology. *Journal of Clinical Monitoring and Computing*, *13*(3), 52–71. https://pubmed.ncbi.nlm.nih.gov/10271518/

Sequoia Project. (2016). HIMSS17 cross organizational patient identity management: Challenges and opportunities. https://sequoiaproject.org/wp-content/uploads/2017/02/2017-02-22-HIMSS-2017-Patient-Matching-Challenges-and-Opportunities-v001.pdf

Sylvia, M. (2020). The population health data model. In Population Health Management Learning Series. ForestVue Healthcare Solutions.

Umansky, D. (2019). Doctor asks for your Social Security number. *Consumer Reports*. https://www.consumerreports.org/personal-information/if-doctor-asks-for-social-security-number/

World Health Organization. (2017). Social determinants of health. Author. http://www.who.int/social_determinants/sdh_definition/en/

Analytic Methods

CHAPTER 19

Overview of Analytic Methods Used in Population Health Management

Martha Sylvia, PhD, MBA, RN

Absent the pressure that "analytic" rigor brings, we settle for muddled results of insufficient weight to settle disagreements, let alone influence policy and practice.

—Fred Brancati, MD, MHS

EXECUTIVE SUMMARY

The population health process critically depends on the ability of analytics to inform each phase. When providing care to individuals, clinicians use data points about patients to make diagnoses and determine appropriate treatments. At the population level, data points that are aggregated into analyzable data structures are necessary to understand health determinants and determine the appropriate interventions for improving outcomes. Multiple analytic methods are applied to turn these data into information and insights.

This chapter provides an overview of the most often used analytic methods in population health analytics and describes their appropriate and common use in the population health process. Further chapters provide details about the techniques used in these methods as well as case studies that showcase examples of their use in population-based strategies.

LEARNING OBJECTIVES

At the end of this chapter, the learner will be able to:

1. Identify analytic methods commonly used in population health management.
2. Associate key analytic methods with the relevant population health process phase.

Introduction

Each phase of the population health process (see Chapter 2) requires certain analytic methods in order to glean insight and understanding in executing in that phase. For the purposes of this section, analytic methods refer to the calculations, statistics, and models developed from data that facilitate the transfer of data to knowledge and wisdom. Although some methods can be used in multiple phases of the population health process, many are primarily used in specified phases and are key to gleaning the necessary insights within a phase. For example, in the *assess* phase, understanding univariate analysis of the mean and distribution of blood pressure within a group of people with hypertension allows for an understanding of how many patients have a blood pressure reading over the desired limit as well as the severity of the highest blood pressure readings.

This chapter provides an overview of analytic methods commonly executed in each phase of the population health process. A description of the methods are provided and framed within the phases. In subsequent chapters within this section, details of selected methods are provided with examples and case studies. Section 7 of the textbook focuses on analytic products such as population assessment and population segmentation and their application in each phase of the population health process.

Analytic Methods

Analytic methods in population health draw from multiple disciplines. Determination of calculations and statistical modeling draw heavily from data-driven disciplines, including biostatistics, epidemiology, finance, economics, actuarial science, and public health. Decisions about data sources, variables representing health determinants and outcomes, the correlation of variables, and structuring of data models are informed by clinical disciplines like medicine, nursing, psychology, and pharmacology as well as the disciplines of sociology, environmental science,

nutritional science, and more. Each discipline has its own set of analytic methods. Population health analytic methods draw on the symbiotic relationship among all involved disciplines to apply methods that are specific and crucial to executing on the population health process.

The next sections will highlight the most commonly used methods describing techniques as well as their use in the population health process with a summary provided in **Table 19.1**.

Univariate Statistics

Univariate statistics explore distributions, means, and proportions of one variable in isolation. As stated above, variables of interest represent health determinants and health outcomes. Before an understanding of the relationships between variables can be explored in higher-level methods, each variable must be understood in and of itself. For instance, the relationship between rates of cancer and living in a certain Zip Code cannot be explored until there is an understanding of the rate of the cancer within the population separately of the proportion of people living in each Zip Code.

Dichotomous variables (two possible values) and *categorical* (a limited and fixed number of values) are usually described by reporting the percentage of people falling into each possible value. For instance, the percentage of people with a clinically determined high body mass indicator (BMI) versus a low BMI would describe the dichotomous variable of "High BMI." To report income level in categories, the percentage of people in each income category would be derived (e.g., 10% earning "0–$30,000," 20% earning "$31,000 to $40,000," etc.).

Continuous variables (having an infinite number of values between any two values) are best described by looking at the distribution of the values, the mean, and the median. The distribution is best presented as a visualization using a histogram or box plot that can be annotated to show the mean and median. **Figure 19.1** shows the distribution of BMI in a population of patients with diabetes using a box plot and a histogram.

Table 19.1 Analytic Methods and Their Use in Population Health

Analytic Method	Definition	Population Health Phase
Univariate descriptive statistics	Calculations using one variable, such as proportions, distributions, means and medians	*Assess phase* to describe determinants of health and outcomes of interest *Development phase* to aid in developing the details of the intervention
Bivariate statistics	The use of statistical tests to determine the relationship between two variables and how they compare with each other	*Assess and focus phases* to determine the relationship between health determinants and outcomes between two groupings *Monitor phase* as part of risk adjustment to aid in the determination of which variables should be used as risk adjusters
Incidence and prevalence	Calculation of the proportion of people with a new illness (incidence) and the total proportion of people with the illness (prevalence)	*Assess phase* to understand and monitor the new onset and existing rates of acute and chronic illness
2×2 table analyses	A table structure used to analyze the relationship of two dichotomous variables by analyzing sensitivity, specificity, positive predictive value, and negative predictive value	*Focus phase* to determine the link between health determinants and outcomes *Predict phase* to validate and evaluate the performance of risk-prediction models
Number needed to treat	A method to estimate the number of enrolled and engaged patients necessary to achieve desired outcomes of the intervention	*Develop phase* to determine the number of patients for programs and interventions
Risk adjustment	Mathematical techniques used to control for observable differences between patients that are unrelated to the outcome of interest	*Assess phase* to understand the impact of unique determinants of health on outcomes *Develop phase* to adjust for illness burden in payment incentive programs *Monitor phase* to isolate the impact of an intervention on its desired outcome
Predictive modeling	Statistical modeling techniques used to assign a probability of an adverse event or to estimate the result of an outcome of interest for individuals across an entire population	*Predict phase* to develop or select a model to predict the adverse outcome that a population health program is seeking to mitigate *Implement phase* to operationalize the risk-prediction model and use the results to select and rank patients for intervention
Prescriptive modeling	Computational techniques to transform knowledge about a topic into a set of rules and optimization techniques that maximize benefits while managing trade-offs	*Develop phase* to optimize intervention staffing, resources, and workflow in order to achieve desired results *Implement phase* to operationalize the risk prescriptive model and apply to decision-making in real time

(continues)

Table 19.1 Analytic Methods and Their Use in Population Health   (continued)

Analytic Method	Definition	Population Health Phase
Data mining	A combination of probability methods with decision theory used to identify patterns in data that can minimize errors and variation	*Assess phase* to discover patterns in data that were unknown and not hypothesized with the goal of gleaning insights about a population *Develop phase* to aid in decision support for interventions
Machine learning	The use of a computer to identify patterns in data to make accurate predictions about outcomes	*Predict phase* to predict the adverse outcome that a population health program is seeking to mitigate *Develop phase* to incorporate into interventions in order to predict the results of multiple and varying clinical pathways or other workflows
Natural language processing	The interpretation of text data into meaningful and analyzable data points using linguistic science	*Assess, focus, develop, implement*, and *monitor phases* used at any point in the population health process to make analyzable data points out of unstructured text data
Statistical process control	The use of statistical methods to monitor metrics over evenly distributed time intervals.	*Monitor phase* to ensure intervention processes are working as planned and that outcomes are progressing towards desired targets

Univariate statistics can be used throughout the population health process but are mainly used in the assess phase to describe characteristics and health determinants and to begin to understand the drivers of outcomes within populations and subgroups. Univariate statistics can also be used in the intervention phase when developing the intervention. Detailed information about selected populations are often needed to develop an intervention to ensure tailoring to population needs. For instance, it is important to describe the age distribution of an intervention targeted toward improving diabetes outcomes because patients of working age may have different access requirements than patients of retirement age.

Bivariate Statistics

Bivariate statistical techniques expand on univariate techniques by examining the relationship between two variables instead of just one. In population health analytics, the most common application of bivariate statistics is the comparison of the mean or proportion of a variable representing a determinant of health or health outcome between two cohorts within a population. For instance, in trying to understand whether patients with diabetes in one region have better diabetes-related outcomes and less hospitalizations than in another region, we could compare the mean hemoglobin A1C and mean number of hospitalizations between the two groups.

Certain statistical tests can be used to determine whether the differences in means and proportions are statistically significant. Correlational statistics are used to determine whether there is any association between two variables. Student's t-test is used to examine differences in means and depends on the assumption that the continuous variable is normally distributed. The chi-square test is used to examine the differences in proportions between two different groups (not the same group at different points in time). When continuous data are not normally distributed or proportions are measured in

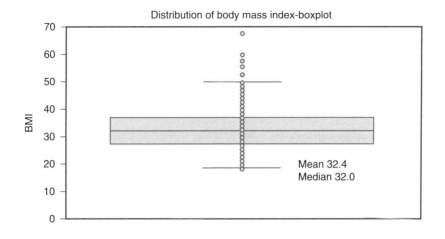

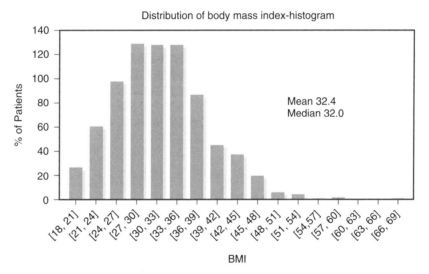

Figure 19.1 Display of Continuous Variable.

the same group, nonparametric statistical tests are used because they do not depend on the assumption of normality of data and, in the case of proportions, do not require independence between the two groupings.

Bivariate statistics are mainly used in the assessment and focus phases of population health to determine the relationship of health determinants and outcomes between two groupings of patients. They are also used as part of risk adjustment to help determine which variables should be used as risk adjusters. For example,

to know if age should be used to risk adjust, the mean difference in age can be tested statistically to see if the differences are significant and therefore warrant adjustment for age differences in an outcome. There are many resources available for learning more about bivariate statistical testing. Here are some: *Basic Biostatistics: Statistics for Public Health Practice, Second Edition*, by B. Burt Gerstman; *Biostatistics for Population Health: A Primer*, by Lisa M. Sullivan; *Principles and Applications of Biostatistics*, by Ray M. Merrill.

Epidemiological Methods

Epidemiological methods used frequently in population health management include the measurement of incidence and prevalence as a way to surveil chronic and acute illnesses and other phenomena of interest. Two-by-two tables are used in epidemiology to evaluate the association between risk factors and an outcome by determining sensitivity, specificity, positive predictive value, and negative predictive value. The tables are also an important methodology in population health to understand the association between health determinants and outcomes of interest. These tables can also be used to validate and evaluate the performance of risk-prediction models. Registries are another method of surveillance used in population health to monitor key indicators and outcomes in populations of interest. Surveillance is primarily used in the *assess* phase while two-by-two tables can be used in the *focus* phase to understand the links between health determinants and outcomes as well as in the *predict* phase as a tool in the development and testing of risk-prediction models.

When implementing population health interventions, it is important to understand the minimum number of participants needed in the intervention to achieve a desired outcome. A determination of the number needed to treat (NNT), using methods similar to those used in epidemiological research, culminates in an estimate of the number of patients needed to achieve a desired outcome in an intervention. NNT analyses are used in the *develop* phase of the population health process when planning the intervention and estimating the number of patients needed to ultimately be enrolled and engaged.

Epidemiological methods applied in population health management are described in detail in Chapter 20.

Risk Adjustment

Risk adjustment uses mathematical techniques to adjust for the effect of multiple health determinants on outcomes of population health to measure the individual impact of each determinant while accounting for the effects of others. Multiple measurable and unmeasurable factors are related to health outcomes. If one were to create an algebraic formula for outcomes, it would look something like this:

> Outcomes = *f*(intrinsic patient-related factors, environmental factors, socioeconomic factors, treatment effectiveness, quality of care, random chance)
>
> (Iezzoni, 2013)

Risk-adjustment methods can be used in the *assess* phase to tease out the impact of individual indicators on health outcomes, in the *develop* phase to adjust for severity of illness in payment incentive programs, and in the *monitor* phase to measure the impact of interventions on improving outcomes. Risk adjustment is critical in programs that pay for value where it is imperative to adjust for factors other than the initiative on outcomes. It is easy to imagine the downfall of a value-based incentive program for providers with no adjustment for the level of illness severity among patients when distributing payments. Chapter 21 details the methods and important points to understand when applying risk adjustment.

Predictive and Prescriptive Modeling

Risk-prediction models are data-driven, decision support tools that estimate an individual's future potential healthcare costs and utilization and allow for identification of the population likely to be at highest cost or highest utilization in subsequent years using predictors from a previous time period (Knutson, Bella, Llanos, & Martin, 2009). Risk-prediction models are developed using information known about the determinants of health in a population to predict outcomes such as hospitalizations, emergency department visits, readmissions, and costs. There are many different types of statistical models used for risk prediction, the most common being logistic and linear regression.

Prescriptive analytics uses computational logic that are techniques to leverage implicit and explicit knowledge about a topic transformed into a set of rules and optimization techniques that seek to maximize benefits while managing resource trade-offs (Brethenoux & Idoine, 2018). Together, predictive and prescriptive analytics determine what is likely to happen and what can be done to make a desirable outcome occur. Prescriptive analytics draws from clinical understanding of treatment processes and in some cases, the field of operations research, which is the science of providing a quantitative basis for complex decisions. Chapter 22 details the methods and important points to understand when developing, choosing, and applying regression-based risk-prediction and prescription analytic models.

Data Mining and Machine Learning

Data mining (DM) is a broad term encompassing analytic methods used to identify relationships in data that give insight into individual preferences and especially what someone might do in a given scenario based on decision theory (Finlay, 2014). DM combines probability methods with decision theory by identifying patterns in data that can minimize errors and variation when relying on clinical decision-making alone. DM uses *parametric* (dependent on normally distributed data) and *nonparametric* (not dependent on normally distributed data and instead using methods such as ranking, clustering, and medians) techniques for analyzing data.

Machine learning (ML) describes machines that mimic cognitive functions that humans associate with the mind such as learning and problem-solving. In ML, a programmed computer has the ability to learn from patterns in data to make accurate predictions about outcomes of interest. Although data mining and machine learning use similar methods, in ML has greater reliance on the computer to recognize patterns.

Chapter 23 provides in-depth information about DM and ML methods and applications.

Natural Language Processing

Using the science of linguistics and cognition, natural language processing (NLP) is a methodology used to translate text-based, nonstructured written information into discrete, analyzable data points. This is a critical capability for population health analytics because much of the documentation at the point of healthcare delivery for patients is in text notes and unstructured data fields. This translation allows a deeper understanding of the complexity of the individual, the health system, and provider factors that drive healthcare outcomes. NLP is used in all steps of the population healthcare process where analytics are limited because of an overabundance of unstructured text data. Chapter 23 provides detailed information about NLP methodologies.

Statistical Process Control

Applying univariate statistical techniques in combination with the calculation of confidence limits, statistical process control (SPC) allows for close examination of process and outcome measures while the intervention is underway. This close scrutiny supports quality improvement during the intervention to correct processes and workflow, thereby ensuring desired outcomes are achieved.

SPC plots measures of interest over evenly distributed time intervals (most commonly weekly, monthly, and quarterly) to examine changes in key intervention metrics. SPC charts use principles of statistics to create measures of variation that allow distinguishing between common cause variation, that which occur as part of normal everyday processes, and special cause variations that occur as a result of intentionally working to change the metric as is done in population health interventions. Chapter 24 provides detailed information about SPC methodologies.

Conclusion

A robust program of analytics is critical to achieving success in population health management. Methods are wide and varied, depending on the population health phase. Univariate and bivariate statistics are used throughout all phases to aggregate data into distributions, averages, medians, and proportions and to make comparisons between groups. Epidemiological surveillance techniques are used to assess populations and identify focus areas and to support the development of risk prediction and adjustment. Risk prediction is used to identify individuals likely to have adverse outcomes and prescriptive analytics is applied to identify the pathway to achieving desired results. Statistical process control is used to monitor the processes and outcomes of interventions as they are being delivered. Sophisticated techniques like data mining, machine learning, and natural language processing are used throughout the process to achieve advanced analytic goals.

The most commonly used analytic methods are summarized in terms of where they optimize the population health process. The list is not exhaustive. Depending on the organization, the way populations are defined, and overarching goals, other analytic methods may also be applied.

Study and Discussion Questions

- Why is an understanding of analytic methods important for all stakeholders involved in population health management programs?
- In thinking about a healthcare organization in which you work, have worked, or plan to work, what are the capabilities around executing population health analytic methods? What needs to be done to improve these capabilities?

Resources and Websites

Centers for Disease Control and Prevention. (2006, October). *Principles of epidemiology in public health practice: An introduction to applied epidemiology and biostatistics* (3rd ed.). https://www.cdc.gov/csels/dsepd/ss1978/index.html

American Statistical Association: https://www.amstat.org/

McGready, J. (n.d.). *Biostatistics in public health specialization.* https://www.coursera.org/specializations/biostatistics-public-health

Academy Health: www.academyhealth.org

References

Brethenoux, E. & Idoine, C. (2018, October 25). *Combine predictive and Prescriptive techniques to solve business problems.* Gartner Research. https://www.gartner.com/en/documents/3891993/combine-predictive-and-prescriptive-techniques-to-solve-

Finlay, S. (2014). *Predictive analytics, data mining and big data* (pp. 1–20). Palgrave Macmillan. https://link.springer.com/chapter/10.1057%2F9781137379283_1

Iezzoni, L. (2013). *Risk adjustment for measuring health care outcomes* (4th ed.). Health Administration Press. http://www.r2library.com/resource/title/9781567934373

Knutson, D., Bella, M., Llanos, K., & Martin, L. (2009, August). *Predictive modeling: A guide for state Medicaid purchasers.* Center for Health Care Strategies. https://www.chcs.org/media/Predictive_Modeling_Guide.pdf

CHAPTER 20

Epidemiological Methods

Martha Sylvia, PhD, MBA, RN

Its methods may be scientific, but its objectives are often thoroughly human. [Reference to the science of epidemiology]

—Alex Broadbent, University of Johannesburg, 2011

EXECUTIVE SUMMARY

The onslaught of data availability, especially longitudinal data points over time, reflecting health indictors and outcomes for large populations affords opportunities to monitor and surveil populations like never before. When applied to population health analytics, epidemiological methods can identify early indicators of the onset of disease states and chronic conditions, the potential for poor outcomes in those having chronic illness, and expected needs for healthcare resources. Armed with these techniques, there is enormous opportunity to intervene.

Epidemiological methods inform polices, programs, prevention, disease and chronic condition treatment, and understanding of the mechanisms of disease and chronic conditions. Population health and epidemiology overlap tremendously because both seek to understand the determinants of health and their relationship to health outcomes. Epidemiology is traditionally thought of as a field of research, although healthcare organizations apply these methods in practice to achieve successful results in population health management programs.

LEARNING OBJECTIVES

At the end of this chapter, the learner will be able to:

1. Identify epidemiological methods used in population health analytics.
2. Use epidemiological methods to answer questions of importance in population health management.
3. Describe the ways in which epidemiological methods are used as the basis for more complex population health analytic methods.
4. Apply epidemiological methods appropriately in the population health process.

Introduction

Population health management draws on many disciplines to accomplish the Triple Aim mandate. This chapter focuses on the discipline of epidemiology and its analytics methods, which form the basis for answering questions of interest in population health management.

Epidemiology is "the study of how disease is distributed in populations and the factors that influence or determine the distribution" (Celentano & Szklo, 2019). Epidemiological methods allow the ability to understand the "distribution of health outcomes" within a population, one of the main components of the definition of population health management (Kindig & Stoddart, 2003).

In addition, epidemiological methods form the basis of and are used to validate more complex analytic methods in population health, including risk adjustment and predictive modeling. By applying epidemiological methods to population-based analyses, we can create longitudinal storage of data points in registries and data models; describe the incidence and prevalence of conditions of interest along with their complications and comorbidities; measure key outcomes and link those outcomes health determinants and risk factors or to processes within interventions to determine what works; risk adjust quality, cost and utilization measures for contracting, payment, and evaluative purposes; and develop and validate risk-prediction models.

Surveillance

Surveillance is an important public health concept and analytical methodology applied in population health analytics and is defined by the World Health Organization as the "[continuous], systematic collection, analysis and interpretation of health-related data [needed for] the planning, implementation, and evaluation of public health practice" (n.d., para. 1).

Surveillance is accomplished by monitoring key indicators, including mortality or death rates and morbidity or the number or proportion of individuals experiencing similar disabilities or illnesses.

In population health analytics the epidemiological surveillance techniques most commonly used are monitoring incidence and prevalence and registries. Monitoring incidence and prevalence allows the identification of new onset and newly identified chronic illness, comorbidities, and complications such as diabetes, as well as onset of acute illnesses that are preventable through population health interventions such as influenza. Registries are used to collect important outcome-based data points for defined populations of interest, usually those with chronic illness or within a particular group at risk of adverse outcomes.

Incidence and Prevalence

When applied to population-based indicators, incidence and prevalence enable insights into the onset, duration, and interrupters of disease processes. *Incidence* is defined as the number of newly identified people with a condition divided by the number of people at risk for that condition over a period of time. Note in the calculation of incidence that once a person gets the condition, he or she is removed from the total number at risk in ongoing measurement of incidence.

Prevalence is the total number of people with a condition divided by the total number of people at risk for the condition over a period of time. The difference between the two is that incidence represents newly identified, and prevalence is the total number of newly identified and existing people with the condition. Unlike the calculation of incidence, the denominator for the calculation of prevalence over multiple time points cumulatively counts the number at risk.

Table 20.1 depicts an example of calculating incidence and prevalence using influenza as the condition of interest. In this example, data were collected for population of 25,369 adults 65 and older in one county who were at risk for developing influenza. Note in this example that those who get influenza are assumed to leave the population at risk in the following month. The denominator for the incidence calculation changes each

Table 20.1 Example of Incidence and Prevalence Calculations

Month	Total Population at Risk (a)	Number of New Cases (b)	Total Number of Cases (c)	Incidence per Thousand = (b ÷ a) * 1,000	Prevalence per Thousand = (c ÷ 25,369) * 1,000
August	25,369	0	0	0	0
September	25,369	30	30	1.18	1.18
October	25,339	50	80	1.97	3.15
November	25,289	120	200	4.75	7.88
December	25,169	140	340	5.56	13.40
January	25,029	110	450	4.39	17.73
February	24,919	80	530	3.20	20.89
March	24,839	50	580	2.01	22.86

month, but the denominator for the prevalence calculation is always the entire original population of 25,369 people at risk for influenza.

Figure 20.1 Depicts the concepts of incidence and prevalence applied to the practice of population health analytics using chronic illness as an example. The left side of the pot depicts the ways in which people with new incidence of a chronic condition are identified in population health management either by a new diagnosis of a condition or by new attribution to a defined

population, healthcare system, provider, or payer. People with the condition leave the pot by dying, by being cured (which may or may not be possible depending on the condition), or by losing attribution.

To illustrate, a provider organization contracts with a health plan to manage a population of people with diabetes. Every month, a process is undertaken to identify new patients diagnosed with diabetes at the provider organization who are managed by that health plan. These patients

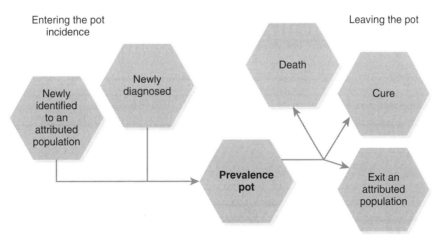

Figure 20.1 Applying the Prevalence Pot Concept in Population Health Management.

are not new to the providers practice but are newly diagnosed with the disease and therefore enter the prevalence pot. In addition, the health plan identifies newly enrolled patients every month and appropriately attributes those with diabetes to the provider organization. These patients are new to the attributed population of patients with diabetes but not newly diagnosed with diabetes. They also enter the prevalence pot.

There is no cure for diabetes, therefore patients cannot leave the prevalence pot through cure. Patients can leave the prevalence pot when they die or are no longer attributed to the provider organization.

Registries

With the widespread use of electronic medical records (EMRs), the ability to collect comprehensive clinical information in an organized and systematic way is better than it has ever been. Registries are organized systems for collecting, storing, retrieving, analyzing, and disseminating information on individual persons who have either a particular disease, a risk factor for disease, or prior exposure to circumstances known to cause adverse health effects (Agency for Healthcare Research and Quality, 2014). Although the EMR is an ideal source of data for registries, any available data sources can be used as long as they contain necessary data points that can be organized at a person level.

There are many types of registries, including those for public health surveillance such as immunization and flu registries, for tracking safety and adequacy of drugs and devices like those in state drug-monitoring programs, and for monitoring health services outcomes like the American Joint Replacement Registry (https://www.aaos.org/registries/registry-program/american-joint-replacement-registry/). In countries where there are universal healthcare systems, robust registries monitor entire populations because data are readily available. The Danish National Registry is a great example (https://econ.au.dk/the-national-centre-for-register-based-research/danish-registers/the-national-patient-register/).

The most commonly used types of registries in population health management are those that measure risk factors for chronic conditions and those that measure clinical outcomes and complications of chronic conditions. Some EMRs have built in the ability to easily configure registries with readily extractable data. Absent this ability, analysts can design and create a registry.

Whether configuring or designing, all registries share common design characteristics. First, the grouping of individual patients who will be included in the registry must be defined using data-based definitions of inclusion and exclusion criteria. For example, a provider practice might define everyone in a diabetes registry as any person who has had a visit with that practice in the preceding 5 years, having a diagnosis of type 2 diabetes on the EMR problem list, age 18 or older, and excluding anyone who has only had gestational diabetes.

Second, unique individuals must be able to be distinguished in the registry. This is easier to accomplish within a single EMR because there is usually one identifier per person who remains the same over time. However, it is more difficult to accomplish when using multiple and varied data sources with multiple identifiers for the same person.

Next, the time frame for collecting measures on a person level is determined. Time frames can vary, depending on the use case for the registry, the frequency with which the system can collect and store data points, and the need for timely monitoring. A registry to monitor outcomes for people with diabetes would likely only need monthly or quarterly measurement points as compared to a registry for people experiencing a viral outbreak who may require weekly or monthly measurement.

Once a method is determined for assigning identification numbers to unique people over time, data points must be defined in terms of their reference to a person at a certain point in time. For instance, a blood pressure result for a person within a monthly hypertension registry may be defined as the most recently available reading for the person in the particular month, even if the reading is 3 months old. Alternatively, it could be defined as the "best" reading within a particular time period. Every measurement within a registry must have a clear definition in terms of how it relates to the person and to the time period for which it is associated.

Clinicians and business leads define outcomes and health determinants of interest that will be collected in the registry. The selection of these elements depends on the purpose of the registry. Wherever possible, measures are standardized and common measures across conditions or risk factors conform to consistent definitions. This is difficult to accomplish in the United States with its vast number of data sources and value-based programs with differing data and metric definitions.

Wherever possible, definitions of data points within a registry should use standardized data elements for comparability across registries and organizations. Examples of standardized data elements include *International Classification of Diseases ICD-10* codes, current procedural terminology, National Drug Code, and others. Data contextualizers that use these types of elements such as diagnosis-related groups and hierarchical condition categories are also considered standardized ways to define data elements.

The outcomes measured within a registry are determined by the purpose of the registry. A registry of patients with diabetes would collect indicators such as measures of blood sugar control, risk factors for poor outcomes, comorbid and complicating conditions, and healthcare utilization and cost. On the other hand, a registry of children with asthma might focus on indicators of asthma control, access to pertinent medications, care coordination, family support, and emergency department utilization.

There are many examples of registries in research and practice. The weblinks and resources at the end of this chapter provide some good examples.

Linking Outcomes to Determinants and Interventions

In population health management it is imperative to understand what factors are impacting health-related outcomes, cost, and utilization. In population health terms, these are the *determinants of health*. Ideally, these factors are isolated so that each individual contribution can be understood, but this is not always possible. Recall from Chapter 2 that health determinants come in many forms, including social, economic, policy, environmental, and more. Health determinants can also be interventions that are applied within a population to improve an outcome. Health determinants and their associated outcomes are measured by data points, and epidemiological methods allow for the analysis of the impact of the determinants on outcomes of interest. Two-by-two table analyses are the mechanism by which sensitivity, specificity, and positive and negative predictive value can be evaluated.

Two-by-Two Table Analyses

Proportions are widely used for measures of population health, and the two-by-two table is a basic methodology and building block for more complex analyses. Two-by-two tables are designed to evaluate the ability of a test or other indicator to predict its intended outcome. For example, in population health, prediction of costs or utilization are used to identify patients for interventions to prevent high costs or hospital admissions. A two-by-two table analysis is a basic methodology used to determine how well that prediction performs in meeting program objectives.

To best structure the two-by-two table, a data set is arranged with three variables: the patient identifier, a 1 = yes, 0 = no indicator of whether that patient was predicted to be at risk of the outcome and a 1 = yes, 0 = no indicator of whether that patient incurred the outcome. It is important to number the yes's as "1" and the no's as "0" so that the yes's can be counted for the prediction

Table 20.2 Example Data Structure for Creating a Two-by-Two Table

Patient ID	Predicted Risk for Hospitalization	Hospitalization Event	Quadrant Placement in Two-by-Two Table
E000124	0	1	Lower left
E000129	0	1	Lower left
E000137	0	1	Lower left
E000126	0	0	Lower right
E000128	0	0	Lower right
E000132	0	0	Lower right
E000134	0	0	Lower right
E000136	0	0	Lower right
E000125	1	1	Upper left
E000130	1	1	Upper left
E000135	1	1	Upper left
E000123	1	0	Upper right
E000127	1	0	Upper right
E000131	1	0	Upper right
E000133	1	0	Upper right

*1 = yes and 0 = no

Reproduced from Sylvia, M. (2020). Epidemiological principles. *In Population Health Management Learning Series*. ForestVue Healthcare Solutions.

and the outcome as the count of the patients who were predicted and the count of patients with the outcome (**Table 20.2**).

The data set is analyzed to create the two-by-two table. **Table 20.3** depicts an example of a two-by-two table setup with results determined from the data set in Table 20.2. The four squares are set up with the predictor along the vertical edge (in this case, prediction of a hospitalization) and the occurrence of the outcome (in this case, a hospitalization) on the horizontal edge. The top left corner contains *true positives*, or the count of patients who were predicted to have a hospitalization and actually had the hospitalization. The right top corner contains *false positives*, or the count of patients who were predicted to have a hospitalization but did not. The lower left corner contains *false negatives*, or the count of patients who were

not predicted to have a hospitalization but did actually have the hospitalization; the lower right quadrant contains *true negatives*, or the count of patients who were not predicted to have the hospitalization and did not. Each person can only be counted in one of the four quadrants—in other words, a person cannot be counted in more than one quadrant. Table 20.2 indicates the quadrant placement for each patient.

There are four important measures that can be determined using a two-by-two table analysis: sensitivity, specificity, positive predictive value, and negative predictive value. **Table 20.4** describes these measures and the importance of each to decision-making in population health management programs. Table 20.3 shows the calculation of these measures using the data provided in Table 20.2.

Table 20.3 Two-by-Two Table and Indicators to Evaluate Predictive Accuracy

		Hospitalization		
		Hospitalization Occurred	Hospitalization did not Occur	
Hospitalization Prediction	**Predicted to Have Hospitalization**	n = 3 **True Positive (TP)**	n = 4 **False Positive (FP)**	*PPV = TP/(TP + FP)* = 43%
	Not Predicted to Have Hospitalization	n = 3 **False Negative (FN)**	n = 5 **True Negative (TN)**	*NPV = TN/(TN + FN)* = 38%
		Sensitivity = TP/(TP + FN) = 50%	*Specificity = TN/(TN + FP)* = 56%	

Reproduced from Sylvia, M. (2020). Epidemiological principles. *In Population Health Management Learning Series.* ForestVue Healthcare Solutions.

When setting up two-by-two table analyses, it is important to understand positive and negative outcomes and what constitutes a "yes" or a "1" value in the data and what constitutes a "no" or a "0" value in the data. This is where it is critical to comprehend how language and double negatives in definitions are translated in data terms. For instance, having a hemoglobin A1c (HbA1c) value of < 9 is considered a desirable outcome, however, if the variable to represent this outcome uses a value of "1" to indicate that the HbA1c is > 9, it is important to realize that the value is indicating the undesirable as opposed to the desirable outcome. The case study at the end of the chapter points out the importance of this nuance in greater detail.

Number Needed to Treat

When planning for successful outcomes in population health interventions, it is important to know the number of people who need to be included in the intervention to be successful.

The number needed to treat (NNT) analysis is an epidemiological method that is typically used in pharmacological and other types of treatment research to determine the number of people who need to be treated for one to benefit. The NNT approach can be applied in planning for population health interventions to estimate the number of engaged patients needed to achieve desired outcomes.

An analysis of the NNT is important when determining the number of patients needed to receive an intervention to achieve a desired target, usually some type of utilization or cost measure. A target can be set in different ways. One way to set a target is by using previous results achieved for the intervention that may be published in research or an industry white paper or in the form of a guarantee of a target as part of a proposal to undertake the intervention.

To determine the *target rate* (also sometimes referred to as *expected rate*) for patients receiving an intervention, the NNT calculation requires careful consideration of the outcome being measured (e.g., admissions, readmissions, falls), the likelihood of occurrence of the outcome

Table 20.4 Two-by-Two Table Calculations and Their Importance in Population Health Management

Concept	Definition	Formula*	Importance in Population Health Management
Sensitivity	The probability someone with a condition was correctly predicted as having the condition	TP / (TP + FN)	Sensitivity and specificity are most often used to determine the ability of a predictor to identify those with an outcome. They exist in an inverse relationship: when sensitivity increases, specificity decreases, and vice versa. When the implementation cost of a population health program is low, such as educational materials for people with chronic illness, high sensitivity is desired because a wide net will be cast to catch all possible patients with the chronic condition without as much concern for those who do not have the condition. Where the desire is to deliver an intervention to only those with the chronic condition, then a higher specificity is desired (ScienceDirect, n.d.-b).
Specificity	The probability someone without a condition was correctly predicted as not having the condition	TN / (TN + FP)	
Positive predictive value (PPV)	The probability someone predicted as having a condition actually had the condition	TP / (TP + FP)	PPV is important in determining whether predictions are useful in an intervention. PPV assesses the occurrence of the outcome and asks whether that outcome was predicted to occur (ScienceDirect, n.d.-a). A high PPV is desired when large numbers of patients are identified for an intervention based on prediction of an adverse outcome. A high PPV ensures that those who are likely to have the outcome receive the intervention designed to prevent that adverse outcome. As an example, a high PPV is desired when identifying patients for care management programs designed to prevent hospital admissions.
Negative predictive value (NPV)	The probability someone predicted as not having a condition did not actually have the condition	TN / (TN + FN)	NPV is important to consider when an intervention is costly to deliver and when withholding intervention can also lead to costly and severe adverse outcomes. When the desire is to ensure that interventions are not delivered to those who do not require them, a high NPV is desired (Umberger, Hatfield, & Speck, 2017). An example where a high NPV is indicated is in identifying participants for end-of-life care.

*TP = true positives; FP = false positives; TN = true negatives; FN = false negatives

(e.g., a "never event" like a medication error is less likely to occur than a hospital admission), and the timing of the outcome in relation to the delivery of the intervention (e.g., the flu season is at its peak within months of the availability of the influenza vaccine where the timing of a patient to experience a gap in taking medication varies from the time of a medication therapy consultation).

The calculation of NNT requires a trade-off decision between the numbers an intervention can afford to treat and the desired outcome. For example, in a cohort of patients with substance use, the current admission rate is 15% with an average admission cost of $20,000. A proposed behavioral health program shows evidence of achieving a two-percentage-point decrease in the admission rate. In a population of 100 patients receiving the program, the reduction in admissions would result in 2 less admissions (at 15% of 100, there are 15 admissions. With a reduction of 2 percentage points the rate reduces to 13% which is 13 admissions), for a savings of $40,000. However, in a population of 500 patients, there would be 10 fewer admissions (at 15% of 500, there are 75 admissions. With a reduction of 2 percentage points, the rate reduces to 13% which is 65 admissions) for a savings of $200,000. It would cost substantially more to deliver the intervention to 500 patients than

to 100 patients. The number needed to treat is optimized by weighing savings against the cost to deliver the behavioral health program for the number of patients.

The concept of NNT used in the business setting is derived from a research definition of the number of people who would need to receive an intervention in order to prevent one adverse event with a smaller NNT having a greater effectiveness (Wiley Clinical Healthcare Hub, 2007).

The NNT is calculated by taking the inverse of the absolute difference in the rate that is expected for the outcome in those who receive an intervention and the rate in that group had the intervention never been offered. In the preceding example, the expected rate of admissions with the intervention is 13%, and the rate if no intervention is offered is 15%. The absolute difference in the rates is $0.15 - 0.13 = 0.02$. The NNT is $1/.02$ or 50. This means that 50 patients would need to be in the intervention to avoid one admission. If the goal is to achieve $200,000 in savings from the intervention and each admission amounts to $20,000 in savings, then 500 patients would need to receive the intervention.

NNT calculators are available online—for example, clincalc.com and graphpad.com. The NNT provides a simple yet powerful assessment of the likelihood of benefit or return on investment from a population health intervention.

Applied Learning: Case Study

A large accountable care organization (ACO) in the United States began a program to monitor the incidence and prevalence of diabetes in its attributed population. The organization created a data set that was updated every month and tracked the number of people in the entire ACO, the number of people newly identified with diabetes, the total number of people with diabetes, and the incidence and prevalence of diabetes.

The first column in **Table 20.5** shows that the number of people in the health plan fluctuates each month with slow but steady increases until January, when there is a large increase in attributed patients. The next two columns show the number of newly identified patients and total number of patients with diabetes. *Identified* means that a diagnosis code was detected either in the EMR or in administrative claims data that indicated the person had diabetes.

The values for the newly identified patients and total number of patients with diabetes fluctuate monthly based on the number of people with diabetes who (1) leave the attributed population, (2) enter the attributed population, (3) are newly diagnosed with diabetes, or (4) die, although the reasons are not distinguishable in this figure. The incidence is calculated by dividing the number of newly identified people

(continues)

Table 20.5 Calculations of Diabetes Incidence and Prevalence in the ACO

Month	Total ACO Population	Number of People Newly Identified with Diabetes	Total Number of People with Diabetes	Incidence per Thousand	Prevalence per Thousand
July	85,369	101	8,700	1.18	101.91
August	87,245	88	8,801	1.01	100.88
September	88,332	95	8,865	1.08	100.36
October	89,112	82	8,911	0.92	100.00
November	88,699	113	9,002	1.27	101.49
December	91,345	110	9,200	1.20	100.72
January	98,446	150	9,310	1.52	94.57
February	99,223	168	9,421	1.69	94.95
March	99,478	170	9,543	1.71	95.93
April	99,697	121	9,643	1.21	96.72
May	100,234	113	9,710	1.13	96.87
June	100,466	98	9,804	0.98	97.59

with diabetes by the total ACO population in each month; the prevalence is calculated by dividing the total number of people with diabetes by the total ACO population in each month. The counts and calculations are adapted from the true epidemiological definition of incidence and prevalence in order to glean similar insights in this at-risk population.

The incidence and prevalence of diabetes is displayed graphically in **Figure 20.2** to show the fluctuation over time in new diagnoses of diabetes and the entire population with diabetes. The data show that, although there is a drop in the prevalence of diabetes in January, there is also a large spike in the incidence of diabetes at the same time—and the incidence rate remains high until April of the year. The prevalence rate drops in January but slowly begins to rise toward the prevalence in December. Data points outside of this analysis but available within the ACO show that there is a large increase in attributed patients in January that makes the denominator for the prevalence larger and thus the prevalence per thousand decreases. However, there is evidence that there were also many newly identified patients with diabetes between January and April as the patients new to the ACO began to access healthcare services for their diabetes.

The ACO wanted to understand whether its patients who were newly identified with diabetes over the year were compliant with their medications in the 3 months after being identified with diabetes compared to those who had existing diabetes during the year. This would assist them in understanding how to better target patients with diabetes for the medication therapy management intervention. If newly identified patients with diabetes are less compliant with their medications, then the ACO could automatically refer newly identified patients with diabetes for a medication therapy management intervention focused on medication adherence.

Compliance was defined as having a *medication possession ratio* (MPR) (a ratio of the day's supply for a medication to the total days prescribed) of $\geq$ 80%. The aggregated data set in **Figure 20.3** is used to

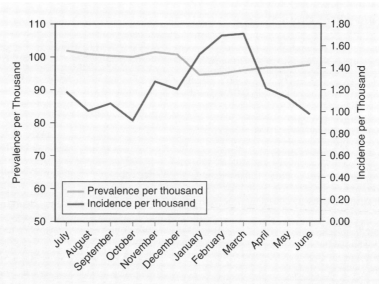

Figure 20.2 Incidence and Prevalence of Diabetes Over the Fiscal Year.

Reproduced from Sylvia, M. (2020). The population health data model. In *Population health management learning series.* ForestVue Healthcare Solutions.

Total number of people with diabetes	Number of people newly identified with diabetes	Number of people with existing diabetes	Number of people newly identified with diabetes with MPR ≥ 80 during the 3 months after identification	Number of people with existing diabetes with MPR ≥ 80 during the months of the period
11,732	1409	10,323	1212	6266

		MPR		
		MPR ≥ 80%	**MPR NOT ≥ 80%**	**Total**
Diabetes identification	**Newly identified**	1212	197	1,409
	Not newly identified (existing)	6266	4057	10,323
	Total	7478	4254	**11,732**

Sensitivity = 1212/7478 = 16%

Specificity = 4057/4254 = 95%

Positive predictive value = 1212/1409 = 86%

Negative predictive value = 4057/10,323 = 39%

Figure 20.3 Aggregated Data Set and Two-by-Two Table for Determining Whether Newly Identified Patients with Diabetes have Lower Medication Adherence.

(continues)

Applied Learning: Case Study *(continued)*

complete a two-by-two analysis. (Note that these counts are aggregated over the entire year as opposed to the monthly data set in Figure 20.3 and therefore cannot be directly calculated).

The two-by-two analysis is set up to answer the question, "Is being newly identified with diabetes associated with whether the patient will have an MPR ≥ 80%?" If being newly identified with diabetes is a good determination of an MPR ≥ 80%, then there is *no need* for the medication therapy management intervention in this group.

The sensitivity is 16%, meaning that of those who were newly identified, 16% have an MPR ≥ 80%. The specificity is 95%, meaning that when patients are not newly identified (have existing diabetes), 95% do not have an MPR ≥ 80%. The positive predictive value (PPV) is 86%, meaning that of everyone who has an MPR ≥ 80%, 86% were newly identified. The negative predictive value is 39%, meaning that of those who are not newly identified (they have existing diabetes), 39% do not have an MPR ≥ 80%. A high PPV ensures that those who are likely to have the outcome receive the intervention designed to prevent that adverse outcome.

The decision to implement the medication therapy management intervention is more heavily dependent on the PPV because the focus is to ensure that those that are more likely to *not* have an MPR ≥ 80% receive the intervention. Because the PPV is 86% in determining the favorable outcome of having an MPR ≥ 80%, the ACO decided *not* to provide the intervention to those newly identified with diabetes.

Conclusion

Surveillance is an important technique used in population health analytics and is achieved through the epidemiological methods of registries and measurements of incidence and prevalence. Together these techniques support monitoring the health determinants and health outcomes of targeted patient populations over time.

Two-by-two table analysis and the concepts of sensitivity, specificity, positive predictive value, and negative predictive value provide important methods to assess the relationship between health determinants and health outcomes and also to evaluate the effectiveness of risk-prediction models to identify future adverse outcomes. The NNT analysis ensures that an adequate number of patients are engaged in the intervention so that overall population outcomes are achieved.

As healthcare organizations strive to improve the health of their populations at risk, epidemiological methods are a critical tool for the population health analytic toolbox.

Study and Discussion Questions

- How can the concepts of incidence and prevalence be used to understand the onset of new chronic illness and existing chronic illness in a provider organization's patient panel?
- How would you design a registry to monitor health determinants and outcomes in a federally qualified health center or other clinic established to care for the underserved?
- What use cases exist in population health analytics for reporting and understanding each of the following concepts?
  - sensitivity,
  - specificity,
  - positive predictive value, and
  - negative predictive value.

Resources and Websites

National Institutes of Health. (n.d.). List of registries: https://www.nih.gov/health-information/nih-clinical-research-trials-you/list-registries

Agency for Healthcare Research and Quality. (n.d.). Computerized disease registries: https://digital.ahrq.gov/key-topics/computerized-disease-registries

What is epidemiology? (n.d.). Chapter 1 in *The British Medical Journal*. https://www.bmj.com /about-bmj/resources-readers/publications/epidemiology-uninitiated/1-what-epidemiology

Open Source Epidemiologic Statistics for Public Health. (n.d.). https://www.openepi.com/Menu/OE_Menu.htm

PHF. (n.d.). *Principles of epidemiology in public health practice* (3rd ed.). http://www.phf.org/resourcestools/Pages/Principles_of_epidemiology_3rd_edition.aspx

References

Agency for Healthcare Research and Quality. (2014, April 30). *Registries for evaluating patient outcomes: A user's guide* (3rd ed.). Author. https://effectivehealthcare.ahrq.gov/products/registries-guide-3rd-edition/research

Celentano, D. D., & Szklo, M. (2019). *Gordis epidemiology*. Elsevier Press.

Kindig, D. A., & Stoddart, G. (2003, March 1). What is population health? *American Journal of Public Health, 93*, 380–383. https://doi.org/10.2105/AJPH.93.3.380

ScienceDirect. (n.d.-a). Positive and negative predictive values—An overview [pdf]. Amsterdam, Netherlands: Elsevier. https://www.sciencedirect.com/topics/nursing-and-health-professions/positive-and-negative-predictive-values/pdf

ScienceDirect. (n.d.-b). Sensitivity and specificity—An overview. https://www.sciencedirect.com/topics/medicine-and-dentistry/sensitivity-and-specificity

Sylvia, M. (2020). The population health data model. In *Population health management learning series*. ForestVue Healthcare Solutions.

Umberger, R. A., Hatfield, L. A., & Speck, P. M. (2017). Understanding negative predictive value of diagnostic tests used in clinical practice. *Dimensions of Critical Care Nursing, 36*(1), 22–29. https://doi.org/10.1097/DCC.0000000000000219

Wiley Clinical Healthcare Hub. (2007, July 23). How results are presented (2): risks, ratios, NNT and NNH. *Prescriber, 18*(8), 21–26. https://doi.org/10.1002/psb.62

World Health Organization. (n.d.). Public health surveillance. https://www.who.int/immunization/monitoring_surveillance/burden/vpd/en

CHAPTER 21

Risk Adjustment

Martha Sylvia, PhD, MBA, RN

No one who brings ordinary powers of observation to bear on the sick and maimed, can fail to observe a remarkable difference in the aspect of cases, in their duration and in their termination in different hospitals.

—Florence Nightingale (1863)

EXECUTIVE SUMMARY

No matter how the financial pie is split, there is only a finite amount of dollars available to pay for health care. An equitable system of distribution is one that provides access to healthcare services for those who need it when they need it. To achieve equity in health care, alignment is necessary to ensure that health insurers, healthcare systems, and providers are not incentivized to turn away the sickest and most vulnerable members of society. Risk adjustment is a method to achieve this alignment and to facilitate equitable provision of healthcare services.

Risk adjustment is important because it facilitates fair distribution of healthcare resources by allowing for more resources to be directed towards patients who need them. Because of risk adjustment, at-risk entities can offer more intensive services and programs for those who need and will benefit from them. In comparing performance of at-risk entities and providers, risk adjustment allows for greater homogeneity among the comparisons. It smooths out differences in outcomes such as costs that result from factors other than the lever that is being measured. For instance, when measuring differences in admissions among the patients of different providers, the impact of age on the likelihood of an admission needs to be removed.

A lack of risk adjustment can lead to perverse incentives for healthcare provision, unfair distribution of healthcare resources, and a lack of understanding of the true determinants of healthcare outcomes. Before risk adjustment, health plans denied coverage and charged higher premiums to sicker people, and at-risk providers avoided providing care for them (Bertko, 2016).

LEARNING OBJECTIVES

At the end of this chapter, the learner will be able to:

1. Define risk adjustment concepts.
2. Explain the ways in which risk adjustment is used in population health analytics.

Introduction

Because risk adjustment is a way of controlling for observable differences between patients when paying for the health care of those patients, it is widely used in population health management. Although used for many different purposes in the population health process, it is mainly used to set payments to health plans to reflect the expected cost of providing health insurance to their members. In other applications, governments, health plans, and other payers in health care will also apply risk adjustment when paying for value (versus paying for services rendered); when measuring outcomes and comparing health systems and providers; and when measuring the impact of population health interventions (Schokkaert & Van de Voorde, 2009; Schone, Brown, & Goodell, 2013).

This chapter will introduce the concept of risk adjustment and important considerations for risk-adjustment methodology. A case study is used to apply these concepts in population health analytics.

Defining Risk Adjustment

When referring to the process of *risk adjustment*, the term can take on multiple meanings. Sometimes it is referencing the medical diagnosis coding that is used in calculating a risk score for individuals or aggregates of members in a health plan. For example, a Medicare Advantage plan often has a strategy to ensure that the diagnosis codes assigned to members in its health plan accurately reflect the complexity of illness of those members. When working toward this strategy, we might refer to the process of achieving accurate coding as *risk adjustment*. In this chapter, the focus is on the analytic methodologies used in risk adjustment.

From an analytics methodology perspective, risk adjustment is the practice of applying statistical techniques to account for differences within and between population cohorts that are unrelated to the outcome of interest (Iezzoni, 2013). Risk adjustment is of utmost importance in population health when determining value-based payments, contracting risk arrangements, and measuring the success of interventions. In population health, the most common applications of risk adjustment are to utilization metrics such as admissions, readmissions, and emergency department visits; quality indicators such as hospital-acquired infection rates, hemoglobin A1C levels in patients with diabetes, and blood pressure readings in patients with hypertension; and costs.

To determine success in these measures, they are best compared within and between cohorts when the impact of factors that are not readily changeable but have an impact on measure results can be eliminated. For example, when comparing readmission rates between hospitals, the Centers for Medicare and Medicaid Services (CMS) apply risk-adjustment techniques to mitigate the effect of age, clinical risk factors, and other known risk factors on the readmissions measure.

Risk-Adjustment Factors

Many factors can be used for risk adjustment, depending on the use case. Patient factors can include age, gender, and race or ethnicity; as well as disease conditions, multimorbidity, frailty, functional status, social factors, financial status, and educational level. Environmental factors include air and water quality and seasonal effects. Health system factors include access to care, rural versus urban healthcare delivery, and more. Any of the multitude of health determinants can be considered in risk-adjustment methods (Sylvia, 2018).

The choice of variables to be used in risk adjustment strongly depends on the availability, completeness, and accuracy of data to represent risk-adjustment factors. The CMS and commercial health plans usually create risk-adjustment variables from enrollment and administrative claims data sources. Alternatively, a provider organization may use risk-adjustment factors created from variables in the electronic medical record. As population health management initiatives partner more with communities, other data sources could also provide value such as health information exchanges and local health department data.

Large-scale payers and integrated healthcare systems have established standardized systems for risk adjustment. Age and gender are the most commonly used factors. Variables based on diagnostic information usually use some type of data contextualizer to group diagnosis codes into meaningful clinical categorizations. Some common methods are hierarchical condition categories (HCCs), adjusted clinical groups (ACGs), and diagnosis-related groups (DRGs). When diagnosis information from medical claims are not available, pharmacy-based data contextualizers like the ACG Pharmacy Morbidity Groups also can be used to create diagnosis variables. Episodes of care can also be used to risk adjust and use groupers such as episode treatment groups (Juhnke, Bethge, & Mühlbacher, 2016).

Indirect and Direct Risk Adjustment Methods

Indirect risk adjustment is used for population health management purposes. Using this method, the experience of a larger reference population is applied to a smaller subgroup of interest. It is most commonly applied by comparing an actual value of an outcome to the expected based on the larger reference population (Diener-West & Kanchanaraksa, 2008). For example, the actual costs in one provider's panel of patients with diabetes might be $10,000 per year. An expected cost could be calculated in a larger reference population that spans all providers and may be larger or smaller than the actual costs in this one provider's patient panel.

This method can be illustrated in an example of an analysis to compare the healthcare spending of the patient panels for two accountable care organizations (ACOs), ACO1 and ACO2 (**Table 21.1**). In this example, ACO1 has a patient panel of patients who are younger, have less morbidity, and have better living conditions than ACO2; their healthcare expenditures are also less than ACO2. In comparing the performance on healthcare expenditures without risk adjustment, it could be determined that ACO1 performs better than ACO2. However, using the reference population that includes all possible ACOs to account for age, gender, multimorbidity, and living conditions, ACO2 is performing better than ACO1 because its actual expenditures are less than its expected expenditures after risk adjustment.

Direct risk-adjustment methods use the experience of subsets of a population to determine expected values in a larger population. These methods are commonly used in reporting vital statistics and in other epidemiological applications but are not commonly used in population health management (Diener-West & Kanchanaraksa, 2008).

Table 21.1 Risk-Adjustment Example

Measure	ACO 1	ACO 2
Mean age	64.5	72.3
% Female	52.3	56.2
Multimorbidity score (higher is worse)	5.6	7.8
Average ranking of area deprivation index (ADI) of neighborhood (higher is worse) (University of Wisconsin, n.d.)	35.2	54.2
Unadjusted mean per member per year costs (actual costs PMPY)	$5,368	$6,109
Expected costs after adjusting for age, gender, multimorbidity, and ADI	$4,859	$6,234
Ratio of actual costs to expected costs	1.10	0.98

Concurrent and Prospective Risk Adjustment

Concurrent or *retrospective* risk-adjustment methods use information from the current year to determine the outcome in the current period. The same time frame is used to collect information to calculate the risk-adjustment score and to determine a risk-adjusted payment. Concurrent risk adjustment is advantageous when there is limited information about a patient before the current year and when the current year provides the most accurate and abundant information available. Concurrent risk adjustment is the most accurate in its ability to assign risk and is preferred for comparative performance of results (Iezzoni, 2013).

An example of concurrent risk adjustment is seen in the methodology that the U.S. government uses to risk adjust payments to insurers who offer health plans under the Affordable Care Act (ACA). ACA health plans are prohibited from denying coverage or charging higher premiums to health plan members who are sicker, and the plans are incentivized to do so through premium and cost-sharing subsidies. These financial payments are calculated using a method of concurrent risk adjustment. One set amount of funds is provided across all health plans to deliver healthcare services for insured members. In the same year in which the member is insured and financial incentive is provided, a risk score is calculated based on multiple factors, including age, gender, morbidity level, and the type of health plan in which the member is enrolled. The program transfers money among ACA plans within a state in such a way that insurers with sicker patients receive higher payments than insurers with healthier patients (American Academy of Actuaries, 2016).

Prospective risk-adjustment methods use information from the current year to predict an outcome in a future time period. Prospective risk adjustment is often used to project payments in risk arrangements for a future time period, often

a year. One major advantage of prospective risk adjustment is that it allows for stability in budgeting for healthcare service payments. For instance, if a risk-bearing entity knows the payment it will receive for its population in a subsequent year, healthcare services and benefits can be provided within a known supporting revenue stream. A substantial disadvantage to prospective risk adjustment is that the factors that are used to risk adjust can change between when a risk score is calculated and when payment is received. Thus, the need for resources can be higher in the subsequent time period.

As an example of prospective risk adjustment, CMS's HCC model is used for risk adjustment in Medicare Advantage managed care health insurance programs. Each year CMS informs Medicare Advantage plans of risk-score calculations, explanations of factors used to calculate risk scores, and the capitation rate that will be used for the subsequent year's payment. Risk scores are calculated in a base year to estimate Medicare benefit costs for the following year using demographic, disability, geographic, living situation, and morbidity information (Centers for Medicare and Medicaid Services, 2014).

Risk adjustment is key to determining payments in value-based arrangements and measuring the performance of population health interventions at multiple levels and points of delivery. There are multiple methods and considerations for risk adjustment and instructional resources available for executing these methods (Iezzoni, 2013; Sylvia, 2018).

Communicating and Reporting Risk-Adjustment Results

The results of risk adjustment are commonly reported by showing the actual outcome results both with and without risk adjustment as in Table 21.1. The ratio of actual to expected (also called *observed to expected*) reports the results in one figure and is expressed as the actual result divided by the expected result after risk adjustment. A ratio of <1 means that the grouping is performing better than expected, a ratio of 1 means that the grouping is performing as expected, and a ratio of >1 means that the grouping is performing worse than expected.

Applied Learning: Case Study

A rural clinically integrated network (CIN) of multiple independent provider groups formed to improve outcomes for those with chronic illness in a Midwestern area in the United States. Through clinical integration, the providers have formed a team accountable for quality and cost outcomes in a population of patients with diabetes, congestive heart failure, and chronic obstructive pulmonary disease. The CIN will secure and fund services and resources to improve outcomes. As an example of shared resources, the entire CIN will use the same telehealth services to monitor chronic illness indicators, intervening before acute care services are needed for acute exacerbations. These types of interventions will prevent acute and long-term complications and reduce unnecessary healthcare utilization and costs.

The CIN expects to see shared savings as a result of their efforts to improve outcomes and has asked the analytic team to develop a method of risk adjustment to fairly distribute the savings among the participating provider groups. The CIN has agreed on a method of assigning risk scores to individual patients that accounts for the level of illness burden.

As a first step, the analyst assembles a patient-level data set with some patient characteristics and the fields needed for risk adjustment, which are the actual costs and the risk score. Next, the analyst uses the entire population in the CIN to determine the expected costs for each risk score increment and assigns the expected costs to each patient according to their risk score. The example of this data set with the actual and expected costs is in **Table 21.2**.

Table 21.2 Risk-Adjustment Patient-Level Data Set

ID	Age	Sex	Provider	Risk Score	Actual Costs ($)	Expected Costs ($)
11011	32	F	1	3	1,571	5,100
11012	32	F	10	2	133	3,500
11013	55	M	4	1	0	2,000
11014	60	F	3	3	6,385	5,100
11015	58	F	2	3	484	5,100
11016	77	M	7	5	1,453	9,200
11017	32	F	8	2	1,527	3,500
11018	4	F	4	4	4,374	6,850
11019	59	F	5	4	7,291	6,850
11020	33	M	2	1	0	2,000
11021	84	M	3	4	15,200	6,850
11022	64	M	8	3	345	5,100
11023	47	F	5	4	10,722	6,850

(continues)

(continues)

Applied Learning: Case Study *(continued)*

Table 21.2 Risk-Adjustment Patient-Level Data Set *(continued)*

ID	Age	Sex	Provider	Risk Score	Actual Costs ($)	Expected Costs ($)
11024	58	F	4	4	11,074	6,850
11025	26	F	2	5	16,164	9,200
11026	72	F	5	5	37,142	9,200
11027	34	M	9	4	8,694	6,850
11028	58	F	3	3	1,437	5,100
11029	27	F	2	3	568	5,100

The analyst then calculates the average actual costs and average expected costs for each provider to calculate the average to expected ratio. **Table 21.3** shows the result of that analysis. Graphical display of the results shows those provider groups who are over and below 1, which is where the actual costs would equal the expected.

These ratios can be used to distribute shared savings as a multiplier. Providers whose ratio is less than 1 are efficient and would receive a higher proportion of the shared savings than providers whose ratio is greater than 1. **Table 21.4** shows one way in which this can be calculated by multiplying the average expected payment per provider without risk adjustment and then multiplying by the inverse of the ratio to get the risk-adjusted payment. Any leftover funds could go into a shared CIN account for adjustments

Table 21.3 Actual to Expected Ratios by Provider

Provider	Count of Patients	Average Actual Costs ($)	Average Expected Costs ($)	Actual/Expected Ratio
1	4,010	2,051	2,127	0.96
2	2,099	2,446	2,583	0.95
3	1,683	2,913	3,251	0.90
4	1,563	2,224	2,076	1.07
5	1,280	2,638	2,022	1.30
6	1,237	2,352	2,524	0.93
7	1,206	2,756	2,326	1.18
8	1,010	2,278	2,172	1.05
9	857	2,892	2,629	1.10
10	823	2,156	2,054	1.05

in future time periods or for mutual investments. If the risk-adjusted sum of all payments goes over the budgeted amount, an across-the-board reduction can be made. Note that the payment analysis in Table 21.4 does not make an adjustment for the number of patients per provider.

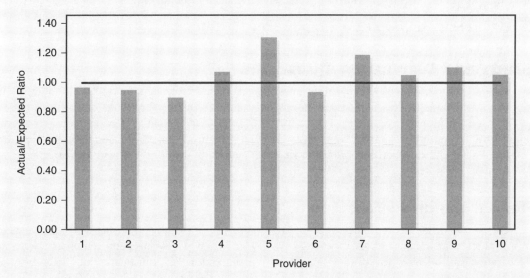

Reproduced from Sylvia, M. (2020). Risk adjustment. In *Population health management learning series.* ForestVue Healthcare Solutions.

Table 21.4 Calculating Risk-Adjusted Payments per Provider

Provider	Count of Patients	Actual or Expected Ratio	Average Expected Payment per Provider	Risk-Adjusted Payment per Provider ($)
1	4,010	0.96	100,000	103,707
2	2,099	0.95	100,000	105,596
3	1,683	0.90	100,000	111,607
4	1,563	1.07	100,000	93,358
5	1,280	1.30	100,000	76,649
6	1,237	0.93	100,000	107,282
7	1,206	1.18	100,000	84,391
8	1,010	1.05	100,000	95,367
9	857	1.10	100,000	90,915
10	823	1.05	100,000	95,245

Reproduced from Sylvia, M. (2020). Risk adjustment. In *Population health management learning series.* ForestVue Healthcare Solutions.

Conclusion

Risk adjustment is an important analytic capability for population health management. Health determinants differ among individuals, patient panels, and entire populations. These factors, which unintentionally impact health outcomes, are important to measure and adjust for when measuring intervention effects and clinician performance in population health management and to ensure equitable distribution of healthcare funds.

Study and Discussion Questions

- Why is risk adjustment an important analytic methodology for population health management?
- What factors are important to consider when risk adjusting outcomes for provider payment purposes?
- What factors are important to consider when risk adjusting the results of an evaluation of population health interventions?
- Identify available data sources that can be used to define risk-adjustment variables.

Resources and Websites

Centers for Medicare and Medicaid Services. (n.d.). Risk adjustment. https://www.cms.gov /Medicare/Health-Plans/MedicareAdvtgSpecRate Stats/Risk-Adjustors

American Health Information Management Association. (n.d.). Documentation and coding practices for risk adjustment and HCCs. https:// bok.ahima.org/doc?oid=302516#.XpJPoPhKiUk

References

American Academy of Actuaries. (2016, April). Insights on the ACA Risk Adjustment Program. Author. https:// www.actuary.org/sites/default/files/files/imce/Insights _on_the_ACA_Risk_Adjustment_Program.pdf

Bertko, J. (2016, March 29). What risk adjustment does—The perspective of a health insurance actuary who relies on it. HealthAffairs. https://www.healthaffairs.org/do/10.1377 /hblog20160329.054175/full/

Centers for Medicare and Medicaid Services. (2014). Risk adjustment. In *Medicare Managed Care Manual.* https://www.cms.gov/Regulations-and-Guidance /Guidance/Manuals/Internet-Only-Manuals-IOMs-Items /CMS019326

Diener-West, M., & Kanchanaraksa, S. (2008). The direct and indirect methods of adjustment. http://docplayer.net /39859756-The-direct-and-indirect-methods-of-adjustment -marie-diener-west-phd-sukon-kanchanaraksa-phd -johns-hopkins-university.html

Iezzoni, L. I. (Ed.). (2013). *Risk adjustment for measuring healthcare outcomes.* Health Administration Press.

Juhnke, C., Bethge, S., & Mühlbacher, A. C. (2016). A review on methods of risk adjustment and their use in integrated healthcare systems. *International Journal of Integrated Care, 16*(4). https://doi.org/10.5334/ijic.2500

Nightingale, F. (1863). Notes on hospitals. Longman, Green, Longman, Roberts, and Green.

Schokkaert, E., & Van de Voorde, C. (2009, March). Direct versus indirect standardization in risk adjustment. *Journal of Health Economics, 28*(2), 361–374. https://doi .org/10.1016/j.jhealeco.2008.10.012

Schone, E., Brown, R., & Goodell, S. (2013, July 1). The synthesis project risk adjustment: What is the current state of the art and how can it be improved? Robert Wood Johnson Foundation. https://www.rwjf.org/en/library /research/2013/07/risk-adjustment---what-is-the-current -state-of-the-art-and-how-c.html

Sylvia, M. L. (2018). Risk adjustment. Pp. 337–348 in M. L. Sylvia & M. F. Terhaar (Eds.), *Clinical analytics and data management for the DNP* (2nd ed.). Springer Publishing Company.

University of Wisconsin. (n.d.). Neighborhood atlas. School of Medicine and Public Health. https://www .neighborhoodatlas.medicine.wisc.edu/

CHAPTER 22

Predictive and Prescriptive Analytics

Martha Sylvia, PhD, MBA, RN

An unsophisticated forecaster uses statistics as a drunken man uses lampposts—for support rather than for illumination.

—Andrew Lang

EXECUTIVE SUMMARY

When the topic of population health management and analytics arises, one of the most common discussions revolves around predictive analytics. Using mathematical theory and data to estimate outcomes that cannot be immediately measured, predictive analytics is touted as the answer to addressing health needs in populations and improving outcomes when the need is to identify future at-risk beneficiaries (Brown, 2018). Similarly, prescriptive analytics, which moves the question of predictive analytics from "What will happen" to "What should be done," is seen as the pinnacle of analytic capabilities for which many healthcare organizations strive. While predictive and prescriptive analytics provide great value in population health, they represent a key analytic capability in a multitude of tools needed to achieve success.

It is important to proceed on the journey to predictive and prescriptive analytic capabilities with thoughtfulness, caution, and, most importantly, with knowledge about the considerations for introducing predictive and prescriptive analytics into clinical and other programs. Although these models identify patients who may benefit, they come with trade-offs such as falsely identifying those who will benefit (false positives) and removing people who might benefit (false negatives). These concepts are important to understand in population health where the desire is to efficiently match people to appropriate interventions and achieve the best outcomes without leaving anyone behind.

LEARNING OBJECTIVES

At the end of this chapter, the learner will be able to:

1. Identify methods used in the development of risk-prediction models.
2. Interpret validation results for risk-prediction models.
3. Distinguish between predictive and prescriptive modeling.
4. Describe applications of predictive and prescriptive modeling in population health.
5. Summarize key decision points for using predictive and prescriptive models in practice.

Introduction

Even those healthcare systems that would likely be deemed lower on the analytics capabilities hierarchy have introduced and practiced some level of predictive modeling. Healthcare systems relying on Excel spreadsheets and manual reporting without any type of data warehouse structure now have the ability to use risk-prediction tools that come with their electronic medical record (EMR) software. Healthcare systems with more analytic resources, data warehouses, supportive population health analytic infrastructure, and automated analytic processes have moved toward robust programs of predictive and even prescriptive modeling to improve patient care.

Examples of risk-prediction and prescriptive uses in health care include:

- using hospitalization data to predict sepsis, ventilator-associated pneumonia, and risk for readmission;
- using health plan data to predict members who may benefit from care management for chronic conditions, medication therapy programs, end-of-life care, and specialized condition management clinics; and
- using outpatient provider and community data to prescribe the best way to schedule appointments based on clinician capabilities, community bus routes, and person-level characteristics.

This chapter focuses on the inner working engine of risk-prediction and prescriptive models. Risk-prediction models that use linear and logistic regression are the subject of this chapter, whereas methods that use machine-learning and pattern-based methods are the subject of Chapter 23, "Advanced Analytic Methods." Whether a healthcare organization chooses to develop its own program of modeling, purchase capabilities within its EMR system, or purchase them from vendors, there are key concepts about the development and validation of risk-prediction and prescription models that are necessary for making these decisions. This chapter focuses on those key decision points and the tools necessary to make informed choices.

Risk Prediction

To achieve the goals of reduced utilization and costs, one approach is to apply intensive interventions to all patients who meet certain algorithmic criteria. However, because a small number of patients are responsible for a majority of hospitalizations and healthcare costs, an alternative approach is to provide the recommended level of care to all patients and identify any subgroup of patients who are at high risk for adverse outcomes so that more intensive interventions can be applied to meet the needs of the highest-risk patients. To do the latter, valid and reliable risk-prediction modeling is needed.

Risk-prediction models in health care are data-driven, decision-support tools that estimate an individual's future potential healthcare costs and utilization. They allow for identification of the subgroupings of a population likely to be at highest cost or utilization in subsequent years using predictors from a previous time period (Knutson, Bella, Llanos, & Martin, 2009). Historically, predictive models have been applied to payer administrative data, although new models of healthcare delivery across payers, clinicians, health settings, and geographic locations lend themselves to population-level identification and risk stratification of people with chronic illness across multiple health plans and data sources using a patient-centered approach.

Risk-prediction modeling is preferred to a method of identifying high-risk patients that is based on some type of threshold or cut point for one or multiple variables, such as all patients with greater than $10,000 in costs, with more than six emergency department visits or HbA1c greater than 9. These types of threshold-based criteria are biased because they select only outliers for intervention and select patients who are likely to regress to the mean in future years. Regression to the mean is a phenomenon in which outliers in a current period are likely to be similar to the average of the group in a future period without any intervention at all. Risk-prediction modeling is preferred over threshold-based models to prevent selection bias and regression-to-the-mean effects (Cousins, Shickle, & Bander, 2004).

Methods Used in the Development of Risk-Prediction Models

This chapter focuses on the commonly used analytic methods used to develop risk-prediction models of logistic and linear regression, also referred to as *multivariate statistical models*. These methods are considered hypothesis based in that predictors are selected based on research showing their impact on outcomes or from analytics demonstrating the correlation between predictors and an outcome (Dankers, Traverso, Wee, & van Kuijk, 2018). During the assessment phase of population health analytics, relationships between health determinants and health outcomes are discovered. These relationships are used to develop risk-prediction models by assigning health determinants as predictors in a model used to predict a related outcome.

When developing risk-prediction models, it is useful to follow a logical sequence such as the following:

- define the population in which risk will be predicted,
- identify the predictor variables,
- define the outcome variable,
- determine the time frame for predictors and the outcome,
- apply the appropriate statistical modeling technique,
- derive outputs, and
- validate the risk-prediction model.

Each step will be reviewed in more detail.

Define the Population

It is important to know the entire population at risk for adverse outcomes and to define that population in terms of inclusion and exclusion criteria in data terms. The defined population is one of concern for a healthcare organization at risk for outcomes, which is usually quality, utilization, or costs. Populations for risk-prediction models can be defined at the macro level or *whole population* representing people across the spectrum from wellness to end of life (Jeffery et al., 2019).

This type of population definition is most often used when a payer or accountable care organization (ACO) is the stakeholder in risk prediction. For example, an ACO would be interested in understanding who is at highest risk for a hospital admission in its entire attributed Medicare population.

Subgroupings of whole populations can also be used to develop risk-prediction models. Segments of the population can be defined in many ways, such as those with a certain chronic condition, residing within a certain community, or receiving primary care from a particular provider or health system. For example, it is common to run interventions that are designed to prevent adverse outcomes in patients with particular chronic conditions such as diabetes, congestive heart failure, or chronic obstructive pulmonary disease because the clinical care guidelines and outcomes are unique to these particular conditions. Risk-prediction models can be developed within these special subgroupings to tailor and deliver the appropriate intensity of intervention to those with the condition at varying risk levels.

When developing risk-prediction models, it is important to develop the model in a population or subgroup as similar as possible to that in which it will be applied in practice. For example, if the intention is to prevent newborn admissions to the neonatal intensive care unit for babies born to mothers in Medicaid, then the population used to develop the risk model would be all women of childbearing age in Medicaid or all pregnant women of childbearing age in Medicaid, depending on the chosen predictors and time periods.

Identify the Predictor Variables

Data inputs or predictors for risk-prediction models are grounded in health determinants that are known to affect health outcomes. Domains for these data inputs may include demographics, morbidities, genetics, relationships with family and communities, economic indicators, and environmental factors. Important determinants of health include factors that predispose, enable, or reinforce behaviors contributing to health risk; individuals' own perception of health risk; the physical and sociocultural environment in which individuals live and work; the macroeconomy of public policy, media, and economy; and the performance of healthcare systems (Jeffery et al., 2019).

In reality, many of these ideal factors are not measurable in practice, therefore risk-prediction models perform best when maximizing available data points in these domains. Risk-prediction factors most commonly used include demographic factors of age, gender, race or ethnicity and less commonly education, geographic location, and income; morbidity factors derived from diagnosis codes in administrative claims data, hospital admission data and less often electronic medical records; utilization data such as hospital admissions and days spent in the hospital, emergency department visits, and readmissions derived from administrative claims data; and less commonly lab values (Jeffery et al., 2019). Other supplemental data sets can include social and behavioral, consumer, social media, and self-reported data (see Chapter 9, "Grouping, Trending, and Interpreting Population Health Data for Receptivity, Engagement, and Activation").

Although integrated data sources are the ideal for model inputs, many health systems do not yet have access to data that are integrated across payer, provider, and other sources; nor do they have the database structure required to make these integrated data available for the operational work of running risk-prediction models in practice. Payer data, which can include any combination of medical and pharmacy claims payment; enrollment; health risk assessment; and lab data, remains a ready and useful source of inputs for risk prediction for population health initiatives.

Identify the Outcome Variable

The outcome used in risk-prediction modeling is also informed by the assessment of the relationship between health determinants and health outcomes, but, more important, the outcome is something that will be prevented. Population health interventions aim to prevent adverse outcomes such as hospitalizations, emergency department visits, high costs, and poor-quality indicators. To prevent them, they first need to be predicted. There needs to be an understanding of who in the population is more likely to experience the poor outcome so that an intervention can prevent it from occurring.

The selection of the outcome is also informed by problems in the business of health care. Assessing populations to identify opportunities for cost savings, more efficient utilization, and better indicators of quality usually stems from a problem identified in one or more of these indicators when running the business of healthcare delivery. For instance, a provider organization who receives payments for keeping blood pressure levels within a certain range for patients with hypertension may notice that payments have decreased because more patients with hypertension are experiencing high blood pressure. This problem, which is identified in running the business, becomes one that will benefit from a prediction of hypertensive patients to better prevent this outcome.

Outcome variables commonly used in risk-prediction modeling include hospitalizations within varying time frames such as 6 months or 1 year, readmissions within 30 days, emergency department visits, high costs, long hospitalization length of stay, admission to specialized settings such as rehabilitation or psychiatric care facilities, and poor-quality indicators such as insufficient blood glucose control in people with diabetes or poor oxygen saturation in people with chronic obstructive pulmonary disease.

Determine the Time Frame for Predictors and the Outcome

Predictive models are useful because they utilize indicators or predictors from a current point in time to predict a future outcome. Because time frames differ depending on the use case, it is important to understand the timing between the predictors and the outcome in order to set time parameters. A predictive model using indicators from a current inpatient stay to predict sepsis will have different time parameters than a model designed to predict a person having a hospitalization from administrative claims data. Once time parameters are understood, data from the current time period are organized into variables that will be used to predict the outcome in the future time period. When developing risk-prediction models, data are available for both time periods and the variables are created appropriately from each.

An important consideration regarding time frames is that the closer the time frame between the predictors and the outcome, the better the prediction. Predicting whether a hospitalization will occur in the next week based on today's available data holds a much different window of time to intervene than predicting whether the hospitalization will occur within the next year. Most prediction models used in population health management predict an outcome within the upcoming year. This allows time to outreach, secure engagement, deliver interventions, and prevent adverse outcomes in those identified as high risk. However, many interventions require shorter time frames such as preventing a readmission within 30 days. The use case will dictate the necessary time period between the prediction and outcome.

Apply the Appropriate Statistical Modeling Technique

Logistic Regression

Logistic regression is the most commonly used regression-based statistical technique for risk-prediction modeling in population health applications. Logistic regression methods are used to predict a dichotomous outcome, such as the occurrence of a hospitalization, and produce individual-level probability scores representing the likelihood from 0% to 100% that the person will have the outcome.

The following formula represents the mathematical equation for logistic regression. Y is the outcome and is equal to the log odds of the outcome and is converted to a probability. Each X

on the right side of the equation represents a predictor variable, and its associated β represents the weight of the predictor toward the probability of the outcome being predicted. Logarithmic conversions are necessary to derive the predicted probability, but the ability to do the conversion is not necessary to understand the concepts of how logistic regression models work (Sylvia, 2020):

$$\log\left\{\left(\frac{Probability\ (Y=1)}{Probability\ (Y=0)}\right)\right\} = \beta_0 + \beta_1 X_1 + \beta_2 X_2 + \dots\dots\dots + \beta_p X_p$$

Linear Regression

Linear regression methods predict continuous outcomes such as costs, number of hospitalizations, or a particular value for a quality measure and produces individual level estimates of the outcome. Linear regression methods are used less often for population health management applications because the goal is not to identify individual-level estimates but to instead identify groupings of individuals at risk for surpassing a particular threshold of an indicator. For instance, there is more of an interest in predicting a person as potentially high cost than predicting what their individual costs will actually be. Occasionally, linear regression will be used to predict the estimate and a cutoff will be applied to the predicted estimate to identify those who are predicted to be above a threshold. For instance, linear regression could be used to predict the cost estimate and then a dichotomous indicator would be created to identify those above or below a specified cost threshold.

The following formula represents the mathematical equation for linear regression. Y represents the outcome and is the estimated value for the outcome. Each X on the right side of the equation represents a predictor variable, and its associated β represents the weight of the predictor toward the value of the outcome being predicted (Sylvia, 2020).

$$\text{Estimate } [Y] = \beta_0 + \beta_1 X_1 + \beta_2 X_2 + \dots\dots\dots + \beta_p X_p$$

Derive the Output of the Risk-Prediction Model

From the mathematical equations for logistic and linear regression, outputs are derived at the person level. Logistic regression produces a probability of 0% to 100% that a person will have the adverse outcome. Linear regression produces an estimate of the result (Sylvia, 2018).

Outputs are derived by placing individual values for each input variable in the equation, applying the β weights, and carrying out the equation to get the estimate. For example, in this equation, the probability of an admission is determined by the following equation:

$$\text{Log odds of admission} = -5.678 + 5.523 \,(\text{age}) + 2.120 \,(\text{chronic conditions})$$

where

Age: ≥ 65 years old $= 1$; < 65 years old $= 0$
Chronic conditions: $\geq 5 = 1$; $< 5 = 0$

To convert this to a probability of admission for a 70-year-old person with eight chronic conditions:
Calculate log odds:

$$\text{Log odds of admission} = -5.678 + 5.523(1) + 2.120(1) = 1.965$$

Convert to odds by taking e to the power:

$$e^{1.965} = 7.13$$

Convert to probability:

$$\text{Probability} = 7.13/1 + 7.13 = 88\%$$

The risk score for this patient is 0.88 or an 88% probability of having an admission (Sylvia, 2018).

Validate the Model

Whether performing logistic or linear regression, risk-prediction models should undergo multiple iterations of testing using development and testing data sets. Bootstrapping is one method of calculating hundreds or thousands of iterations of a result to determine the confidence in results.

Bootstrapping can be performed to get multiple replications of other validation statistics like the C statistic described in the next section (Harrell, Lee, & Mark, 1996; Steyerberg et al., 2001).

Validation Methods for Logistic Regression

Whether developing an in-house predictive model or purchasing, a predictive model can be validated using data in the organization in which it will be operationalized. Three methods commonly used to validate the performance of logistic regression-based, risk-prediction models are discrimination, bootstrapping, and calibration.

Discrimination measures the model's ability to separate members with different responses and at its foundation uses two-by-two tables to measure sensitivity, specificity, positive predictive value, and negative predictive value. Recall from Chapter 20 the definitions of each and the situations in which it is desirable to maximize each. To create two-by-two tables and make these calculations, a cutoff point of the risk-prediction score is made to dichotomize the prediction. For instance, a probability of greater than 80% may be considered high risk and below 80% considered low risk. The outcome is also dichotomized into whether it does or does not occur.

The goal in most population health initiatives is to select individuals with the highest risk for an adverse outcome and intervene to prevent it from occurring. Discrimination is determined for this purpose by using the C statistic or "area under the operator receiving curve." It represents the probability that an individual who actually has the outcome will have a higher predicted risk than the individual who does not actually have the outcome. It measures the ability of the model to rank individuals from high to low risk but not the accuracy of the actual individual-level predicted risk (Harrell et al., 1996). The C statistic ranges from 0.50 or 50% where the model is no better than chance alone; to 100%, where the model predicts with complete accuracy (Pencina & D'Agostino, 2015). A C statistic greater than 0.70 indicates adequacy for use in population health management programs, with higher values indicating better performance.

Calibration is used to evaluate the agreement of predicted probability with the observed probability. One way to calibrate is to create bins of probability scores (quartiles work well) and compare them with the observed outcome results looking for similarities in the averages.

Examples of the application of these techniques are provided in the case study.

Validation Methods for Linear Regression

Linear regression–based models use the R^2 statistic to measure model performance. The R^2 statistic represents the amount of variance explained by a linear regression model and is expressed as a percentage. A value of 100% indicates that the model perfectly predicts the outcome, and a value of 0% means there is no relationship between the predictors and the outcome. The R^2 statistic indicates the ability of the entire model to predict the outcome and not the ability of each individual predictor.

The R^2 statistic should be interpreted with great care when used in population health management. R^2 cannot convey the relationship between two variables and, more importantly, a single outlier observation can have a large effect on the R^2 statistic. Typically, R^2 results in risk-prediction models used in population

health management can be as low as 15%. This is why risk-prediction models that produce a point estimate of an outcome like the predicted costs or predicted number of hospitalizations are seldom used for targeting participants for intervention in population health management interventions.

The mean absolute prediction error (MAPE) estimate is a less-known indicator of predictive accuracy and is defined as the ratio of the sum of the individual absolute values of the prediction error to the sample size. Prediction error is the difference between the predicted value and the actual value by individual. The MAPE is difficult to compare across prediction models because it is not expressed in a standardized scale; generally, however, the smaller the MAPE, the more accurate the prediction (Sylvia, 2020).

Assessing a Risk-Prediction Model for Use in Practice

Whether an organization has developed its own risk-prediction model or is purchasing a risk-prediction model to operationalize in practice, a core set of criteria should be assessed based on model-development procedures and parameters as well as organizational capabilities. These criteria are summarized in **Table 22.1**.

Table 22.1 Checklist for the Assessment of Risk-Prediction Models

Domain and Question	Acceptable Criteria
Population Used for Development	
Is the population in which the model was developed reflective of the population in which it will be implemented?	The development population should be similar in important characteristics to the population in which it will be used.
Data Inputs	
Are the data sources appropriate for the data input?	Data sources used appropriately represent the data input concept (e.g., hospital admissions are sourced from administrative claims data).

(continues)

Table 22.1 Checklist for the Assessment of Risk-Prediction Models *(continued)*

Domain and Question	Acceptable Criteria
Data Inputs	
Are the data inputs used for the model available, accessible, and appropriately structured in the organization in which the model will be developed?	The data inputs required to run the model must be available to the organization that will implement the model. The inputs must be accessible and structured so that the risk-prediction model can easily accept them.
Predictive Accuracy	
How do the developers substantiate consistency of model performance across multiple data sets?	The predictive model should have been tested in multiple iterations of testing data sets using a technique like bootstrapping or similar method.
Is the predictive accuracy reporting appropriate for the type of model?	Logistic regression models should report discrimination statistics of sensitivity, specificity, positive predictive value, negative predictive value, and the C statistic as well as calibration results.
	Linear regression methods should report the R^2 statistic and the mean absolute prediction error.
	The developer should explain the results of these statistics in the context of the use case for using the model in the organization.
Purpose of the Score	
Do the risk model, time frames, and score produced match the purpose in which they will be used?	The intent of the intervention, the type of model, and the time frame for the prediction need to be compared to the organizational use case for appropriateness. For instance, in a care-transition program to prevent readmissions, the prediction model should predict readmissions using logistic regression within 30 days of a previous hospital admission.
Feasibility of Operationalizing the Model	
Can this model be implemented in this organization?	Feasibility is one of the most important considerations, and criteria include:
	■ transparency of model inputs and outputs such that all stakeholders understand how to implement,
	■ clinician buy-in for using the model,
	■ information technology and analytic people resources to
	• automate the model,
	• make outputs available at the point of care in decision-support and patient care technology, and
	■ the data infrastructure to readily and regularly automate model inputs.

Applied Learning: Case Study

Diabetes-Specific Risk Prediction of Hospitalization in a Primary Care Health Improvement Initiative

Martha Sylvia, PhD, MBA, RN

Sarah Kachur, PharmD, MBA, BCACP

Yanyan Lu, MS

Shannon Murphy, MA

This case study was implemented as part of an initiative to improve the care of patients with diabetes. The work was sponsored by a large health plan with patients spanning multiple primary care providers in a risk arrangement incentivizing Triple Aim outcomes of high-quality health care and positive patient experiences at a reasonable cost. The health plan supported the providers in identifying patients with diabetes who were at high risk of adverse outcomes and most amenable to the intervention.

To identify high-risk patients, a diabetes-specific predictive tool that estimates the risk of subsequent year all-cause hospitalization using administrative healthcare data in combination with lab data was created. The model was designed to predict all-cause hospitalization in patients with diabetes using a population of patients with diabetes spanning multiple health plans, combining claims data with lab vendor data, using methodology that supports care-management processes, using clinical predictors that are impactful by the care-management team, using risk stratification to select patients for tiered levels of intervention, and culminating in the implementation of the risk-prediction tool in practice.

Development of the Predictive Model

Identification of Patients with Diabetes

Patients who were enrolled in any of the available health plans were included if they were 18 or older and had at least 1 day of enrollment in the predictor year and the outcome year. A diagnosis of diabetes was determined if there were an occurrence of at least one diabetes code from the *International Classification of Diseases, 10th Revision, Clinical Modification* (ICD-10-CM) or one from the National Drug Code for diabetes medication in the predictor year. Patients who were identified with gestational diabetes, steroid-induced diabetes, or polycystic ovaries were excluded. ICD-10 diagnoses for lab and radiology services or durable medical equipment were excluded for identification purposes to avoid rule-out diagnoses.

Outcome and Predictor Variables

The outcome variable for the logistic regression model was an indicator of any admission in year 2. All-cause admissions to acute-care inpatient facilities were used, excluding admissions to skilled nursing and psychiatric facilities.

Predictor variables were identified from year 1 data. Exploratory data analysis was conducted to determine the definitions of predictor variables. Continuous predictors were converted to categorical predictors for ease of interpretation in the logistic model, based on either clinical meaning or the ability to achieve an even distribution of values. Only 30% to 60% of patients had a value for the lab-based predictors depending on the type of lab test. To keep the information for those in which lab predictors were available, a missing value category was created for each variable.

Results

Predictive Model and Validation

A multivariate logistic regression model was built to predict the likelihood of hospitalization in year 2 using predictors from year 1. Model performance was evaluated using discrimination, which was measured by the bootstrap-determined C statistic and calibration. The C statistic was 0.75 with and

(continues)

Table 22.2 Outcome Year Admissions and Costs for Estimated Probability Quartiles

Quartile	N	Mean Predicted Score	Number (%) with ≥ One Admission in Outcome Year	Number (%) of Total Admissions in Outcome Year	Mean Costs per Person in Outcome Year
q1	2,419	0.425	1,001 (41.8%)	2,368 (65.3%)	$28,190
q2	2,419	0.186	475 (19.7%)	716 (19.8%)	$13,310
q3	2,419	0.110	282 (11.7%)	370 (10.2%)	$7,830
q4	2,419	0.065	134 (5.6%)	171 (4.72%)	$4,328

without bootstrapping. Sensitivity, specificity, and positive predictive value were calculated at the specific cut points of the estimated probability score. Using a risk score of 0.3 or higher, 18% of the entire eligible study population would be identified as high risk for hospitalization. The sensitivity, specificity, and positive predictive value achieved at a cut point of 0.3 are 44%, 88%, and 48%, respectively.

Table 22.2 shows the results of using calibration to further validate the model. In this table, the entire population used for developing the model is split into four quartiles of equal counts of patients in order of their risk score. The mean predicted score in each group is compared to the percent with ≥1 admission in the outcome year. The mean predicted score matches closely with the percent with ≥1 admission, thus validating the model's performance. The percent of total admissions in the outcome year and mean costs are added for supplemental information.

Application of the Predictive Model in Practice

The diabetes care pilot project aimed to transform the delivery of health care for people with diabetes with a focus on self-management support and integrated primary care delivery. The beta coefficients created during the development phase of the predictive model were applied to the most current administrative data of patients for the health plan. Diabetic patients at high risk for hospitalization were selected for the pilot. *High risk* was defined as a predictive score of ≥ 0.25 based on the distribution of scores for patients with diabetes, considerations for program capacity, and the percentage of patients expected to engage in the program once identified. **Figure 22.1** shows the distribution of risk scores for the health plan, all patients with diabetes, and those patients selected for the pilot. The risk score ranges from 0 to 1, with 1 representing a 100% chance of being hospitalized in the next year.

Table 22.3 shows demographic and clinical characteristics of the overall population with diabetes and the cohort of patients with diabetes who receive primary care at the pilot sites. The characteristics are compared between the overall and pilot group and between those at high risk with a score above 0.25 and those at medium to low risk. An analysis of the characteristics of the high-risk pilot population whose results are in column 3 indicate that the model appropriately identifies patients with diabetes who are older, have complex chronic illness, and have opportunities for reducing hospitalizations and emergency department visits and improving treatment for their diabetes.

Patient Characteristics

For detailed patient characteristics, see Table 22.3.

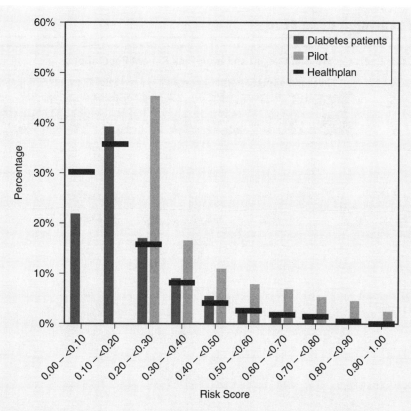

Figure 22.1 Risk Score Distribution.

Table 22.3 Characteristics of Overall and High-Risk Patient Populations

Characteristic	Overall Population with Diabetes		Pilot Provider Group Cohort	
	High Risk >.25 (n = 3923)	*Medium-Low Risk (n =11,772)*	*High Risk >.25 (n = 401)*	*Medium-Low Risk (n = 811)*
Age: mean (SD)	55.27 (16.0)	49.49 (14.5)	57.38 (15.0)	52.57 (14.7)
Age over 65: number (%)	1,067 (27.2%)	1435 (12.2%)	123 (30.7%)	139 (17.1%)
Female: n (%)	2,432 (62.0%)	7262 (61.7%)	266 (66.3%)	554 (68.3%)
Diabetes complications: n (%)	1,820 (46.4%)	1950 (16.6%)	202 (50.4%)	164 (20.2%)
Coronary artery disease: n (%)	1,450 (37.0%)	734 (6.2%)	166 (41.4%)	49 (6.0%)
Congestive heart failure: n (%)	791 (20.16%)	128 (1.09%)	87 (21.7%)	8 (1.0%)

(continues)

Table 22.3 Characteristics of Overall and High-Risk Patient Populations *(continued)*

Characteristic	Overall Population with Diabetes		Pilot Provider Group Cohort	
	High Risk >.25 (n = 3923)	*Medium-Low Risk (n =11,772)*	*High Risk >.25 (n = 401)*	*Medium-Low Risk (n = 811)*
Hypertension: *n* (%)	3,342 (85.2%)	6978 (59.2%)	360 (89.8%)	539 (66.4%)
Kidney disease: *n* (%)	890 (22.7%)	344 (2.9%)	105 (26.2%)	25 (3.0%)
Depression: *n* (%)	573 (14.61%)	644 (5.4%)	43 (10.72%)	44 (5.4%)
Chronic condition count: mean (SD)	6.17 (3.2)	2.42 (2.0)	6.43 (2.9)	2.79 (1.9)
Total drug count: mean (SD)	16.34 (8.2)	7.96 (5.5)	16.57 (6.7)	9.05 (5.6)
Diabetes medication possession ratio: mean (SD)	0.76 (0.28)	0.77 (0.29)	0.76 (0.27)	0.81 (0.25)
Hemoglobin A1c: mean (SD)	7.4 (2.1)	7.2 (1.8)	7.8 (2.2)	7.4 (2.0)
Primary care visits: mean (SD)	4.1 (4.6)	1.8 (2.5)	5.8 (4.4)	3.1 (2.9)
Any inpatient admission: *n* (%)	2057 (52.4%)	543 (4.6%)	226 (56.4%)	26 (3.2%)
Any emergency department visit: *n* (%)	2710 (69.1%)	2834 (24.1%)	263 (65.6%)	208 (25.6%)
Total annual cost of care: mean (SD)	$31,674 ($42,039)	$5159 ($8437)	$33,072 ($37,063)	$4,699 ($5,831)

Prescriptive Analytics

Whereas predictive analytics tells us what can happen with a probability representing the likelihood of something happening, prescriptive analytics understands the factors involved in what can happen and understands the weights of the factors involved. Prescriptive analytics is considered more powerful because it provides the ability to specify a desirable outcome and prescribes the action necessary to achieve that outcome (Insights

Analytics, n.d.). The volume and velocity of data about people from sources like personal devices and social media in combination with data and information from healthcare records facilitates the ability to move into the realm of prescriptive analytics in health care.

Ideally, predictive and prescriptive analytics work together to first identify "What is likely to happen?" and then use prescriptive analytics to determine and answer the question, "What should be done?" or "What can we do to make

X happen?" Prescriptive analytics uses computational logic, which is a technique to leverage implicit and explicit knowledge about the topic, and is transformed into a set of rules and optimization techniques that seek to maximize benefits while managing resource trade-offs (Brethenoux & Idoine, 2018). Together, predictive and prescriptive analytics encompass the analytic techniques discussed previously.

Prescriptive Analytics Methodologies

Methodological approaches for achieving prescriptive analytics are either rules based or use optimization techniques. Rules-based methods use organizational and industry knowledge and create structured rules applied to data (Brethenoux & Idoine, 2018). In the delivery of healthcare services, this could mean applying evidence-based clinical care guidelines to the treatment of chronic conditions but could also extend to the analysis of patient flow through the healthcare system, incorporating understanding of how clinical care services need to be delivered along with information about transportation systems and patients' ability to access services. The expertise and knowledge in rules sets are owned by clinical and business leaders and are structured in a way that they can be changed as needed. The technical ownership of rules sets lie in an informational technology department where they can be made operational and available at point-of-care decision-making.

Optimization techniques are grounded in operational research methods that use advanced analytical techniques to make optimal solutions for complex decisions. Simulation is an optimization technique that imitates real-life situations, weighing alternative conditions and courses of action (Brethenoux & Idoine, 2018). In health care, the development of simulation analyses requires business and clinical knowledge that can inform the development of the specific scenarios and constraints on certain decision-making within the scenario to maximize the solution. For instance, when determining which interventions

might best meet the needs for those with complex multimorbidity, the interventions of nurse care management, a specialty chronic care clinic, or home-based medical care could each be tested as options for interventions. Constraints on those options could be the cost for staff and resources to implement, the number of patients who could be served, and expected outcomes for each intervention. The optimal solution would be one in which all three are maximized.

In one application of prescriptive analytics, researchers sought to move from generic diabetes care guidelines to personalized diabetes management using information from EMRs. The researchers divided individual patient's medical history into distinct lines of pharmaceutical therapy and modeled outcomes resulting in a prescriptive algorithm providing personal treatment recommendations. The algorithm prescribed the regimen with the best predicted outcome in HbA1c (a measure of blood sugar control in patients with diabetes) and provided predicted improvement in HbA1c. The result of the work was a dashboard displaying the recommendation algorithm and an improvement in HbA1c levels when applied (Bertsimas, Kallus, Weinstein, & Zhuo, 2017).

Factors to Consider When Implementing Predictive and Prescriptive Analytics

Introducing predictive and prescriptive analytics into the work of population health management requires a strategic and thoughtful approach. A substantial investment is required in terms of changing organizational culture, ensuring that the organization has the right skill sets and knowledge in its people, procuring the necessary software, determining ways to operationalize results, and fully dedicating the people and tools to this effort. Specific considerations include the organizational culture in support of advanced analytic methods, organizational resources, and the determination of whether to build or buy solutions.

Organizational Culture for Advanced Analytic Applications

Most healthcare organizations are comfortable with using analytic reporting to understand the financial accounting for business viability, management reporting to understand volume and timeliness of services, and perhaps using risk-prediction models for a specific clinical scenario. However, most healthcare organizations are not at the point where analytics determine on a large scale what services they will provide and when, who they will provide services to, and how they will deliver those services. Clinicians know best treatment and care practices and methods to apply evidence-based care at the patient level, tailoring evidence to meet the needs of individual patients. Analytics driven business and clinical decisions may be viewed as less optimal and challenging to the patient–clinician relationship in healthcare organizations. When taking on an analytic approach using prediction and prescription, it is important to take clinicians and business stakeholders on the entire journey to empower the culture necessary for success.

Organizational Resources

Developing and implementing an operational program of predictive and prescriptive analytics requires investment in data infrastructure, tools, and people to do the work. Data infrastructure needs to be standardized with longitudinal person-centric data points represented in a robust, regularly updated data model in a data warehouse. Data-management, querying, and mining tools are required as well as specialized statistical, simulation, and other software. The data infrastructure and tools cannot be functional without the people with the skill sets and knowledge to be able to run them and include, developers, programmers, data analysts, and data scientists. Subject matter experts for the data sources, clinical care, and business expertise are also necessary.

Build versus Buy

The assessment of organizational culture and resources will require thoughtfulness about which capabilities to build internally and when to seek out external expertise through vendors and partnerships. Healthcare delivery organizations are not designed to double as analytic powerhouses. Over the years, health plans have developed greater capacity in each resource area, but few healthcare organizations hold all of the needed capabilities in-house. Robust execution of predictive and prescriptive analytics requires a mix of purchasing or partnering for specialized services and developing internal capabilities.

Conclusion

Imagine giving clinicians a list of patients at high risk of hospitalization and leaving the determination of how to prevent admissions for multiple patients to them amid their daily work of caring for individual patients or vice versa, informing clinicians of what they can do to prevent admissions without knowing who is at risk. Predictive and prescriptive analytics work best together by accurately forecasting poor outcomes and determining optimal interventions to use for the course of action. To robustly operationalize these advanced analytic techniques and integrate them into point-of-care decisions, a comprehensive strategy that considers organizational culture, resources, and the right mix of build versus buy technology is needed.

Study and Discussion Questions

- Consider the specialization of a healthcare organization in which you work or are familiar. How could this organization benefit from predictive analytics? From prescriptive analytics? What challenges would need to be overcome?

- How can the results of predictive and prescriptive analytics be integrated into point-of-care decision-making?
- What might be some reasons not to move forward with implementing predictive and prescriptive analytics into healthcare delivery?

Resources and Websites

Healthcare Data and Analytics Association: https://www.hdwa.org/

Healthcare Information Management Systems Society, Analytics: https://www.himssanalytics.org/

Health Catalyst: https://www.healthcatalyst.com /predictive-analytics, https://www.healthcatalyst .com/prescriptive-analytics-improving-health-care

References

Bertsimas, D., Kallus, N., Weinstein, A. M., & Zhuo, Y. D. (2017). Personalized diabetes management using electronic medical records. *Diabetes Care, 40*, 210–217. https://doi.org/10.2337/dc16-0826

Brethenoux, E., & Idoine, C. (2018). Combine predictive and prescriptive techniques to solve business problems. Gartner Research. https://www.gartner.com /en/documents/3891993/combine-predictive-and -prescriptive-techniques-to-solve-

Brown, M. S. (2018, July 30). Predictive analytics terms business people need to know (no hype allowed). *Forbes.* https://www.forbes.com/sites/metabrown/2018/07/30 /predictive-analytics-terms-business-people-need-to -know-no-hype-allowed/#7f29de913d43

Cousins, M. S., Shickle, L. M., & Bander, J. A. (2004, July 5). An introduction to predictive modeling for disease management risk stratification. *Disease Management, 5*(3), 157–167. http://www.liebertonline.com/doi/abs/10 .1089/109350702760301448

Dankers, F. J. W. M., Traverso, A., Wee, L., & van Kuijk, S. M. J. (2018, December 22). Prediction modeling methodology. Pp. 101–120 in *Fundamentals of Clinical Data Science.* https://doi.org/10.1007/978-3-319-99713-1_8

Insights Analytics. (n.d.). Prescriptive analytics: A model future in healthcare. https://insightsanalytics.com/2019 /04/prescriptive-analytics-in-healthcare/

Jeffery, A. D., Hewner, S., Pruinelli, L., Lekan, D., Lee, M., Gao, G., Holbrook, L., & Sylvia, M. (2019, April). Risk prediction and segmentation models used in the United States for assessing risk in whole populations: A critical literature review with implications for nurses' role in population health management. *JAMIA Open, 2*(1), 205–214. https://doi.org/10.1093/jamiaopen/ooy053

Knutson, D., Bella, M., Llanos, K., & Martin, L. (2009, August). *Predictive modeling: A guide for state Medicaid purchasers.* Center for Health Care Strategies. https://www .chcs.org/resource/predictive-modeling-a-guide-for-state -medicaid-purchasers/

Pencina, M. J., & D'Agostino, R. B. D. Sr. (2015, September 8). Evaluating discrimination of risk prediction models: The C statistic. *Journal of the American Medical Association, 314*(10), 1063–1064. https://doi.org/10.1001 /jama.2015.11082

Sylvia, M. L. (2018). Predictive modeling. In M. L. Sylvia & M. F. Terhaar (Eds.), *Clinical analytics and data management for the DNP* (2nd ed., pp. 361–372). Springer Publishing Company.

Sylvia, M. L. (2020). Predictive modeling using logistic and linear statistical modeling techniques. In *Population health management learning series.* ForestVue Healthcare Solutions.

CHAPTER 23

Advanced Analytic Methods

Martha Sylvia, PhD, MBA, RN

Medical thinking has become vastly more complex, mirroring changes in our patients, our healthcare system, and medical science. The complexity of medicine now exceeds the capacity of the human mind.

—Obermeyer and Lee (2017)

EXECUTIVE SUMMARY

Now more than ever the opportunity exists to make sense of the voluminous and complex data used to make accurate and efficient healthcare decisions. Health care has experienced the ability of computerized systems to diagnose complex medical conditions, provide sustaining life support, calculate medication dosages, predict adverse outcomes, and provide pathways to increase the likelihood of desirable results.

Artificial intelligence (AI) is making its way into healthcare operations with uses in optimizing workflow, scheduling patients and clinical staff, and marketing to potential patients. Clinical applications of artificial intelligence are even more exciting with the ability to interpret and diagnose conditions from radiology results in partnership with clinicians, monitor patient conditions such as blood glucose levels in patients, provide automatic medication dosing of insulin based on the results, and measure population health risk and segment populations to receive appropriate interventions.

There is much more work to be done to fully capture the advantages of AI in health care. Restrictions on the use of data, data quality, siloed healthcare systems, lack of interoperability, challenges with workflow integration, workforce education, and oversight and regulation are just some of the barriers to achieving uses seen in other disciplines such as astrophysics and consumer marketing. Yet AI strategies have the potential to improve care delivery and outcomes for patients and relieve the cognitive burden causing unprecedented burnout in clinicians across health care.

LEARNING OBJECTIVES

At the end of this chapter, the learner will be able to:

1. Distinguish key terms used in pattern-based risk modeling.
2. Describe the process of knowledge discovery in databases.
3. Identify common machine-learning techniques applied in population health analytics.
4. Describe natural language processing methods.

Introduction

This chapter focuses on advanced analytical techniques applied to what are considered big data in terms of large volume, variety, velocity, and veracity. Knowledge discovery in databases provides a process to approach such methods and results in knowledge acquisition that is useful and valuable for healthcare delivery and improving outcomes. Here the focus is on pattern-based techniques used in data mining and falling under the broad terminology of artificial intelligence and machine learning. Classification and clustering are two commonly used methods forming the basic underlying techniques for even more advanced applications.

Natural language processing (NLP) is a special advanced analytic technique used in health care to make data points from the vast amounts of written text in clinical notes and other documentation. NLP is critical to improving data-based modeling and decision-making because it deciphers written text into analyzable data, adding to our understanding of health determinants and outcomes in population health analytics.

Knowledge Discovery in Databases

Knowledge discovery in databases (KDD) is the entire process of identifying valid, novel, potentially useful, and ultimately understandable information from data. Although the effort results in knowledge generation from data, remember that KDD remains a process and is described as such. Recognizing KDD as a process allows for a systematic methodology for addressing important problems in health care using large volumes, varieties, and velocities of data (Fayyad, Piatetsky-Shapiro, & Smyth, 1996). The framework combines knowledge about any database used, domain knowledge, and a set of user-defined biases that provide the focus. The output is discovered knowledge that can be directed to the user or back to the system as domain knowledge (Frawley, Piatetsky-Shapiro, & Matheus, 1992). **Figure 23.1** displays the KDD process, which is defined by the following steps:

1. In the selection step, it is necessary to understand the data, the domain, and the goal of the process from the customer's viewpoint.

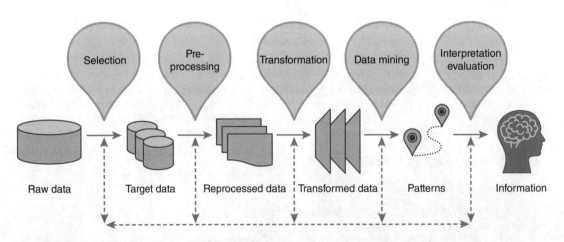

Figure 23.1 Process of Knowledge Discovery in Databases.

Data from Fayyad, U., Piatetsky-Shapiro, G., & Smyth, P. (1996). From data mining to knowledge discovery in databases. *AI Magazine, 17*(3), 37–54. https://ojs.aaai.org/index.php/aimagazine/article/view/1230

A target data set is formed that focuses on a subset of variables or samples of the data in which knowledge discovery will be undertaken.

2. In the preprocessing step, data are cleaned, unnecessary data are removed, rules are applied for missing data, and time sequencing is arranged.

3. During transformation, data reduction takes place and depends on the goals of the knowledge discovery use case.

4. Data mining encompasses exploratory analysis, methods, model selection, and applying data analysis and discovery algorithms that result in pattern recognition or modeling of the data. There are multiple types of methods used in the data mining step. Data mining will be explored in more detail in this chapter.

5. Interpretation and evaluation lead to the acquisition of knowledge that is gained when patterns and modeling exceed an informative threshold that is user oriented, domain specific, and determined by criteria set by the user.

Data Mining

Data mining (DM) is part of KDD and, as a broad term, encompasses analytic methods used to identify relationships in data that give insight into individual preferences and what might occur in a given scenario based on decision theory. DM combines probability methods with decision theory by identifying patterns in data that can minimize errors and variation when relying on clinical decision-making alone (Fayyad et al., 1996).

Data mining is a broad term that encompasses analytic methods used to identify relationships in data that give insight into individual preferences, especially what someone might do in a given scenario based on decision theory (Finlay, 2014). DM combines probability methods with decision theory through identifying patterns in data that can minimize errors and variation

when relying on clinical decision-making alone (Chen & Fawcett, 2016). DM relies on the KDD framework and process of information extraction from raw data.

Several data models are used to mine data and are described in greater detail by Chen and Fawcett (2016), including the following:

- Decision trees, or the categorization of decisions into one or more algorithms that link(s) the populations to their outcomes.

- Linear regression (single or multiple), or the development of a linear equation to determine the degree to which the predictor variables result in a particular outcome.

- Cluster data models, or the grouping of data that is determined to be similar in nature to one another.

- Neural networks, or the training of an algorithm to perform one or more inter-related tasks based upon multiple training examples.

- Expert-based systems, or the replication of expert-based human decision-making in the form of algorithms that may be inter-related.

- Support vector machines, or algorithms that apply classification and regression analysis to data in a supervised learning model.

- Rough sets/rough set theory, or sets of data that help reduce uncertainty in decision-making by assigning upper and lower approximations for each rule.

- Genetic algorithms, or the sequencing of data based on like characteristics and founded in the principles of genetics and natural selection.

- Bayes classifiers, or a method to minimize the probability of misclassifying data.

Data-mining techniques are used to support and improve medical diagnosis assignment, determine medical treatment, reduce adverse events such as drug interactions, and predict adverse health outcomes. A big advantage of DM is improvement in diagnostic accuracy and timeliness by managing a large amount of data efficiently. To perform data mining well requires enormously large databases to develop a model and define patterns. Therefore, DM techniques are often restricted to certain conditions or scenarios. In addition, although linkages are identified between decisions and patterns, the reasoning for the linkages cannot be discerned and requires additional understanding and context (Chen & Fawcett, 2016).

Data-Mining Examples

In one example, data-mining techniques were used to identify patient and support system factors associated with mobility improvement in home care and identify patterns of factors associated with improvement or lack of improvement in mobility. Data were used from Medicare-certified home healthcare agencies to place patients into groups based on mobility scores at admission. Discriminative pattern mining was used to determine patterns associated with improvement or no improvement of mobility within levels of mobility status (independent, device needed, supervision needed, two levels of chairfast, and bedfast). Patterns and therefore factors related to improvement differed among mobility levels. For instance, for patients using a device, those most likely to improve were younger, postsurgical, needed infrequent assistance, and had adequate support. Armed with this information, home health agencies can improve mobility by direct resources appropriately (Dey et al., 2015).

In another example, data mining was used to understand patterns of multimorbidity in older adults in the United States so that decision-making about provision of healthcare services and interventions could be better informed and the impact of multimorbidity could be better understood. In this study, multiple analytic methods—including regression, decision trees, random forest, and support vector machine—were applied using the KDD process to diagnoses from administrative claims data to create classifications of morbidity groupings, predict them, and determine their impact on important population health utilization and cost outcomes. These additional analyses confirmed that the presence of chronic illness and higher

counts of chronic illness were significantly related to hospital length of stay. In addition, morbidity clusters and gender were associated with in-hospital death. These results also showed that age, gender, length of stay, in-hospital death, and multiple chronic illness are critical predictors of hospital costs, thus making the case for intervening to reduce hospitalizations, length of stay, and death occurring in the hospital (Al-Shanableh, Al Diabat, & Mafraq-Jordan, 2019).

Artificial Intelligence

Artificial intelligence incorporates multiple methods used in data mining with the goal of having computers exhibit or simulate intelligent behavior. AI systems range from those that attempt to accurately model human reasoning to solve a problem, to those that ignore human reasoning and exclusively use large volumes of data to generate a framework to answer questions of interest, to those that attempt to incorporate elements of human reasoning but do not require accurate modeling of human processes. Often, the terms *artificial intelligence* and *machine learning* are used interchangeably, but machine learning is considered a component of artificial intelligence. The term *artificial intelligence* is often used when marketing or selling machine-learning methods while the term machine learning is used by analysts involved in the development, methods, and techniques (Sylvia, 2020). In addition, when referring to machine learning in partnership with human review and applied context, the term *human-guided machine learning* is often used.

AI can provide significant benefit to health care in supporting decisions considered "dull" or repetitive such as continuous monitoring with notification alerts; "detailed," needing to evaluate vast amounts of data to make a decision, like using multiple sources of information to make the best treatment recommendation; and "dear," or expensive to be executed manually when automation can provide instant response, as in interpreting radiologic results (Kuhnen, 2018). **Figure 23.2** depicts some of the areas of AI where health care

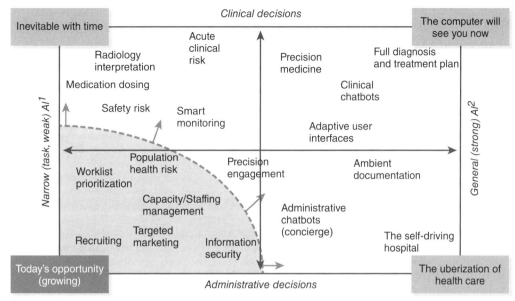

Figure 23.2 The Landscape for Artificial Intelligence Applications.

Reproduced from Kuhnen, G. (2018). *The decision machine: Analytics and the rise of AI.* https://www.advisory.com/en/topics/classic/2018/09/the-decision-machine-analytics-ai-1

is capitalizing on its abilities and the vision for future applications.

The National Academies of Medicine identified ways in which AI is changing health and healthcare delivery and summarized these use cases in **Table 23.1**.

Machine Learning

Machine learning (ML) is a component of AI in which a programmed computer has the ability to learn from patterns in data to make accurate predictions about outcomes of interest. Learning by a computer is particularly valuable where human expertise does not exist or when humans are unable to explain their expertise and therefore a computer program cannot be directly written from the human perspective. ML is also helpful when the problem to be solved changes over time or across circumstances—for example, human behaviors (Alpaydın, 2014). Machine learning

is a method of data mining using pattern-based methods to achieve knowledge acquisition in the KDD process.

Pattern recognition is the prominent activity of machine learning and is the automated recognition of patterns and regularities in data through the use of computer algorithms and making use of these patterns through classification or clustering techniques. Two of the most common pattern-recognition techniques are classification and clustering. While there are many different methods to achieve each of these techniques, there are basic underlying principles for each method.

Classification and Clustering Pattern-Based Techniques

Classification is a form of supervised learning in which the learning algorithm seeks to learn from a set of labeled examples or patients represented

Table 23.1 Examples of AI Applications

Use Case or User Group	Category	Examples of Applications	Technology
Patients and families	Health monitoring Benefit–risk assessment	Devices and wearables Smartphone and tablet apps, websites	Machine learning, NLP, speech recognition, chatbots
	Disease prevention and management	Obesity reduction Diabetes prevention and management Emotional and mental health support	Conversational AI, NLP, speech recognition, chatbots
	Medication management	Medication adherence	Robotic home telehealth
	Rehabilitation	Stroke rehabilitation using apps and robots	Robotics
Clinician care teams	Early detection, prediction, and diagnostics tools	Imaging for cardiac arrhythmia detection, retinopathy Early cancer detection (e.g., melanoma)	Machine learning
	Surgical procedures	Remote-controlled robotic surgery AI-supported surgical road maps	Robotics, machine learning
	Precision medicine	Personalized chemotherapy treatment	Supervised machine learning, reinforcement learning
	Patient safety	Early detection of sepsis	Machine learning
Public health program managers	Identification of individuals at risk	Suicide risk identification using social media	Deep learning (convolutional and recurrent neural networks)
	Population health	Eldercare monitoring	Ambient AI sensors
	Population health	Air-pollution epidemiology Water microbe detection	Deep learning, geospatial pattern mining, machine learning
Business administrators	*International Classification of Diseases, 10th Rev. (ICD-10)* coding	Automatic coding of medical records for reimbursement	Machine learning, NLP

Business administrators	Fraud detection	Healthcare billing fraud Detection of unlicensed providers	Supervised, unsupervised, and hybrid machine learning
	Cybersecurity	Protection of personal health information	Machine learning, NLP
	Physician management	Assessment of physician competence	Machine learning, NLP
Researchers	Genomics	Analysis of tumor genomics	Integrated cognitive computing
	Disease prediction	Prediction of ovarian cancer	Neural networks
	Discovery	Drug discovery and design	Machine learning, computer-assisted synthesis

Matheny, M., Israni, S. T., Ahmed, M., & Whicher, D. (Eds.). (2019). *NAM special publication: Artificial intelligence in health care: The hope, the hype, the promise, the peril.* National Academy of Medicine. https://nam.edu/wp-content/uploads/2019/12/AI-in-Health-Care-PREPUB-FINAL.pdf. Reprinted with permission from the National Academy of Sciences, Washington, DC.

by input data such as demographics and labels such as diagnoses, as well as generalize to new examples. In classification, the classes are predefined. An example of this is the identification of disease conditions in radiographs where multiple radiology scans for a disease condition are entered into an algorithm that, based on the learnings from this input, can indicate whether a new scan is indicative of the same condition.

Clustering is a form of unsupervised learning where the learning algorithm does not have a set of labeled examples and instead groups examples or patients by some shared commonality. Clusters do not have predefined classes. One use of clustering could be to identify patients who should have been assigned into hierarchical condition categories for risk adjustment in a Medicare Advantage plan but do not have the proper diagnosis code billed in administrative claims data.

Figure 23.3 compares and contrasts classification and clustering methods. As an example, to make this comparison more applicable, objects could be thought of as people, classes can be thought of as groupings of people into categories like having an emergency department (ED) visit, and attributes are data points about the people.

In classification, the goal is to predict classes from given properties and attributes about objects. Classification is commonly used to predict a dichotomous class. In the example, a set of classification criteria would be provided to assign people as having an ED visit, and the goal of the classification algorithm would assign ED visit occurrence based on the attributes provided. Classes are predefined in classification methods (Fayyad et al., 1996; Sylvia, 2020; Wang, 1999).

In clustering, the goal is to identify similar groups of objects to place into classes, which are not predefined but discovered. Using the example, attributes of patients would be examined for patterns or clusters to create classes with the expectation that classes would define groups

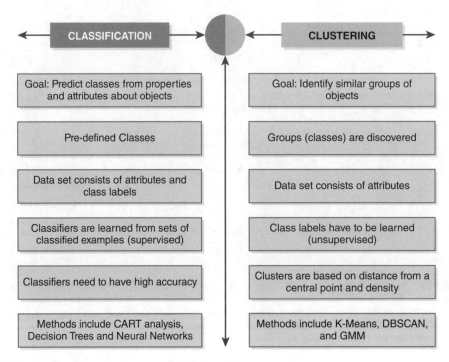

Figure 23.3 Classification and Clustering Method Comparison.

Reproduced from Sylvia, M. (2020). Predictive modeling using pattern-based methods. In *Population health management learning series*. ForestVue Healthcare Solutions.

of patients who perhaps have similar ED use patterns.

The data set used in classification contains attributes and class labels at the object level, whereas in clustering the data set only contains attributes. In classification, classifiers, and assignment of classification for new objects are learned from sets of examples already classified, which is considered *supervised* learning. In clustering, classifiers and assignment is learned, considered *unsupervised* learning. Classifier example sets used in classification methods need to have high accuracy because they are already defined. In clustering, the clusters are built based on the distance between individual data points and a central point of a density of data points (Frawley et al., 1992; Sylvia, 2020; Wang, 1999).

Classification methods include classification and regression trees, decision trees, and neural networks. K-means is probably the most well-known clustering algorithm. Density-based spatial clustering of applications with noise, and

Gaussian mixture models are also clustering methods (Bishop, 2006; Wang, 1999).

Illustrative Example of Classification and Clustering

This example uses a condensed data set with few variables to demonstrate the techniques of classification and clustering. (In reality, these analyses use large volume data sets). The variables in this data set follow.

- Patient_id: a unique identifier for each patient
- Age: age in years
- Chronic Conditions: the number of chronic conditions for each patient
- Medications: the number of medications for each patient
- Admissions: an indicator of whether each person did (=1) or did not (=0) have an admission. (Note that this variable is used only in the classification example).

Classification

In this example, a classification method is used from the data in **Table 23.2** to create an algorithm that classifies by whether or not they will have an admission. Input variables for this classification algorithm are continuous variables as opposed to dichotomous or binary. Using this data set, age, the count of chronic conditions and the number of medications are the variables considered to be *attributes* in the model. In reality, additional attributes could be used, but more attributes increase the complexity of the resulting classification algorithm. The *admission* variable is the *class label* in the model.

To create the classifications, the statistical software uses many iterations to optimize the pathways. The classification model learns the algorithm from these data with class label assigned and associated with attributes. The model could then be used to determine whether people who do not already have an assigned class label are likely to experience an admission. The depth of

Table 23.2 Structure of Classification and Clustering Data Set

Patient_id	Age	Chronic Conditions	Medications	Acute Admission
119	69	3	1	0
122	32	0	1	0
125	68	6	7	1
126	1	0	0	0
128	44	0	0	0
129	11	0	0	0
130	9	0	0	0
133	69	5	0	1
135	9	0	4	0
137	8	0	0	0
138	52	0	1	0
141	86	2	0	0
145	26	0	2	0
130	9	0	0	0
133	69	5	0	1
135	9	0	4	0
137	8	0	0	0
138	52	0	1	0
141	86	2	0	0
145	26	0	2	0

Reproduced from Sylvia, M. (2020). Predictive modeling using pattern-based methods. In *Population Health Management Learning Series*. ForestVue Healthcare Solutions.

the branches is only as deep as the number of attributes provided.

Figure 23.4 displays the resulting classification algorithm. The algorithm is initiated at the highest level with the result of the class label variable. In this data set were 5,758 people; 5.8% of them had an admission. The attribute with the most contribution to the likelihood of having an admission is the chronic condition count that is the next level in the algorithm. Examining to the far right, 534 of the people have greater than four chronic conditions and 30% of them have an admission for a total of 160 admissions. Progressing down the same path on the algorithm, there are 239 people with greater than four chronic conditions and age 73 and older, and 36.4% of them have an admission. This part of the pathway in the algorithm indicates that those with more than four chronic conditions, 73 and older capture the highest proportion of admissions. With this information, such an algorithm could be used in practice to target those 73 and older with more than four chronic conditions in order to prevent an admission.

Clustering Methods Example

This example uses a clustering analysis to create subgroupings of patients, based on the data in Table 23.2 (absent the admission variable). This analysis shows how patients can be observed to fall into recognizable patterns based on attributes. This type of clustering analysis uses a popular method called *k-means* with continuous variables as inputs.

The k-means method is based on calculating the distances between data points for each person in the sample population, to the center points, or centroids, of each subgroup of data points. Using statistical techniques designed to optimize the number of clusters and use-case–based judgment, an analyst decides on the number of clusters in which to separate patients. The k-means method is an iterative process that starts with a random assignment of people to subgroups, or *clusters*,

and then calculates distances between data-point coordinates by person, repeatedly adjusting the cluster assignments until an optimal convergence of clusters is achieved.

In this analysis, the number of clusters for assignment is four. The graph in **Figure 23.5** shows each cluster number on the *x*-axis with each data point representing a person and his or her distance from the centroid of the cluster. A value of zero means that the person is at the center. The units for the distance are standardized and interpreted in relationship to one another. The data table shows number of people and the average of each attribute. These values are reviewed by the analyst and clinician to determine whether the cluster assignments are reasonable.

These clusters do seem to produce different sets of people who would benefit from unique and different healthcare interventions. For instance, in cluster 3 the average age is 14, with no conditions and minimal medications. It is likely this group would need only some type of preventive intervention. Cluster 1—with an average age of 57, two conditions, and five medications—may benefit from disease management and medication therapy management (Sylvia, 2020).

Machine Learning in Practice

Applications of machine learning in healthcare settings are in the exploratory and investigative stages. Most examples are in the published research and have not yet been translated into practice. One reason for the slowness to adopt is the lack of robust data structures and knowledgeable analysts within healthcare organizations to operationally support these types of models. In addition, there are concerns that algorithms may mirror human biases in decision-making, further perpetuating disparities in healthcare delivery and outcomes (Char, Shah, & Magnus, 2018).

In one interesting application of ML, researchers correlated Google reviews of nursing

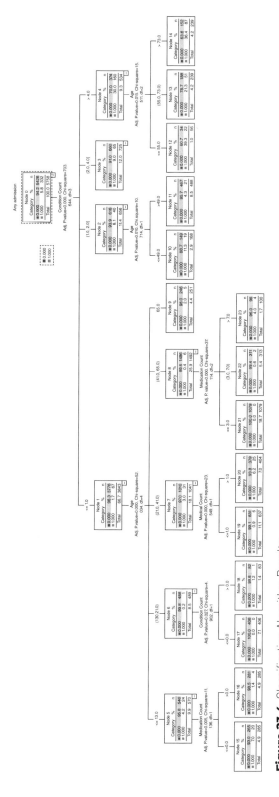

Figure 23.4 Classification Algorithm Results.

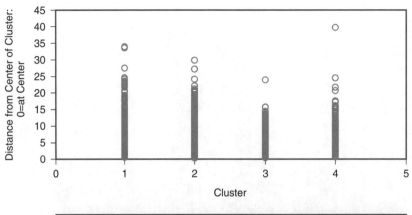

Cluster	1	2	3	4	All
Number of People	2087	1046	1368	1257	5758
Average Age	57	76	14	36	46
Average Number of Conditions	2	4	0	1	1
Average Number of Medications	5	1	2	2	3

Figure 23.5 Clustering Results.

Reproduced from Sylvia, M. (2020). Predictive modeling using pattern-based methods. In *Population health management learning series*. ForestVue Healthcare Solutions.

homes with CMS Medicare inspection results of nursing homes using the publicly available Nursing Home Compare data set to determine the extent to which the reviews reflect quality of care and the presence of elder abuse. They developed an algorithm that could be used going forward to detect elder abuse and to assess the quality of care in nursing homes based with high precision and when significant numbers of reviews are available (Mowery, Andrei, Le, Jian, & Ward, 2016). In other examples, machine-learning techniques are applied to big data in intensive care units to determine patient acuity, assign resources, deliver appropriate interventions, and monitor results (Ghassemi, Celi, and Stone, 2015).

In a clinically operational application of ML, a behavioral health management service provider used machine-learning tools to analyze more than 30 different data sources and 400 variables to improve care coordination for patients with serious mental illness in combination with physical illnesses (Bresnick, 2017). These examples highlight the enormous potential of ML to drive desirable healthcare outcomes.

Validation of Machine-Learning Methods

Validation of a pattern-based model broadly means determining whether the model is behaving as expected, given the knowledge of the real-world phenomenon being modeled. The analyst and clinician work together to determine whether the results make sense given their knowledge of the data, population, and clinical reality.

Cross-validation is the process of using multiple iterations of the data in development and testing data sets to ensure consistency of results and then to validate classification and clustering methods. Classification algorithms can be validated by methods used for logistic regression if the class prediction is dichotomous. Chapter 22, "Predictive and Prescriptive Analytics," describes these methods. Clustering methods should verify that the model has *converged*, meaning that the cluster assignments on the two last iterations of the model are the same or very close to the same. Other more complex statistical techniques may also be used to select the best clustering method by optimizing the cluster assignment with respect to proximity to cluster centers.

Assessing Machine-Learning Methods for Use in Practice

Validation uses statistical methods to determine the accuracy of machine-learning models, although there are other considerations besides statistical accuracy when determining whether to use risk-prediction models in practice. It is also important to understand whether implementation will be feasible in a particular healthcare organization and, even more important, whether their implementation will actually lead to improved patient outcomes. Many factors determine whether models will result in positive changes in outcomes, including a clinician's capacity to formulate a responsive action, weigh the risks and benefits, and execute action; and a patient's capacity to adhere to the clinical recommendations (Shah, Milstein, & Bagley, 2019).

The purpose of the model should be evaluated in terms of whether the model is addressing the identified need and in a way that will feasibly impact the desired outcome. For instance, previous examples identified that a pattern-based model could effectively reduce clinician time in reviewing hundreds of radiology scans, thus meeting the need of reducing unnecessary tasks. When considering the purpose, the ability to determine the net incremental value of taking plausible alternative actions must be considered by assessing the number of actions the care team can take, the cost and efficacy of those actions, and the chance that the patient will follow the recommended action (Shah et al., 2019).

Machine-learning models need to be transparent in that the healthcare providers who are expected to use the model should be able to understand the factors being used for prediction or the *attributes* and should have a high-level understanding of how the model is developing its conclusions. This is important in gaining clinician buy-in for using the technology. The model developer should report the methods and results of evaluating the performance of the model in a way that can be understood by and instill confidence in all stakeholders. Models should also provide actionable information.

Perhaps most difficult to achieve is the ability to run the model in an operational way within an organization. Predictive models remain highly dependent on high-quality, readily available data; when implemented in an organization having missing or poor-quality data, the accuracy of the models are eroded (Peterson, 2019). To implement these types of models, data must be readily available, structured in a way that supports the model, available with the appropriate frequency, and obtainable at the point of care in which it will be used. In addition, operationalizing these types of models requires a commitment from information technology resources for automating processes and moving models into the transactional systems of care delivery—most commonly, the electronic medical record (EMR).

The U.S. Food and Drug Administration (FDA) has developed a framework for approving machine-learning models as a medical device termed *Software as a Medical Device* (SaMD) that sets expectations for developers of machine-learning models to meet transparency requirements and monitor the performance of models as a medical device. SaMDs are considered medical devices because they intend to treat, diagnose, cure, mitigate, or prevent disease or other conditions. The FDA has already approved several machine-learning SaMDs that have algorithms that are considered to be "locked" before marketing as opposed to those whose algorithms may change after going to market (U.S. Food and Drug Administration, 2019).

When deciding to implement machine learning, checking whether the model has had or is undergoing an approval process with the FDA is a good idea; if not, reviewing the FDA guidelines when assessing a model could be quite helpful. The FDA has developed a model for good machine-learning practices, depicted in **Figure 23.6**, which is based on general

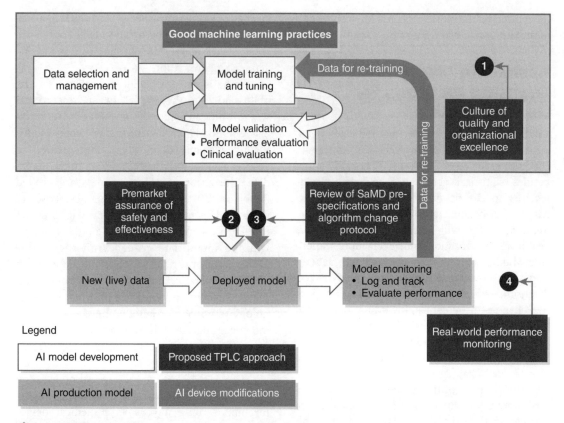

Figure 23.6 Good Machine-Learning Practices Framework.

U.S. Food and Drug Administration. (2019, April 4). *Proposed regulatory framework for modifications to Artificial Intelligence/Machine Learning (AI/ML)-based Software as a Medical Device (SaMD)—Discussion paper and request for feedback.* https://www.regulations.gov/document/FDA-2019-N-1185-0001

principles that balance benefits and risks and strive to provide safe and effective SaMDs.

Natural Language Processing

Natural language processing is grounded in linguistic science, whose purpose is to be able to characterize and explain linguistic observations, including the cognitive side of how humans acquire, produce, and understand language; the relationship between uttered language and the world; and the linguistic structures by which language communicates (Manning & Schutze, 2003). NLP is a theory-driven set of computational techniques for the automatic

analysis and representation of human language (Cambria & White, 2014). IBM, a well-known provider of NLP services in health care, defines NLP as the "parsing and semantic interpretation of text, which allows systems to learn, analyze, and understand human language" (Jones, 2019). In healthcare applications, NLP is mainly used to make analyzable data points out of unstructured or free text data.

Despite progress in documenting healthcare transactions in electronic medical records, a plethora of information remains that was collected at points of care that remain in unstructured text fields in the form of clinical notes, assessments, radiologic and other reports, electronic communications, and more. Nearly 80% of all data in health care is unstructured and unused in population health analytics after it is created (Kong, 2019). The average clinical note is 150 times as large as an average EMR record (Dow, 2018). In addition, patient-generated, unstructured data exist in multiple online applications, especially in social media. Thus, there is great potential in gleaning insights from unstructured data using NLP.

NLP can be used to detect nonclinical factors such as instability in housing, food insecurity, lack of social support, and other health determinants that are more likely to result in a higher need for healthcare resources. Social determinants of health are more likely to be found in an unstructured format and harder to access (Kent, 2018).

Implementing NLP as a competency in population health analytics requires a uniquely different skill set, knowledge base, and tools than are used in a typical healthcare analytics environment. At its basic level, NLP requires an understanding of free text in general and the particular form used in documentation. The use of NLP software requires a technical "training" of the software to the documentation for which it will be used. NLP software applies probabilistic modeling to text to get to the most likely meaning from that text. The ideal analytical skill sets for NLP include a combination of linguistics and data engineering.

Low-level NLP tasks include the following.

- *Sentence boundary detection*: the ability to determine the start and end of a sentence. Items such as abbreviations, titles, and items in a list can complicate delineation of boundaries.
- *Tokenization*: identifying individual structures within sentences such as words and punctuation. In health care, tokens often contain characters used as boundaries like hyphens, slashes, and quotations.
- *Part-of-speech assignment to individual words (POS tagging)*: the ability to link a word to a part of speech based on its definition and the context within which it is used. For instance, the word *order* can be a noun when used to reference a physician's order or a verb when

used to reference informing a patient of the order of events for a procedure.

- *Morphological decomposition*: breaking down complex words into their meaningful parts. The task of *lemmatization* may be used, which is the process of converting a word to its root by removing suffixes. For example, *neurodegenerative* can be broken down into the meaningful parts of *neuro-*, *-generative*, and *de-*.
- *Shallow parsing* or *chunking*: identification of phrases from constituent POS tagged tokens. The process identifies particular parts of sentences and links them to higher order units with distinct grammatical meaning. For example, "out of bed."
- *Problem-specific segmentation*: placing text into meaningful groups or sections like "Symptoms" or "Family History" (Nadkarni et al., 2011).

Higher-level tasks are use-case specific and include spelling and grammatical error identification and recovery, categorization of words and phrases (e.g., *diabetes* into *chronic diseases*), negation and uncertainty identification, word-sense disambiguation, determination of relationships between entities or events, temporal inferences, and the identification of problem-specific information with transformation into a problem-specific structured form (e.g., *microalbuminuria* into *kidney disfunction* (Nadkarni et al., 2011).

Symptom identification and management, the underpinning of *symptom science* are important in achieving positive outcomes for people with chronic and acute illness but are often difficult to detect in data if not assigned a diagnosis code in billing or administrative data. In multiple-use cases, NLP has been used to analyze symptom information from free text in the EMR in people with heart disease, mental illness, multiple sclerosis, influenza, inflammatory bowel disease, cancer and more. In addition, symptom science using NLP has been deployed to prevent adverse outcomes such as adverse drug events, admissions, and readmissions (Koleck, Dreisbach, Bourne, & Bakken, 2019).

Conclusion

Advanced analytic methods have the potential to disruptively change the way health care is delivered. The knowledge discovery in databases framework provides an organized set of steps to follow when embarking on the data-mining journey. Pattern-based data-mining methods are referred to as *machine learning* and are applied to expansive data to discover relationships and patterns that may be meaningful in addressing health-related outcomes.

Terminology in pattern-based methods is important to understand especially because terms can have overlapping meanings. Data mining is the component of knowledge discovery in databases, and machine learning is a substantial method of data mining. *Artificial intelligence* and *machine learning* are often used interchangeably, but machine learning is one component of artificial intelligence. *Classification* and *clustering* are two common methods of machine learning.

There are multiple examples or use cases for pattern-based methods in health care. These use cases encompass multiple objectives of the Triple Aim in reducing waste and inefficiency, improving health outcomes and quality, ensuring safe care, enhancing patients' experience, and lowering costs. However, it is important to carefully assess whether to introduce machine-learning interventions into population health management by evaluating size of the data sets, the accuracy of models, and the ability of models to ultimately provide clinically meaningful results.

Study and Discussion Questions

- Consider the specialization of a healthcare organization in which you work or are familiar. How could this organization benefit from machine learning?
- When is it better to use a clustering technique as opposed to a classification technique, and vice versa?
- How can the results of machine learning be integrated into point-of-care decision-making?
- What might be some reasons not to move forward with implementing machine-learning techniques into healthcare delivery?
- What are some ways in which natural language processing could be used to improve patient outcomes?

Resources and Websites

Association for the Advancement of Artificial Intelligence: https://www.aaai.org/

Open AI, a research laboratory whose mission is to ensure that artificial general intelligence benefits all of humanity: https://openai.com:

Gartner, a research and advisory company: https://www.gartner.com/en

University of Minnesota. (2019). Nursing knowledge big data science workgroup and conference: https://www.nursing.umn.edu/centers/center-nursing-informatics/news-events/2019-nursing-knowledge-big-data-science-conference

References

Al-Shanableh, N., Al Diabat, M., & Mafraq-Jordan, A. (2019). Multimorbidity prediction using data mining model. In *World of Computer Science and Information Technology Journal* (WCSIT) (Vol. 9). https://www.researchgate.net/publication/332410956_Multimorbidity_Prediction_Using_Data_Mining_Model

Alpaydın, E. (2014). *Introduction to machine learning* (3rd ed.). MIT Press.

Bishop, C. M. (2006). *Pattern recognition and machine learning*. Springer. https://www.springer.com/gp/book/97803873 10732

Bresnick, J. (2017). Using machine learning to target behavioral health interventions. Health IT Analytics. https:// healthitanalytics.com/news/using-machine-learning-to -target-behavioral-health-interventions

Cambria, E., & White, B. (2014, May). Jumping NLP curves: A review of natural language processing research [Review article]. *IEEE Computational Intelligence Magazine, 9*(2), 48–57. https://doi.org/10.1109/MCI.2014.2307227

Char, D. S., Shah, N. H., & Magnus, D. (2018, March 15). Implementing machine learning in health care-addressing ethical challenges. *New England Journal of Medicine, 378*, 981–983. https://doi.org/10.1056/NEJMp1714229

Chen, L.-Y. A., & Fawcett, T. N. (2016). Using data mining strategies in clinical decision making: A literature review. *Computers, Informatics, Nursing, 34*(10), 448–454. https:// doi.org/10.1097/CIN.0000000000000282

Dey, S., Cooner, J., Delaney, C. W., Fakhoury, J., Kumar, V., . . . , Westra, B. L. (2015). Mining patterns associated with mobility outcomes in home healthcare. *Nursing Research, 64*(4), 235–245. https://doi.org/10.1097/NNR.0000000 000000106

Dow, M. (2018, November 8). Healthcare NLP: Four essentials to make the most of unstructured data. HealthCatalyst. https://www.healthcatalyst.com/insights/healthcare -nlp-4-essentials

Fayyad, U., Piatetsky-Shapiro, G., & Smyth, P. (1996). From data mining to knowledge discovery in databases. *AI Magazine, 17*(3), 37–54. https://ojs.aaai.org/index.php/aimagazine /article/view/1230

Finlay, S. (2014). Introduction. Pp. 1–20 in *Predictive analytics, data mining and big data*. Palgrave Macmillan. https://link. springer.com/chapter/10.1057%2F9781137379283_1

Frawley, W. J., Piatetsky-Shapiro, G., & Matheus, C. J. (1992, Fall). Knowledge discovery in databases: An overview. *AI Magazine, 13*(3), 57. https://ojs.aaai.org/index.php /aimagazine/article/view/1011

Ghassemi, M., Celi, L. A., Stone, & D. J. (2015). State of the art review: The data revolution in critical care. *Critical Care, 19*(118), 1–9.

Jones, M. T. (2019). A beginner's guide to natural language processing. IBM. https://developer.ibm.com/articles/a -beginners-guide-to-natural-language-processing/

Kent, J. (2018). 4 natural language processing use cases for healthcare orgs. Health IT Analytics. https://healthitanalytics .com/news/4-natural-language-processing-use-cases-for -healthcare-orgs

Koleck, T. A., Dreisbach, C., Bourne, P. E., & Bakken, S. (2019, February 6). Natural language processing of symptoms documented in free-text narratives of electronic health records: A systematic review. *Journal of the American Medical Informatics Association, 26*(4), 364–379. https:// doi.org/10.1093/jamia/ocy173

Kong, H. J. (2019). Managing unstructured big data in healthcare system. *Healthcare Informatics Research, 25*(1), 1–2. https://doi.org/10.4258/hir.2019.25.1.1

Kuhnen, G. (2018). *The decision machine: Analytics and the rise of AI*. https://www.advisory.com/en/topics/classic/2018/09 /the-decision-machine-analytics-ai-1

Manning, C. D., & Schutze, H. (2003). *Foundations of statistical natural language processing*. MIT Press. https:// www.cs.vassar.edu/~cs366/docs/Manning_Schuetze _StatisticalNLP.pdf

Nadkarni, P. M., Ohno-Machado, L., & Chapman, W. W. (2011). Natural language processing: An introduction. *Journal of the American Medical Informatics Association, 18*(5), 544–551. https://doi.org/10.1136/amiajnl-2011-000464

Obermeyer, Z., & Lee, T. H. (2017, September 28). Lost in thought—The limits of the human mind and the future of medicine. *New England Journal of Medicine, 377*, 1209–1211. https://doi.org/10.1056/NEJMp1705348

Peterson, E. D. (2019, November 22). Machine learning, predictive analytics, and clinical practice: Can the past inform the present? *Journal of the American Medical Association, 322*(23), 2283–2284. https://jamanetwork .com/journals/jama/article-abstract/2756195

Roski, J., Heffner, J., Trivedi, R., Kukafka, R., & Estiri, H. (2019). How artificial intelligence is changing health and health care. In M. Matheny, S. Israni, M. Ahmed, & D. Whicher (Eds.), *Artificial intelligence in health care: The hope, the hype, the promise, the peril* (pp. 59–88). National Academies of Medicine. https://nam.edu/wp -content/uploads/2019/12/AI-in-Health-Care -PREPUB-FINAL.pdf

Shah, N. H., Milstein, A., & Bagley, S. C. (2019, August 8). Making machine learning models clinically useful. *Journal of the American Medical Association, 322*, 1351–1352. https://jamanetwork.com/journals/jama/article-abstract /2748179

Sylvia, M. (2020). Predictive modeling using pattern-based methods. In *Population health management learning series*. ForestVue Healthcare Solutions.

U.S. Food and Drug Administration. (2019, April 4). Proposed regulatory framework for modifications to Artificial Intelligence/Machine Learning (AI/ML)-based Software as a Medical Device (SaMD)—Discussion paper and request for feedback. https://www.regulations.gov/document/FDA -2019-N-1185-0001

Wang, W. (1999). *Predictive modeling based on classification and pattern matching methods*. https://www.semanticscholar .org/paper/Predictive-Modeling-Based-On-Classification -And-Wang/111a38236108b03413fd2fb0b838723bc6e 6555c

CHAPTER 24

Run Charts and Statistical Process Control

Martha Sylvia, PhD, MBA, RN

If you can't measure it, you can't improve it.

—Peter Drucker

EXECUTIVE SUMMARY

"If we invest in that intervention, how will we know that we're getting results?"
"How is our care management program performing?"
"Are we realizing a return on our investment for the medication therapy program?"

If you have been in a leadership or executive board meeting in any healthcare organization, chances are you have heard one of these questions or one remarkably similar to them. With limited dollars to spend on healthcare interventions, it is important to understand whether chosen initiatives are actually meeting process milestones and achieving desired patient outcomes—all while lowering healthcare utilization and costs. This is a lofty goal, and the questions can be uncomfortable and difficult to answer.

Confidence is gained in answering these questions when a well-planned and well-executed monitoring strategy is ongoing and producing results on a regular basis. Statistical process control is a method used to understand when population health initiatives are stable by running as planned and also understand when intentional improvements are meeting set targets. A monitoring strategy using statistical process control as the methodology prepares the analysts and intervention leadership to make ongoing adjustments to improve or keep processes stable and informs business leaders about the value of investments.

LEARNING OBJECTIVES

At the end of this chapter, the learner will be able to:

1. Identify statistical process control methods used in population health analytics.
2. Use statistical process control methods to monitor metrics of interest in population health.
3. Apply statistical process control methods appropriately in the population health process.

Introduction

Statistical process control (SPC) is a philosophy, a strategy, and a set of methods for the ongoing improvement of systems, processes, and outcomes (Carey, 2003a). It is based on the theory of variation in measurement and facilitates determination of the patterns and magnitude of variation that is needed to be reasonably sure that improvement has actually occurred (Benneyan, Lloyd, & Plsek, 2003). SPC was developed in the 1920s by Walter Shewhart as a way to measure variation in processes and results at Bell Telephone Laboratories. In the late 1990s, it began to be used increasingly in healthcare settings, largely from the work of the Institute for Health Improvement in the work in pursuit of the Triple Aim (Carey, 2003a).

SPC is a key tool used during the monitoring phase of the population health process. This chapter provides a description of process and outcome measures that form the basis of SPC and describes the way in which variation is defined, measured, and used to interpret SPC findings. Run charts are described in this chapter as the precursor to SPC charts and a useful tool to evaluate variation simply and efficiently. Details of SPC charts are provided in terms of development; the steps to making an SPC chart; measurement and interpretation of variation; and application of results of SPC to monitoring population health interventions.

Process and Outcome Measures

Comprehensive monitoring of population health interventions includes the monitoring of both process and outcome measures. It is common to refer to all intervention measures as "outcomes" but there is a difference between the two when doing the work of improving health care. Process measures what is actually done and can be thought of as the intervention itself (Donabedian, 1980). For instance, a medication therapy management intervention may provide a medication review or reconciliation consultation with documentation

or an accountable care organization may waive the patient fee for a preventative visit.

Outcomes represent the impact of interventions on the health status of patients and populations (Donabedian, 1980). Outcomes answer the question, "what is the impact of the intervention on health status, quality, patients' experience of care, and costs and utilization?" or, the Triple Aim. In the previous example, the outcomes that may be impacted by the interventions mentioned may respectively be improved medication adherence or less hospitalizations for preventative conditions. Statistical process control is used to measure both process and outcome measures in population health interventions.

Common and Special Cause Variation

When examining the results of statistical process control, and depending on the question at hand, stability or variation is sought after. When the variation seen in data points over time is steady and is within expected parameters the measures are seen as stable and exhibiting "common cause" variation. With common cause variation a measure is predictable, in that at each interval of time only a relatively small increase or decrease is occurring in the result (Carey, 2003c). This is usually the case when an intervention has been ongoing over a long period of time and has peaked in its ability to make sweeping changes to results. In one example, a program to reduce readmissions using the same targeting and enrollment criteria and same intervention over more than 3 years went from a 10% readmission rate to a 4% readmission rate over the first two years of the program but at each monthly measurement over the past year has stabilized between 3.7% and 4.2%.

With "special cause" variation the measure is notably unstable and changing. Depending on the question at hand, this instability may or may not be desirable (Carey, 2003c). For example, special cause variation is sought after when first implementing a program to reduce readmissions where the desire would be to see decreasing rates of readmissions for those targeted and enrolled in the intervention. Special cause variation is distinguishable from common cause variation through certain criteria that are applied to the pattern and placement of data points when visualized over time. These criteria vary depending on the type of chart used and will be explained in further detail in the next sections.

It is important to understand that special and common cause variation in and of themselves are neither "good" or "bad." It depends on the use case. A population health intervention that has been running for a long period of time with optimal processes and reaching target outcomes is expected to be stable and exhibit common cause variation over time, unless quality-improvement methods are being used to change the intervention. A newly implemented intervention is likely to experience special cause variation as it ramps up, goes through cycles of quality improvement, and reaches outcome targets. However, special cause variation may be undesirable in the first example of a long-term intervention that is considered stable. For example, if a large spike in readmissions from 4% to 10% in one month is realized then that would warrant further investigation to identify the cause.

Run Charts

A graphical display of data points over time—a *run chart*—forms the basis of and is the precursor for SPC charts. Run charts provide a simple way to determine whether a process is performing as expected, outcomes are at target, and improvement is being realized with minimal mathematical complexity. Run charts can be used to display data to make results visible, allow for a temporal view of data, determine whether tested changes are resulting in improvement, and determine whether gains in improvement level out and remain steady (Perla, Provost, & Murray, 2010). The run chart is simple to construct and interpret; can be used with any type of measure data, including counts, percentages, ratios, and more; can be constructed using paper and pencil; and do not require any statistical knowledge or skills making them easy to use but less sensitive than statistical process control (Carey, 2003c).

A run chart is calculated from a data set that contains values of the measure of interest over time. The values represent a summary of the measure. For example, when looking at monthly measures, each month might report a count of patients enrolled or engaged, the percentage of patients who have had a phone call or assessment, an average of a lab result like hemoglobin A1C (HbA1c), or the per thousand admission rate. For population health intervention monitoring, the time interval is most often a month but could be quarters of the year or weeks.

The *x*-axis of a run chart represents the time intervals, and the *y*-axis is the value for the measure of interest. A run chart displays the median (the value at which 50% of values fall above and 50% fall below) of all values included in the run as central point and a way to help in determining variation. A run chart may also contain annotation representing milestones for the intervention and a line representing a target. **Figure 24.1** displays an example of a run chart used to monitor the number of patients enrolled in a program along with the summarized data used for creating the chart.

Interpreting Variation in Run Charts

Determining whether to act on the results presented in the run chart or to proceed as planned and continue to monitor processes and outcomes depends on whether the results indicate special or common cause variation. Based on the definition of a *run*—one or more consecutive data points on the same side of the median—four tests (displayed in **Figure 24.2**) can be used to identify when special cause variation is present in a run chart.

1. *Shift*: six or more consecutive points either above or below the median with points on the median not counted as adding or breaking up the shift.

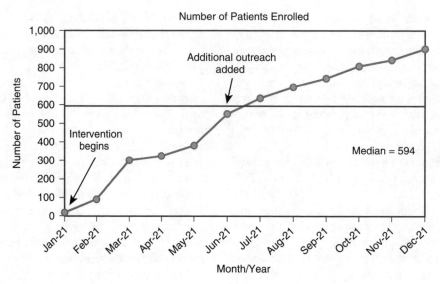

Figure 24.1 Run Chart.

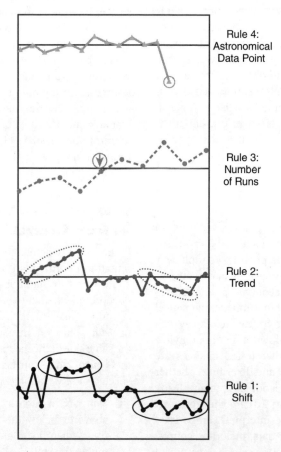

Figure 24.2 Application of Rules to Identify Special Cause Variation in Run Charts.

2. *Trend*: five or more consecutive points all going up or all going down with multiple points in a row with the same value counting as one point in making up a trend.
3. *Number of Runs*: too few or too many runs or crossings of the median, which signifies too much or too little variability. Because the run chart uses the median as its center, when only common cause variation is present, there is a regular cadence at which runs present themselves.
4. *Astronomical point*: a point that is unusually large or small and obviously or blatantly different than the other points (Carey, 2003c; Perla et al., 2010).

Statistical Process Control Charts

Building on the concepts for development of run charts, SPC charts are similar to run charts by plotting measures over regularly spaced time intervals and by distinguishing common cause from special cause variation. The difference is that SPC charts incorporate more rigorous statistical techniques based on the tenets of probability theory and of variation that are used to assess statistically significant changes in determining the presence of special cause variation (Marstellar, Huizinga, & Cooper, 2013).

An SPC chart can use the same data set, chart axes, and time-series data points as a run chart, although there are differences to the setup of an SPC chart that make it more rigorous. The SPC chart uses the mean, or the arithmetic average of each data point in the series for the centerline, as opposed to the median in a run chart. The SPC chart also contains and upper (UCL) and lower (LCL) control limit that adds sensitivity and power and allows for additional tests for special cause variation. Note that the UCL and LCL are not the same as the confidence limits of a distribution; instead, they represent the limits of a measure over time because they are calculated using the differences in aggregated measures over points

in time (Carey, 2003b). Calculation of the UCL and the LCL depends on the type of SPC used.

SPC charts are beneficial in that they:

- identify intervention effects on measurable process and outcome measures in real time as much as possible;
- provide evidence of impact on health outcomes, quality, utilization, and cost absent the ability to undertake lengthy, resource intensive program evaluations;
- avoid the lack of statistical power issues that could result from small sample sizes;
- can be used to assess the measurement of events that rarely occur such as falls (Sherry & Sylvia, 2018).

Interpreting Variation in SPC Charts

When examining SPC charts for special cause variation, a set of rules is applied to the graphical display. The rules are based on the position of the time-series data points in reference to the mean, UCL, and LCL, with special cause variation indicated when:

- one point is outside the upper or lower control limits,
- two of three successive points are on the same side of the center line *and* more than two standard deviations (also known as *sigmas*) from the center line (mean),
- four out of five successive points more than one standard deviation from the mean on the same side of the center line,
- eight successive points on the same side of the center line,
- six successive points increasing or decreasing (a trend), and
- when there is obvious cyclical behavior (see **Figure 24.3**) (Benneyan et al., 2003).

Note that these rules are those commonly applied in health care, but the rules vary depending on the industry and the expert developing them (Benneyan et al., 2003; QI Macros, 2020).

30 Day All Cause Readmission Rate

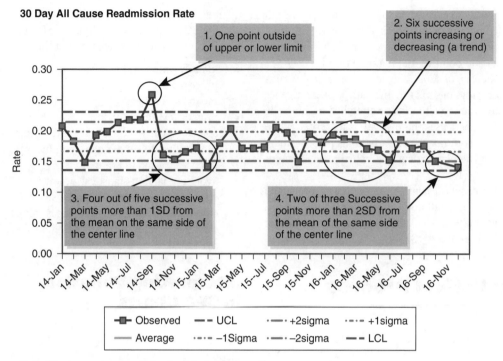

Note: The terms sigma and standard deviation have the same meaning

Figure 24.3 Application of Rules to Identify Special Cause Variation in SPC Charts.

Reproduced from Sherry, M., & Sylvia, M. (2018). Ongoing Monitoring. In M. Sylvia & M. Terhaar (Eds.), *Clinical analytics and data management for the DNP* (2nd ed., pp. 281–301). Springer Publishing Company.

Applied Learning: Case Study

The Steps for Creating SPC Charts

In an accountable care organization (ACO), one of the quality measures used to determine reimbursement of savings to providers is defined by the National Quality Foundation as:

> The percentage of members 18–75 years of age with diabetes (type 1 and type 2) whose most recent HbA1c level during the measurement year was greater than 9.0% (poor control) or was missing a result, or if an HbA1c test was not done during the measurement year. (National Quality Forum, 2017)

To understand if processes are working correctly to measure HbA1c and the outcome of poor control of blood glucose, the ACO will use statistical process control to monitor these results on a monthly basis.

Step 1

The first step in the process is to structure data points representing the measures of "% of patients with diabetes who have had a HbA1c test in the last 12 months" and "% of those patients with diabetes who have been tested during the year with a test result greater than 9.0%" in the desirable time sequence, which is months. See **Table 24.1**. Note that unique observations in this data set are identified by a unique measure and time. Although this data set is created from person-level observations, the data structure to create the charts is not at the person level.

Step 2

In the next step, data points are plotted on a graph where the x-axis represents the time intervals and the y-axis represents the values for the measure using software such as Excel or a statistical software

Table 24.1 Data Set for Creating SPC Chart

Month	% with HbA1c Test	% with HbA1c >9%
January	58	17.1
February	62	17.6
March	64	17.9
April	66	17.2
May	70	16.8
June	68	16.6
July	72	16.2
August	74	15.8
September	76	15.4
October	77	15.2
November	78	15.1
December	79	14.9

package. Ideally, the *y*-axis scale extends on the upper and lower end 20% higher and lower than the highest and lowest value. Adding the median to the graph makes this a run chart. **Figure 24.4** shows the run chart for each measure.

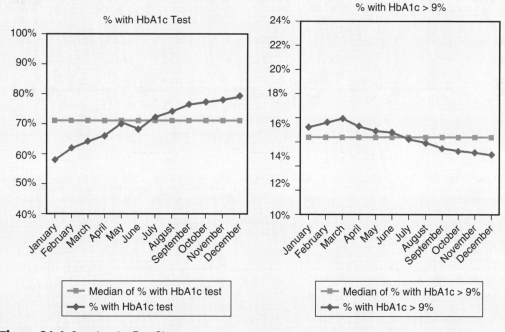

Figure 24.4 Creating the Run Chart.

(continues)

Applied Learning: Case Study *(continued)*

Step 3

In this step, to make the statistical control chart, the median is replaced with the mean, and the UCL and LCL are created. There are many variants of the calculation for the upper and lower control limits based on the type of distribution of the data. This example is using the well-understood textbook definition for standard deviation based on a normal distribution, although when using SPC in practice it is important to review the many SPC publications and resources to identify the best formula for the data (Benneyan et al., 2003). Using the preceding data, the UCL and LCL are calculated by first determining the standard deviation for the series using the following steps:

1. Determine the mean of the distribution (the simple average of the numbers).
2. Then for each number, subtract the mean and square the result.
3. Then determine the mean of the squared differences calculated in step 2.
4. Finally, take the square root of the mean of the squared differences; this is the standard deviation or SD (Math is Fun, 2017).

After calculating the standard deviation, the limits for one, two, and three SDs are calculated. The calculation for three SDs plus or minus the mean represents the UCL and LCL.

   Figure 24.5 displays an example of these calculations for the measure of the percentage of patients who have had an HbA1c test. Although there are many types of SPC charts and methods for calculating the upper and lower control limits that vary mainly based on the data type used for the measure (e.g., counts,

Month	% with HbA1c Test	Mean of % with HbA1c Test	Absolute Value of (Value – Mean) Squared	LCL % with HbA1c Test	UCL % with HbA1c Test	Lower 1 SD % with HbA1C Test	Upper 1 SD % with HbA1C Test	Lower 2 SD % with HbA1C Test	Upper 2 SD % with HbA1C Test
January	58%	70.3%	0.0152	50.7%	89.9%	63.8%	76.9%	57.3%	83.4%
February	62%	70.3%	0.0069	50.7%	89.9%	63.8%	76.9%	57.3%	83.4%
March	64%	70.3%	0.0040	50.7%	89.9%	63.8%	76.9%	57.3%	83.4%
April	66%	70.3%	0.0019	50.7%	89.9%	63.8%	76.9%	57.3%	83.4%
May	70%	70.3%	0.0000	50.7%	89.9%	63.8%	76.9%	57.3%	83.4%
June	68%	70.3%	0.0005	50.7%	89.9%	63.8%	76.9%	57.3%	83.4%
July	72%	70.3%	0.0003	50.7%	89.9%	63.8%	76.9%	57.3%	83.4%
August	74%	70.3%	0.0013	50.7%	89.9%	63.8%	76.9%	57.3%	83.4%
September	76%	70.3%	0.0032	50.7%	89.9%	63.8%	76.9%	57.3%	83.4%
October	77%	70.3%	0.0044	50.7%	89.9%	63.8%	76.9%	57.3%	83.4%
November	78%	70.3%	0.0059	50.7%	89.9%	63.8%	76.9%	57.3%	83.4%
December	79%	70.3%	0.0075	50.7%	89.9%	63.8%	76.9%	57.3%	83.4%
Mean of Squared Differences		0.0043							
Square Root		0.0654							
1 Standard Deviation		0.0654							
2 Standard Deviation		0.1307							
3 Standard Deviation		0.1961							

Figure 24.5 Calculating Upper and Lower Control Limits.

ordinal, interval, ratio), the general rule for UCLs and LCLs is that they represent three standard deviations above and below the mean of the time series of values (Sherry & Sylvia, 2018). Note that even though this example is showing the same value for the control limits and SD calculations, in reality these would be recalculated and applied retrospectively with each month of new data.

Step 4

In this final step, the final version of the statistical control chart is created by adding the upper and lower confidence limits and lines representing one and two standard deviations above and below the mean to the chart and changing the median to the mean. The final charts are displayed in **Figure 24.6**.

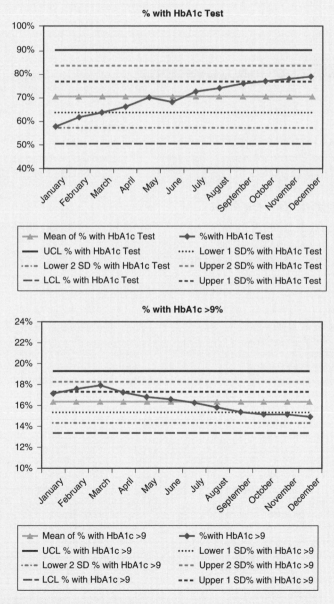

Figure 24.6 Statistical Process Control Charts.

Conclusion

Statistical process control is a relatively simple way of monitoring process and outcome measures of importance to population health interventions. SPC charts plot measures over regular time intervals and use a set of rules to identify common cause variation that represents stability in an intervention and special cause variation that represents a change in the intervention. Variation rules are applied to the patterns and placement of the time series to measure values in relationship to the mean and the upper and lower control limits.

When used to monitor population health interventions, statistical process control methods provide answers to the following questions:

"If we invest in that intervention, how will we know that we're getting results?" "How is our care management program performing?"

"Are we realizing a return on our investment for the medication therapy program?"

Study and Discussion Questions

- Referencing the charts in Figure 24.6, identify instances of common and special cause variation.
- How can run charts and statistical process control be used to understand the ability of an intervention to have its desired impact?
- How would you know if an intervention is having an impact by examining a statistical process control chart?
- How could you use the results of run charts and statistical process control to set targets for a population health intervention?

Resources and Websites

Institute for Health Care Improvement (n.d.), Quality improvement essentials toolkit. http://www.ihi.org/resources/Pages/Tools/Quality-Improvement-Essentials-Toolkit.aspx

The American Society for Quality (ASQ): https://asq.org/

References

Benneyan, J. C., Lloyd, R. C., & Plsek, P. E. (2003). Statistical process control as a tool for research and healthcare improvement. *BMJ Quality & Safety, 12*(6), 458–464. https://doi.org/10.1136/qhc.12.6.458

Carey, R. G. (2003a). Preface. Pp. xvii–xxi in R. G. Carey (Ed.), *Improving healthcare with control charts*. American Society for Quality. http://asq.org/quality-press/journal/index.html?item=H1165&author=Raymond+G.+Carey

Carey, R. G. (2003b). Control chart theory simplified. Pp. 13–26 in *Improving healthcare with control charts*. American Society for Quality.

Carey, R. G. (2003c). Basic SPC concepts and the run chart. In *Improving healthcare with control charts* (pp. 3–12). American Society for Quality.

Donabedian, A. (1980). *Basic approaches to assessment: Structure, process, and outcome*. Health Administration Press.

Marstellar, J., Huizinga, M. M., & Cooper, L. A. (2013, March). Statistical process control: Possible uses to monitor and evaluate patient-centered medical home models. Agency for Healthcare Research and Quality. https://pcmh.ahrq.gov/page/statistical-process-controlpossible-uses-monitor-and-evaluate-patient-centered-medical-home

Math Is Fun. (2017). *Standard deviation formulas*. https://www.mathsisfun.com/data/standard-deviation-formulas.html

National Quality Forum. (2017). Comprehensive diabetes care: Hemoglobin A1c (HbA1c) poor control (>9.0%). http://www.qualityforum.org/QPS/MeasureDetails.çaspx?standardID=1225&print=0&entityTypeID=1

Perla, R. J., Provost, L. P., & Murray, S. K. (2010). The run chart: A simple analytical tool for learning from variation in healthcare processes. *BMJ Quality & Safety, 20*(1), 46–51. https://doi.org/10.1136/bmjqs.2009.037895

Q I Macros. (2020). Control chart rules. https://www.qimacros.com/control-chart/stability-analysis-control-chart-rules/

Sherry, M., & Sylvia, M. (2018). Ongoing Monitoring. In M. Sylvia & M. Terhaar (Eds.), *Clinical analytics and data management for the DNP* (2nd ed., pp. 281–301). Springer Publishing Company.

Sylvia, M. (2020). Introduction to Population Health Analytics. In *Population health management learning series*. ForestVue Healthcare Solutions.

SECTION VII

Analytics Support for the Population Health Process

CHAPTER 25

Assessing Populations

Martha Sylvia, PhD, MBA, RN
Ines Maria Vigil, MD, MPH, MBA

Diagnosis is not the end, but the beginning of practice.

—Martin H. Fischer

EXECUTIVE SUMMARY

The population health assessment is a fundamental building block of any population health project. The time spent on assessing the population sets the stage for a successful population health project outcome and has the potential to generate more insights than can be acted on at one time. A thoughtful approach to assessing the experience, health, cost, and utilization of populations can quickly advance organizations into data-driven decision-making, a culture of health, and financial profitability.

Population health analytics is a valuable tool to identify actionable insights from what are often considered complex and multifaceted healthcare challenges. Assessing population health precedes the analytic steps of and defines the analyses for the allocation of scarce resources and the calculation of a financial return on investment, and significant time must be given to this activity to ensure downstream success. In addition, an effective population health assessment warrants thorough preparation, dedicated time, critical thinking, and an understanding of the healthcare landscape that contributes to the needs of the populations of interest.

Traditional cost and utilization analyses often stop short of providing information on determinants, health outcomes, and actionable data outliers, whereas population health assessments dive deeper into understanding the underlying causes of behavior, lifestyle, and social factors that contribute to improved and worsened health outcomes that drive cost and utilization. It is not uncommon for traditional cost and utilization analyses to identify an emerging trend in the data that, on closer inspection, proves to represent appropriate utilization and cost of a condition whose severity or prevalence is increasing over time. Where traditional cost and utilization analyses may assist in explaining the rising cost of care, it is population health assessments that identify insights in the data that can be transformed into actionable solutions in the form of targeted lists of patients that warrant one or more evidence-based interventions to mitigate risk.

LEARNING OBJECTIVES

At the end of this chapter, the learner will be able to:

1. Describe the framework for assessing populations.
2. Evaluate the steps for assessing populations.
3. Identify the relationship between health determinants and health outcomes.
4. Determine the use of evidence in supplementing a population assessment.
5. Distinguish the characteristics of ideal opportunities to favorably impact outcomes.

Introduction

U.S. healthcare delivery organizations, payers, governments, and other independent organizations regularly monitor pertinent health indicators and resource utilization (Kruse, Stein, Thomas, & Kaur, 2018; Mo, Choi, Li, & Merrick, 2004; Murray et al., 2012, 2018; Reschovsky, Hadley, O'Malley, & Landon, 2014). An unexpected rise or fall in these indicators often triggers the need to understand more deeply the unique characteristics of the affected population and the health determinants that impact care, cost, and utilization. Population health assessments are best suited to pinpoint the underlying causes of unexpected changes, predict future unexpected changes, and guide population health teams to develop evidence-based interventions to address the underlying causes and prevent future unexpected changes.

The population health assessment hones in on the health determinants, which are driving cost and utilization within subgroupings of the population and their relationship to health-improvement opportunities (Curtis, Fry, Shaban, & Considine, 2017; Kaplan, Spittel, & David, 2015; Hawe & Potvin, 2009; Pettit, 2002). The PopHealth Troika (PHT) introduced in Chapter 31, "Building a Team Culture for Population Health," works collaboratively with care teams and organizational leaders to make recommendations for addressing identified opportunities in actionable subgroupings of populations of interest. For the purposes of this chapter and going forward, a comprehensive population health assessment is a written and

oral presentation of the *assess* and *focus* phases introduced in Chapter 2, "Guiding Frameworks for Conceptualizing Population Health Analytics," using storytelling techniques to disseminate the results and to gather stakeholder support for addressing these opportunities.

This chapter outlines the process to identify the types of challenges in health care that lead to the need for a population health assessment, defines the data and nondata elements necessary for the assessment, and details the process steps required to comprehensively assess a population's health to identify opportunities for health improvement. In addition, this chapter introduces the concept of person-centered analytics as a best practice when assessing the health of a population.

Framework for Assessing Populations

A population health assessment stems from the identification of problems in health care. Healthcare delivery organizations, payers, governments, and other independent organizations regularly monitor pertinent health indicators and resource utilization. Indicators that are out of expected ranges are the frontline of problem identification. An unexpected rise in hospital admissions for people with chronic illness, an increase in readmissions for patients having orthopedic surgeries, an increasing incidence of people identified with heart disease; or a large proportion of children with emergency department visits for uncontrolled asthma are all examples of unexpected results in monitored measures that identify a problem. These are the types of problems that benefit from a population-based approach to understanding the link between health determinants and these undesirable outcomes in aggregate.

Once the problem has been clarified, the population assessment process is activated. The population assessment process has five steps, and even though they are meant to take place in order, there is fluidity and flexibility between steps with multiple iterations before getting to identified opportunities. **Figure 25.1** lists each step, and the remainder of this section will describe the steps in detail.

Defining Determinants and Outcomes

Determinants

A multitude of determinants impact health-related outcomes. The selection of health determinants begins with data that are readily available. In healthcare organizations, the most commonly available sources of data are from administrative claims (enrollment, medical, and pharmacy), the electronic medical record, and lab data. These sources of data are used to select health determinants that are suspected of impacting outcomes based on the problem identified. For instance, if the problem was that people with chronic illness

were having an increase in hospital admissions, then selected health determinants might include the type and number of chronic conditions, complications and comorbidities, frailty, measures of medication adherence, indicators of access to care, and care-coordination markers.

Once sources of internal data are exhausted, sources of health determinants outside the healthcare organization are considered. The county health rankings (Robert Wood Johnson Foundation, n.d.) provide a structure for understanding and selecting health determinants outside of those available for clinical care. Chapter 7, "Social and Behavioral Data," describes social determinants of health data and the drivers of poor outcomes that are based on a model of community health that emphasizes the many factors that influence how long and how well we live. The rankings use more than 30 measures that help communities understand how healthy their residents are today (health outcomes) and what will impact their health in the future (health factors) (Givens, Gennuso, Jovaag, Van Dijk, & Johnson, 2019). Additional sources of external data can be considered, including a variety of self-reported, consumer, social media, and social and behavioral determinants of health data. More details on the definitions, applications, and examples can be found in Chapter 9, "Grouping, Trending, and Interpreting Population Health Data for Receptivity, Engagement, and Activation."

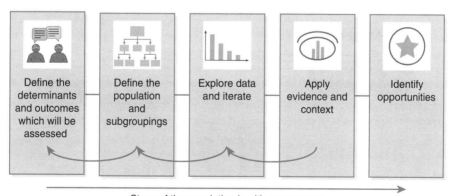

Figure 25.1 Steps of the Population Assessment.

Reproduced from Sylvia, M. (2020b). The population health assessment. In Population health management learning series. ForestVue Healthcare Solutions.

Outcomes

Outcomes measure the impact of health determinants on health status, quality, patients' experience of care, utilization, and costs. Selected outcomes depend on the initially identified problem. In the problem of increased hospital admissions for those with chronic illness, the outcome would likely be the hospital admission rate and the percentage of individuals who have any hospitalization. In **Figure 25.2**, outcomes are defined as length of life and quality of life. Intervening outcome measures may also be selected. These are measures that precede high cost or utilization. For instance, in the case of patients with diabetes, a prolonged high level of hemoglobin A1c (HbA1c) may be identified before any hospitalization occurs. It would be worthwhile to also look at the impact of health determinants on HbA1c in this scenario. When considering intervening outcomes, the difference between health determinants and outcomes can sometimes overlap. It is important that PHT members engage in dialogue and agree when defining outcomes and

health determinants. Chapter 24, "Run Charts and Statistical Process Control," and Chapter 28, "Monitoring and Optimizing Interventions," provide more information about outcome measures.

Defining the Population and Subgroupings

The population health assessment begins by defining the population in terms of variables and criteria applied to values. The definition and criteria relate back to the identified problem. In the earlier example, people with chronic illness were having higher hospitalizations, so the population might be defined as "adults with chronic illness who had a hospitalization over the past year" or the assessment may start with "all adults with certain types of chronic illness like diabetes, chronic obstructive pulmonary disease, and coronary artery disease. When the understanding of the problem is minimal, the population definition is defined broadly to allow for filtering and comparisons among subgroups. When the problem is

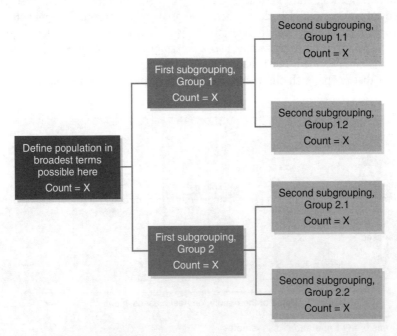

Figure 25.2 Defining the Population and Subgroupings.

understood in more detail, the population for the assessment can be narrowed—for instance, when it is known that patients with sickle cell disease are having higher numbers of emergency department visits following the closing of the specialty clinic where they previously received care.

Developing findings is usually accomplished by creating subgroupings of the population. For instance, in the example of those with chronic illness, population subgroupings may be created based on age, chronic condition type, medication adherence rate cut points, or other criteria, depending on findings during the assessment. When defining the population, a diagram is helpful for collaboration and mutual understanding around the criteria for forming the population and subgroupings like the one in Figure 25.2. Supporting text with further descriptions can be added as annotation. It is helpful to provide the estimated or actual count of people who fall into the entire population and subgroupings in each box.

Understand that some iteration with the data in the entire population may be necessary before defining the subgroupings. It is OK to formulate the subgroup descriptions as information becomes clearer in the data about the best way to divide the population. The subgrouping decisions are usually made based on findings about the relationship between health determinants and outcomes.

Data Exploration and Iteration

Data exploration and iteration is perhaps the longest step. The PHT, consisting of the analyst, business, and clinical experts, work together to look at data. The process begins by analyzing means and proportions for each health determinant and then moves to analyze the relationships between health determinants and health outcomes in the whole population and comparisons between subgroupings. Analytic methods are mainly univariate and multivariate statistics. Many analytic tools are used in this step, including graphing, geomapping, and visualization software; appropriate data contextualizers; and statistical software.

It is important to be patient in this step and plan to spend a substantial amount of time together reviewing data points and brainstorming information. The analyst is the data expert and guides the clinical and business leader to ask questions that can be answered with the data. The business leader understands strategy and priorities, contracting, legal agreements, resources, and culture around addressing findings in the data and provides guidance on the path forward. The clinical leader understands clinical care and the way to apply data for clinical decision-making at the aggregate and person level, and he or she can put findings into the context of clinical strategy and priorities.

The evolution of this part of the process is moving to the focus phase of the population health process in which the drivers of outcomes are clarified and the PHT focuses on the extent to which health determinants are impacting outcomes. More attention is given to cost and utilization drivers within subgrouping and the relationship to health-improvement opportunities.

Application of Evidence and Context

The data available to assess populations and subgroupings usually only allow a limited understanding of the impact of health determinants on outcomes of interest. When data at the person-level are unavailable, it is helpful to seek out other sources of information that can help provide context and further understanding. Other sources of evidence and information include peer-reviewed journal articles, professional organizations such as the American Diabetes Association and the Centers for Disease Control and Prevention, private and public sources of health-related data like the county health rankings (Robert Wood Johnson Foundation, n.d.), and organizational consortiums that share data such as Vizient (n.d.), a member-driven healthcare performance improvement organization. **Table 25.1** displays some of the sources and types of evidence that are useful in supplementing the population assessment.

Table 25.1 Sources and Types of Evidence Used in Assessing Populations

Source of Evidence	Types of Evidence Identified	Useful Website
Google Scholar	Systematic reviews, clinical guidelines, peer-reviewed literature	https://scholar.google.com/
PubMed: biomedical literature	Systematic reviews, clinical guidelines, peer-reviewed literature	https://pubmed.ncbi.nlm.nih.gov/
Cumulative Index to Nursing and Allied Health Literature	Systematic evidence reviews, clinical guidelines, peer-reviewed literature	https://health.ebsco.com/products/the-cinahl-database
Cochrane Library	Systematic reviews	https://www.cochranelibrary.com/
Agency for Healthcare Research and Quality	Clinical guidelines and recommendations, industry publications and white papers	https://www.ahrq.gov/prevention/guidelines/index.html
National Guideline Clearinghouse	Clinical guidelines	https://health.gov/node/160
American Association of Family Physicians	Clinical guidelines and recommendations	https://www.aafp.org/patient-care/browse/type.tag-clinical-practice-guidelines.html
Other professional organizations such as the American Diabetes Association or the American Heart Association	Clinical guidelines and recommendations	https://www.diabetes.org/ https://www.heart.org/
U.S. Food and Drug Administration	Information on approval of medical devices, drugs, vaccines, and biologics	https://www.fda.gov/home
Google	Systematic reviews, clinical guidelines, peer-reviewed literature, industry publications and white papers, popular literature	https://www.google.com/

Reproduced from Sylvia, M. (2020a). Evidence-based practice. In *Population health management learning series.* ForestVue Healthcare Solutions.

Sources and Types of Evidence Used in Assessing Populations

Opportunity Identification

The PHT works through all findings to determine the most important connections between health determinants and outcomes. These connections culminate in opportunities to address the relationship and prevent undesirable outcomes. The opportunities are considered within the context of the feasibility for addressing them.

Opportunities in which resources cannot be identified or where the capacity of the organization is not able to address them, are put aside in favor of those that are feasible. A win–win occurs when the most impactful opportunity is also largely feasible to translate into practice. **Figure 25.3** shows a compelling way to present opportunities to stakeholders. All findings culminate in a story (see Chapter 29, "Storytelling with Data") that is told to stakeholders using easy-to-understand data visualizations, compelling them to prioritize and assign resources to act.

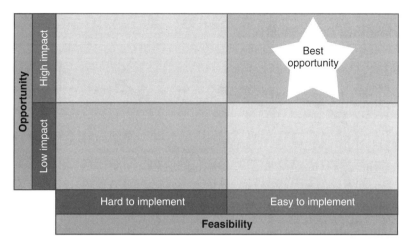

Figure 25.3 Optimal Opportunities.

Reproduced from Sylvia, M. (2020b). The population health assessment. In *Population health management learning series.* ForestVue Healthcare Solutions.

Applied Learning: Case Study

This case study provides additional context for the case studies in Chapter 22, "Predictive and Prescriptive Analytics," and Chapter 28, "Monitoring and Optimizing Interventions," by reviewing a modified version of a population assessment that would lead to the predictive model developed in Chapters 22 and 28.

Define the Problem

A large health plan with patients spanning multiple primary care providers is administering a risk arrangement with several of the provider groups. The goals of the risk arrangement are to identify one or more Triple Aim (Berwick, Nolan, & Whittington, 2008; Institute for Healthcare Improvement, n.d.) opportunities to perform high-quality health care with a positive patient experience at a reasonable cost. The health plan has requested that hospital admissions and costs for patients with diabetes be part of the selected monitoring and performance metrics. **Figure 25.4** shows that month-over-month costs consistently rose in year 2 when compared to year 1. These rising costs are identified to be driven by the hospital admission rate, which rose in tandem with costs. Average costs per member per month went from $397 to $426, and hospital admissions per thousand increased from 25.0 to 27.0. The health plan and the provider group collaborated to form a population health team similar to the PopHealth Troika introduced in Chapter 31, "Building a Team Culture for Population Health," consisting of an analyst from the health plan, a provider leader from the groups at risk, and a provider representative leading the contract from the health plan.

Define the Determinants and Outcomes

Combining the data from the health plan and the lab vendor, the PHT planned the health determinants and outcomes used for the analysis. Health determinants were defined in terms of broader categories of demographics, geographic regions, illness burden, risk factors, and medication adherence. Outcomes were defined in terms of utilization and costs with an interest in also examining HbA1c levels, which serve as both an indicator of outcomes and an outcome itself—that is, as a leading indicator of avoidable utilization or inappropriate costs. **Figure 25.5** shows the variables, data sources, time periods, and values that will be aggregated at the person level to create the data set used to assess the population of patients with diabetes.

(continues)

Applied Learning: Case Study *(continued)*

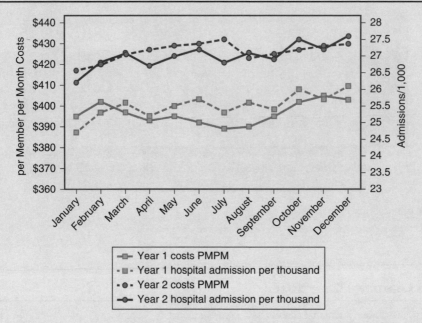

Figure 25.4 Hospital Admissions and Costs in Patients with Diabetes.

	Variables	**Data source**	**Time period**	**Values**
Determinants demographics and provider group	• Age • Gender • Race • Provider group	Insurance eligibility	As of 12/31/2020	• 0–100 • 1 = Male, 0 = Female • CMS race codes • 1 through 3 groups
Determinants illness burden	• # Chronic conditions • Chronic and mental health condition indicators	Medical claims Diagnosis codes grouped by conditions	If the condition was ever coded between 1/1/19 and 12/31/20	• 0–20 • 1 = Yes, 0 = No for hypertension, hyperlipidemia, complications, mental health condition
Determinants medication adherence	• Proportion of days covered • Medication gaps	Pharmacy claims NDC Codes grouped by condition	Calendar year 2020	• 0–100% • 0–12
Intervening outcome HbA1c	• HbA1c % • HbA1c > 9%	Lab vendor data	Last value in calendar year 2020	• 5.0–18.0 • 1 = Yes, 0 = No
Outcomes	• Admissions • Total costs	• Administrative claims grouped into admits • Administrative claims summed by costs	Calendar year 2020	• 0–60 • $0–$1,000,000

Figure 25.5 Health Determinants and Outcomes for Assessing the Population of Patients with Diabetes.

Identify the Population and Subgroupings

Patients who were enrolled in the health plan were included if they were 18 or older and had at least 6 months of enrollment during calendar year 2020. A diagnosis of diabetes was determined if there was an occurrence of at least one Diabetes International Classification of Diseases, 10th Revision, Clinical Modification (ICD-10-CM) code or one National Drug Code for diabetes medication in the predictor year. Patients who were identified with gestational diabetes, steroid-induced diabetes, or polycystic ovaries were excluded. ICD-10 diagnoses for lab and radiology services or for durable medical equipment were excluded for identification purposes to avoid rule-out diagnoses. The PHT decided to subgroup the population by provider groups and the presence of any hospital admission. The subgroupings were formed so they would be mutually exclusive.

Figure 25.6 demonstrates the way data can be subgrouped to identify populations.

Explore Data and Iterate

The PHT worked together to explore the data and determine pertinent results that are worth understanding further. They performed univariate statistics on each variable to look at distributions and compare these distributions among provider groups and among those who did and did not have an admission. After a great deal of iteration, the data were summarized by the analyst and are shown in **Table 25.2**. The highlighted boxes are those in which the team spent more time in the focus phase of the analysis.

Application of Evidence and Context

The data available to assess the population are limited in the context of understanding the impact of other health determinants on the outcomes of interest. In addition to other evidence reviewed, the PHT accessed data from the county health rankings (Robert Wood Johnson Foundation, n.d.) to supplement findings. The county health rankings and road maps are based on a model of community health that emphasizes the many factors that influence how long and how well we live. The rankings use more than 30 measures that help communities understand how healthy their residents are today (health outcomes) and what will

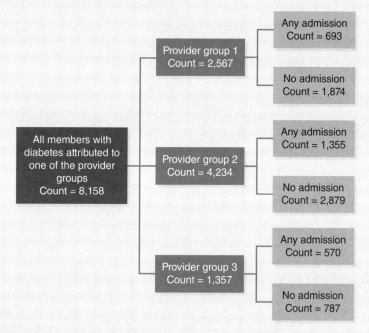

Figure 25.6 Population and Subgroupings for Assessing the Population of Patients with Diabetes.

(continues)

Table 25.2 Population and Subgroupings for Assessing the Population of Patients with Diabetes

	Provider Group 1			Provider Group 2			Provider Group 3		
	Overall	With Admission	No Admission	Overall	With Admission	No Admission	Overall	With Admission	No Admission
Female %	56.0%	57.8%	55.2%	58.0%	56.7%	59.2%	54.0%	56.1%	52.3%
Race									
% White (non-Hispanic)	68.0%	62.9%	69.9%	57.6%	48.9%	61.7%	38.0%	34.0%	40.9%
% Black (non-Hispanic)	18.0%	24.8%	15.5%	29.0%	37.5%	25.0%	51.6%	55.6%	48.7%
% Asian/Pacific Islander	10.6%	8.3%	11.4%	5.2%	4.6%	5.5%	1.2%	1.0%	1.3%
% Hispanic/Latino	3.4%	4.0%	3.2%	8.2%	9.0%	7.8%	9.2%	9.4%	9.1%
% American Indian/Alaska Native	0.0%	0.0%	0.0%	0.0%	0.0%	0.0%	0.0%	0.0%	0.0%
% Other, Missing, Unknown	0.0%	0.0%	0.0%	0.0%	0.0%	0.0%	0.0%	0.0%	0.0%
	100.0%	100.0%	100.0%	100.0%	99.9%	100.0%	100.0%	100.0%	100.0%
% w Hypertension	64.0%	85.4%	56.1%	67.2%	79.0%	61.7%	72.0%	83.6%	63.6%
% w Hyperlipidemia	52.3%	66.2%	47.2%	54.4%	73.4%	45.5%	57.6%	77.2%	43.5%
% w Diabetes Complication	32.6%	51.5%	25.6%	39.1%	55.2%	31.5%	48.0%	72.1%	27.9%
% w any Mental Health Condition	14.8%	26.4%	10.5%	15.1%	24.4%	10.7%	20.2%	30.8%	12.5%
Mean (SD) Proportion of Days Covered for Diabetes Medication	87.8% (0.27)	82.2% (0.25)	92.2% (0.28)	82.3% (0.29)	78.9% (0.26)	85.6% (0.30)	67.8% (0.28)	58.2% (0.26)	75.2% (0.29)
% with any Diabetes Medication Gap	5.6%	7.8%	4.8%	7.8%	9.8%	6.9%	19.7%	25.3%	15.6%
% with any Admission	27.2%			32.3%			48.9%		
% with HbA1c > 9	28.3%	32.4%	67.6%	30.0%	35.6%	64.4%	35.6%	67.8%	32.2%
Mean (SD) HbA1c	7.2 (1.4)	8.1 (1.8)	6.7 (1.1)	7.5 (2.2)	8.3 (1.9)	6.5 (1.3)	8.1 (2.7)	9.8 (1.9)	7.7 (1.3)
Mean (SD) Total Costs	$18,886 ($22,356)	$25,332 ($29,566)	$6,789 ($8,587)	$19,678 ($23,948)	$26,948 ($28,993)	$7,432 ($9,856)	$22,456 ($27,678)	$31,879 ($41,356)	$10,878 ($15,356)

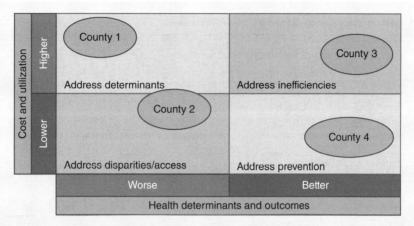

Figure 25.7 Comparison of Health Determinants and Outcomes Among Provider Groups.

Reproduced from Sylvia, M. (2020b). The population health assessment. In *Population health management learning series*. ForestVue Healthcare Solutions.

impact their health in the future (health factors) (Population Health Institute, 2020). The data are available by county, and all persons in the population were assigned counties based on their home address in the health plan enrollment file.

The admission and cost data were aggregated at the county level, and the grid in **Figure 25.7** was created using four statistics: admission rate and average costs (both derived from administrative claims data) and health determinant and health outcome ranking (calculated by the county health rankings) (Robert Wood Johnson Foundation, n.d.). The grid separates the four counties where most of the population lives into quadrants based on the level of utilization and costs and the rankings. The PHT worked together to determine the most important factors to analyze based on the quadrant in which the county was assigned. When costs are higher but rankings are lower, then it is important to identify and address health determinants that may serve as underlying causes. When costs are lower and rankings are lower, there may be an issue with access to healthcare services. When costs are higher and rankings are higher, an analysis should be undertaken to determine whether inefficiencies in care delivery exist. Finally, the desired outcome is when rankings, cost, and utilization are all in the lower right-hand quadrant.

Opportunity Identification

The PHT worked together to identify opportunities based on the analysis. Remember that this case study is showing a limited portion of the work and data review that goes into a population assessment. It is meant to highlight the process but not encompass the complete set of analyses that go into summarizing findings and identifying opportunities. Based on the results included in the assessment, the following pertinent findings are listed. Once agreed on, the PHT uses storytelling techniques to disseminate findings in the organization.

Findings and Recommendation Highlights

- Provider group 3 has noticeably more patients with poor outcomes, higher morbidity, more gaps in medication adherence, and health disparities. Recommendations can include:
  - checking the analysis to ensure the population is properly risk-adjusted.
  - setting up a meeting with the provider group to understand its practice, neighborhood, community, practice workflows, and quality-improvement efforts; and
  - collaborating with the practice to set up a pilot program that includes self-management support techniques and medication management to be tested with provider group 3.
- The health plan would benefit from undertaking further analysis to understand any inefficiencies and waste in population subgroupings living in county 3. Recommendations can include:
  - a provider practice variation analysis, including a review of pricing and volume changes over time;

(continues)

Applied Learning: Case Study *(continued)*

- medical policies and benefit changes that may be out-of-date or inconsistently followed by the providers in the practice;
- a review of any quality incentive revenue that the practice may be missing by not identifying known gaps in care quality in a timely manner or for patients who may have been lost to follow-up; and
- a review of medication fill rates, medication counts, and any lapses in adherence of patients predicted to be at high risk of an avoidable hospital admission or emergency department event.
- The health plan and provider would benefit from working together to develop strategies for addressing health determinants, health disparities and access issues, especially for those living in counties 1 and 2. Recommendations can include:
  - providing a list of community organizations that provide a variety of services that address social and economic disparities,
  - collaborating to provide safe and timely transportation to and from outpatient medical services, and
  - access to behavioral and social care management services.

Conclusion

Selecting a framework, defining populations, exploring the data, and applying the evidence-based learnings are all key elements of assessing populations to identify actionable opportunities to improve patient experience and health outcomes and to reduce avoidable cost. Aligning the insights gleaned from a population health assessment with the goals of the organization, the care team, or the patient (or all three) provides a clear path to action through the development and implementation of evidence-based interventions that address the underlying causes of the problem to solve. Population health teams like the ones introduced in Chapter 31, "Building a Team Culture for Population Health," are perfectly suited to learn, propagate, and apply the stepwise population health assessment process outlined in this chapter.

This chapter provides an outline for a population health assessment that defines the population health phases of *assess* and *focus* introduced in Chapter 2, "Guiding Frameworks for Population Health Analytics," identifies when a population health assessment is warranted and characterizes the data and nondata elements needed in a stepwise phased approach using person-centered analytics. Also provided is information on techniques used to disseminate results and the importance of gathering feedback and support to build the business case for pursuing the next step in the process and the development and implementation of targeting criteria and algorithms to identify patients with rising or predicted risk of an avoidable healthcare event.

Study and Discussion Questions

- What are the key considerations when assessing populations?
- Discuss the relationship between health determinants and health outcomes using real-life examples.
- Identify an appropriate use of evidence as part of a population assessment.
- What are the characteristics of ideal opportunities to address in population health management?

Resources and Websites

Association of State and Territorial Health Officials (ASTHO). (2009, August). Public health data sources and assessment tools: A resource compendium to measure access and health disparities. Arlington, VA: ASTHO.

Centers for Disease Control and Prevention (CDC). (n.d.). Other resources for completing health assessments. https://www.cdc.gov/publichealthgateway/cha/resources.html

National Institutes of Health & Agency for Healthcare Research and Quality. (n.d.). R. M

Kaplan, M. L. Spittel, & D. H. David (Eds.), Population health: Behavioral and social science insights. https://www.ahrq.gov/sites/default/files/publications/files/population-health.pdf

RCHN Community Health Foundation. (n.d.). Population health resources. https://www.rchnfoundation.org/?p=4893

Robert Wood Johnson Foundation. (n.d.). 2020 county health rankings and roadmaps. https://www.countyhealthrankings.org/

References

Berwick, D. M., Nolan, T. W., & Whittington, J. (2008). The triple aim: Care, health, and cost. *Health Affairs, 27*(3), 759–769. https://doi.org/10.1377/hlthaff.27.3.759

Curtis, K., Fry, M., Shaban, R. Z., & Considine, J. (2016, September 20). Translating research findings to clinical nursing practice. *Journal of Clinical Nursing, 26*(5–6), 862–872. https://onlinelibrary.wiley.com/doi/full/10.1111/jocn.13586

Givens, M., Gennuso, K., Jovaag, A., Van Dijk, J. W., & Johnson, S. (2019). *2019 County Health Rankings Key Findings Report.*

Hawe, P., & Potvin, L. (2009). What is population health intervention research? *Canadian Journal of Public Health, 100*(1), 18–114. https://doi.org/10.1007/bf03405503

Hewlett-Packard. (2004). Carly Fiorina speech: Information: the currency of the digital age. http://www.hp.com/hpinfo/execteam/speeches/fiorina/04openworld.html

Institute for Healthcare Improvement. (n.d.). The IHI Triple Aim. http://www.ihi.org/Engage/Initiatives/TripleAim/Pages/default.aspx

Kaplan, R. M., Spittel, M. L., & David, D. H. (2015). Population health: Behavioral and social science insights. National Institutes of Health.

Kruse, C. S., Stein, A., Thomas, H., & Kaur, H. (2018). The use of electronic health records to support population health: A systematic review of the literature. *Journal of Medical Systems, 42*(11). https://link.springer.com/article/10.1007%2Fs10916-018-1075-6

Mo, F., Choi, B. C. K., Li, F. C. K., & Merrick, J. (2004). Using Health Utility Index (HUI) for measuring the impact on health-related quality of Life (HRQL) among individuals with chronic diseases. *The Scientific World Journal, 4*, 746–757. https://www.hindawi.com/journals/tswj/2004/183434/

Murray, C. J. L., Mokdad, A. H., Ballestros, K., Echko, M., Glenn, S., Olsen, H. E., Mullany, E., Lee, A., Khan, A. R., Ahmadi, A., Ferrari, A. J., Kasaeian, A., Werdecker, A., Carter, A., Zipkin, B., Sartorius, B., Serdar, B., Sykes, B. L., Troeger, C., Murray, C. J. L. (2018, April 10). The state of US health, 1990–2016: Burden of diseases, injuries, and risk factors among US states. *Journal of the American Medical Association, 319*(14), 1444–1472. https://doi.org/10.1001/jama.2018.0158

Murray, C. J. L., Vos, T., Lozano, R., Naghavi, M., Flaxman, A. D., Michaud, C., Ezzati, M., Shibuya, K., Salomon, J. A., Abdalla, S., Aboyans, V., Abraham, J., Ackerman, I., Aggarwal, R., Ahn, S. Y., Ali, M. K., AlMazroa, M. A., Alvarado, M., Anderson, H. R., Lopez, A. D. (2012). Disability-adjusted life years (DALYs) for 291 diseases and injuries in 21 regions, 1990–2010: A systematic analysis for the Global Burden of Disease Study 2010. *The Lancet, 380*(9859), 2197–2223. https://www.thelancet.com/journals/lancet/article/PIIS0140-6736(12)61689-4/fulltext

Pettit, J. (2002). Managing the most expensive patients. *Harvard Business Review, 2*(6), 304–315.

Population Health Institute. (2020). County health rankings. University of Wisconsin; https://uwphi.pophealth.wisc.edu/chrr/

RCHN Community Health Foundation. (n.d.). Population health resources. https://www.rchnfoundation.org/?p=4893

Reschovsky, J. D., Hadley, J., O'Malley, A. J., & Landon, B. E. (2013, July 5). Geographic variations in the cost of treating condition-specific episodes of care among Medicare patients. *Health Services Research, 49*(1), 32–51. https://onlinelibrary.wiley.com/doi/abs/10.1111/1475-6773.12087

Robert Wood Johnson Foundation. (n.d.). 2020 county health rankings and roadmaps. https://www.countyhealthrankings.org/

Sylvia, M. (2020a). Evidence-based practice. In *Population health management learning series*. ForestVue Healthcare Solutions.

Sylvia, M. (2020b). The population health assessment. In *Population health management learning series*. ForestVue Healthcare Solutions.

Vizient. (n.d.). Member-driven healthcare performance improvement. https://www.vizientinc.com/

CHAPTER 26

Targeting Individuals for Intervention

Martha Sylvia, PhD, MBA, RN

There is always a path to our target; the problem is to discover it!

—Mehmet Murat ildan

EXECUTIVE SUMMARY

A small percentage of individuals account for a large portion of healthcare spending. According to a study by the Kaiser Family Foundation, the top 5% of individuals account for 50% of healthcare spending, and the top 20% account for 80% (Kaiser Family Foundation, 2019). The crux of improving health outcomes while reducing healthcare costs and utilization is the ability to identify these small groups of high-needs patients, intervene to prevent avoidable utilization, and strive for a more normally distributed curve of healthcare spending (Pearl & Madvig, 2020). It is common to look retrospectively at the cohort accounting for high healthcare spending in past time periods and analyze descriptive information about those high-expenditure cohorts as a way to characterize and prevent future outcomes. However, a historical view is not enough to identify those who will benefit from interventions designed to prevent poor outcomes. In large part, this is related to the finding that less than 50% of past high healthcare utilizers will remain as such seven months later and less than 30% will remain high utilizers after a year (Johnson et al., 2015).

Accurately targeting individuals for intervention requires a balance between preventive and precision techniques. The former uses probabilistic techniques to deliver an intervention across an entire population at risk to minimize the percentage of people who have poor outcomes, and the latter closely targets intervention to those who are at risk but are also determined by a set of criteria to benefit from the intervention. Where the science of targeted interventions in precision medicine is more advanced in diseases such as cancer and hemophilia, interventions are targeted based on discernable biomarkers. However, for chronic illnesses like cardiovascular conditions, precision techniques are not advanced or readily applicable at all (Psaty, Dekkers, & Cooper, 2018). In these conditions, a rigorous process of risk-prediction modeling, population stratification and segmentation, and identifying individuals for appropriate intensity of interventions is an efficient way to achieve Triple Aim objectives in populations.

Introduction

Healthcare organizations progress through levels of maturity in the methods they use for targeting individuals for intervention. First attempts usually involve lists of people who are currently high cost or have high hospital admissions, readmissions, or emergency department visits that are usually provided by some type of financial or actuarial analysis. Next, a referral system may be used where providers refer patients to interventions. As organizations evolve, they develop competency to use data to predict future outcomes of whole populations, regardless of their previous healthcare utilization; stratify populations based on their risk of adverse outcomes; and segment populations to appropriate interventions.

Previous chapters in this textbook have laid the foundation for developing and implementing targeting methods in population health. This chapter brings together an understanding of population health data sources and structures, risk-prediction modeling, population assessment, and linkages between health determinants and health outcomes to explain the application of identifying, stratifying, and segmenting populations for intervention.

Population Identification

Population identification refers to the process of delineating the population in its entirety prior to considering risk-prediction scoring, stratification, segmentation, or patient identification. In the broadest sense of the term, populations are defined as whole populations whose constituents include everyone across the health spectrum of wellness to illness (Jeffery et al., 2019). Examples of whole populations include all members of a health plan or accountable care organization, all people living in a geographic region, or all employees. Populations may also be defined by narrower criteria such as everyone in a certain age group, with a certain health condition (or absent a health condition), or a certain socioeconomic status. Population health recognizes that people may identify with multiple groups, so individuals may belong to many different populations and subgroupings (Fabius, 2021).

Populations are defined by using multiple data sources at a person level. Data sources vary depending on the type of healthcare organization and the data available within the organization and the data obtained by the organization through partnerships. For instance, health insurers have internal administrative claims data generated from payment transactions of healthcare services but may also obtain data from provider electronic medical records (EMRs) and from laboratory vendors. Conversely, providers have internal EMR data but may obtain administrative claims data from health insurers. In this text, Section 2, "Data Sources," describes data sources in detail, and Chapter 13, "The Population Health Data Model," describes the organization of data at the person level in support of defining populations of interest.

Risk Prediction

Risk prediction is the process of using analytic techniques to estimate an individual's future potential for a poor health outcome, high healthcare utilization, or excessive costs based on individually assigned values for a selection of health determinants. (Risk-prediction modeling is explained in detail in Chapter 22, "Predictive and

Prescriptive Analytics.") The result of risk prediction is assignment of a score to every individual in the population that indicates that individual's risk of the outcome as a probability or an estimate of the outcome as a point value. The majority of risk-prediction models used in population health produce a probability score assigned at the individual level, and the remainder of this chapter will use this same probability score for the application of risk-prediction scores. Risk prediction assigns a score to individuals in an entire defined population; it does not indicate which individuals should receive certain interventions.

Population Risk Stratification

Risk stratification is usually based on dividing a population based on a risk score, prior utilization of services, or specific health conditions such as diabetes or blood pressure. The idea is that costs and utilization can be predicted and prevented based on stratification using a hierarchy of risk scoring. There is a presumption of homogeneity in risk stratification such that all persons that fall above a certain risk score are similar in terms of their personal characteristics and their likelihood to benefit from intervention (Long et al., 2017). Risk stratification is typically exemplified through a population health pyramid like the one shown in **Figure 26.1**. This figure depicts the process where a whole population is defined, and risk scores are assigned that represent the probability of having an adverse event in the future like a hospitalization or of being high cost. The population is then stratified according to cut points of the risk score.

When using risk-stratification techniques, the next step would be to understand the characteristics of the population at each level to determine which interventions might be appropriate for each level of risk. For example, when the population is defined as everyone within a health plan and stratified by the risk score, members with the lowest risk likely have no health conditions and benefit from health promotion activities, whereas the 10% at the highest level will likely have multiple health conditions and impact from other health determinants and benefit from intensive interventions such as chronic

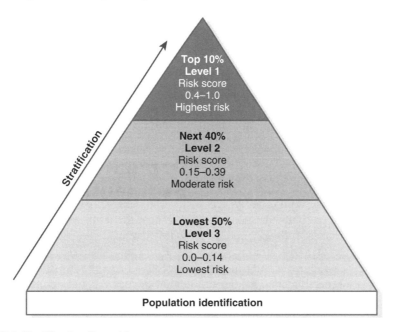

Figure 26.1 Risk-Stratification Pyramid.

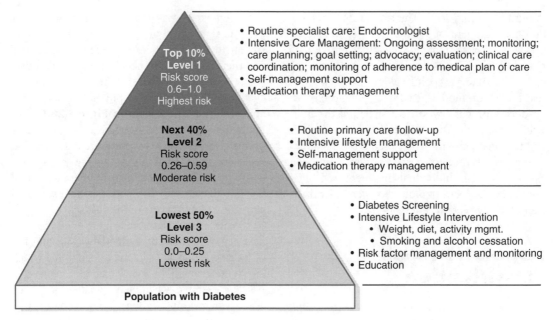

Figure 26.2 Risk Stratification and Intervention Assignment for People with Diabetes.

Reproduced from Sylvia, M. (2020). Targeting for population health interventions. In *Population health management learning series*. ForestVue Healthcare Solutions.

care management. **Figure 26.2** shows the risk stratification pyramid for an entire population of people with diabetes along with the recommended interventions at each level based on an estimate of needs at each risk level. Notice that the risk score distribution at each level of risk progresses by incrementally increasing the risk-score cutoff value.

Risk stratification is usually based on a predictive modeling score as opposed to a cut point from a measure in a current time period such as identifying those with high hospital admissions, emergency department visits, or high costs. This is because methods based on current utilization and costs often select outliers for intervention who are likely to "regress to the mean" in future years—meaning that absent any intervention at all, the patient is likely to have less cost and utilization in a future period (Cousins, Shickle, & Bander, 2002).

In another example of a risk-stratification model, the population was defined as "All patients aged 65 and older at a general internal medicine practice enrolled in the same health plan." A risk score was generated that assigned each individual in the population a probability of being within the top 5% of the highest-cost patients in the next year. Patients within the top 18% of risk scores

were assigned as high risk (Sylvia et al., 2006). An intervention was delivered to high-risk patients that included assignment to a specially trained nurse who partnered with patients' primary care physicians to complete specialized patient assessments, design mutually agreeable care plans, set patient goals, and monitor progress toward goals (Sylvia et al., 2008). The key to success of the interventions was identification of appropriate individuals who would most benefit from the resource intensive intervention.

Population Segmentation

Although the terms *risk stratification* and *segmentation* may often be used interchangeably, there is a difference between the two approaches to matching patients with interventions. Segmentation divides a patient population into distinct groups, each with specific needs, characteristics, or behaviors, which allows care delivery and policies to be tailored for these groups (Vuik, Mayer, & Darzi, 2016). Population segmentation is driven by the goal of grouping individuals in a population by the care they need and how often they will need it. It involves separating the highest-risk patients into subgroups with similar healthcare needs. Key to segmentation modeling is the ability to account for the unique factors that drive an individual's healthcare needs (Long et al., 2017). Risk-prediction scores may or may not be used for population segmentation.

A workgroup convened by the National Academies of Medicine has published a method that uses a novel taxonomy to assign individuals within whole populations into mutually exclusive clinically actionable segments to inform care and workflow decisions using data that are readily available to healthcare leaders (Long et al., 2017). Most healthcare organizations have diagnosis and procedure data available to them and can contextualize these data to create clinically meaningful segmentation categorizations. The segmentation model in **Figure 26.3** expands the clinical taxonomy to include additional determinants of health in the realm of functional, social, and behavioral

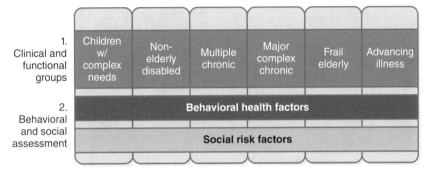

Note: For this taxonomy, functional impairments are intrinsically tied to the clinical segments.

Clinical Group	Features
Children with complex needs	Have sustained severe impairment in at least four categories together with enteral/parenteral feeding or sustained severe impairment in at least two categories and requiring ventilation or continuous positive airway pressure[A]
Non-elderly disabled	Under 65 years and with end-stage renal disease or disability based on receiving Supplemental Security Income
Multiple chronic	Only one complex condition and/or between one and five noncomplex conditions[B,C]
Major complex chronic	Two or more complex conditions or at least six noncomplex conditions[B,C]
Frail elderly	Over 65 years and with two or more frailty indicators[D]
Advancing illness	Other terminal illness, or end of life

[A] Categories for children with complex needs are: learning and mental functions, communication, motor skills, self-care, hearing, vision.

[B] Complex conditions, as defined in (Joynt et al., 2016), are listed in Table 2-1.

[C] Noncomplex conditions, as defined in (Joynt et al., 2016), are listed in Table 2-1.

[D] Frailty indicators, as defined in (Joynt et al., 2016), are gait abnormality, malnutrition, failure to thrive, cachexia, debility, difficulty walking, history of fall, muscle wasting, muscle weakness, decubitus ulcer, senility, or durable medical equipment use.

(Long et al., 2017)

Figure 26.3 Example Segmentation Model for Whole Populations.

Long, P., Abrams, M., Milstein, A., Anderson, G., Apton, K. L., Dahlberg, M. L., & Whicher, D. (Eds.). (2017). *NAM special publication: Effective care for high-need patients: Opportunities for improving outcomes, value, and health.* National Academy of Medicine. https://nam.edu/wp-content/uploads/2017/06/Effective-Care-for-High-Need-Patients.pdf. Reprinted with permission from the National Academy of Sciences, Washington, DC.

factors. Patients are first assigned to a clinical segment based on the medical needs driving costs and are subsequently assessed for behavioral health issues and the need for social services to determine specific intervention elements (Long et al., 2017).

Segmentation methods are often uniquely tailored to the healthcare organizations that design and use them. Even when using an evidence-based method published in the literature, organizations will need to adjust the methodology based on what works for them. This is because the success of segmentation models in terms of improved patient outcomes and lowered utilization and costs depends on patients' willingness to engage in interventions, the amenability of patients' conditions and circumstances to the intervention, and the level of infrastructure and capabilities within the healthcare organization to provide the care and services needed by patients within the designated segments (Jean-Baptiste, O'Malley, & Shah, 2017). Data used for segmentation can be both qualitative and quantitative. For instance, an organization may use a qualitative provider assessment of amenability for an intervention in combination with quantitative data that identify social determinants of health, multimorbidity, and other pertinent health determinants.

Although there is no consistent set of groupings used in segmentation models across healthcare organizations, a set of commonly used segments include:

- the frail elderly,
- advanced illness requiring palliative care or hospice care services,
- acute illness requiring transitional care services,
- being homebound,
- comorbid medical conditions such as diabetes and congestive heart failure,
- comorbid medical and mental health conditions,
- chronic care rising risk,
- disability, and
- end-stage renal disease (O'Malley et al., 2019).

Single disease conditions are not recommended for segmentation because they fail to address the complexity within individuals, their environment, and the underlying causes of their healthcare needs (O'Malley et al., 2019). In addition, the data sources and the way that data are combined to define segments depends on the healthcare organization. For instance, a health plan may use a procedure code in authorization data (used in health plans to approve payment for medical services) or medical claims to identify hospice services, whereas a provider organization may use a referral for hospice care found in the EMR.

Applied Learning: Case Study

An integrated health system consisting of five hospitals, 89 primary care physicians, and a Medicare Advantage (MA) health plan sought to take a population health approach to managing its population of MA members 65 and older. This case study describes the process from data sources to linking individuals to interventions.

In the first step of the process, the population is identified. **Figure 26.4** shows the data sources that are available for population health analytics in this integrated health system at the top level and include medical and pharmacy claims data, MA enrollment data, EMR data, laboratory data, and area deprivation index (ADI) data (see Section 2, "Data Sources," for more information about data sources). The data are then processed through data contextualizing software to generate variables of interest at the person level (refer to Section 3, "Data Contextualizers," for more information on applying context to data). There are many data fields processed into person-level variables. For the purposes of this initiative, the contextualized data points of interest are a score predicting the risk of a hospitalization in the next 12 months, an indicator of hospice or palliative care services, the number of chronic conditions, indicators of frailty, indicators of disability, and the ADI score, which is a national percentile rankings at the census block group level from 1 to 100, with higher numbers indicating higher levels of disadvantage and therefore probable health disparities in a neighborhood (University of Wisconsin, 2015).

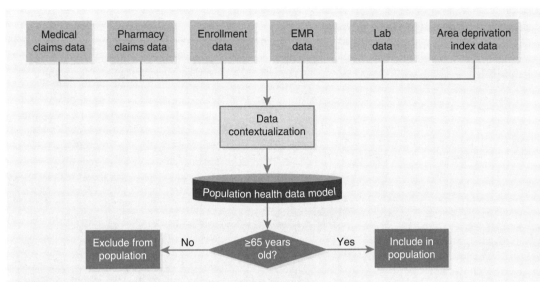

Figure 26.4 Case Study Population Identification.

In the next step, the identified population of MA members 65 and older are assessed for the value of their individually assigned scores for high risk of hospitalization in the next 12 months. Those with a risk score of under 0.40 or a 40% probability or less of having a hospitalization in the next month are triaged to receive outreach about available services and reminders for annual preventive care appointments. Those with a risk score of ⩾ 0.40 will be segmented into smaller groupings for targeted interventions. This step is outlined in **Figure 26.5**.

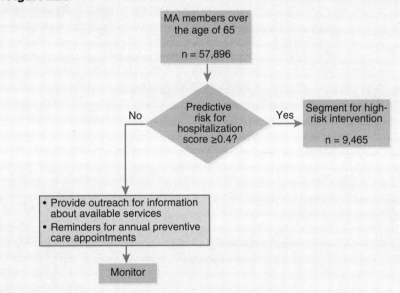

Figure 26.5 Case Study Risk Stratification.

(continues)

Applied Learning: Case Study *(continued)*

The next step is to segment the high-risk subpopulation into segments for intervention and is depicted in **Figure 26.6**. This segmentation methodology is a tailored approach based on available evidence and the capabilities of this integrated healthcare delivery organization (Long et al., 2017; Zhou, Wong, & Li, 2014). The segmentation model creates mutually exclusive groupings by assigning patients to segments starting with the highest-need segments and incrementally assigning unique segments based on morbidity, disability, and the potential for social care needs. This is only one example of applying a segmentation model. Remember that a segmentation model must consider data availability, the needs of the patient population based on a population assessment (see Chapter 25), and the capabilities of the organization.

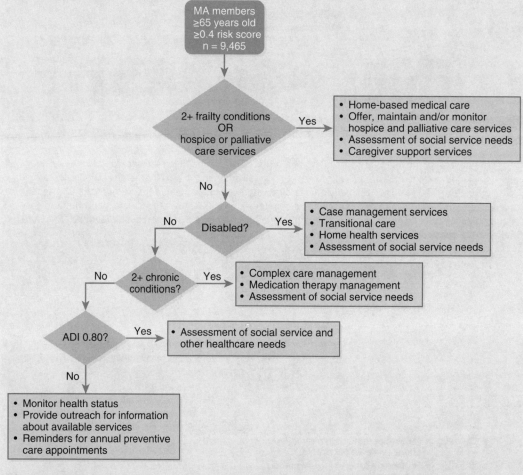

Figure 26.6 Case Study Population Segmentation and Assignment of Individuals to Interventions.

Conclusion

Appropriate targeting of individuals for population health interventions is essential to achieving successful outcomes. If done well, the patients who are identified to benefit are linked to meaningful interventions, their lives are improved, and limited healthcare resources are wisely allocated. Risk prediction is a tool that assigns risk scores to individuals, and it represents the likelihood of experiencing an adverse outcome. These risk scores can then be used to stratify populations according to increasing levels of risk as a way to offer more resource intensive interventions to those at greater risk of poor outcomes. Segmentation builds on the methods of risk prediction and stratification by grouping patients according to their expected need for healthcare services and amenability offerings. Well-designed targeting processes in population health optimize available data and organizational capacity when delivering interventions to patient populations. Combined with other methods to intervene, monitor progress, and measure performance, targeting is an opportunity to set the stage for an effective population health project that is tailored to the unique needs of the populations identified.

Study and Discussion Questions

- What are the key considerations when targeting individuals for intervention?
- What are the differences and similarities between risk stratification and risk segmentation?
- What is the role of risk-prediction scoring in risk stratification and segmentation?
- Why is it valuable to use segmentation methodologies?

Resources and Websites

Centers for Disease Control and Prevention. (n.d.). What is population health? Population Health Training: https://www.cdc.gov/pophealthtraining/whatis.html

National Committee for Quality Assurance. (n.d.). Population health resources: https://www.ncqa.org/videos/what-is-population-health -management/?utm_source=google&utm _medium=cpc&utm_campaign=php2020 &gclid=EAIaIQobChMIhdODi9a76gIVDI3I Ch0fVQCvEAAYASAAEgLsa_D_BwE

Health Information and Management Systems Society (HIMSS). Resources: https://www.himss .org/

References

Cousins, M. S., Shickle, L. M., & Bander, J. A. (2002). An introduction to predictive modeling for disease management risk stratification. *Disease Management,* 5(3), 157–167. http://www.liebertonline.com/doi/abs/10 .1089/109350702760301448

Fabius, R. J. (2021). The population health promise. In B. Nash, D. A. Skoufalos, R. J. Fabius, & W. H. Oglesby (Eds.), *Population health: Creating a culture of wellness* (3rd ed., pp. 3–22). Jones & Bartlett Learning.

Jean-Baptiste, D., O'Malley, A. S., & Shah, T. (2017, December 1). Population segmentation and targeting of health care resources: Findings from a literature review. Mathematica. https://www.mathematica.org/our-publications-and -findings/publications/population-segmentation-and -targeting-of-health-care-resources-findings-from-a -literature-review

Jeffery, A. D., Hewner, S., Pruinelli, L., Lekan, D., Lee, M., Gao, G., Holbrook, L., & Sylvia, M. (2019, April). Risk prediction and segmentation models used in the United States for assessing risk in whole populations: A critical literature review with implications for nurses' role in population health management. *JAMIA Open,* 2(1), 205–214. https://doi.org/10.1093/jamiaopen /ooy053

Johnson, T. L., Rinehart, D. J., Durfee, J., Brewer, D., Batal, H., Blum, J., Oronce, C. I., Melinkovich, P., & Gabow, P. (2015, August). For many patients who use large amounts of health care services, the need is intense yet temporary. *Health Affairs, 34*(8), 1312–1319. https://doi.org/10.1377/hlthaff.2014.1186

Kaiser Family Foundation. (2019, January 16). How do health expenditures vary across the population? https://www.kff.org/slideshow/how-health-expenditures-vary-across-the-population-slideshow/

Long, P., Abrams, M., Milstein, A., Anderson, G., Apton, K. L., Lund Dahlberg, M., & Whicher, D. (Eds.). (2017). Effective care for high-need patients: Opportunities for improving outcomes, value, and health. National Academy of Medicine. https://nam.edu/wp-content/uploads/2017/06/Effective-Care-for-High-Need-Patients.pdf

O'Malley, A. S., Rich, E. C., Sarwar, R., Schultz, E., Cannon Warren, W., Shah, T., & Abrams, M. K. (2019, January 1). How accountable care organizations use population segmentation to care for high-need, high-cost patients. *Issue Brief, 2019*, 1–17. https://pubmed.ncbi.nlm.nih.gov/30645057/

Pearl, R., & Madvig, P. (2020, January–February). Managing the most expensive patients. *Harvard Business Review*. https://hbr.org/2020/01/managing-the-most-expensive-patients

Psaty, B. M., Dekkers, O. M., & Cooper, R. S. (2018, August 28). Comparison of 2 treatment models: Precision medicine and preventive medicine. *Journal of the American Medical Association, 320*, 751–752. https://doi.org/10.1001/jama.2018.8377

Sylvia, M. L., Griswold, M., Dunbar, L., Boyd, C. M., Park, M., & Boult, C. (2008, February 16). Guided care: Cost and utilization outcomes in a pilot study. *Disease Management, 11*(1), 29–36. https://doi.org/10.1089/dis.2008.111723

Sylvia, M. L., Shadmi, E., Hsiao, C.-J., Boyd, C. M., Schuster, A. B., & Boult, C. (2006, February 8). Clinical features of high-risk older persons identified by predictive modeling. *Disease Management, 9*(1), 56–62. https://doi.org/10.1089/dis.2006.9.56

University of Wisconsin. (2015). Neighborhood Atlas. https://www.neighborhoodatlas.medicine.wisc.edu

Vuik, S. I., Mayer, E. K., & Darzi, A. (2016, May). Patient segmentation analysis offers significant benefits for integrated care and support. *Health Affairs, 35*(5), 769–775. https://doi.org/10.1377/hlthaff.2015.1311

Zhou, Y. Y., Wong, W., & Li, H. (2014, Summer). Improving care for older adults: A model to segment the senior population. *The Permanente Journal, 18*(3), 18–21. https://doi.org/10.7812/TPP/14-005

CHAPTER 27

Analytics Supporting Population Health Interventions

Ines Maria Vigil, MD, MPH, MBA

Better health for all Americans depends on focusing our efforts where they're needed most.

—Tom Frieden (as cited in Centers for Disease Control and Prevention, 2013)

EXECUTIVE SUMMARY

Population health analytics are an important part of developing and deploying cost-effective, cost-efficient, evidence-based clinical, and administrative interventions. Data and analytics can be used to support various activities throughout the life cycle of an intervention and can serve as important indicators of success. From assisting teams to understand the magnitude of a problem to solve to developing performance measures, population health analytic methods and process can be an effective way to bring structure and order to developing and measuring interventions to improve patient experience, health outcomes, and cost.

Several elements of successful population health interventions using analytics are covered in this chapter along with examples, best practices, and pitfalls to avoid. Developing and implementing population health interventions that transform the way health care is delivered to achieve the Triple Aim require the following already be in place, and the analytics covered in this chapter highlight the way in which these elements can be moved into a practical application:

- person-centric population data model,
- data asset management model,
- data analytics maturity model, and
- population health management and analytics process.

To be successful in supporting interventions, the learner must draw from earlier chapters in this book. The goal of this chapter is to put into practice all previous learnings, including moving a data model into practice, developing a data workflow from a clinical or administrative workflow, and various data checks along the way to ensure the data flow and process are working correctly. These processes are in addition to applying population health analytic methods to define the problem using data, developing predictive analytics to support patient interventions, and developing monitoring and performance metrics already covered in previous chapters.

LEARNING OBJECTIVES

At the end of this chapter, the learner will be able to:

1. Discuss the types and timing of analytics that are needed to support the development, implementation, and monitoring of interventions.
2. Distinguish system-level interventions from other approaches of addressing healthcare problems in practice.
3. List the steps required to ensure the analytics to support the deployment of population health interventions are high quality, evidence based, cost effective, and cost efficient.

Introduction

Population health analytics can be infused within every step along one or more care pathways, the care continuum, or one or more interventions and enables the tracking and monitoring of the population health stepwise process. Moving from population health concepts and methodologies into their practical application requires a data infrastructure, analytic capabilities, and a process to deploy population health methods to be in place before embarking on supporting clinical and administrative interventions. This is to ensure the data that are needed are available, that all precalculations and transformations to the data are transparent all the way to the data source, and to provide clarity to the process for the population health team. Once in place, the population health team, like the PopHealth Troika described in previous chapters and later in Chapter 31, "Building a Team Culture for Population Health," can confidently apply population health analytic methods and techniques to effectively develop, monitor, and report results to support population health interventions.

Numerous frameworks for deploying population health in organizations exist, most focusing on the population health team's activities at the point-of-care delivery, and with many relying on a data infrastructure, model, and capability to already exist. This chapter focuses on deploying the analytics necessary to support interventions and also outlines the analytics required to check the data infrastructure, model, and capabilities to ensure proper upstream analytic functioning. Also included are approaches to develop effective population health interventions, best practices, and pitfalls to avoid when using analytics to develop and deploy interventions, along with additional resources for engaging clinicians and patients.

Defining Population Health Intervention Analytics

Summarizing several evidence-based publications that discuss population health interventions, population health interventions can be defined as policies, programs, and actions that address health risks by addressing underlying behavioral, lifestyle, social, economic, and environmental conditions (Cantor, Haller, & Greenberg, 2018; Hawe & Potvin, 2009; Smith, Wallace, O'Dowd, & Fortin, 2016). Given this definition, this text offers a definition of population health intervention analytics as the analytic support of the development and application of population health interventions to identify, stratify, measure, and report outcomes on behavioral, lifestyle, social, economic, and environmental health determinants.

In the second edition of *Population Health: Creating a Culture of Wellness*, David Nash and colleagues outline several successful models of population health in action, many of which are outlined later in this chapter (Nash, Skoufalos, Fabius, & Oglesby, 2021). A common theme across the successful models outlined in Nash's textbook is the importance of employing system-level thinking when developing and implementing population health programs and interventions. The text goes further to recognize the need for health systems to track improvements made over time, use evidence-based medicine to inform care delivery, and endorse metrics that are transparent in their design, calculations, and comparisons. Nash introduces the importance of applying systems thinking to the development of population health interventions, outlining three core categories, including macro, meso, and micro levels of intervention and measurement of outcomes.

- *Macro or systems-level interventions* occur at the level of organizations and governments through the development of policies, procedures, practice guidelines, tools, programs, and services. An example of a macro-level intervention and outcome:
  - The child, adolescent, and adult immunization schedule for healthcare providers from the Centers for Disease Control and Prevention (CDC, 2020).
  - Outcome measures include broad goals that summarize an improvement such as the reduction in the number of all-cause hospitalizations per 1,000 patient days in children, adolescents, and adults because of vaccine administration (Bruhn et al., 2017).
- *Meso or clinician practice-level interventions* address practice design (singular versus multidisciplinary), workflows, technology, and capabilities. An example of a meso-level intervention and outcome:
  - a primary care practice group's application of the CDC's child, adolescent, and adult immunization schedule for healthcare providers via patient vaccination reminders in the electronic medical record (EMR) (CDC, 2020; Hofstetter, Larussa, & Rosenthal, 2015).
  - Outcomes measures include goals that represent trends in best practices or need such as a list of the clinicians in the practice ranked lowest to highest in their rates of up-to-date vaccination of children, adolescents, and adults after inclusion of patient vaccination reminders in the EMR (Hofstetter et al., 2015).

- *Micro or patient-level interventions* incorporate patient needs, preferences, lifestyle, and care-seeking behaviors. An example of a micro-level intervention and outcome:
  - Improving uptake of the CDC's child immunization schedule for healthcare providers via focused and improved provider communication and patient education (Chung, Schamel, Fisher, & Frew, 2017).
  - Outcomes measures include goals that are relevant to hands-on care such as the major influencers of trust in their provider and communication on immunization decision-making among U.S. parents of young children (Chung et al., 2017).

This application of organizing interventions and outcomes into discreet macro, meso, and micro levels supports a methodological approach to defining the data and analytics needed to support the efforts. In addition, it furthers the concept that system-level, clinician-level, and patient-level interventions can and are often interrelated, and a greater impact can be achieved when the interventions are cohesively developed. This type of organized intervention and analytic approach also connects the big picture to its parts and represents the multiple perspectives that may influence the outcomes (Best et al., 2003; Cabrera, Colosi, & Lobdell, 2008).

The Benefits of Effective Analytics to Support Population Health Interventions

The time spent planning before a single analysis is done cannot be underestimated. Thoughtful discussion and planning to clearly articulate the population health problem to solve, the goals of intervening, populations of interest, and effective and evidence-based ways to intervene are all required for analytics to effectively identify opportunities for improvement to support the development and implementation of population health programs and interventions. In Chapter 25, "Assessing Populations," Figure 25.1 outlines the process steps to successfully identify opportunities to improve the patient experience, health outcomes, and cost.

Effective planning and development can provide a narrative to the population health project and a call to action to garner support for data-driven decision-making using population health analytics. Effective development of interventions using analytics can also be used to standardize workflows, organize analyses, and promote the adoption of population health concepts and methodologies such as those described in Chapter 21, "Risk Adjustment," Chapter 22, "Predictive and Prescriptive Analytics," and Chapter 23, "Advanced Analytic Methods."

Population Health Interventions Using Analytics: The Basics

Several requirements must be in place to effectively support the development and implementation of population health interventions: a population health data model, a data infrastructure, analytic capabilities, a population health framework or process model, and a team-based population health culture.

A Population Health Data Model, Infrastructure, and Analytic Capabilities

The implementation of population health concepts and methodologies requires a data model, infrastructure, and analytic capabilities. It is important to have transparent data when supporting clinical and administrative interventions such that the data can be traced from an opportunity for improvement all the way to the source data that contributed to the finding. This sets up a strong foundation for all analytics that are performed thereafter, that the data needed are available, and that all precalculations and transformations to the data are transparent such that updates to

definitions and maintenance of programming code can be performed easily. More detailed information on data models and infrastructure can be found in Section 4, "Creating the Population Health Data Model," and Section 5, "Data Infrastructure." In addition, understanding an organization's capabilities to perform descriptive, diagnostic, predictive, and prescriptive analytics will define the type and maturity of the analytics that can be used to support interventions. For more information on building analytic capabilities, see Chapter 30, "Assessing Organizational Capabilities for Population Health Analytics," and Chapter 32, "Skills Assessment of Population Health Analysts."

A Population Health Framework or Process Model

Population health interventions are best supported by analytics when a population health framework or process model is adopted to guide the activities of the project team. Various frameworks and models exist and are outlined in Chapter 2, "Guiding Frameworks for Population Health Analytics." Utilizing a population health framework or process model allows team members to reach agreement on the approach, methods, and expectations. It also outlines the steps for the team to understand when the development of an intervention is complete and when the process enters a maintenance or optimization phase for the project. It is important to follow a stepwise approach to enable the population health team to follow along the process and to set expectations for next steps.

A Team-Based Population Health Culture

Developing a population health team and team-based culture is critical in successfully supporting data-driven decision-making in population health interventions with analytics. More detail on effective population health teams can be found in Chapter 31, "Building a Team Culture for Population Health." The combination of various skill sets, experience, and knowledge enhances the development of interventions, provides a basis for incorporating multiple perspectives, and boosts the productivity of any one individual working alone.

Elements of Successful Population Health Analytics Using Analytics

Depending on the type of population health problem to solve, the various interventions, and their respective metrics, a combination of the following elements will be included in the population health analyses. All are core to population health and overlap with other disciplines, including but not limited to public health, medical economics, and actuarial analytics. Core to population health management is the application of these elements to identify opportunities for improvement to achieve the Triple Aim (Berwick, Nolan, & Whittington, 2008). **Table 27.1** outlines the elements to be included in support of the development and implementation of population health interventions.

The table puts together all elements discussed in greater detail throughout this textbook with the goal of weaving together the various concepts, methods, and analyses into the practical application of developing and implementing population health

Table 27.1 Analytic Elements to Support Population Health Interventions

Element Name	Element Description	Important Considerations
Know the Population	Analysis includes a summary of the total population, various subsets, demographics, preferences, behaviors in accessing care, health determinants, trends, benchmarks, utilization, and cost.	A decision tree indicating the total population and its various subset populations can assist in framing the opportunities for improvement. Refer to the example in Chapter 25, "Assessing Populations," Figure 25.2, "Defining the Population and Subgroupings."
Define the Intended Outcome	Defining the outcome as improvement in the patient experience, the health outcomes, or the total cost of care.	Several frameworks reference the Triple Aim (Berwick et al., 2008) and emphasize the importance of defining the outcome of interest before embarking on analyses. Refer to Chapter 2, "Guiding Frameworks for Population Health Analytics," for more detail.
Research the Evidence Base	Conduct a review of the evidence-based, medical peer-reviewed literature to identify effective interventions.	This body of evidence also provides analytic methods, monitoring metrics, and analytic pearls, including power of studies, confidence intervals, p-values, and study limitations. Refer to Section 3, "Data Contextualizers," and Chapter 25, "Assessing Populations," for more detail.
Know the Data Variables	Understand all data variables along with their respective numerators, denominators, inclusions, exclusions, definitions, and calculations.	Transparency and documentation are key. When identifying risk and translating it into an opportunity to intervene, the input data must be visible to the end user. Refer to Section 2, "Data Sources," and Section 3, "Data Contextualizers" for more detail.

(continues)

Table 27.1 **Analytic Elements to Support Population Health Interventions** *(continued)*

Element Name	Element Description	Important Considerations
Know the Data Sources	Be able to trace all data variables to their respective data sources and understand any precalculations, transformations, completeness, accuracy, and timeliness.	Governance and documentation are key. Partnership between information technology (IT) and analytics is essential to ensuring the level of data governance exists to communicate the availability, quality, and accuracy of needed data. Refer to Section 2, "Data Sources," Section 3, "Data Contextualizers," and Section 5, "Data Infrastructure," for more detail.
Know the Population Data Model	Be familiar with the population health data model, how data variables are related to one another, the various data joins, and definitions.	Without a population health data model, analysis will be disparate, inconsistent, and inaccurate and may lead to errors in findings and conclusions. Refer to Section 4, "Creating a Population Health Data Model," for more detail.
Know the Intervention Team	Get to know the team deploying the intervention and the members' challenges, barriers, actions, and motivations.	Personalizing the intervention to care teams and patients increases engagement, collaboration, communication, and feedback. Refer to Chapter 33, "Clinical Workflow Transformation," for more detail.
Map the Intervention Workflow	Understand and map the care team workflow used to deploy the intervention, the process for documentation, and the process for follow-up, task closure, and case closure.	Observe the care team through several workflows from start to finish and document the steps taken in order of occurrence as a conceptual model. Refer to Chapter 12, "Creating the Population Health Data Model," and Chapter 33, "Clinical Workflow Transformation," for more detail.
Map the Data Workflow	Understand and map the logical model of the data, marking where in the intervention workflow the data applies in the conceptual model.	Document the logical model alongside the conceptual model, marking where the data are unavailable, inaccurate, or incomplete, along with proposed solutions for how to resolve if possible. Refer to Chapter 12 "Creating the Population Health Data Model," for more detail.
Data Filters, Slicers, and Dicers	List all data filters, slicers, and dicers that will be used to add context to the data, noting where a calculation is present and documenting its formula and any references to evidence-based literature or methods.	Many filters, slicers, and dicers are commonly repeated within organizations. It saves time to include the organization's commonly used filters, slicers, and dicers to ensure consistency and to avoid having to go back to include at a later date. Refer to Section 2, "Data Sources," and Section 3, "Data Contextualizers," for more detail.

Data Definitions	Document all data definitions, noting where a calculation is present, and document its formula and any references to evidence-based literature or methods.	Different combinations of data variables can create multiple definitions for what appear to be similar, such as the definition of a readmission within 7, 14, or 30 days. Changing one element of timing, inputs, or age can change the definition and must be documented separately. Refer to Section 2, "Data Sources," and Section 3, "Data Contextualizers," for more detail.
Data Input Validation	Develop data quality and integrity checks at the data source to ensure high performance of data prototypes, algorithms, precalculations and calculations.	Partner with IT to develop audit scripts to ensure data completeness, accuracy, and timeliness. Refer to Section 5, "Data Infrastructure," for more detail.
Data Output Validation	Run multiple analyses to ensure the data workflow, filters, and definitions are producing reasonable results. Review programming code and refine.	Review data output with population health team members and check results against benchmarks, historical data, and other completed analyses. Refer to Chapter 16, "Data Management and Preparation," for more detail.
Risk Assessment, Adjustment, and Stratification	Assess the risk of future worsened patient experiences, worsened health outcomes, inappropriate and avoidable utilization, and inappropriate and avoidable cost. Adjust analyses and stratify by risk type, score, and actionability. Align each stratified subpopulation to a proposed evidence-based intervention.	Assess data to appropriately apply analytical techniques, particularly the data infrastructure and techniques required to perform advanced analytics. Refer to Chapters 19 to 24 in Section 6 "Analytic Methods," Chapter 10 "Grouping, Trending, and Interpreting Population Health Data for Assessing Risk and Disease Burden" and Chapter 25, "Assessing Populations," for more detail.
Interventions: Health Education, Health Literacy, Care Coordination, Clinical Care Management, Transitional Care, Advance Care Planning, Medication Therapy Management, Behavioral Health, Community Health Outreach, Etc.	Review evidence-based medical literature to understand programmatic workflows, data sources, data-capture methods, and analytic methods used to quantify and qualify results and comparisons, along with study limitations. Review recommendations for existing and proposed interventions.	A wealth of information exists in the evidence-based medical literature. Meta-analysis and reviews of existing publications over time are more robust than case studies. Refer to Section 3, "Data Contextualizers," and Section 6, "Analytic Methods."
Interventions: Personalized Care Plans and Goal Setting	Work closely with the care team implementing the intervention to identify the presence and documentation of care plans and care goals for patients. Review documentation to determine ability to monitor and report and adjust documentation to capture if not available initially.	Personalized care plans and goal setting are demonstrated to increase patient and clinician engagement, increase the effectiveness of interventions, and link actions to results (Bodenheimer & Handley, 2009; Pearson, 2012; Strecher et al., 1995). Refer to Chapter 33, "Clinical Workflow Transformation," for more details.

(continues)

Table 27.1 Analytic Elements to Support Population Health Interventions · *(continued)*

Element Name	Element Description	Important Considerations
Resource Allocation	Analytics to support the effective allocation of often scarce resources includes calculating the average cases or services per person per day, month, quarter, or year; and incorporating the results into several analytic scenarios that enable the population health team to recommend cost-effective and cost-efficient staffing ratios.	Setting performance targets are highly dependent on the resources available to deploy the intervention. Resources can be people, technology, supplies, and services. It is important to understand the limitations that a lack of appropriate resources can have on the implementation of interventions (Fuchs, Lane, McGuire). Refer to Section 3, "Data Contextualizers," for more details.
Leading Indicators, Lagging Indicators, Monitoring Measures, Performance Measures, Observed to Expected Ratios, Patient Experience Outcomes, Health Improvement Outcomes, Financial Improvement Outcomes	Develop numerators, denominators, inclusions, exclusions, algorithms, process measures, and outcomes measures that reflect the intent and track performance against the intended outcomes of each intervention implemented. Draw from the review of the clinical evidence-based medical literature and leading best practices in analytic methods.	Commonly thought of as the foundation of population health analytics, developing measures to track productivity and performance is one of many areas where analytics can best support population health interventions. Refer to Section 6, "Analytic Methods," and Chapter 28, "Monitoring and Optimizing Interventions," for more details.
Feedback Loop	Regularly review analytic outputs and results for insights, findings, and trends. Work collaboratively with care teams implementing interventions to provide and receive feedback to refine the data model, algorithms, and results.	Best practices exist to engage clinicians implementing interventions and to optimize population health interventions for success. Refer to Chapter 33, "Clinical Workflow Transformation," for more details.

interventions. The elements are ordered as they would be completed in the process to develop and implement a clinical or administrative intervention. Many of the chapters in this book are represented in the table, and specific chapters are called out in the "Important Considerations" column in the table.

Approaches to Developing Effective Interventions Using Population Health Analytics

Multiple approaches can be taken when working in a population health team to identify opportunity, develop effective interventions, allocate resources

to deliver the interventions, and track performance. The approach selected will be unique to the population health project team, and no approach is better than any other. In addition, the approaches outlined in the following can be used in combination with others, and a thoughtful approach to identifying the problem to solve and the interventions needed to address the problem can contribute significantly to clearly articulating the work for the team, building the business case for need, and telling a consistent story of progress and results.

One approach outlined earlier is to identify the level of intervention as *macro* or *systems level*, *meso* or *clinician practice level*, or *micro* or *patient level*. The most impactful intervention or set of interventions considers all levels of interventions and are often needed to address the most widespread and complex healthcare challenges.

Another approach is outlined in Section 3, "Data Contextualizers," and takes the approach of identifying the outcome of interest as outlined by the Triple Aim (Berwick et al., 2008) as:

- enhancing the experience and outcomes of the patient,
- improving the health of the population, and
- reducing per capita cost of care for the benefit of communities.

This approach considers the intended outcome and guides the population health team to consider all interventions that are likely to achieve the desired result.

A third approach can be aligned with an area of focus, also outlined in Section 3, "Data Contextualizers," as disease, intervention, utilization, cost, health disparities, community, or patient preference drivers. This is a common approach in which a specific clinical expertise is available and driving the project such as specialty-driven projects of diabetes, cardiovascular disease, and orthopedics. Also favored by most health insurance plans, this approach considers all aspects of care, including clinical outcomes and financial impact.

Refer to Section 3, "Data Contextualizers," and Chapter 29, "Storytelling with Data," for specific examples, evidence-based medical literature, and additional resources of the approached summarized above.

Best Practices and Pitfalls to Avoid

Numerous best practices and pitfalls to avoid exist when developing and implementing population health interventions. As population health aims to address the underlying cause of disease and worsening health outcomes in populations, more current research seeks to understand the connections between social inequities and their impact on the overall health and well-being of the population. As outlined in previous chapters, several best practices have been identified and are summarized in the following. These best practices can also help avoid pitfalls because missing one or more elements can easily derail a population health project and project team. The importance

of the following elements in the design and implementation of population health interventions cannot be understated:

- leadership and accountability;
- alignment of mission, goals, and approach;
- clearly stating the problem to solve using population health analytics;
- defining the population and population subsets;
- developing intervention and analytic workflows;
- mapping conceptual and logical models to workflows;
- using decision trees to capture decision-making in the analyses;
- researching the evidence-based medical literature for effective interventions, recommendations, and analytic methodologies;
- defining and documenting the data, data sources, and monitoring and performance metrics early in the development of population health interventions to ensure mutual understanding of the goals and limitations of each intervention;
- engaging care teams that will implement the interventions in their development;
- clearly articulating the actions believed to generate the greatest impact and results;
- monitoring process and outcomes measures simultaneously; and
- building in flexibility to course correct and adapt the intervention to optimize engagement and success.

The following studies highlight additional best practices, cautions, and considerations when developing population health interventions.

In 2013, Bahaudin Mujtaba and colleagues summarized the successes, cautions, and considerations associated with implementing employer-based health and wellness programs to improve employee satisfaction and health outcomes and to address rising healthcare costs in "A Review of Employee Health and Wellness Programs in the United States" (Mujtaba, Cavico, & Wayne, 2013). The review provides a comprehensive list of best practices and pitfalls to avoid when developing legal, ethical, and effective wellness programs to employees.

- Include aspects to increase self-motivation, goal setting, and persistency of action in interventions.
- Create a "fun" workplace culture to increase engagement and participation among employees.
- Review the federal and state statutory and regulatory definitions and laws associated with administering programs.
- Review the legal, ethical, and practical ramifications of interventions when applying requirements and options for participation such as the Americans with Disabilities Act.
- Consider the use of incentives and disincentives when developing interventions such as gift cards, lowered health insurance premiums, and access to health products or services.
- Avoid any direct or indirect discrimination when creating or implementing interventions.
- Make sure health-related rewards or penalties do not exceed 30% of the cost of the employee's health coverage (as required by the Affordable Care Act).
- Do not tie an employee's pay to any healthcare issue.
- Provide alternatives and exemptions for persons who cannot participate or meet certain intervention requirements because of underlying medical reasons.
- Do not request health records before extending an offer of employment or make decisions on employment based on a person's ability or willingness to participate in interventions.
- Keep all healthcare information strictly confidential.
- Create committees to implement and oversee interventions.
- Implement interventions gradually and seek feedback to inform upstream activities.

The American Hospital Association's January 2011 report, "A Call to Action: Creating a Culture of Health" (AHA, 2020) shares several examples of the hospital industry implementing population health interventions to improve patient experience and health outcomes and to reduce the financial burden of avoidable or unnecessary healthcare cost and utilization. The researchers highlight several recommendations and actions to consider when developing and implementing interventions, including partnering with the community, serving as a role model of health for the community, creating a culture of healthy living, providing a variety of program offerings, including positive and negative incentives to increase participation and improve outcomes, tracking participation and outcomes, measuring for return on investment, and focusing on sustainability.

Additional considerations are detailed in the Agency for Healthcare Research and Quality's (AHRQ) 2015 report "Population Health: Behavioral and Social Science Insights" related to social and behavioral determinants of health. The report details the importance of considering for intervention the drivers of social inequities, primarily socioeconomic status, and geographic location to address health inequities. Also recommended as a best practice is the consideration of enhancing access to economic resources, improving neighborhood and housing conditions, providing interventions that address the accumulation of adversity over a patient's lifetime, investing in early childhood interventions, and addressing the residual effects of race and systemic racism (Kaplan, Spittel, & David, 2015).

Use Cases for Applying Analytics to Support Population Health Intervention Development

Many use cases for the development of population health interventions are available throughout this textbook and are best reviewed in the context of their chapters. Additional considerations to apply when reviewing the case studies included in this textbook include the following:

- What are the major cost drivers in this population?
  - Price, volume, and disparity

- What are the highest priority needs for this population?
  - Improve the experience, health outcomes, access to care, and financial impact
- What types of interventions would you implement?
  - Macro, meso, micro versus goal-oriented versus area of focus
- How would you deliver those interventions?

- By phone, face-to-face, integrated into care, and so on
- What other tools would you need?
  - Incentives, policies, technology, and so on
- What other information do you need?

Refer to Section 3, "Data Contextualizers," and Chapter 33, "Clinical Workflow Transformation," for case studies to apply the following questions for consideration.

Conclusion

Developing and implementing population health interventions requires a combination of elements that infuse analytics throughout. Analytics is a vital component of developing effective, efficient, and evidence-based interventions to improve patient experience, health outcomes, and cost. This chapter outlined the elements that can be used to support a population health team to identify opportunity and support the development and deployment of successful population interventions. Additional information is provided to guide learners on how to order their activities when participating in population health teams and when

developing solutions to challenging and complex population health problems. Several best practices are shared and cover a wealth of information too large for this chapter to cover in detail the legal, ethical, and practical considerations to make in avoiding negative ramifications for an otherwise well-intentioned intervention. Referencing other chapters throughout this textbook, this chapter aimed to bring together the concepts, methods, and examples presented in previous chapters and throughout the literature to portray the practical role that population health analytics can serve to improve health, track progress, and report results.

Study and Discussion Questions

- What are other examples of interventions that build on one another at the meso, macro, and micro levels of intervention?
- Discuss the advantages and disadvantages of having or not having a facilitator role when working to develop interventions in teams.

- Select one case study in the textbook that does not have an intervention articulated and apply the information outlined in this chapter to define the intervention and its considerations. Discuss with others.

Resources and Websites

Advisory Board. (2017, September 12). 5 key considerations for measuring the ROI of your care management interventions. https://www.advisory.com/research/care-transformation-center/care-transformation-center-blog/2017/09/measuring-roi

American Hospital Association. (2020). A call to action: Creating a culture of health. https://www.aha.org/ahahret-guides/2013-01-09-call-action-creating-culture-health#:~:text=In%20 2010%2C%20as%20an%20extension,Health%20 For%20Life%3A%20Better%20Health.&text =The%20Committee%20has%20developed%20 a,creating%20a%20culture%20of%20health

Arora, R., Boehm, J., Chimento, L., Moldawer, L., & Tsien, C. (n.d.). Designing and implementing Medicaid disease and care management programs: A user's guide. Rockville, MD: Agency for

Healthcare Research and Quality. https://www
.ahrq.gov/patient-safety/settings/long-term-care
/resource/hcbs/medicaidmgmt/index.html

Cantor, J., Haller, M. R., & Greenberg, M. E.
(2018, January). Rising risk: An overview of identification and intervention approaches. Boston,
MA: JSI Research & Training Institute. https://
publications.jsi.com/JSIInternet/Inc/Common
/_download_pub.cfm?id=19182&lid=3

Ditton, M. (2018). Goal-setting worksheet. http://
www.goalsettingbasics.com/support-files/goal
_setting_worksheet.pdf

National Institutes of Health (NIH) & Agency for
Healthcare Research and Quality (AHRQ). (n.d.).
R. M Kaplan, M. L. Spittel, & D. H. David (Eds.),
Population health: Behavioral and social science
insights. https://www.ahrq.gov/sites/default/files
/publications/files/population-health.pdf

References

Agency for Healthcare Research and Quality. (2015, July).
Population health: Behavioral and social science insights.
https://www.ahrq.gov/sites/default/files/publications/files
/population-health.pdf

American Hospital Association (AHA). (2020). A call to action:
Creating a culture of health. https://www.aha.org/ahahret
-guides/2013-01-09-call-action-creating-culture-health

Berwick, D. M., Nolan, T. W., & Whittington, J. (2008,
May–June). The Triple Aim: Care, health, and cost.
Health Affairs, 27(3), 759–769. https://doi.org/10.1377
/hlthaff.27.3.759

Best, A., Moor, G., Holmes, B., Clark, P. I., Bruce, T.,
Leischow, S., Buchholz, K., & Krajnak, J. (2003). Health
promotion dissemination and systems thinking: Towards
an integrative model. *American Journal of Health Behavior*,
27(Suppl. 3), S206–S216. https://pubmed.ncbi.nlm.nih
.gov/14672381/

Bodenheimer, T., & Handley, M. A. (2009, August). Goal-
setting for behavior change in primary care: An exploration
and status report. *Patient Education and Counseling*, 76(2),
174 180. https://doi.org/10.1016/j.pec.2009.06.001

Bruhn, C. A. W., Hetterich, S., Schuck-Paim, C., Kürüm,
E., Taylor, R. J., Lustig, R., Shapiro, E. D., Warren, J. L.,
Simonsen, L., & Weinberger, D. M. (2017). Estimating
the population-level impact of vaccines using synthetic
controls. *Proceedings of the National Academy of Sciences of
the United States of America*, 114(7), 1524–1529. https://
doi.org/10.1073/pnas.1612833114

Cabrera, D., Colosi, L., & Lobdell, C. (2008, August). Systems
thinking. *Evaluation and Program Planning*, 31(3), 299–
310. https://doi.org/10.1016/j.evalprogplan.2007.12.001

Cantor, J., Haller, R., & Eliana Greenberg, E. (2018, January).
Rising risk: An overview of identification and intervention
approaches. JSI Research & Training Institute. https://
publications.jsi.com/JSIInternet/Inc/Common
/_download_pub.cfm?id=19182&lid=3

Centers for Disease Control and Prevention. (2013, November
21). *CDC report documents health disparities*. https://www
.cdc.gov/media/releases/2013/p1121-health-disparities.html

Centers for Disease Control and Prevention. (2020). Immunization schedules. https://www.cdc.gov/vaccines/schedules
/index.html

Chung, Y., Schamel, J., Fisher, A., & Frew, P. M. (2017, July
28). Influences on immunization decision-making among
US parents of young children. *Maternal and Child Health
Journal*, 21(12), 2178–2187. https://doi.org/10.1007/s10995
-017-2336-6

Dykes, B. (2012, October 25). 31 essential quotes on analytics
and data. Analytics Hero. http://www.analyticshero.com
/2012/10/25/31-essential-quotes-on-analytics-and-data/

Hawe, P., & Potvin, L. (2009, January 1). What is population
health intervention research? *Canadian Journal of Public
Health*, 100, 18–114. https://doi.org/10.1007/bf03405503

Hofstetter, A. M., Larussa, P., & Rosenthal, S. L. (2015).
Vaccination of adolescents with chronic medical conditions:
Special considerations and strategies for enhancing
uptake. *Human Vaccines and Immunotherapeutics*, 11(11),
2571–2581. https://doi.org/10.1080/21645515.2015
.1067350

Kaplan, R. M., Spittel, M. L., & David, D. H. (Eds.). (2015).
Population health: Behavioral and social science
insights. National Institutes of Health. https://www
.ahrq.gov/sites/default/files/publications/files/population
-health.pdf

Mujtaba, B. G., Cavico, F. J., & Wayne, T. H. (2013, August).
A review of employee health and wellness programs in the
United States. *Public Policy and Administration Research*, 3.
https://www.iiste.org/Journals/index.php/PPAR/article
/view/5331

Nash, D., Skoufalos, A., Fabius, R. J., & Oglesby, W. H.
(2021). *Population health: Creating a culture of wellness*.
Jones & Bartlett Learning.

Pearson, E. S. (2012, April). Goal setting as a health behavior
change strategy in overweight and obese adults: A
systematic literature review examining intervention
components. *Patient Education and Counseling*, 87(1),
32–42. https://doi.org/10.1016/j.pec.2011.07.018

Smith, S. M., Wallace, E., O'Dowd, T., & Fortin, M. (2016,
March). Interventions for improving outcomes in patients
with multimorbidity in primary care and community
settings. *Cochrane Database of Systematic Reviews, 2016*.
https://doi.org/10.1002/14651858.CD006560.pub3

Strecher, V. J., Seijts, G. H., Kok, G. J., Latham, G. P., Glasgow,
R., DeVellis, B., Meertens, R. M., & Bulger, D. W. (1995,
July 1). Goal setting as a strategy for health behavior
change. *Health Education & Behavior*, 22(2), 190–200.
https://doi.org/10.1177/109019819502200207

CHAPTER 28

Monitoring and Optimizing Interventions

Martha Sylvia, PhD, MBA, RN

It is not the strongest of the species that survives, nor the most intelligent, but the one most responsive to change.

—Charles Darwin (Wei, 2015)

EXECUTIVE SUMMARY

Interventions in population health management are dynamic and complex and are often developed and deployed in stages. Interventions often start with a development phase and are typically not considered fully operational until protocols are optimally functioning. To understand the effectiveness and efficiency of interventions delivered daily at the point of care, several considerations are necessary, such as:

- the evolutionary nature of population health interventions,
- the significant investment of funding and resources to intervene to prevent disease and morbidity,
- the interactions between health determinants and poor outcomes,
- the need to understand value in the near term,
- the requirement for pragmatic solutions that are delivered in real-time, and
- the identification of actionable opportunity.

Flexible, defendable, and deeply reflective methods are required in a program of ongoing monitoring and optimization. With these principles in mind, value is understood in a near real-time frame, measured through ongoing monitoring of significant program metrics, and optimized by structured and intentional stakeholder collaboration.

LEARNING OBJECTIVES

At the end of this chapter, the learner will be able to:

1. Compare and contrast monitoring and evaluation methods.
2. Identify stakeholder roles and need for information when monitoring and optimizing population health interventions.

3. Apply the concepts of evidence-based practice and quality improvement to monitoring and optimizing population health interventions.
4. Define basic population health monitoring metrics.
5. Discuss components of the optimization process.

Introduction

As an intervention progresses from initiation to steady state, monitoring ensures that the intervention is being delivered as intended and that progress is being made toward achieving desired outcomes. During this "Monitor and Optimize" phase (as outlined in Chapter 2, "Guiding Frameworks for Population Health Analytics"), all stakeholders have a role in reviewing and interpreting reporting about the interventions. With a population health approach, staff work to deliver interventions through direct patient care and are able to monitor reports focused on the numbers of patients receiving the intervention and whether the cohorts they have direct responsibility for are receiving each component of the intended intervention. Managers and directors are analyzing reports of the entire cohort eligible for the intervention to ensure that targets for enrollment and engagement are achieved and that, once engaged, patients' intended intervention components are optimized. Executive-level leaders are monitoring process and outcomes metrics on a regular basis for the overall intervention to ensure targets are achieved and results articulated (Sylvia, 2020).

This chapter describes the multiple vantage points for the ongoing near real-time monitoring of results of population health interventions with examples of the types of reporting needed to meet the expectations of frontline staff, key stakeholders, and executives. Intervention monitoring is framed within the context of quality improvement and evidence-based practice (EBP) processes. Process and outcome measures of interest to population health interventions are suggested along with a case study. The focus of the chapter is on the analytics to support monitoring and optimization; it does not cover organizational approaches to achieving desired results

such as the system-level requirements to support population health as outlined in Chapter 33, "Clinical Workflow Transformation."

Monitoring versus Evaluation

Monitoring population health interventions involves continuously collecting and analyzing data to determine how well an intervention is performing against expected results. Intervention monitoring measures performance incrementally in real time, and it allows for frequent program adjustments to be made. Monitoring population health interventions answers the following types of questions:

- Is the intervention being delivered according to protocol?
- Is the protocol stable and free of errors?
- Does the intervention deliver the intended protocol components consistently and dependably?
- Is there variation in delivering the protocol between staff members, clinicians, sites, and so on?
- Are targets for performance and outcomes being met? (World Health Organization, 2016)

Evaluation, on the other hand, uses quasi-experimental research-derived techniques to discover evidence for causal relationships between the intervention and outcomes. It is a systematic investigation of the merit, worth, or significance of an intervention, and it has evolved as a discipline with definitions, methods, approaches, and applications to diverse subjects and settings (Koplan, Milstein, & Wetterhall, 1999). Steps of the evaluation process include engaging stakeholders, describing the intervention, designing the methods of the evaluation, gathering credible evidence, justifying conclusions, and sharing lessons learned (Centers for Disease Control and Prevention, 2015).

Evaluation of population health interventions ideally takes place 1 to 3 years following their commencement. Key methodological components used to evaluate population health interventions include the following:

- Identification and use of a comparison group that closely resembles the intervention group to provide a counterfactual estimate for the expected difference in outcomes had the participants not been exposed to the intervention.
- Propensity score matching of intervention and comparison group membership, which is a statistical technique used to ensure that the comparison group is just as likely to receive the intervention as the intervention group, and that the distribution of baseline characteristics is similar between groups, thus mitigating confounding of results.
- A difference-in-difference design in which the pre- and post-intervention differences in outcomes are evaluated and compared between the two groups.
- Timing adjustments for ramp-up and fully functioning intervention periods (Murphy, Hough, Sylvia, Dunbar, & Frick, 2018).

Evaluating population health interventions can be cumbersome, resource intensive, and time prohibitive for most healthcare delivery organizations. Analysts with the required knowledge, education, training, and skill sets to undertake population health intervention evaluation may not be available within many healthcare organizations, smaller organizations may not have the population cohort sizes needed to meet evaluation criteria, and the needed funding may not be allocated to hire the consultants equipped with the skill to perform these types of evaluations. Yet these organizations still desire to implement population health methods, understand the impact of their efforts to implement an EBP and get results to ensure the delivery of high-quality, low-cost, and personalized care.

This chapter offers a tested and effective way for these organizations to participate in and benefit from the available methodologies for measuring performance and have selected methods that consider the speed at which these organizations make decisions and the overwhelming need for practical solutions. The editors of this textbook think that when population health interventions are accompanied by well-designed monitoring programs using statistical process control (SPC) and target-setting, that intensive and more long-term measurement and evaluation efforts are likely to confirm the findings of the monitoring program in terms of realization of quality, utilization, and cost outcomes. In addition, the methods proposed in this chapter allow staff to deploy interventions that course correct based on initial findings, make changes to workflows along the way to remove barriers, and tailor the experience to the needs of the populations intervened. Therefore, in the majority of situations, the results of a strong monitoring program can be used to optimize and determine the value of population health interventions.

Stakeholder Roles and Information Needs for Monitoring and Optimization

The need for information and type of reporting required during the monitoring and optimization phases of population health vary depending on the stakeholder's role, responsibility and accountability for intervention results, and levers used to optimize interventions. **Table 28.1** describes each in more detail.

Those who are responsible for directly interacting with patients need information about their individual patients and their responsibilities when delivering the intervention. For instance, for a medication therapy management intervention, the pharmacist who is providing counseling needs to know the patients for which they have provided services and those next in line, the patients who are at each point in the process of outreach, engagement, and follow-up, and progress toward targeted results.

Table 28.1 Stakeholder Roles, Reporting Needs, and Intervention Levers for Optimization

Role	Responsibility and Accountability for Results	Reports Needed	Optimization Levers
Outreach staff	Responsible for a targeted amount of outreach attempts and following outreach protocols	Run charts and SPC of outreach and enrollment rates Lists of patients eligible for outreach	Recommends outreach protocol changes to program leadership
Intervention staff (frontline professional staff delivering the intervention to individual patients)	Responsible for engagement rates, delivering intervention per protocol, and following up with assigned individual patients with undesirable outcome results	Run charts and SPC of engagement rates, process, and outcome rates Lists of assigned patients with individual outcome results	Designs, obtains approval, and implements intervention protocol changes
Managers (of outreach and intervention staff)	Accountable for following outreach and intervention protocols across all staff reporting to them Responsible for process and outcome results	Run charts and SPC of engagement rates, process, and outcome rates. Reporting filtered by staff–patient assignments	Designs, obtains approval, and implements protocol changes across all protocols for which staff members are responsible
Program directors	Accountable for outcomes across entire intervention Accountable for adherence to intervention protocols	Run charts and SPC of engagement rates, process, and outcome rates at the level of the intervention	Oversees intervention budget, allocates intervention resources, provides direction for intervention optimization, approves protocol changes
Executive-level managers (e.g., chief executive officer, chief medical officer, chief financial officer)	Accountable for organizational key performance metrics Accountable for return on investment for population health interventions	Key performance indicators (outcome measures) compared to target	Allocates resources for interventions and decides on intervention sustainability

Reproduced from Sylvia, M. (2020). Monitoring and optimizing population health interventions. In *Population health management learning series*. ForestVue Healthcare Solutions.

Managers and directors need similar information although with patients aggregated according to the leaders' scope of responsibility. Reporting may require a breakdown of results by staff person. Executives are monitoring key process and outcome measures at the level of the overall intervention, its cost to deliver, and its resource allocation.

Patient-level reports, dashboards, run charts, statistical process control, and benchmarking are proposed as the ideal methodology for ongoing monitoring of population health intervention metrics. These methodologies allow for a continuous quality-management feedback loop in which data are continuously analyzed as compared to expectations and shared with quality-improvement teams for continuous improvement of ongoing program processes.

Monitoring and Optimization in the Context of Evidence-Based Practice and Quality Improvement

The concepts of evidence-based practice and quality improvement are applied when monitoring and optimizing population health interventions. The evaluation step of EBP described in Chapter 2 directly applies to monitoring and optimization in population health. During the development phase of the population health process, metrics are defined. Metrics can be directly linked back to the findings of the population's *assess* and *focus* phases outlined in Chapter 2, "Guiding Frameworks for Population Health Analytics." For instance, a finding that people with diabetes who have high hemoglobin A1c (HbA1c) laboratory values (an indicator of prolonged poor glucose control) are more frequently admitted to the hospital for complications of their conditions may result in an intervention that targets people with diabetes and poor glucose control. Based on the reason for delivering this intervention, two of the outcome measures should focus on lowering HbA1c and reducing hospital admissions. This ensures that the intervention is addressing the problem identified at the onset of the process. This concept of tying outcome measures back to the identified problem and reason for the intervention is key to monitoring the results of population health interventions.

There are various models of quality improvement. For the most part they all share the same common components and basic process. For the purposes of this text, an accelerated and iterative derivative of the commonly used Plan Do Study Act (PDSA) model is referenced and is referred to as Rapid Cycle Performance Improvement (RCPI). **Figure 28.1** lays out the PDSA cycle as it applies

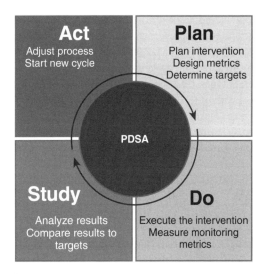

Figure 28.1 PDSA Cycle for Population Health Monitoring and Optimization.

Modified from Langley, G. L., Nolan, K. M., Nolan, T. W., Norman, C. L., & Provost, L. P. (2009). *The improvement guide: A practical approach to enhancing organizational performance* (2nd ed.). Jossey Bass.

to population health monitoring and optimization. During the *plan* phase, the process for delivering the intervention is planned and includes everything from identifying people for intervention to completing intervention delivery. Monitoring metrics and target goals for the metrics are also defined in the planning phase. In the *do* phase, the intervention is delivered, and monitoring metrics are reported. In the *study* phase, the population health team analyzes results, compares results to targets, and determines adjustments that need to be made to intervention processes. The *act* phase entails adjusting processes to achieve desired goals; once enacted, the process starts over (Langley, Nolan, Nolan, Norman, & Provost, 2009).

This process can be exemplified using the previous scenario where an intervention is designed to lower HbA1c and reduce admissions. In the *plan* phase, one intervention could be to outreach to targeted patients, complete a primary care visit, develop a patient-centric plan of care with goal setting, and assign a care manager to assist the patient in meeting care-planning goals. Each process of the intervention includes methods of outreach, which ensures each component is delivered as intended and determination of patient goal achievement is planned. In addition, process and outcome measures are developed. For instance, a process measure might be the percentage of outreached patients who complete a care plan; an outcome measure would be the percentage of targeted patients who experience a hospitalization. In the *do* phase, dashboards are created to monitor process and outcome measures, using the techniques of run charting and statistical process control (see Chapter 24, "Run Charts and Statistical Process Control"). In the *study* phase, all stakeholders review the results and come to consensus on recommended changes to process. For instance, if the percentage of patients completing a care plan is less than expected, then a change could be made to the modality for completing the care plan such as allowing portions to be completed electronically versus manually. Finally, the *act* phase involves implementing the process change and moving into another PDSA cycle.

RCPI is an evolution of the PDSA cycle where incremental changes are made, results are measured and evaluated, and the process is completed. The cycle focuses on action rather than planning under the assumption that stakeholders in the intervention have the knowledge and aptitude needed to be successful (Terhaar, 2021). The key to success in RCPI is determining the timing of the cycles, which can be measured in terms of hours, days, weeks, or months, depending on the processes being evaluated. For instance, changes to the scripts used by outreach workers can be adjusted based on daily monitoring of rates of agreement to engage in the intervention by targeted patients. Changes to the steps of the outreach process may need a longer turnaround time to adjust and monitor if system reconfiguration and compliance or other approvals are needed.

Metrics

Process metrics are considered leading indicators of intervention results and measure what is actually done in the intervention to enable desired results. Outcomes are considered lagging indicators because changes in outcomes follow changes in process measures. Outcomes measure the impact of the intervention on health status, quality, and patients' experience of care, utilization, and costs. More information about process and outcome measures is provided in Chapter 24, "Run Charts and Statistical Process Control."

Interventions use a set of metrics that are organized to assess and improve results with a core, parsimonious group of measures providing a quantitative indication of intervention progress; areas for improvement; and outcome impact (National Academies of Medicine, 2016). Well-designed metrics are developed with the initial population health assessment in mind and are tailored to the relationship between health determinants and poor outcomes identified in the *focus* phase of the population health process (see Chapter 2 "Guiding Frameworks for Population Health Analytics," and Chapter 25, "Assessing Populations"). For instance, if the *focus* phase identified that poor medication adherence was related to increased hospital admissions, then the intervention would be designed to improve medication adherence, and key metrics would include the medication possession ratio (MPR) adherence measure and the rate of hospital admissions. Targets would be set to raise the MPR and lower admission rates.

Intervention stakeholders work together to develop a core set of intervention metrics that will be monitored throughout the program and used to optimize the intervention and ensure outcomes are achieved. The chosen metrics are grounded in the philosophy of selecting a core set of measures that identify adherence and variation from protocols, indicate when processes may not be working as intended or achieving desired results, measure the impact of interventions on pertinent outcomes derived from the *assess* and *focus* phases of the population health process, and are assigned reachable yet challenging goals in athe form of target values. **Table 28.2** provides examples of population health intervention metrics in each identified area and can be used as a starting point for tailoring metrics for population health interventions.

Table 28.2 Basic Metrics Used for Population Health Monitoring

Metric	Measure	Type	Common Data Source	More Information
Outreach number or rate	% of targeted patients who have a completed contact for enrollment into the intervention	Process	Electronic medical record	Targeted patients are those who are matched to specific interventions (see Chapter 26, "Targeting Individuals for Intervention"). Outreach is a process used to inform targeted patients about the intervention and gain their commitment to participate. The contact is complete when the outreach staff is able to complete the entire outreach protocol with a patient.
Enrollment number or rate	% of outreached patients who agree to receive the intervention	Process	Electronic medical record	Enrollment in an intervention is the patient's commitment to participate.
Engagement number or rate	% of enrolled patients who have met criteria for engagement	Process	Electronic medical record	An example of criteria would be a certain amount and type of contacts or completion of a care plan with goal setting.
Rate of receipt of key intervention components	% of engaged patients receiving critical component of the intervention	Process	Electronic medical record	Each intervention consists of key components that are crucial to achieving successful outcomes. For instance, a medication therapy management (MTM) program requires a medication reconciliation consultation meeting certain requirements. Key components are identified and measured to ensure intervention processes are received by patients according to protocols.
Rate of goal obtainment for clinical indicators	% of engaged patients meeting targets for critical clinical component of the intervention	Outcome	Electronic medical record or administrative claims data	Each intervention consists of key clinical indicators with targets. For instance, an intervention for patients with diabetes may aim to achieve blood glucose control measured by HbA1c values achieving a target of less than 8%. An MTM program may set medication adherence targets at greater than 80%. Depending on the type of intervention, key clinical outcomes are identified and measured.

(continues)

Table 28.2 Basic Metrics Used for Population Health Monitoring *(continued)*

Metric	Measure	Type	Common Data Source	More Information
Emergency department visit rates	% of engaged patients with an ED visit and the ED visit rate per thousand rate in engaged patients	Outcome	Administrative claims data	When patients are receiving needed care and services ED visits should be avoidable especially when related to chronic conditions.
Inpatient admissions rates	% of engaged patients with an inpatient admission and the ED visit rate per thousand rate in engaged patients	Outcome	Administrative claims data	When patients are receiving needed care and services hospital admissions should be avoidable especially when related to chronic conditions.
Readmission rates	% of engaged patients with a readmission and the readmission rate per thousand in engaged patients	Outcome	Administrative claims data	Some population health programs are designed to specifically address transitions of care, often after an inpatient admission. Unplanned readmissions are unnecessary admissions occurring within 30 days of a previous inpatient admission.
Total cost of care	Average costs per member per month of engaged patients	Outcome	Administrative claims data	When population health interventions are performing as expected and utilization goals are met, total cost of care is often lowered.

Optimizing Population Health Interventions

The concept of RCPI previously described in the chapter forms the basis for optimization in population health interventions. Although the input of all stakeholders is solicited, the optimization team includes those accountable for the intervention at an organizational level, staff management, and those who are working on the frontlines to outreach, enroll, engage, and deliver interventions to patients. This team regularly monitors reporting related to its role and optimization levers and collaboratively reviews results to identify issues, develop solutions, and implement adjustments to the intervention. The team does this through multiple cycles of rapid process improvement.

Large-scale interventions administered to high volumes of patients or across multiple sites are more vulnerable to problems of variability in the way that the intervention is delivered, have many more stakeholders invested in successful results, and require a more formal structure for optimization processes. When delivering large-scale interventions, it is a good idea to have an optimization team comprising representatives from each role and the intervention site. In addition, the optimization team will include stakeholder leadership across all sites and any other pertinent members. The optimization team meets regularly to review intervention-level reporting, compares the results of process and outcome measures to set targets, and addresses variance in process and outcome measures among sites.

Regardless of the size of the intervention, the membership of the optimization team should consider these questions:

1. Who knows the work?
2. Who will be impacted?
3. Who would be a good champion or representative for other teammates?
4. Who has approval and who has veto power?
5. Who has the authority to make changes to make things work?
6. Who are the formal and informal leaders?

Applied Learning: Case Study

This case study extends on the case study presented in Chapter 22, "Predictive and Prescriptive Analytics." Recall from the case study that a predictive model was developed to identify people with diabetes who were at risk of having a hospital admission. The predictive model was validated, the risk-score distribution was presented, and the differences in characteristics between high- and medium- to low-risk cohorts was presented. In this phase of the case study, the patients identified as high risk in the pilot site's cohort are being outreached and targeted for the intervention that focuses on self-management support and integrated primary care delivery with the outcome goal of increasing the percentage of patients with an HbA1c value of less than 9% and decreasing the percentage of patients with an all-cause hospital admission.

The intervention allows for a 12-week ramp-up period for outreaching, enrolling, and engaging patients. During this time, the focus is on getting as many targeted patients to engage as possible. The process measures during this time focus on this part of the intervention protocol, and the optimization team meets regularly to review the data and adjust the protocol as necessary.

Figure 28.2 shows the results of outreach for each week. Each week, the number of unique targeted patients outreached for intervention is shown. An outreach is defined as a completed outreach attempt in which the outreach worker was able to complete the entire outreach protocol with the patient. The target number of members for outreach in each week is 52, and the median number outreached in a week is 49. The outreach workers were only able to surpass the target number in weeks 8 and 9. The optimization team will address this challenge and review the outreach protocol with outreach workers to determine what adjustments can be implemented.

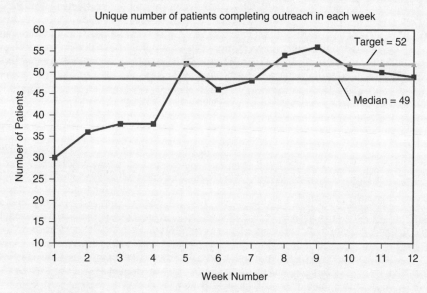

Figure 28.2 Case Study Run Chart of Outreached Patients for 12-Week Ramp-Up.

(continues)

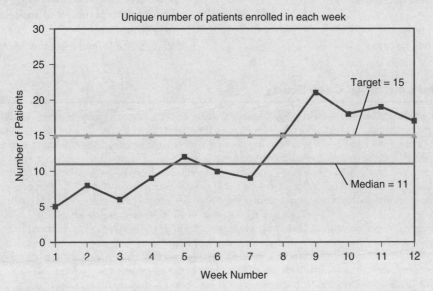

Figure 28.3 Case Study Run Chart of Enrolled Patients for 12-Week Ramp-Up.

Figure 28.3 shows the results of enrollment for each week, including the number of unique outreached patients enrolled for intervention. Enrollment is defined as a commitment on the part of patients that they will participate and engage in the intervention. The target number of members for enrollment in each week is 15, and the median number enrolled in a week is 11. The enrollment process is considered optimum after week 8 because weeks 9 through 12 are above the target, and the run chart shows that the five points from months 8 through 12 are consistently above the median (see run chart variation interpretation in Chapter 24, "Run Charts and Statistical Process Control").

Figure 28.4 shows the results of engagement for each week. Each week, the number of unique enrolled patients engaged in the intervention is shown. Engagement is defined as completing an interview and initial intake assessment with an assigned intervention provider. Because the engagement activities occur after outreach and enrollment, the targets will probably not be achieved before the sixth week of the 12-week ramp-up period. The number of engaged patients has steadily increased since the commencement of the intervention, with weeks 10 through 12 at or above the target number. The optimization team plans to continue to monitor progress without adjustments to the protocols.

As the intervention moves from the ramp-up phase to fully operational phase, the team monitors process and outcome measures. Measurement is now monitored monthly beginning at the first month after the ramp-up phase. This is a cumulative measure, which means that once a person is in the denominator, he or she remains in the denominator. The same is true for the numerator; once a patient in the denominator completes the requirements for care planning and goal setting, he or she remains in the numerator. **Figure 28.5** shows the run chart of the results of one of the process measures, which is the percentage of engaged patients who complete a care plan and set personal health-related goals.

The first patients completed this entire process in April of the intervention year. The optimization team closely monitored results and was concerned with the dip in the percentage that occurred in November. As it turned out, this dip was a result of previously engaged patients disenrolling from the intervention. Still, the target seemed out of reach for the intervention because the target was well above the rate achieved throughout the year. On further interviews with intervention staff, the optimization team learned that a patient

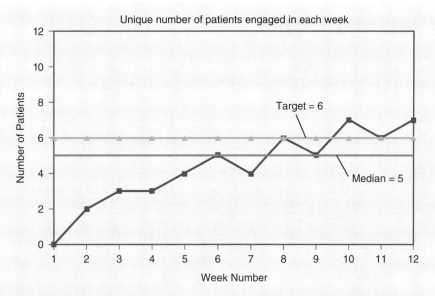

Figure 28.4 Case Study Run Chart of Engaged Patients for 12-Week Ramp-Up.

is not considered in the numerator until every item on the care plan is complete and a total of three patient health goals are set. The intervention staff was unable to meet all of these requirements for patients in the intervention because patients often became overwhelmed with the idea of aspiring to three goals instead of one at a time. In December, the protocol was changed to require only one personal health-related goal.

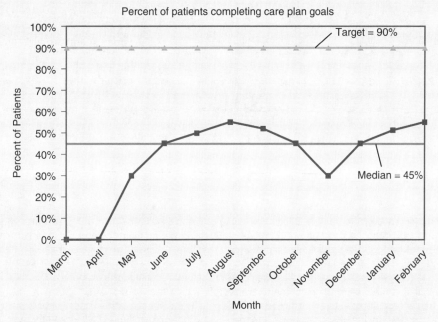

Figure 28.5 Percentage of Engaged Patients Completing Care Plans and Personal Health Goal Setting.

(continues)

Applied Learning: Case Study   (continued)

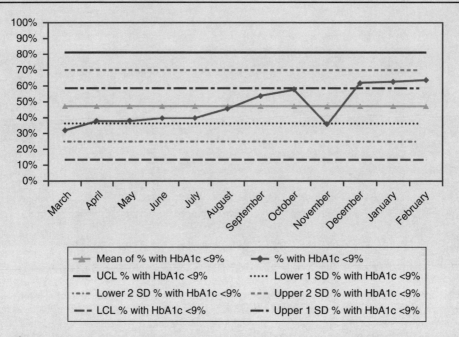

Figure 28.6 Percentage of Patients with an HbA1c < 9%.

During the operational phase of the intervention, outcome measures are also monitored. One clinical outcome for the intervention is the percentage of engaged patients with a recent HbA1c measure less than 9% (lower HbA1c levels indicate better prolonged blood glucose control for patients with diabetes). This is also a cumulative measure, which means that once a person is in the denominator, he or she remains in the denominator. A patient is in the numerator if his or her last recorded HbA1c level is less than 9%. **Figure 28.6** shows the SPC chart of the percentage of engaged patients with an HbA1c < 9%. The month of November shows the same dip in the percentage seen in the process measures because of patient disenrollment. However, absent that dip, there is an upward trend in this clinical outcome measure. The optimization team plans to monitor this outcome measure and is confident at the end of the first year that overall this clinical outcome is headed in the right direction and that blood glucose control is improving in the patients receiving the intervention.

The primary utilization outcome is the percentage of engaged patients with any hospitalization, which is also a cumulative measure. **Figure 28.7** shows the SPC chart of the percentage of engaged patients with a hospitalization. These results provide convincing evidence that the intervention is having the intended impact of reducing hospitalizations because the trend in the percent of patients with an admission decreased from June to December; the months of September through December show four out of five successive points more than one standard deviation from the mean on the same side of the center line (see SPC variation interpretation in Chapter 24 "Run Charts and Statistical Process Control").

At the executive level, *key performance indicators* (KPIs) are reported for the intervention. Two of the KPIs for this intervention are the outcome measures of percent of engaged patients with an HbA1c < 9% and the percentage of patients with a hospital admission. The executive team has set targets for these KPIs based on the finding of special cause variation over program duration. The KPI is set to green if favorable special cause variation is identified, to yellow if there is confidence that special cause variation will be achieved within 2 to 3 months, and to red if there is a lack of confidence that special cause variation will be achieved. The KPI reporting to executives for February is shown in **Figure 28.8**.

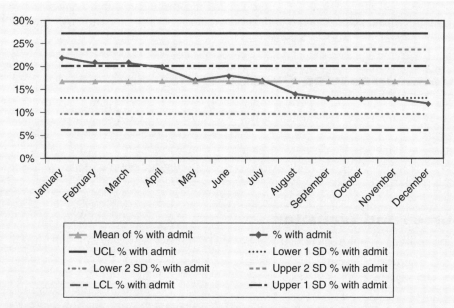

Figure 28.7 Percentage of Patients with a Hospitalization.

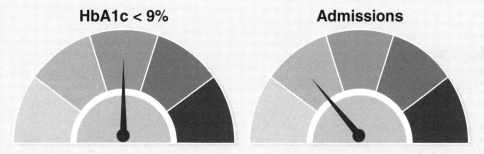

Figure 28.8 Executive-Level KPI Reporting.

Reproduced from Sylvia, M. (2020). Monitoring and optimizing population health interventions. In *Population health management learning series*. ForestVue Healthcare Solutions.

Conclusion

When executed in a structured and methodical way, monitoring process and outcome measures using run charts and SPC along with ongoing optimization cycles provides a clear lens to the value of population health interventions. Monitoring and optimization processes are closely aligned with evidence-based practice and quality-improvement methods that have been used in health care for decades. Multiple stakeholders are invested in the success of population health interventions with varying needs for information and ability to adjust intervention protocols and practices. Population health analytics and the monitoring metrics and performance measurement outlined in this chapter focus on the tailoring of information to stakeholder needs using established measures and methods. Equipped with the right information and ability to improve interventions, stakeholders work collaboratively as members of an optimization team to realize value in population health interventions.

Study and Discussion Questions

- Why does the type of reporting vary based on the role of the stakeholder in the intervention?
- What are the differences between process and outcome measures? Why are both needed? What is the purpose of each?

- What is the best way to ensure that population health interventions achieve desired outcomes?
- How do the concepts of evidence-based practice and quality improvement apply to monitoring and optimization of population health interventions?

Resources and Websites

Institute for Healthcare Improvement: IHI.org

Agency for Healthcare Research and Quality Guidelines and Measures: https://www.ahrq.gov /gam/index.html

Agency for Healthcare Research and Quality Tools and Resources for Research, Quality Improvement and Practice: https://www.ahrq.gov/ncepcr /tools/index.html

U.S. Department of Health and Human Services Health Resources and Services Administration (HRSA), Quality Improvement: https://www.hrsa .gov/sites/default/files/quality/toolbox/508pdfs /qualityimprovement.pd

References

Centers for Disease Control and Prevention. (2015). Evaluation. Workplace health promotion. https://www .cdc.gov/workplacehealthpromotion/model/evaluation /index.html

Koplan, J. P., Milstein, R. L., & Wetterhall, S. F. (1999, September 17). Framework for program evaluation in public health. *Morbidity & Mortality Weekly, 48*(RR11), 1–40. https:// www.cdc.gov/mmwr/preview/mmwrhtml/rr4811a1.htm

Langley, G. L., Nolan, K. M., Nolan, T. W., Norman, C. L., & Provost, L. P. (2009). *The improvement guide: A practical approach to enhancing organizational performance* (2nd ed.). Jossey Bass.

Murphy, S. M. E., Hough, D. E., Sylvia, M. L., Dunbar, L. J., & Frick, K. D. (2018, February 8). Key design considerations when calculating cost savings for population health management programs in an observational setting. *Health Services Research, 53*(51), 3107–3124. https://doi.org /10.1111/1475-6773.12832

National Academies of Medicine. (2016). Metrics that matter for population health action: Workshop summary. https://

www.nap.edu/catalog/21899/metrics-that-matter-for -population-health-action-workshop-summary

Sylvia, M. (2020). Introduction to population health analytics. In *Population health management learning series.* Charleston, SC: ForestVue Healthcare Solutions.

Terhaar, M. F. (2021). Methods for translation. In K. M. White, S. Dudley-Brown, & M. F. Terhaar (Eds.), *Translation of evidence into nursing and healthcare* (3rd ed., pp. 173–198). Springer Publishing Company.

Wei, J. (2015). It is not the strongest of the species that survive—Charles Darwin. DUE. https://due.com/blog/not -strongest-species-survive-charles-darwin/#:~:text =%E2%80%9CIt%20is%20not%20the%20strongest, one%20more%20responsive%20to%20change.%E2 %80%9D&text=This%20quote%20from%20Charles%20 Darwin,out%20and%20pursue%20their%20dreams.

World Health Organization. (2016). *Monitoring and evaluating digital health interventions: A practical guide to conducting research and assessment.* https://apps.who.int/iris/bitstream /handle/10665/252183/9789241511766-eng.pdf

CHAPTER 29

Storytelling with Data

Mary Terhaar, PhD, RN, ANEF, FAAN

Stories bring brains together.

—Paul J. Zak (2013)

EXECUTIVE SUMMARY

The most effective leaders, businesspeople, artists, advocates, politicians, teachers and scientists share the ability to tell a great story (Gallo, 2016): not just a funny one or one that is spectacularly uncommon, but a story that conveys meaning along with information, a story that connects to the audience, or a story that triggers a deep and personal response. Such storytelling creates an advantage for anyone who shares it and everyone who hears it. Mastery of storytelling is worth the effort to learn and worth the time to craft.

The discipline of population health is complex, its concepts and methodologies complicated, and its analytics routinely produce extensive and diverse data on which to build a compelling story. The storytelling challenge associated with population health is to use powerful analytics in ways that are easily understood, engaging, and useful for the public. Keep in mind that a story without data is no more persuasive than data without a story.

The purpose of this chapter is to guide development of storytelling skills that can be applied to the practice of population health. In support of that goal, this chapter is designed to help create the story that supports analysis, engages the audience, amplifies impact, and contributes to a lasting understanding of key points. This chapter will help build capability and comfort as a storyteller. Strategies that can be used to overcome factors that interfere with stakeholders' reception, retention, and appreciation of analytics work will be presented. These strategies will be especially useful when presenting data to those who may be mathematically anxious or numerically challenged or do not speak the language of population health. Best practices for telling stories and the kinds of devices and strategies that help to increase impact will be presented. At the close, population health stories will be provided to demonstrate application of key concepts.

LEARNING OBJECTIVES

At the end of this chapter, the learner will be able to:

1. Discuss the role of story in society.
2. Explain the ways storytelling affects the brain.
3. Identify the basics of good story.

4. Describe the structure and attributes of effective stories.
5. Describe the devices practiced by effective storytellers.
6. Explore the elements of effective story.
7. Explore use of storytelling to create credible narrative in population health.
8. Develop a plan to apply storytelling to presentation of analysis and results.

Introduction

The Role of Stories in Society

By nature, humans are social organisms. We live in community and are profoundly interdependent. Flow of information enhances both chances of survival and quality of life (Zak, 2013). Throughout human history, stories have been told around campfires, at court, and at watercoolers as a means to share important information. Consider these messages: "Beware of the wooly mammoth!" "Hercules is strong and moral. He is a hero." "Get ready, a storm is coming." "You really need to wash your hands!" Stories have been told in petroglyphs and hieroglyphs; in print, music, dance, theater, and film; person to person, generation to generation, and face to face; by letter or text, phone, and Internet.

Storytelling and narratives are especially well suited to communication between experts and nonexperts in large measure because of the ability of the story to persuade and influence (Dahlstrom, 2014). Consider social media, lay media, and the arts where well-told stories can carry a message broadly and quickly to create strong, lasting impressions. Scientists, politicians, and business leaders have used stories to great advantage: consider Super Bowl advertising and TED talks. Storytelling is a tool that can be deployed to teach, disseminate science, and explain complexities to the benefit of society (Martin & Miller, 1988).

Imaging studies have established that the average person will experience a similar neural response to a challenging computational problem as he or she would to the threat of actual physical harm (Stoet, Bailey, Moore, & Geary, 2016). As a result, the value of the data that scientists and analysts produce and the analyses conducted can be hijacked by the human tendency to avoid and oppose threatening stimuli. Because storytelling is a means to overcome this all-too-human *fight-or-flight response*, it has the potential to enhance the impact of any population health analyses. It is an effective way to increase audience members' contextualization, understanding, and retention of complicated and important findings. Effective storytelling can reach audiences that are broader and more diverse than the collection of analysts, scientists, clinicians, administrators, and policy practitioners who make up the population health community.

Well-told stories are important in society for two main reasons (Zak, 2014). First, impactful stories seize and hold the attention of the target audience and bring that audience into the world of the characters. Second, a well-told story can form a bridge from analyses to impact. Stories can link those who operate comfortably in the land of data with those who rely on data and analytics to improve performance and outcomes.

How Stories Affect the Brain

A well-told story impacts body chemistry and brain function. Any story that triggers emotion releases hormones in the listener that create feelings and experiences that link the audience to the storyteller (Zak, 2013, 2014, 2015).

Oxytocin and Tender Stories

Story can be constructed to stimulate oxytocin production that, in turn, creates empathy. The audience will identify with the storyteller and characters in well-told story. Oxytocin, which is commonly associated with labor, childbirth, and bonding between mother and child has also been associated with trustworthiness, generosity, charity, and compassion. Warm and fuzzy stories can stimulate oxytocin, which can lead to strongly positive affective states (Zak, 2014). These stories can create connection between storyteller and audience and thus make the content more memorable. In this situation, the audience identifies with the storyteller; imaging studies reveal neural functions that mirror those of the storyteller. This can have powerful impact.

Dopamine Epinephrine, Endorphins, and Humorous or Engaging Stories

Humorous and intriguing storytelling stimulates the release of dopamine, epinephrine, and endorphin and increases attention and the retention of information. Here, too, imaging studies of the audience are remarkably similar to those of the storyteller. This experience of mirroring will advantage both teller and audience by increasing comprehension and retention. Because dopamine generates focus and motivation, it keeps the audience in the game (TEDx Talks, 2017). Storytellers who can trigger dopamine have an advantage in conveying their message.

Humor triggers laughter, which stimulates the release of dopamine, epinephrine, and endorphins that, in turn, increase creativity, relaxation, and focus (TEDx Talks, 2017; Zak, 2014). So, while adding humor makes a story more enjoyable and fun, it also makes the message more relatable and memorable. For these concrete reasons, humor increases the impact of the message.

Cortisol and Adrenaline and Scary Stories

Story can also be constructed to stimulate fear and anxiety. A scary or frightening story is powerful in its own way. It triggers cortisol and adrenaline, which can raise attentiveness. Both can create feelings of intolerance and impatience. Concurrent with generating a sense of urgency, cortisol and adrenaline reduce creativity and impair memory. They can trigger systems 2 thinking (the fight-or-flight response) that is well suited to situations of imminent threat (think of a fire or an oncoming car) but poorly suited to solving complex problems that demand systems 1 thinking (deliberate reason and critical analysis) (Khaneman, 2011).

Although a scary story may command attention that is positive, it can interfere with retention at the same time. For that reason, frightening stories need to be carefully used and thoughtfully placed in relation to the intended message.

The Basics of Storytelling

Just as with teaching, writing, and public speaking, stories with the greatest impact are achieved by beginning with the end in mind (Bowen, 2017). Reverse design makes the best story, just like reverse engineering makes the highest-quality systems. So the storyteller needs to consider the message intended and then construct the story to achieve that end.

The previous section detailed the process by which a good story creates in the audience a strong physiologic and neurologic connection to the message. More than simply conveying content, good storytelling couples fact and data with softer information like emotion and empathy, which increase the probability of persuasion, retention, and action.

Story can communicate the strengths, values, and accomplishments of the business beyond any organization to influence or increase its audience or customer base. It can introduce outsiders to the unique perspective and strengths that define the work of the group and in so doing can attract business. Story performs well in advertisement because it can carry a complete message to a target group (Villaire, 1992).

Within an organization, story is particularly well suited to communicating values and building culture. It can help individual players appreciate the many ways their contributions add to the success of the organization to benefit the community or society as a whole (Zak, 2014). In this way, story can increase engagement, a sense of commitment, pride, and affiliation in a workforce (Benner, 1992).

Best Practices of Effective Storytellers: Structure and Attributes of Effective Stories

Many time-tested practices can increase the clarity and impact of a story. These practices are described in the following section; examples from literature and media are provided.

Know Your Audience

A strong message is designed with a specific audience in mind. When speaking to colleagues, it may be reasonable to expect familiarity with the vocabulary and basic concepts. When speaking to audiences outside one's discipline, this expectation can prove fatal.

The effective storyteller understands the gap between the target audience's understanding and the baseline knowledge, attitudes, and effect of the audience. Strong story lays a foundation, including basic language, concepts, context, and application of the message. Age, gender, education, discipline, role, and lived experience all influence receptivity and readiness to the message.

Provide a Compelling Opening to Create Connection

Good story wastes no time in grabbing its audience (Monarth, 2014). Within the first 30 seconds in a good talk, in the first paragraph of a good book, in the first few images of a good film, the master storyteller has the audience in the palm of his or her hand. Good story begins with a clear statement of intent as to what will be understood at its end or it creates anticipation and curiosity to continue (Wiggins & McTighe, 1998).

Consider the opening lines of popular books:

- "All happy families are alike; each unhappy family is unhappy in its own way." (*Anna Karenina*—Tolstoy, 1887)
- "In my younger and more vulnerable years my father gave me some advice that I've been turning over in my mind ever since. Whenever you feel like criticizing anyone, he told me, just remember that all the people in this world haven't had the advantages that you've had." (*The Great Gatsby*—Fitzgerald, 1925)
- "This is my favorite book in the world though I've never read it." (*The Princess Bride*—Goldman, 1973)
- "Mr. and Mrs. Dursley of number four, Privet Drive, were proud to say that they were perfectly normal, thank you very much." (*Harry Potter and the Philosopher's Stone*—Rowling, 1997)
- "You better not tell nobody but God." (*The Color Purple*—Walker, 1982)

Consider these openings of memorable speeches.

- "Fans, for the past two weeks you have been reading about the bad break I got. Yet today I consider myself the luckiest man on the face of the earth. I have been in ballparks for seventeen years and have never received anything but kindness and encouragement from your fans. Look at these grand men. Which of you wouldn't consider it the highlight of his career to associate with them for even one day?" (Gehrig, 1939)
- "I am the first accused." (Mandela, 1964)
- "We meet at a college noted for knowledge, in a city noted for progress, in a state noted for strength, and we stand in need of all three, for we meet in an hour of change and challenge, in a decade of hope and fear, in an age of both knowledge and ignorance. The greater our knowledge increases, the greater our ignorance unfolds." (Kennedy, 1962)

Each opening grabs the audience immediately, invites curiosity, invokes emotion, or creates in the audience a connection with or empathy for the storyteller. Strong openings may shock or soothe, tease or foreshadow, disarm or create closeness. For these reasons, they are memorable.

It is a challenge to find opening lines that contain numbers and data. This is an indicator of territory to be won by analysts and population health experts with important stories to tell. Here are two that may satisfy these criteria:

- "It was a bright cold day in April, and the clocks were striking thirteen." (*1984*—George Orwell)
- "124 was spiteful." (Toni Morrison's *Beloved*).

In the first example, Orwell uses numbers to clearly and briskly establish that something is not right. The reader is drawn in and anticipates something to come. If just one number can accomplish all that, then numbers can add impact and clarity to many more stories when they are thoughtfully integrated.

In the second example, Morrison creates curiosity and draws the reader in. Whereas numbers can be used to add clarity and increase understanding in storytelling, they can depersonalize in real life. Morrison conveys this with urgency.

Make the Body as Powerful as the Opening

Once the story has activated attention and curiosity, it needs to sustain and amplify interest as well as understanding. It needs to be detailed and complete and may employ humor, imagery, anecdote, or data to accomplish its purpose. Each can clarify, verify, and amplify the intended message.

Edit and Refine

All art is about the countless decisions that influence the final product. Just as painters select canvases, working media, colors, and style to present their thoughts, so too the storyteller chooses the language and pace and makes important decisions about what to include as essential and what to omit.

Think of the points in a story as though they were pieces of art in a museum. There is only so much space, and the curator must make important decisions about what to display and what to remove. The storyteller must curate the collection of thoughts to achieve the desired impact. Each element included in the story must represent a message, a point, a desired action. The following paragraphs describe the devices of impactful stories that can be applied to population health analytics storytelling.

Close with Precision

Every word counts. Creating a strong last impression is key for retention and application. The storyteller may recreate a connection to the opening, provide a summary, share a reflection, or forecast a future. Each option is intended to reinforce connection and persuasion toward acceptance and retention of the key takeaway point at the core of the story.

Perfect Practice

Everyone has story in them, but not everyone is comfortable telling stories. So the best way to prepare is to practice. Practice with colleagues. Invite feedback. Edit again. Add emphasis. Curate your thoughts. All can be accomplished through practice and will hone the message.

The Devices of Impactful Story

In addition to the structure of story, interest can be fanned, and impact enhanced by using some devices that are familiar from literature but less commonly encountered in scientific work. These include humor, imagery and anecdote. Visual artifacts like social math and infographics are useful in making connections to current knowledge and projections to meaning and application.

Humor

Humor adds richness to story. It is defined as "the quality of being amusing or comic" (Dictionary .com, n.d.-a). For scientists, humor may be unfamiliar or uncomfortable largely because we lack practice. Scientists and analysts have worked diligently to create strong, evidence-based logic for every assertion. Humor has a different foundation and form. The important consideration with humor is that it must relate precisely to the message and amplify or clarify the story. If not, it may well detract from the impact of the story. Well-selected story will complement and enhance the message and impact.

Mark Twain (1897) explained there are three different aspects of funny stories. The humorous story, he says, is uniquely American—brisk in pace and reliant on the quality of its telling far more heavily than on construction and delivery. The latter two, he asserted, are far less challenging to write.

Still, humor is a spice that is best saved for select uses. Inappropriately applied, humor offends and creates distance. It can impair receptivity in the audience and so is to be used with judgement, respect, and practice.

Anecdote

Anecdote is defined as a short, entertaining story (Dictionary.com, n.d.-b). Anecdotes can briskly hold attention and convey rich and complex information. They are particularly effective for creating empathy and identification with the character of interest. Well told, anecdote transports the audience as though they were captured in the moment within the story.

Consider your experience when you are viewing a movie and become frightened or anxious. This same connectedness with content can be accomplished with population health stories when anecdote is well constructed and well used. **Figure 29.1** provides an example of a powerful anecdote, one well suited to conveying a complex message that might ordinarily trigger avoidance. It tells a population health story that can reach the intended audience to great effect and to the benefit of many.

Imagery

Imagery in narrative enhances clarity of message as well as retention. *Imagery* refers to text "that evoke(s) sense-impressions by literal or figurative reference to perceptible or 'concrete' objects, scenes, actions, or states" (Baldick, 2001, p. 121). Visual imagery helps create a precise picture in the mind's eye. Other forms of imagery create a sense or feeling. In all its forms, imagery complements and amplifies understanding of a message.

My beloved daughter, Chelsea Marie Heptig, died on May 3, 2002 at 8:50 a.m. She was 2 weeks shy of her senior prom, one month shy of her 18th birthday, and 7 weeks away from high school graduation. She was my very best friend.

On April 26, 2002, she had an argument with her boyfriend and went to talk to a friend who gave her ecstasy. I got a call from the police that she was in the hospital from a drug overdose and arrived to find her unconscious and having powerful seizures. It was horrific! They induced a coma to stop the seizures.

She never came out of the coma . . . instead her internal organs stopped functioning . . . one by one.

For a week we prayed, cried, begged, promised, and hoped. I washed her body, combed her hair, and massaged her feet. She had a high temperature, was hooked up to machines, was breathing through a respirator. My little girl was losing the battle. First her lungs, her brain, her kidneys, her bowels . . . everything was slowly deteriorating. She was in a vegetative state.

We took her off life support . . . she breathed for 8 minutes and died at 8:50 a.m. Me, her mom, her dad, her brother . . . we will never be the same. My heart was crushed that day.

I have shared her personal story with thousands of high school and college students in hopes that they think about the consequences of their actions when they are confronted with drugs.

Chelsea also would not have died if a phone call were made sooner to the police. . . . I also talk about that. If you see a friend acting sick, make a call.

Figure 29.1 The Compelling Anecdote.

As with all writing techniques and all storytelling, imagery is best constructed by beginning with the end in mind.

Consider the exact impression you intend to create and then work to make it happen. In the case of the spoken word, images come from vivid descriptions, which include small and potent details. In the introduction to her novel *To Kill a Mockingbird* (Lee, 1960), which can be found online, Harper Lee creates a strong, clear, and detailed narrative of the feel of the town in which her story is told. She paints a canvas on which to convey the complexity and completeness of the story she tells.

Elements of a Successful Story

Dating back as far as Aristotle, carried to the pulpit by numerous preachers, and commonly repeated by expert public speaker Dale Carnegie; clergy, orators, advocates, and educators have been encouraged to consistently "Tell the audience what you are going to say, say it; then tell them what you've said" (Quote Investigator, 2017). The plan identifies three parts of a story that are useful to bear in mind when constructing and telling memorable narrative.

A more detailed framework provided by German playwright Gustav Freytag identifies seven phases in a well-told story (1894). Originally developed to teach the structure for writing plays, the pyramid provides clear guidance for any storyteller. Because of its granularity, the framework helps the storyteller avoid omitting important information and experience.

Exposition is the first phase. Here the goal is to capture the audience's attention. The storyteller may open with a quote, as seen in the chapters of this book. They may create an exciting moment, a frightening or disturbing one, or a shocking one or they may create an emotional link with the audience. The objective is to pique interest and engage the target audience.

Consider the opening lines of good books or opening scenes of great movies. In both, the audience is drawn in, and an atmosphere is created that foreshadows or portends what is to come.

Rising action is the second phase. Here the goal is to add detail and create distress. This can be accomplished be sharing a vignette or personal experience that allows the storyteller to generate sympathy, empathy, or identification. The data from analyses, which may be baseline data or background information, can be joined to the narrative to deepen understanding and connection with key points.

Complication follows. In film or the theater, this is the point at which the central character faces a challenge. Here the goal is to create a question about what happens next, about what the outcome will be.

Climax is the fourth phase. This is the occasion of greatest tension and uncertainty. Here the storyteller wants to use the connection established with the audience to create a deep understanding with the central character.

Reversal is the point in the story where the central character's condition is changed, often becoming worse—too often, irreversibly so.

Falling action is the point in the story where the central character's characteristics cause personal loss. Here the goal is to show the unintended consequences of actions taken with which the audience can readily identify. The goal is to expose vulnerability and teach lessons of loss.

Denouement is the final point in the story in which stability is lost or new equilibrium attained. One can learn from the experience of the story and achieve a higher level of function or the challenge can remain unmet and the lesson remain unlearned.

In this framework, there are two points of inflection, two points that change the course of the story and the trending direction of the line. The first is the *inciting incident* or the distress. This is the event that changes the arc of the story or the course of history. The second is the *resolution*, which represents the intervention or action that produces the final result or state. This could be an invention, innovation,

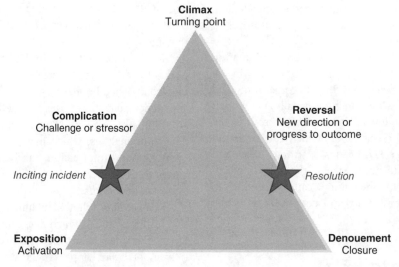

Figure 29.2 The Freytag Pyramid (1863).

Modified from Freytag, G. (1894). *Freytag's technique of the drama, an exposition of dramatic composition and art by Dr. Gustav Freytag: An authorized translation from the sixth German edition by Elias J. MacEwan, M.A.* (3rd ed.). Scott, Foresman and Company.

intervention, or policy and is a point of interest in population health.

This phased construction is presented in **Figure 29.2**. Developed as a framework for writing drama, it applies quite effectively to the construction of stories in the domain of population health where the intent is not to exaggerate drama. Quite the opposite, population health stories will be most effective when they create appreciation for the experience, understanding of risk, and exploration of options with the potential to achieve favorable outcomes without hyperbole or overplay of drama.

Visual Storytelling

Visual storytelling helps achieve the goal of explaining rather than exploring a topic. For this reason, it is particularly well suited to the telling of data-rich stories.

Exploratory Data

Exploratory use of data refers to efforts to present the big picture and situate important points in context. Imagine you have 100 oysters and want to tell a story about them (**Figure 29.3**, Knaflic,

Exploratory

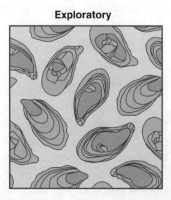

Explanatory

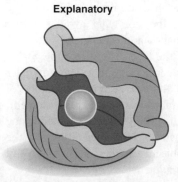

Figure 29.3 Exploratory & Explanatory Data in Story.

2015). You might have 100 different oysters, and you might want to pose 100 hypotheses about them. That analysis and those findings would be exploratory in nature. You zoom in to understand the one oyster and you zoom out to understand the 100. You take the audience with you in your storytelling by zooming out to provide context.

Explanatory Data

Explanatory use of data refers to efforts to present the picture in detail and to create deep understanding in context. Here you have a single oyster (Figure 29.3) and you want to tell a story about that one. You zoom in to understand the one oyster fully, and you take the audience with you.

There are two particularly useful approaches to telling story with data. Both can help connect to the reader and provide context that enriches understanding; both can achieve impact, understanding, and retention. The first is infographics, and the second is social math.

Infographics

An *infographic* is a "visual representation of data, information or knowledge that tells a story through visual communication" (CDC, n.d.-a). Pie charts, bar graphs, line graphs, spider plots, timelines, lists, flowcharts, and visual articles are among the more common forms of infographics.

Much like the storytelling device of imagery, infographics create a memorable and sophisticated understanding of the concept to be conveyed. Not to be confused with imagery, which uses words to create rich sensory impressions in the mind's eye, infographics can present that same data in visual form. This approach has the potential to support integration of complex information and establish deeper understanding of findings (Miciklas, 2012).

The spread of infectious disease is influenced by many variables. Data can predict the number of individuals who would contract illnesses from the first person infected. **Figure 29.4** shows the increase in Covid cases following a motorcycle rally.

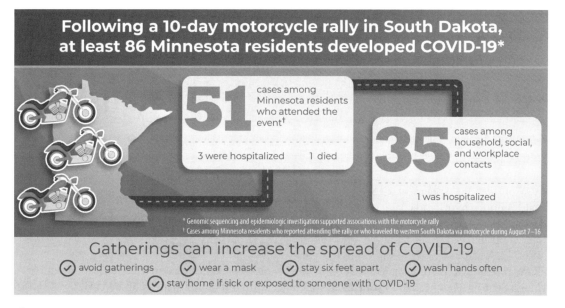

Figure 29.4 Motorcycle Rally and Covid Cases.

Reproduced from Firestone, M. J., Wienkes, H., Garfin, J., Wang, X., Vilen, K., Smith, K. E., Holzbauer, S., Plumb, M., Pung, K., Medus, C., Yao, J. D., Binnicker, M. J., Nelson, A. C., Yohe, S., Como-Sabetti, K., Ehresmann, K., Lynfield, R., & Danila, R. (2020). COVID-19 outbreak associated with a 10-day motorcycle rally in a neighboring state–Minnesota, August–September 2020. *Morbidity and Mortality Weekly Report, 69*(47), 1771–1776. http://doi.org/10.15585/mmwr.mm6947e1

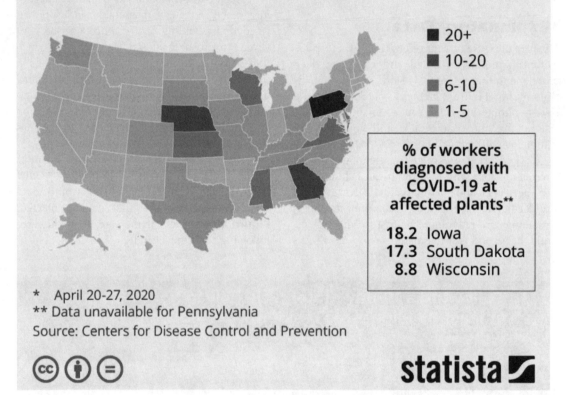

COVID-19 Detected At Meat Processing Plants In 19 States

Number of meat processing plants
reporting COVID-19 cases in U.S. states*

■ 20+
■ 10-20
■ 6-10
■ 1-5

% of workers diagnosed with COVID-19 at affected plants**

18.2 Iowa
17.3 South Dakota
8.8 Wisconsin

* April 20-27, 2020
** Data unavailable for Pennsylvania
Source: Centers for Disease Control and Prevention

statista ◢

Figure 29.5 Infographic of Coronavirus Cases at Meat-Processing Plants.

Consider the spread of COVID-19. Public health entities have worked to present complex data to the public and to policy makers in ways that contribute to understanding and inform action. Infographics have been central to that effort. A granular picture of COVID-19 in the United States is presented in **Figure 29.5**, which illustrates the COVID-19 cases at meat-processing plants in 19 states.

These examples of infographics demonstrate complex data in ways that can be clearly understood. They are easy to read and hard to ignore.

Social Math

Social math is closely related to the infographic. It is used to amplify meaning by creating relatable, memorable connections. The more precisely the storyteller can connect content to existing understanding, the better the impact of the story. This is the focus of social math.

Table 29.1 Steps to Constructing Info Graphics and Social Math Objects

	Step	Detail
1	Understand your message	Begin with an understanding of the message you want to convey that requires a thorough understanding of the content.
2	Know the data forward and backward	Work from the results of your analyses. Determine the most critical and valuable points.
3	Break down the data	Consider the data with respect to time (historical or longitudinal data) or place (geographic distribution).
4	Make the data personable and relatable	Draw correspondence to data with which the audience is familiar. Aim for everyday references as points of reference.
5	Make ironic comparisons	Irony is a device that needs to be used like an expensive spice. It can have great impact when used carefully. It is a powerful memory device and a persuasive tactic in storytelling.
6	Establish connections	Use images and references to which your audience can relate and are likely to remember.
7	Tell the reader what you have said	Circle back around to the key points you intend to make. Assure you provide data and image to support each and every one.

Social math is a practice that uses easy to visualize comparisons to make large numbers comprehensible and compelling. Using social math allows advocates to talk about statistics and data by placing them in a *social* context that provides meaning (Community Change, n.d., para. 1).

Social math is a simple way to make data that include large numbers easier to grasp by relating them to things that we already understand. It is an analogy based on numbers. It is a tool to combine the emotional impact of stories with the power of data. It is a way of presenting numbers in a real-life, familiar context to help people see the story behind them. (Heffernan, 2017).

Consider the information presented in **Figure 29.17** in Case Study 3 of this chapter. A presentation that uses social math provides context to the rate of diabetes using examples that are easily understood and relatable. The association of the size of the population with diabetes to the size of the population in four states easily shows the relativeness of the problem.

A stepwise approach to creating infographics and social math objects is helpful, especially when first attempting these techniques. **Table 29.1** lays out these steps.

Creating a Credible Narrative around Population Health Data and Analytics

Population health is a discipline rich with data. Those who practice it demand data and are prepared and committed to giving them careful consideration. Those who are influenced by data—or need to be—may be less experienced and less committed. They can be expected to require guidance, and telling story with data can provide it.

Credibility is *the quality of being believable or worthy of trust* (Dictionary.com, n.d.-c). Scientists, who prize precision and clarity, have come to face increasing public scrutiny and distrust. Some members of the public worry that scientists create or cite so-called alternative facts and worry that spurious conclusions result in undue influence on policy because of bias introduced by sponsors and industry. To increase public understanding and merit trust, the careful and complete telling of stories accompanied by relatable human experiences and clear, well-presented analytics may prove useful. Stories can convey the nuanced messages the public needs to hear and understand especially in relation to population health.

Planning and Developing a Population Health Analytics Story

Telling a population health story is about creating understanding of the health of a select group of individuals. This is commonly captured in the language of outcomes and big data. Such stories are perfectly suited to the use of narrative, numbers, and images. Arranging the marriage of narrative to analytics can provide a more useful and practical understanding of the magnitude of the population health challenge.

To demonstrate application of the concepts and strategies introduced in this chapter, three case studies will be presented. The first uses visualization software to present data: its purpose is to demonstrate data visualization techniques and the nuances in graphics that lead to differing story lines. The second is abstracted from open access public sources and told as one would share a narrative in print. The third is derived using secondary analysis of proprietary data and presented in the form of slides to be used at a public presentation. Each combines narrative, data, and images with the intent to move the reader to care, remember, or act.

Case Study 1: Storytelling Using Tableau

Courtesy of Jonathan Goodhue.

The way data are presented plays a huge role in the way that information is received. Careful selection of the style and presentation radically affects the impact that data have on an audience. Tableau is a powerful software tool that facilitates visualizing data; it can be used to select the best way to share data based on the message to be received.

Consider data about driving in the United States. If the concern is about fatalities, there are several ways to present information about collisions that can affect how the story progresses. **Figure 29.6** shows all fatal collisions and highlights the fact that the majority of collisions were not by speeders. The letters represent different states, and the visualization shows that the story is the same across all states: The majority of collisions are experienced by nonspeeders.

The states in Figure 29.6 are sorted descending by the number of fatal collisions and answers the question, "Which state has the highest amount of fatal collisions?" In this case, state A is first. If the question is, "Which state has the highest ratio of speeders to drivers?" the data could be put into descending order by the number of speeders. This is shown in **Figure 29.7**, where state K has the highest number of speeders in fatal collisions.

Maps in Tableau are easy to make and are valuable for storytelling. **Figure 29.8** shows the density of the percentage of drivers involved in fatal collisions who were speeding across the United States. If the story more closely focuses on speeding across the United States and related fatalities, then this may be a more effective presentation.

One look reveals that speeding is a concern in most states across the country, though seemingly less so in states such as New Mexico and Nebraska. The right combination of visuals can convey a lot of different information. For this reason, it is important to make careful selections to be sure the desired story is told.

The way data are presented plays a critical role in how they are received. Being able to display information in a manner that is accessible and easily visualized goes a long way. Data visualization software like Tableau is immensely powerful in ensuring that a data story unfolds quickly and completely.

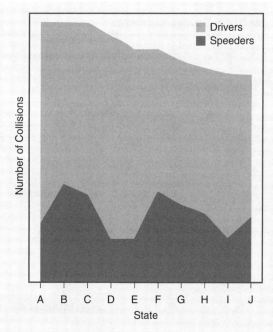

Figure 29.6 Drivers Involved in Fatal Collisions.

Data from Chalabi, M. (2014). *Dear Mona, which state has the worst drivers?* FiveThirtyEight. https://fivethirtyeight.com/features/which-state-has-the-worst-drivers

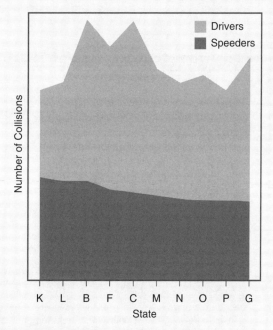

Figure 29.7 Drivers Involved in Fatal Collisions per Billion Miles Driven, Sorted Descending by the Number of Speeders.

Data from Chalabi, M. (2014). *Dear Mona, which state has the worst drivers?* FiveThirtyEight. https://fivethirtyeight.com/features/which-state-has-the-worst-drivers

(continues)

Case Study 1: Storytelling Using Tableau *(continued)*

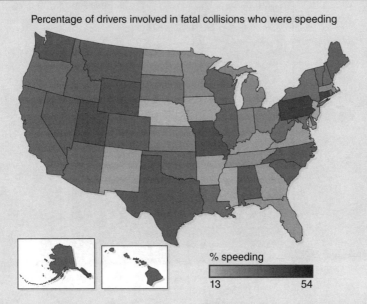

Percentage of drivers involved in fatal collisions who were speeding

Figure 29.8 Geomap Showing Density of the Percentage of Drivers Involved in Fatal Collisions Who Were Speeding.

Data from Chalabi, M. (2014). *Dear Mona, which state has the worst drivers?* FiveThirtyEight. https://fivethirtyeight.com/features/which-state-has-the-worst-drivers

Case Study 2: Storytelling from Open Access Public Sources

The opioid crisis is an extremely complex population health story that can be effectively told using data, image, and story. The more society understands this problem, the more fully it will grasp its scope and impact and the more likely effective interventions can be developed and implemented.

The Opening That Grabs the Reader

The scale of the opioid problem in the United States is stunning. More than 130 people die every day from overdoses of opioids such as fentanyl and heroin and other prescription pain relievers. That is an increase of greater than 1,000% per year since 1980 (Schnell, 2019). During 2018, some 10.3 million Americans acknowledged misusing prescription opioids (U.S. Department of Health and Human Services, n.d.). The epidemic of misuse costs the United States $78.5 billion a year (Addiction Center, n.d.).

This story begins with a hook (a strong and clear statement that draws readers in and leaves them wanting more). It incorporates data and foreshadows what is to come. A recent survey reveals some 69% of Americans could understand how a person might become accidentally addicted (American Pharmacists Association, 2017). Of note is that locations where opioids are more routinely prescribed are also areas where more opioid deaths are more commonly reported (Schnell & Currie, 2018).

At the annual meeting of the American College of Physicians in 2019, one physician opened his remarks about the crisis with this challenging statement to his colleagues. "Responsibility for the problem and its solution rests with us all." Controversial, direct, and engaging, the opening in **Figure 29.9** foreshadows his major thesis.

Increasing Action and Complication

The story can be told effectively using a combination of anecdote and data. In the case of the opioid crisis, there is no shortage of unsettling and heartbreaking stories.

I actually don't blame the pharmaceutical companies (for the opioid crisis), I blame our healthcare system, which left an opening for industry, and they took the opening.

—Charles Reznikoff, MD

Figure 29.9 The Engaging Opening.

Reproduced from Frieden, J. (2019, April 14). *Don't just blame drug companies for the opioid crisis—Healthcare system 'left an opening for industry,' expert says.* https://www.medpagetoday.com/meetingcoverage/acp/79220

The Compelling Anecdote: One Person's Experience

Here one 22-year-old tells a story of addiction and abuse that is at once persuasive and credible. Her story develops the complexity of the problem and engages the audience. Her story connects with the brain, stimulating oxytocin and empathy. She is relatable in ways that no one wants to acknowledge. Her story, at once memorable and distressing, is presented in **Figure 29.10**.

Abbey Zorzi, 22 (in her own words)

Everyone knows what a drug addict looks like, right?

I used to picture an addict as someone under a bridge with a needle in his arm. The end of addiction might look that way, but it sure doesn't begin like that. I never pictured myself as a drug addict until I became one as a teenager.

I'm 22 now, and I've been clean for a little over 2 years. My experiences inspired me to become an addiction specialist, and I came to the Fred Rogers Archive to learn what Mister Rogers had to say on the topic of addiction.

I found a 1971 article by Fred Rogers called "Children and Magic and Drug Abuse." While reading this article, I felt emotionally connected to his words. My struggles mirrored much of what he wrote. I'm sharing my story to help adults and young people understand that addiction doesn't always look like we think it does.

As a child, I had a loving family, a love of competition and sports, and good grades. My future was looking bright. What could possibly go wrong?

Like any teenager, I wanted to fit in with kids my age. Going to parties and drinking alcohol was the norm in high school. Everyone else was doing it. Why shouldn't I? During my freshman year I discovered that the euphoria from alcohol beat the adrenaline rush from making a game-winning shot in basketball. Alcohol became a security blanket for me. It covered up the self-confidence problems that I had secretly felt my whole life. I didn't think alcohol was a problem. Life continued to go on as I drank it away. This was just the beginning of a long, miserable journey.

When I had my wisdom teeth removed as a sophomore in high school, the doctor prescribed Vicodin for the pain. I didn't know much about drug addiction or what drugs could do to a person's body. I took more Vicodin than the doctor prescribed. I went through two bottles of the stuff in just one week. When I ran out, I started to have frequent headaches and cravings.

Friends of mine told me where I could buy narcotics so I wouldn't have to keep going through withdrawal. I started to buy Vicodin off the streets. I continued to chase the high because I loved the way it made me feel. As my tolerance for the Vicodin increased, I needed more and more to get the effect I wanted. I started to use stronger narcotics such as Percocet, OxyContin, Opana, and morphine. When the pills on the street became too expensive, heroin became a viable option.

When I found heroin, I told myself that I'd never inject it because the needles just scared me too much. (My mother used to have to hold me down at the doctor's office when I needed a vaccine.) But my addiction told me otherwise. Not more than two weeks into using the drug, I switched to injecting it.

I thought to myself, "This is what falling in love feels like." Heroin became my best friend, my significant other, and, ultimately, my abusive domestic partner. We had a love–hate relationship. After a week or two of using, I felt trapped and scared. I experienced a moment when I knew in my heart there was no turning back. Heroin had total control over my life, physically and mentally. Once that drug was in me, it told me what to do. I didn't take heroin; heroin took me.

Figure 29.10 The Anecdote: First Person Experience with Addiction—Abbey Zorzi, 22.

Reproduced from Zorzi, A. (2019). *Abbey Zorzi, 22.* https://www.getsmartaboutdrugs.gov/consequences/true-stories/abbey-zorzi-22

(continues)

Case Study 2 *(continued)*

This personal story is powerful as presented in the words of the people affected. The story can be further developed and its relevance expanded by adding data presented in carefully constructed infographics obtained from reliable sources. Such a source might be an experienced analyst in the community or a reliable institution.

The Crisis Over Time

The remarkable rise in use and deaths can be understood to have progressed in three phases. Deaths attributed to use of prescription opioids came first, beginning in the late 1990s and plateauing around 2010. Heroin overdose deaths followed, rose steeply beginning in 2010, and then appeared to plateau in 2016. Finally, deaths attributed to synthetic opioids made up the third wave. Deaths from this crisis continue to rise, destroy lives, command resources, and ruin families. This is the story told by National Vital Health Statistics in **Figure 29.11**.

The Centers for Disease Control and Prevention (CDC) converted these data to a different infographic designed to be more readily understood by the public. The story in **Figure 29.12** is the same, but it is intended for a different and broader audience. The outcome is the same. Some 399,000 people lost their lives to addiction and overdose.

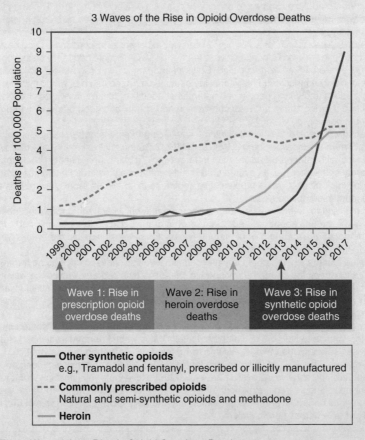

Figure 29.11 Three Waves of the Rise in Opioid Overdose Deaths.

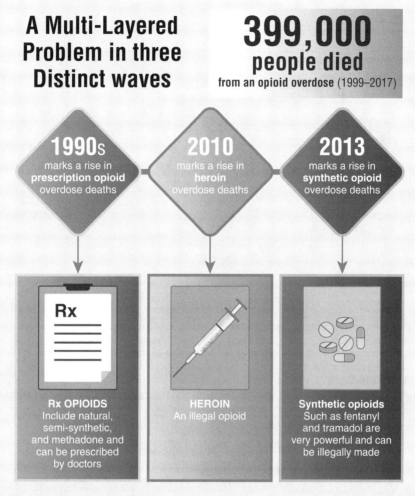

A Multi-Layered Problem in three Distinct waves

399,000 people died from an opioid overdose (1999–2017)

1990s marks a rise in **prescription opioid** overdose deaths

2010 marks a rise in **heroin** overdose deaths

2013 marks a rise in **synthetic opioid** overdose deaths

Rx

Rx OPIOIDS Include natural, semi-synthetic, and methadone and can be prescribed by doctors

HEROIN An illegal opioid

Synthetic opioids Such as fentanyl and tramadol are very powerful and can be illegally made

Figure 29.12 Rise in Opioid Overdose Deaths in America.

Reproduced from Centers for Disease Control and Prevention/National Center for Health Statistics. (n.d.-b). *Opioid overdose: Opioid data analysis and resources.* Retrieved 2018, from https://www.cdc.gov/drugoverdose/data/analysis.html

Impactful Visual Storytelling: Opioids across the United States

Across the nation, the number of communities impacted by the opioid crisis is increasing, and the number of deaths resulting from it continues to rise.

Cool blue areas on the map of the United States report low mortality numbers and those areas in warmer colors—yellow, orange, and red—report higher numbers of deaths. Over time, more communities across the United States report higher numbers of deaths. A visual such as this would be easy to interpret and incredibly distressing to see.

The Story of Opioids across the Globe

The appetite for opioids and the resultant devastation across the globe is remarkable. This is the story told in **Figure 29.13**.

Marry the data in Figures 29.11 through 29.13 to the anecdote in Figure 29.10 and to the concern expressed in Figure 29.9 and you have a fuller and more memorable understanding on which to ground

(continues)

Case Study 2 *(continued)*

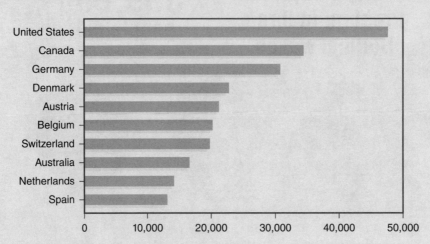

Figure 29.13 Opioid Consumption by Country.

Courtesy of U.N. International Narcotics Control Board.

research, intervention, strategy, and advocacy. Together these components of story create a compelling call to action. That is the point made in **Figures 29.14** and **29.15**.

The Climax of This Story

Neither data nor anecdote indicate that addiction and the resultant deaths have reached a peak or have begun to decline. People are dying, families are suffering, and communities are experiencing great loss.

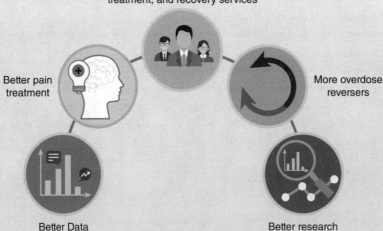

Figure 29.14 Evidence-Based Solutions.

Courtesy of United States Department of Health & Human Services.

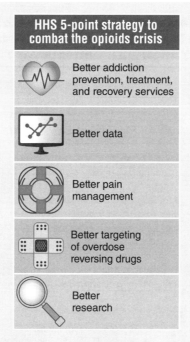

Figure 29.15 Evidence-Based Solutions.

Reproduced from Khanna, G. (2018, February 14). *AHRQ stands ready to assist Secretary Azar in the fight against opioid epidemic* [Blog post]. AHRQ views. Agency for Healthcare Research and Quality. https://www.ahrq .gov/news/blog/ahrqviews/opioid-5-point-strategy.html

Images of the Opioids Crisis

Privacy issues and the need to demonstrate respect for those affected create challenges to the effective use of images in the telling of the story.

This image of a naloxone overdose response kit, which can save lives, tells a positive part of the story. Sadly, it addresses a symptom (overdose) rather than the root cause of opioid deaths. Still, these images add value and clarity to the telling of the story (**Figure 29.16**).

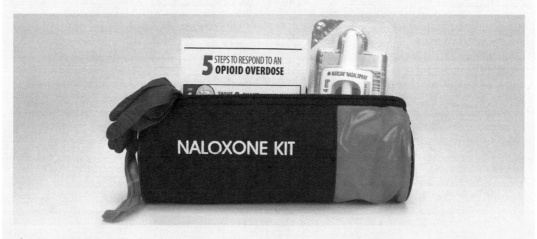

Figure 29.16 Image Used to Tell a Positive Part of the Story.

Case Study 3: Storytelling Using Proprietary Data in the Form of a Slide Presentation: A New Predictive Model to Identify High-Risk Patients with Diabetes

Contributed by Donna Logan

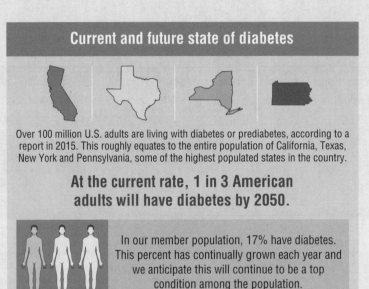

Figure 29.17 The Opening That Grabs the Reader.

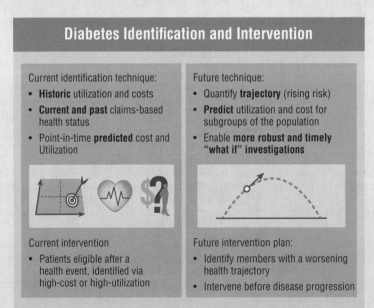

Figure 29.18 Increasing Action and Complication.

New Model to Identify Members for Diabetes Program

New population health model was built and tested on diabetic members in our population. The model performs accurately.

When the model was applied to our current population, we discovered:

- Utilization and cost increases with age, regardless of diabetes diagnosis. However, utilization does not increase until age 35.
- However, using standardized density, we can see when diabetics and nondiabetics utilize the same amount, diabetics are more expensive.
  - **Opportunity:** If there is a gap between the peak of the diabetic curve and the nondiabetic curve, there is an opportunity to intervene and bring the diabetic utilization/cost down.

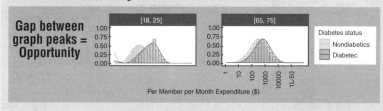

Figure 29.19 The Compelling Anecdote: One Entity's Experience.

New Model to Identify Members for Diabetes Program

When identifying members for a new program focused on identifying those who have an opportunity, we want to focus on the gap between the peaks in the histograms below. From these results we can see there is a divergence from age 18 to age 65.

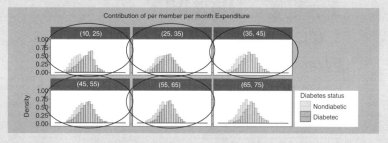

Since utilization increases after age 35 and the difference between diabetic and nondiabetic utilization stops at 65, the ideal age range for the intervention is between 35 and 65.

Question:

- Who would be the perfect candidate for a new diabetes intervention program, aimed at reducing the progression of diabetes and avoid a worsening health state?

Figure 29.20 Infographics that Clarify and Connect.

(continues)

Case Study 3: Storytelling Using Proprietary Data in the Form of a Slide Presentation: A New Predictive Model to Identify High-Risk Patients with Diabetes *(continued)*

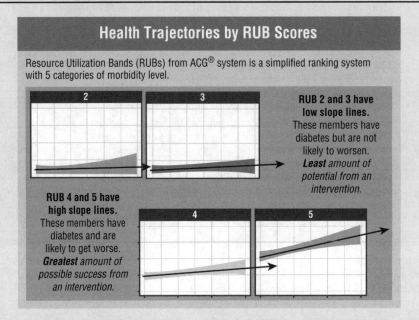

Figure 29.21 The Crisis Over Time.

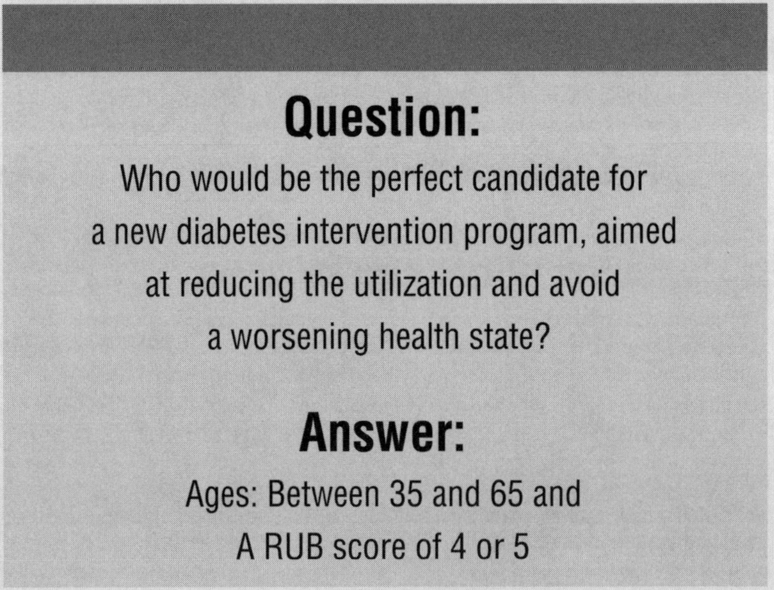

Question:
Who would be the perfect candidate for a new diabetes intervention program, aimed at reducing the utilization and avoid a worsening health state?

Answer:
Ages: Between 35 and 65 and
A RUB score of 4 or 5

Figure 29.22 Interaction with the Audience.

Perfect Practice Makes Perfect

Once the story is constructed and refined, the selected components have been integrated, and it has been carefully reviewed and edited, it is time to rehearse delivery. If the story is to be told on paper, peer review by an unbiased colleague can be helpful. Ask a reader who can represent the intended audience. Ask an experienced colleague. If the story is to be presented orally in public, take time to run through the slides under conditions similar to those in the venue. Here are some other suggestions:

- Invite peer review.
- Go to the back of the room and be merciless.

- If slides are too crowded, remedy the problem.
- If colors do not work, choose others.
- Eliminate redundancies and correct omissions.
- Speak aloud, make notes, monitor timing, and police for nervous patterns of speech ("um" and "uh"). Try the narratives on for size.
- Make sure all words are familiar and comfortable.
- Emphasize or accentuate the important points.

Figure 29.23 contains a review tool that can be used to help ensure satisfaction with decisions about inclusion, exclusion, and emphasis; evaluate story components; and provide constructive criticism to peers.

Well Done	Moderately Done	Needs Improvement	Criteria	Comment
Strength of Storytelling				
☐	☐	☐	Opening is clear and captures attention	
☐	☐	☐	Explicitly states question to be answered	
☐	☐	☐	Defines key concepts and terms	
☐	☐	☐	Uses expository rather than exploratory approach	
☐	☐	☐	Adjusts message to the target audience	
☐	☐	☐	Uses anecdote effectively	
☐	☐	☐	Uses humor effectively	
☐	☐	☐	Uses images effectively	
☐	☐	☐	Highlights important information	
☐	☐	☐	Connects with audience	
☐	☐	☐	Memorable conclusion reinforces key points	
Strength of Analytics				
☐	☐	☐	Uses social math effectively	
☐	☐	☐	Uses infographics effectively	
☐	☐	☐	Eliminates distractions	
☐	☐	☐	Creates a visual hierarchy of information	
☐	☐	☐	Uses critical thinking skills to structure argument	
☐	☐	☐	Simplifies information	
☐	☐	☐	Makes robust use of text	
☐	☐	☐	Breaks down analysis appropriately to tell story	
☐	☐	☐	Makes the message personal	

Figure 29.23 Story Proofing and Evaluation Document.

Conclusion

Those who practice in population health are endowed with an abundance of data. This book describes the logic, process, and tools to manage those data in service of accurate understanding. This chapter explains how one can surround data with compelling story in service of impact and asserts that another set of tools, those of storytellers, strongly complement analytics. Well-crafted and well-told story has the capacity to extend the reach and the impact of science and analytics.

Curating the collection of the analyses and results is essential. There comes a point of diminishing return when adding more data detracts from meaning and memory. So, making good choices about what analyses to report and how to communicate the findings plays a vital role in ensuring the data have their best impact.

The rules of good storytelling encourage you to tell the reader what you plan to say, say it, and then remind them of what you have said. In the case of population health analytics, this practice will help ground the data in story and promote retention of data. It will allow the audience to reflect, connect, and question in support of clear understanding.

Study and Discussion Questions

- What are the components of a great story?
- How can storytelling enhance the impact of population health analytics?
- What are social math and infographics and how do they apply to analytics and population health?
- Describe one benefit of storytelling that would support your work?
- Tell a fascinating story about a recent population health project you have conducted.

Resources and Websites

Center for Teaching. (2020). Understanding by design. Nashville, TN: Vanderbilt University. https://cft.vanderbilt.edu//cft/guides-sub-pages/understanding-by-design/

Few, S. (2004). Perceptual edge. http://www.perceptualedge.com/

Teaching for Enduring Understanding: https://iteachu.af.edu/enduring-understandings/

TEDx Talks. (2017, March 16). The magical science of storytelling | David JP Phillips | TEDxStockholm [Video]. YouTube. https://www.youtube.com/watch?v=Nj-hdQMa3uA

References

Addiction Center. (n.d.). The opioid epidemic. https://www.addictioncenter.com/opiates/opioid-epidemic/

Agency for Healthcare Research and Quality. (2018). AHRQ stands ready to assist Secretary Azar in the fight against opioid epidemic. Agency for Healthcare Research and Quality. https://www.ahrq.gov/news/blog/ahrqviews/opioid-5-point-strategy.html

American Pharmacists Association. (2018, May 11). Nearly one in three people know someone addicted to opioids: APA poll. https://www.pharmacist.com/article/nearly-one-three-people-know-someone-addicted-opioids-apa-poll

Baldick, C. (2001). *The Oxford dictionary of literary terms* (3rd ed.). Oxford University Press. https://www.oxfordreference.com/view/10.1093/acref/9780199208272.001.0001/acref-9780199208272

Bowen, R. S. (2017). Understanding by design. Vanderbilt University Center for Teaching. https://cft.vanderbilt.edu/understanding-by-design/

Centers for Disease Control and Prevention. (n.d.-a). Infographics. https://www.cdc.gov/socialmedia/tools/InfoGraphics.html

Reproduced from Centers for Disease Control and Prevention/National Center for Health Statistics. (n.d.-b). Opioid overdose: Opioid data analysis and resources. Retrieved 2018, from https://www.cdc.gov/drugoverdose/data/analysis.html

Centers for Disease Control and Prevention & National Center for Health Statistics. (n.d.-c). Opioid overdose: Understanding the epidemic. Retrieved 2018, from https://www.cdc.gov/drugoverdose/epidemic/index.html

Chalabi, M. (2014). *Dear Mona, which state has the worst drivers?* FiveThirtyEight. https://fivethirtyeight.com/features/which-state-has-the-worst-drivers

Community Change. (n.d.). *Power from the ground up.* https://housingtrustfundproject.org/campaigns/making-your-case/communication-strategy/being-heard/social-math/

Dahlstrom, M. F. (2014, September 16). Using narratives and storytelling to communicate science with non-expert audiences. *Proceedings of the National Academy of Sciences, 16*(111), 13614–13620. https://www.pnas.org/content/111/Supplement_4/13614

Dictionary.com. (n.d.-a). Humor—defined. https://www.dictionary.com/browse/humor?s=t

Dictionary.com. (n.d.-b). Anecdote—defined. https://www.dictionary.com/browse/anecdote?s=t

Dictionary.com. (n.d.-c). Credibility—defined. https://www.dictionary.com/browse/credibility?s=t

Drug Enforcement Administration. (n.d.). Abbey Zorzi, 22. Get smart about drugs. https://www.getsmartaboutdrugs.gov/consequences/true-stories/abbey-zorzi-22

Firestone, M. J., Wienkes, H., Garfin, J., Wang, X., Vilen, K., Smith, K. E., Holzbauer, S., Plumb, M., Pung, K., Medus, C., Yao, J. D., Binnicker, M. J., Nelson, A. C., Yohe, S., Como-Sabetti, K., Ehresmann, K., Lynfield, R., & Danila, R. (2020). COVID-19 outbreak associated with a 10-day motorcycle rally in a neighboring state–Minnesota, August–September 2020. *Morbidity and Mortality Weekly Report, 69*(47), 1771–1776. http://doi.org/10.15585/mmwr.mm6947e1

Fitzgerald, F. S. (1925). *The great Gatsby.* Charles Scribner's Sons.

Freytag, G. (1894). *Freytag's technique of the drama, An exposition of dramatic composition and art by Dr. Gustav Freytag: An authorized translation from the sixth German edition by Elias J. MacEwan, M.A.* (3rd ed.). Scott, Foresman & Company. https://openlibrary.org/books/OL7168981M/Freytag's_Technique_of_the_drama

Frieden, J. (2019). *Don't just blame drug companies for the opioid crisis.* MEDPAGE Today. https://www.medpagetoday.com/meetingcoverage/acp/79220

Gallo, C. (2016). *The storyteller's secret.* St. Martin's Griffin.

Gehrig, L. (1939) *Farewell to baseball. American rhetoric: Top 100 speeches.* https://www.americanrhetoric.com/speeches/lougehrigfarewelltobaseball.htm

Goldman, W. (1973). *The princess bride: S. Morgenstern's classic tale of true love and high adventure.* Harcourt.

Heffernan, P. (2017, August 10). *Changing minds: Social math, stories and framing* [Blog post]. Change Conversations. https://www.marketing-partners.com/conversations2/changing-minds-social-math-stories-and-framing

Just Think Twice. (n.d.). Get the facts about drugs. https://www.justthinktwice.gov/true-stories/chelsea-marie-heptig-17-ecstasy

Kennedy, J. F. (1962). *John F. Kennedy moon speech.* https://er.jsc.nasa.gov/seh/ricetalk.htm

Khaneman, D. (2011). *Thinking fast and slow.* Farrar, Straus & Giroux.

Khanna, G. (2018, February 14). AHRQ stands ready to assist Secretary Azar in the fight against opioid epidemic [Blog post]. *AHRQ Views.* Agency for Healthcare Research and Quality. https://www.ahrq.gov/news/blog/ahrqviews/opioid-5-point-strategy

Knaflic, C. N. (2015). *Telling story with Dara.* Wiley.

Lee, H. (1960). *To kill a mockingbird.* J. B. Lippincott & Co.

Mandela, N. (1964). *I am prepared to die.* https://www.historyplace.com/speeches/mandela.htm

Martin, K., & Miller, E. (1988). Storytelling and science. *Language Arts, 65*(3), 255–259. http://www.jstor.org/stable/41411379

McCarthy, N. (2020). COVID-19 detected at meat plants in 19 U.S. states. *Statista.* https://www.statista.com/chart/21585/meat-processing-plants-reporting-coronavirus-cases

Miciklas, M. (2012). The power of infographics: Using pictures to communicate and connect with your audience. QUE.

Monarth, H. (2014, March 11). The irresistible power of storytelling as a strategic business tool. *Harvard Business Review* [online]. https://hbr.org/2014/03/the-irresistible-power-of-storytelling-as-a-strategic-business-tool

Morrison, T. (2004). Beloved. Vintage Books.

National Health Care for the Homeless Council. (2017, August). Addressing the opioid epidemic: How the opioid crisis affects homeless populations. https://nhchc.org/wp-content/uploads/2019/08/nhchc-opioid-fact-sheet-august-2017.pdf

Orwell, G. (1949). *1984.* Secker & Warburg.

Quote Investigator. (2017, August 15). Aristotle? Dale Carnegie? J. H. Jowett? Fred E. Marble? Royal Meeker? Henry Koster? Anonymous? https://quoteinvestigator.com/2017/08/15/tell-em/

Rowling, J. K. (1997). *Harry Potter and the philosopher's stone.* Bloomsbury.

Schnell, M. (2019). The opioid crisis: Tragedy, treatments and trade-offs. Stanford, CA: Stanford Institute for Economic Policy Research. https://siepr.stanford.edu/research/publications/opioid-crisis

Schnell, M. & Currie, J. (2018). Addressing the opioid epidemic: Is there a role for physician education? *American Journal of Health Economics, 4*(3), 383–410. https://doi.org/10.1162/ajhe_a_00113

StarkEffects.com (2006.). The humorous story. http://www.starkeffects.com/humor.shtml

Stoert, G., Bailey, D. H., Moore, A. M., & Geary, D. C. (2016, April 21). Countries with higher levels of gender equality show larger national sex differences in mathematics anxiety and relatively lower parental mathematics valuation for girls. *PLoS ONE, 11*(4), e0153857. https://doi.org/10.1371/journal.pone.0153857

TEDx Talks. (2017, March 16). The magical science of storytelling | David JP Phillips | TEDxStockholm [Video]. YouTube. https://www.youtube.com/watch?v=Nj-hdQMa3uA

Tolstoy, L. (1887). *Anna Karenina*. Thomas Y. Crowell & Co.

Twain, M. (1897). How tell a story and others by Mark Twain (Samuel Clemens). Project Gutenberg eBook. http://www.gutenberg.org/files/3250/3250-h/3250-h.htm

U.S. Department of Health & Human Services. (n.d.). Strategy to combat opioid abuse, misuse, and overdose: A framework based on the five point strategy. https://www.hhs.gov/opioids/sites/default/files/2018-09/opioid-fivepoint-strategy-20180917-508compliant.pdf

U.S. Drug Enforcement Administration. (n.d.). Just think twice. https://www.justthinktwice.gov/true-stories/chelsea-marie-heptig-17-ecstasy

Villaire, M. (1992). Patricia Benner: Uncovering the wonders of skilled practice by listening to nurses' stories. *Critical Care Nursing, 12*(6), 82–89.

Walker, A. (1982). *The color purple*. Harcourt Press.

Wiggins, G., & McTighe, J. (1998). Backward design. In G. Wiggins & J. McTighe (Eds.), *Understanding by design* (pp. 13–34). Association for Supervision and Curriculum Development.

Zak, P. J. (2013, December 17). How stories change the brain. *Greater Good Magazine*. https://greatergood.berkeley.edu/article/item/how_stories_change_brain

Zak, P. J. (2014, October 28). Why your brain loves good storytelling. *Harvard Business Review*. https://hbr.org/2014/10/why-your-brain-loves-good-storytelling

Zak, P. J. (2015, January–February). Why inspiring stories make us react: The neuroscience of narrative. Cerebrum. https://www.ncbi.nlm.nih.gov/pmc/articles/PMC4445577/

Creating the Culture in Organizations

CHAPTER 30

Assessing Organizational Capabilities for Population Health Analytics

Martha Sylvia, PhD, MBA, RN
Evelyn Ann Borucki, MHA

Only when we are brave enough to explore the darkness will we discover the infinite power of our light.

—Brown (2010)

EXECUTIVE SUMMARY

Healthcare organizations are facing some of the biggest analytic challenges ever experienced in their histories. Coming out of an intense phase of investment in electronic medical records over the last decade, providers of health care are now challenged with using their data to optimize care delivery and achieve value-based care. This is all during and after the challenges of the COVID-19 pandemic in which the ways people access the healthcare system and health care is delivered are rapidly changing, with patients seeking alternatives to in-person maintenance visits and providers flocking to risk-based contracts in a world of fluctuating fee-for-service revenue (Basu, Phillips, Phillips, Peterson, & Landon, 2020; Preston, 2020).

These changes require healthcare organizations to have robust capabilities in managing and achieving value from their data and analytics programs. Unfortunately, these changes also come at a time when healthcare organizations are in the initial stages of ramping up analytic capabilities, especially in comparison to other industries and with a widening gap between healthcare organizations who are and are not able to invest in required resources. Although 70% of chief information officers in healthcare report having some type of organizationally integrated analytic strategy, the 30% without a strategy report lower levels of executive analytic leadership and enterprise-level data governance; less technical staff such as data architects, visualization developers, data scientists, and extract, transform, and load architects (Hagan, Graves, Kinsella, & Gerhardt, 2019).

The biggest challenges to achieving success in today's healthcare organizational priorities of analytics, artificial intelligence, and consumer engagement technology are related to funding, cultural change, and business processes with executive leadership struggling to make the business case for analytic transformation (Gilbert & Jones, 2019).

For healthcare organizations with a mandate to successfully engage in risk-bearing contracts requiring population-based care initiatives, the ability to assess organizational analytic capabilities accurately and completely is a crucial first step for success. Assessing organizational capabilities leads to a strategic vision and mission for analytics with tactical steps and milestones, the allocation of resources tied to return on investment for analytic expansion, and incremental achievement of analytic maturity.

LEARNING OBJECTIVES

At the end of this chapter, the learner will be able to:

1. Describe a framework for assessing organizational analytic capabilities.
2. Determine important domains for assessment of organizational capabilities for population health analytics.
3. Critique organizational capabilities for population health analytics.

Introduction

No matter where healthcare organizations sit in their journey to achieving advanced maturity for population health analytics, they need a yardstick to help them understand baseline capabilities, set strategies, develop road maps, determine milestones, and measure success. A comprehensive assessment of organizational analytic capabilities with a focus on those competencies specific to population health is the first step. This chapter tailors the review of organizational capabilities for population health analytics within the context of widely accepted and utilized frameworks across industries and within health care. Domains of assessment are specific to population health analytic requirements and are presented in a way that makes them readily applicable. Example application of the domains for assessing population health analytic capabilities are then applied in the form of survey and interview questions.

A Framework for Evaluating Organizational Capabilities

Utilizing a framework to assess an organization's capabilities creates a standardized method to identify specific areas for improvement and potential future strategies within an organization. Frameworks serve as a loose, conceptual outline that can be modified to fit the evaluation of any organization. One notable framework used across healthcare settings for quality and improvement is the Donabedian model.

In 1966, physician and researcher Avedis Donabedian developed the model to classify healthcare measures into structures, processes, and outcomes to examine the quality of healthcare organizations or services (Donabedian, 1980). Structures represent the who and what, including the physical environment and attributes employees bring to an organization. Processes represent the how, when, and what, including workflows and coordination of resources. Both structures and processes contribute to outcomes, which represents the why, including health-related changes, results, and satisfaction. There is overlap between the classifications, which contributes to the flexibility of the model when examining the organizational capabilities.

The structure, process, and outcome model is in alignment with well-known methods of assessing digital, information-technology, and analytics capabilities that follow a "people, process, and technology" scheme born out of process-improvement and information-technology frameworks (Prodan, Prodan, & Purcarea, 2015). The components used to assess capabilities are grounded in these existing frameworks but are tailored to the specific needs of developing organizational analytic maturity for population health analytics with the following domains.

People: individual skills, knowledge, experience are assessed along with the mix within and across teams. Data points include team size, structures supporting interdisciplinary practice, the balance between centralization and decentralization, and diversity.

Organizational culture supporting analytics: organizational social norms both formal and informal that guide the way employees approach their work, address issues at work, interact with others, and measure their success.

Strategic planning and executive engagement: existence and components of an analytic strategic plan with analytics included in an organization-wide strategy, the handling of data as a valuable commodity, and the assignment of ample resources and support for analytic initiatives.

Data sources and structure: data sources, their uses, and their ability to support population health analytic needs, including the structure of data.

Processes supporting analytic workflow: processes support collaboration and interdisciplinary work and manage large- to small-scale analytic projects and requests.

Processes used for data management: processes that support master data management, data governance, data warehousing, and data preparation.

Analytic methods: the capacity for executing analytic methods specific to population health analytics in support of the population health process and the extent to which methods are able to be operationalized in practice.

Analytic tools: data contextualizers and software used to analyze, report and visualize data; includes collaboration and project-management tools.

Value of analytic capabilities: refers to the outcomes and achievements of analytic products.

The capabilities in each domain are discussed in more detail in the following section.

Domains for Assessing Organizational Capabilities

When assessing organizational capabilities, it is important to examine factors within major domains that are important to the success of population health analytics. Each domain listed in the previous section is described in more detail here along with parameters to guide organizations so they might thrive in each realm.

People
Individuals

The structure of an organization revolves around the employed personnel, who heavily influence the work culture. The people of an organization represent the largest asset in many healthcare settings. Evaluating the people of an organization involves gathering information about their individual skills, knowledge, and experience for their position and as an asset to the organization. General information on the backgrounds of the employees working within analytics and supporting analytic infrastructure brings perspective into areas of achieving a diverse workforce and utilizing employee strengths efficiently.

These descriptions may include technical training and certifications or the projects they have completed or are currently developing in their role. Gathering genuine opinions about the organization from working employees provides valuable information. This information should also be compared to the actual job descriptions and examined on their alignment. Chapter 32, "Skills Assessment of Population Health Analysts," of the text provides detailed information for assessing analytic skills and knowledge.

Staffing Structures

In addition to the assessment of analytic personnel, the makeup of the entire stakeholder group for population health analytics is assessed in aggregate and in terms of how teams are structured. Chapter 31, "Building a Team Culture for Population Health," shows that the analyst works as part of the PopHealth Troika (PHT), with the business and clinical leads. In addition, analysts need to partner with technical staff members such as database administrators, data engineers and architects, and project managers.

Tending to diversity within analytic teams is key to successful results and needs to be undertaken intentionally by organizational leadership. Ensuring a diverse analytic workforce gives access to a greater range of talent, provides broader insight into understanding the needs of populations and subgroupings, and makes healthcare organizations more effective, successful, and profitable (Shemla, 2018). Diversity begins by ensuring representation from various cultures as well as race, color, religion, sex, pregnancy, sexual orientation, gender identity, national origin, age, disability, and genetic information. All of these extend to variation in personality and thought styles; cultural backgrounds and geographic locations; language, linguistics and accents; social roles; ideologies; behaviors; life experiences; socioeconomic status; and more (Reiners, 2020; U.S. Equal Employment Opportunity Commission, n.d.).

The analytic structure and bandwidth fall into this realm, assessing the physical infrastructure the analytics departments utilize on a regular basis. This includes elements such as proximity and access to resources to engage with coworkers and complete tasks. Analytic teams might work closely with another department, depending on the extent to which organizations collaborate and value interdisciplinary teamwork, as well as the ways in which data evolve into insights.

The structure of analytic units in healthcare organizations vary across the spectrum of centralized to decentralized. Models that work are blended to organize resources so that they can work across boundaries to gain insights that cannot be developed in silos. The ideal model combines centralized and decentralized functions to:

- accomplish a shared strategic and tactical plan for analytics;
- enable an enterprise view of analytics;
- optimize shared data infrastructure, knowledge sharing, communication, collaboration, and staff development;
- encourage innovation while retaining departmental flexibility;
- make it easier to match the right analyst to the right strategic project; and
- allow quick responsivity of analysts within units (Schlegel & Buytendijk, 2018).

Organizational Culture

Understanding organizational culture involves understanding the collective thought processes that inform behavior consciously and unconsciously. Organizational culture is a factor of the way the organization was originally formed; original founders and executive leadership within the organization; and the shared basic assumptions invented, discovered, or developed by groups as the culture learns to manage problems within and impacting the organization (Schein, 2010). Culture is assessed in terms of a wide range of organizationally experienced social phenomena, including:

- the influence of the individuals founding and leading the organization;
- formal and informal structures;
- characters and norms defined by the organization, including customary dress, language, behavior, beliefs, values, assumptions, symbols of status and authority (for example, parking spaces, lunch with the president, innovation awards);
- myths;
- ceremonies and rituals, and
- modes of deference and subversion (Scott et al., 2003).

These defining characteristics are shared by members of the organization and not necessarily what the individuals within the organization would ascribe to when on their own. For instance, it may be customary to speak English in work meetings, but individuals may speak their native language at home or when talking one-on-one with other staff members who also speak their native language. This alludes to one of the difficulties in changing organizational culture: it is often difficult to determine why certain cultural norms exist and where they originated, and organizational norms can be in conflict with individuals' cultural norms.

The organizational culture in health care for analytics is quite different, depending on the type of organization. Some healthcare organizations are primarily technology-based and ascribe to cultural norms found in other technology-based industries. On the other hand, when analytic departments are within an organization whose primary purpose is to deliver high-quality healthcare services on a budget and to use data as an asset to do so, the organizational culture for information technology, data infrastructure, and analytics exists within the broader healthcare delivery organization. When analytic divisions are within healthcare delivery organizations, there may be a technological subculture within the overall healthcare delivery system culture. In this scenario, analysts usually need to bridge the two cultures to accomplish their work, moving between clinically oriented and technically oriented organizational cultures.

Strategic Planning and Executive Engagement

Distinctive to data-driven population-focused healthcare delivery is the presence of an enterprise-wide strategy that includes a vision along with measurable objectives designed to advance the organization in analytic maturity and ensure success in executing the population health process. Healthcare executives agree that a clear and integrated analytic strategy is necessary, with 70% agreeing that one exists in their organization,

nearly double the agreement in just a 3-year period (Hagan et al., 2019). Health systems with an overarching strategy have a clear path to developing the basic infrastructure needed to support analytics; ensuring highly skilled and knowledgeable analytic executives, leadership, and staff; appropriate levels of investment in analytic resources; and an organizational culture that embraces analytic competency and maturity.

The strategic plan is assessed to determine the extent to which its vision clearly addresses the value of data as an asset and to which analytically related objectives are *specific, measurable, achievable, realistic*, and *time bound* (SMART) (University of Chicago Medicine, 2016). Once it is established that the enterprise-wide strategic plan adequately addresses analytics, departmental goals and objectives are assessed to determine that they also contain SMART objectives and tactics that can be tied back to the organizational strategy. In addition, budget allocation to analytics is assessed to ensure that the appropriate dollars are allotted to achieve analytic strategic objectives.

Data Sources and Structures

It is important to understand the data sources that are available, the ways in which these data sources are used currently, and the level at which data is structured to facilitate ease and flexibility for population-focused analyses. The data sources most commonly used in population health analytics and described in detail in Section 2, "Data Sources," of this textbook include data from medical claims, pharmacies, laboratories, electronic medical records, and social determinants of health sources. Some mix of these foundational data sources available for entire populations forms the basis for understanding health determinants and their link to health outcomes. Beyond these, other data sources can add richer dimension to analyses, including publicly available data measuring social determinants of health, water and air quality, use of community services, and emergency support systems; and data that can be acquired privately such as purchasing patterns, social media usage and interactions, and various survey data.

The ability to readily assemble populations and subgroupings from a person-centered data model, to concisely and consistently match patients by ID numbers, and to accurately and reliably validate the various types of data and information gathered throughout the analytic process are crucial to fully understanding the health risks of a defined population. These data form the infrastructure for the entire population health management program and are the basis of information used in the development of interventions specifically tailored to the needs of the target population. Ideally, data are structured in a population health data model (see Chapter 13, "The Population Health Data Model") after applying robust techniques to ensure data are well prepared and high quality (see Chapter 16, "Data Management and Preparation," and Chapter 17, "Assessing Data Quality").

Processes Supporting Analytic Workflow

The work of analytics for population health is accomplished through interdisciplinary execution of small- to large-scale projects and smaller ad hoc analyses and requests. When done well, analytic workflow takes on a structured process similar to the one depicted in **Figure 30.1**. In this example of analytic workflow, the process begins with a question that will be asked of the data. Next, a plan is devised to determine data sources, analytic methods, and the way in which the results of the analysis will turned into insights. Following the development of a plan, data are acquired and prepared for analysis, and analytic methods are applied. As the process moves toward visualizing data and developing insights, there may be times when previous steps need repeating—for instance, if different or more data are needed or data needs further preparation. The PHT works together in the discovery and insights phase to understand results and their application to the original data question. In the long term, solidified methods are placed into operational workflow

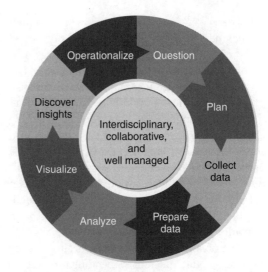

Figure 30.1 Analytic Workflow.

where they support the population health process in action.

Analytic workflow exists within an interdisciplinary and collaborative environment with strong project management support. Specific processes assessed in this realm include:

- the ways in which data-related questions are generated and whether they are congruent with a population health approach to addressing healthcare challenges;
- the use of systematic methods for vetting and prioritizing analytic projects and requests;
- the use of intentional methods of planning for an analysis prior to executing;
- the ease at which data are organized to support analyses at the person level and in aggregate;
- the extent to which data-preparation techniques must be applied by those in an analyst role prior to working on gaining insights;
- the use of processes that support interdisciplinary collaboration;
- the employment of project-management processes that support agile methods, rapid prototyping, and optimal time to insight; and
- the ease with which insights can be operationalized.

Processes Used for Data Management

Data are managed through processes of data governance, master data management (MDM), and data warehousing. The extent to which each of these functions are executed within an organization provides an understanding of the foundation for achieving high levels of analytic maturity.

Data Governance

Data governance is a system of decision rights and accountabilities for information-related processes, executed according to agreed-on models that describe who can take what actions with what information, when, under what circumstances, and using which methods (Thomas, n.d.). It is

> the policies, procedures and processes by which stewardship responsibilities are conceptualized and carried out. Data governance establishes the broad policies for access, management, and permissible uses of data; identifies the methods and procedures necessary to the stewardship process; and establishes the qualifications of those who would use the data and the conditions under which data access can be granted. (Rosenbaum, 2010)

The Data Governance Framework is a logical structure for organizing thoughts and communication for data governance concepts, developed by the Data Governance Institute (DGI). The framework and materials for data governance are adopted widely throughout a variety of industries and is suitable to use as a framework for governing the complexities of healthcare data and population health data in particular. The DGI framework lays out 10 universal components for governing data that can serve as criteria for evaluating data-governance programs for population health (**Table 30.1**). The assessment would determine the existence of each component along with the extent to which each component is performing.

Table 30.1 Components of Data Governance

Domain	Component
Rules and rules of engagement	1. Mission and vision 2. Goals, governance metrics, success measures, and funding strategies 3. Data rules and definitions 4. Decision rights 5. Accountabilities 6. Controls
People and organizational bodies	7. Data stakeholders 8. Data governance office 9. Data stewards
Processes	10. Proactive, reactive, and ongoing data-governance processes

Reproduced from Thomas, G. (n.d.). *The DGI data governance framework.* https://datagovernance.com/

Master Data Management

Master data include all of the data within a healthcare organization and typically refers to that which is core to its business operations and transactions. When referring to MDM for population health data, the focus is on managing data for the purposes of robust analytics at the person level. Chapter 16, "Data Management and Preparation," describes MDM and its components in more detail. A critical component of MDM for population health analytics is the ability to match identities of people, providers, and sites of care across multiple data sources. Once this core competency and the ability to systematically execute are established, top priorities for MDM in population health are:

- optimal preparation of data for population health analytics, including data intake, cleansing, and structuring (see Chapter 16, "Data Management and Preparation");
- the ability to attribute unique people to a unique primary care provider, identify unique providers across multiple disciplines within and across data sources, and attribute unique providers to the larger systems in

which they provide care (clinics, health systems, accountable care organizations, clinically integrated networks, and other at-risk entities); and

- high-quality data.

Chapter 17, "Assessing Data Quality," lays out the details of data quality assessment that should be used to assess organizational capabilities.

Data Warehousing

The ability to collect and manage large volumes of data requires electronic storage with updating capabilities and is best accomplished within a data warehouse. As discussed in Chapter 14, "Options for Warehousing Data for Population Analytics," and Chapter 15, "Process for Warehousing Data for Population Analytics," a data warehouse is a database system used to store, query, analyze, and report current and historical data (Panneerselvam, Liu, & Hill, 2015). It can include the entire system of data to facilitate not only day-to-day operations of the business but also population health analytics (Inmon, 1999). Chapters 14 and 15 lay out ideal options and processes for data warehousing for population health analytics and should be used as a guide for assessing organizational capabilities in this realm. At a high level, components of data warehousing that should be assessed are:

- the existence of a data warehouse structure and its use to create and store the data infrastructure necessary for population health analytics, and
- the extent to which data warehousing processes are optimized for population health analytics.

Analytic Methods

Although the population health process uses a wide assortment of analytic methods, one set of methods are vital to use in certain phases of the process. The assessment of population health analytic methods focuses on the ability of healthcare organizations to apply these certain analytic methods to data, whether they have the ability to do so in-house or use vendors and contractors for portions or all of the techniques. Once it is established that organizations have analytic methods capabilities, it is important to assess whether methods are applied appropriately and optimally to achieve population health objectives. Chapter 19, "Overview of Analytic Methods Used in Population Health Management," provides an overview of analytic methods applied to population health data and recommends their appropriate use in support of the population health process and can be used as a guideline when assessing organizational capabilities for population health analytic methods.

Analytic Tools and Technology

For a healthcare organization and its analytics department, the tools and technology are the resources that shape the structure and processes in a way that facilitates population health analytics. These tools include analytic software for applying methods to data, data contextualizers and groupers, and data visualization and reporting products. The tools and technology assessment determines whether available tools are adequate to achieve population health analytic goals and the extent to which tools are appropriately used and optimized. Specific points of assessment include the following:

- the optimal use of data groupers and contextualizers (Section 3, "Data Contextualizers," describes data contextualizers and their appropriate use and should be used to guide this piece of the assessment);
- The use of the right software for the right analytic method, including the use of querying software for data collection, aggregation, and preparation; the use of data visualization and spreadsheet tools for exploring data distributions and univariate statistics (see Chapter 19, "Overview of Analytic Methods Used in Population Health Management"); the use of statistical software for bivariate, multivariate, and some machine-learning

methods; the use of data visualization tools for self-service analytics, interdisciplinary review of data insights, and dissemination; and appropriate tools for other advanced analytic methods like artificial intelligence, prescriptive analytics, and natural language processing.

Value of Analytic Capabilities

There must be value to investing in programs of analytics for healthcare organizations. Budgeted amounts must be allocated between the systems and providers delivering healthcare services and analytics. To show its value, the work of analytics is realized when interactions between providers and patients are optimized, savings are realized, or costs are reduced by the investment in analytic

strategies. Healthcare organizations that excel in analytics also understand and regularly measure the value of analytics in achieving Triple Aim of better health outcomes and better patient experiences at a lower cost.

Organizational Assessment Tools

An assortment of assessment tools are available in the market for determining organizational analytic capabilities specifically for healthcare organizations. These readily available tools can be used as is or as a starting point for tailoring an organizational assessment to the organization in which it will be used. **Table 30.2** describes some of these tools and provides a link to learn more about them.

Table 30.2 Market-Based Assessment Tools

Tool	Description	Link
Healthcare Information and Management Systems Society (HIMSS) Analytics Model for Analytics Maturity (AMAM)	An assessment tool based on the eight-stage HIMSS AMAM model, which ranges from 0 (no organizations have analytic capabilities) to 7 (organizations optimize advanced data sets and use prescriptive analytics to deliver mass customization of care). The tool is used as part of a toolkit that supports organizations on their journey to achieving stage 7 of the AMAM.	https://www.himssanalytics.org/amam
Center for Care Innovations Analytics Capabilities Assessment	An assessment tool that was developed to address a gap in the safety net for defining and assessing analytics capabilities in health centers and to educate health centers on the complexities of working with data and building a data-driven culture. The tool uses a "people, processes, and technology" framework with capabilities defined as *reactive*, *responsive*, *proactive*, or *predictive*.	https://www.careinnovations.org/resources/analytics-capability-assessment/
The Healthcare Analytics Adoption Model Self-Assessment Survey	An assessment tool based on the eight-level healthcare analytics adoption model. Organizations can determine their level of analytic maturity and identify areas for improvement. The assessment can serve as a baseline for improvement and a way organizations can benchmark themselves against other healthcare organizations.	https://www.healthcatalyst.com/webinar/building-an-analytics-strategy-based-on-the-healthcare-analytics-adoption-model/

(continues)

Table 30.2 Market-Based Assessment Tools   *(continued)*

Tool	Description	Link
The Data Warehouse Institute Analytics Maturity Model and Assessment Tool	This assessment tool is not specific to healthcare organizations. It is based on five stages of analytics maturity defined in order as *nascent*, *preadoption*, *early adoption*, *corporate adoption*, and *mature visionary* with the suggestion that there is a "chasm" between early adoption and corporate adoption. After completion, organizations receive a score of analytic maturity and the ability to benchmark against other organizations by industry and size.	https://tdwi.org/pages /maturity-model/analytics -maturity-model -assessment-tool
ForestVue Organizational Capabilities Assessment	This assessment specifically measures organizational capabilities for population health analytics. See Figure 30.2 and Table 30.3 for more information.	www.forestvue.com

Executing an Organizational Assessment

The best way to undertake an organizational assessment of analytic capabilities for population health is to use a blend of surveying through self-report, direct observation of analytic processes, and targeted follow-up interviews with key stakeholders. Online survey tools such as SurveyMonkey offer a fast, inexpensive, and flexible way to gather initial insights to the questions at hand. In addition, surveys can be administered in a way that the identities of respondents are removed so they are more likely to candidly answer controversial or more difficult questions. **Figure 30.2** shows an example of some survey questions that could be administered to analytic and other staff working directly with data administered using an online survey tool.

The online survey tool is complemented with direct observation of analytic work by the designated assessor. Direct observation involves reviewing samples of analyses performed in population health analytics. A good way to approach

---

Survey Questions

1. What is your title? (open text)
2. How long have you been at Company X? (select one)
   - 0–3 mos
   - 4–6 mos
   - 7–12 mos
   - 1–2 years
   - 3–5 years
   - 6+ years
3. Describe your role and responsibilities (open text)
4. Degrees achieved (check all that apply)
   - High School
   - Technical certificate(s)
   - Associate
   - Bachelors

Figure 30.2 *(continued)*

- Graduate non-degreed
- Masters
- Technical Degree
- Doctoral Degree
5. Discipline of your highest degree:
   - Medical
   - Nursing
   - Information Technology
   - Analytics
   - Social Sciences
   - Basic Science or Engineering
   - Business
   - Allied Health
   - Education
   - Arts, Humanities
   - Other (free text in)
6. Do you analyze data, engineer data, or architect data in your daily work? (select one)
   - Yes
   - No
   - If yes, branch to these questions:

Branch-Analytics Infrastructure Roles/Functions

- Total years of experience in analytics (select one)
  - 0–1
  - 2–3
  - 4–5
  - 5+
- How would you classify yourself? (select all that apply)
  - Business analyst
  - Data and report writer
  - Programmer
  - Data architect
  - Data warehouse analyst
  - Technical analyst
  - Specifications developer
  - Applications developer
  - Software developer
  - Statistician
  - Data Scientist
  - Director/manager of analytic unit
  - Other (provide space to write-in)
- What types of analyses have you performed? (check all that apply)
  - Produce files of individual level data (for example, fields might include patient id number, age, gender, clinical values, utilization values, etc.)
  - Produce summary reports of individual-level data (for instance number of patients meeting certain criteria, percentages, rates)
  - Produce summary reports of individual-level data that describe statistical information for values (e.g., mean, standard deviations, ranges, confidence intervals)
  - Trend analysis (e.g., analyzing financial trends over time)
  - Statistical process control (e.g., analyzing clinical, quality, financial outcomes at multiple points in time to measure quality improvement and monitor ongoing programs)
  - Data mining (extracting relevant information from large, complex data sets)

Figure 30.2 (*continued*)

- Data visualization (communicating information from complex data clearly and effectively through graphical means)
- Evaluation with statistical comparisons of outcomes between groups. (e.g., t-tests, chi-square, other parametric/non-parametric statistics)
- Evaluation with statistical modeling of outcomes comparing between groups. (e.g., simple linear/logistic regression, poisson models, generalized estimating equations, etc.)
- Actuarial modeling (using current financial and utilization information to predict future trends)
- Predictive modeling (using statistical procedures to predict future health status or resource utilization, e.g., GLM, logistic regression, ordinary least squares, recursive partitioning)
- Predictive modeling using other techniques (e.g., machine learning, neural networks)
- What software do you use for analyses? (Rate use as light, moderate or heavy. Leave blank if not used.)
  - SQL
  - Excel
  - Business Objects
  - Cognos
  - Tableau
  - Qlik
  - SAP Business Intelligence Platform
  - SAS
  - SPSS
  - Stata
  - Visual Studio
  - Python
  - R
  - IBM Analytics, Cognos, or Watson
  - Apache Hadoop
  - Apache Spark
  - Minitab
  - MATLAB
  - Natural Language Processing Software (name of software)
    - Include a space to write in software name
  - Google Analytics
  - RapidMiner
  - Alteryx
  - Sisense
  - Looker
  - Zoho Analytics
  - Yellofin
  - Domo
  - GoodData
  - Birst
  - Informatica
  - Other (open ended)
- What data contextualizers do you use for analytics? (Rate use as light, moderate or heavy. Leave blank if not used.)
  - Diagnosis Related Groups (DRGs)
  - Hierarchical Condition Categories (HCCs)
  - Episode Treatment Groupers (ETGs)
  - Adjusted Clinical Groups® (ACGs)
  - Milliman Healthcare Guidelines (HCGs)
  - Cave Grouper™ (CCGroup Marketbasket System)
  - Chronic Disability Payment System (CDPS)
  - LACE score

Figure 30.2 *(continued)*

- Ambulatory Payment Classification (APC)
- Agency for Healthcare Research and Quality Clinical Classifications Software (AHRQ CCS)
- Other (open ended)
- How is the data that you analyze architected and modeled? (select the best choice)
  - Data are not modeled in a specific architecture and when performing an analysis, I code the specific structure of the data set I need from raw data
  - We have multi-faceted data resources ranging from unstructured raw data to semi-structured data tables without planned architecture to data mart(s) to an enterprise data warehouse.
  - We have a data warehouse with a documented data architecture for that data warehouse
  - We have created data models using warehoused data that are accessible through the analytics layer
- Do you have access to a person-level population health data model with person-level descriptors, process, and outcome measures? Y/N
- What data sources have you used at Company X? (Check all that apply)
  - Administrative medical claims data
  - Administrative pharmacy claims data
  - Electronic Medical Record billing data
  - Electronic Medical Record prescription data
  - Electronic Medical Record diagnosis data
  - Electronic Medical Record clinical outcomes data
  - Electronic Medical Record registries
  - Electronic Medical Record lab data
  - Electronic Medical Record social determinants of health data
  - Electronic Medical Record care management process, assessment, care planning data
  - Laboratory vendor data
  - Marketing data
  - Workplace productivity or other employer data
  - Health risk assessments
  - Company X patient-collected data
  - Other (write in)
- Auditing of data processing and product delivery at Company X is achieved through: (select all that apply)
  1. Database user and log information associated with each automated ETL or stored procedure
  2. Procedures tracked through assignment to specific individuals
  3. Manual process logging
  4. Multiple means as listed above
  5. Unsure
  6. Other (write in)
- Most of the data processing that currently takes place is automated or operationalized via the use of Extract Transact Load procedures (ETLs), stored procedures, etc.
  - Y/N /unsure
- High quality data processing standards are assured through: (check all that apply)
  - Monitoring and tracking of automated quality control metrics for each process
  - Process dependencies are tracked and monitored via run statistics to ensure complete process chain compliance
  - Automated email notifications in the event of any process failure
  - Task assignment limited to knowledgeable individuals
  - Data changes affected through transformation are captured and stored in an auditable fashion
  - Unsure
  - Other (write in)
- Accuracy of data content is assured through: (select all that apply)
  - Scheduled periodic review of data dependencies/resources, such as code sets, remain up to date
  - Scheduled periodic review of development code to ensure optimized data
  - Documented quality review of all developed code and final products
  - Data stewards identified for each domain

Figure 30.2 *(continued)*

- Subject Matter Experts (SMEs) identified for each domain
- Data owners identified for each domain
- Peer review during code or other product development
- Formal Quality Assurance testing of code or developed data product
- Fit for purpose requirements documented for each data product developed
- User acceptance testing
- Unsure
- Other (write in)

- Have you worked with data source integration? Y/N
  - Yes
  - No
  - If yes, branch to this question:
    - What is the highest number of data sources you have integrated to produce a single analysis?
      1. 2
      2. 3–4
      3. 5–6
      4. 7–8
      5. 9 or more
    - When integrating data sources, what software do you use?
      1. Microsoft Access
      2. Microsoft Excel
      3. Microsoft SQL
      4. SAS
      5. Python
      6. R
      7. Stata
      8. SPSS
      9. Other

- Do you encounter these data challenges in your work at Company X? (Y/N)
  - Dirty data
  - Incomplete data
  - Lack of data science talent in the organization
  - Company politics/lack of management/financial support for data management team
  - Lack of a clear question to be answered or clear direction to go in with the available data
  - Unavailability of or difficult data to access
  - Lack of, or inadequate, technical resources
  - Data science results not used by business or clinical decision-makers
  - Explaining data analytic methods and results to others
  - Privacy issues
  - Lack of significant domain expert input
  - Lack of documentation for and/or understanding of data assets

- Who are your main customers?
  - My immediate supervisor
  - Department leadership
  - Leadership across multiple departments in my organization
  - Organizational/Executive leadership
  - Leadership across multiple department within Company X
  - Leadership across multiple departments within and outside of Company X
  - Other (open ended)

- As realistically as possible, assign the percent of time per week that you typically devote to any categories listed below:

  Data architecture   _____

  Data engineering   _____

Figure 30.2 *(continued)*

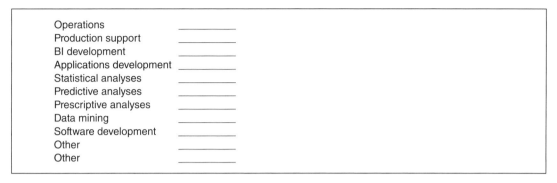

Operations   _____
Production support   _____
BI development   _____
Applications development _____
Statistical analyses   _____
Predictive analyses   _____
Prescriptive analyses   _____
Data mining   _____
Software development   _____
Other   _____
Other   _____

Figure 30.2 Self-Reported Survey Questions Administered to Staff Working with Data.

© ForestVue Healthcare Solutions.

this is to ask analysts to provide a work product of which they are proud and demonstrates what they perceive as the value that analytics provide to the organization. It is acceptable if this work product is not representative of the everyday work that analysts engage in because it also represents potential of the work that could be made operational. In addition, the assessor can gain access to self-service analytic products, operational analytic tools such as targeting algorithms and monitoring metrics, and documentation. Each of these tangible analytic products are reviewed in the context of the applicable domains.

Survey and observation results are followed by targeted stakeholder interviews. The purpose of the interviews is to fill in missing information, provide clarity about concerning or unexpected findings from surveys and observation, and offer key stakeholders an opportunity to provide information otherwise unsolicited until this point. The information gathered from this tactic reveals organizational strengths, opportunities, and areas for growth. These developments lead to further steps of identifying gaps and planning goals to improve the organization.

Although many of the interview questions are tailored to previous findings, a set of standard and icebreaker types of questions is helpful as a starting point. **Table 30.3** displays an example of questions that can be used as a starting point to interviews. In this case, the assessment includes a variety of interviews involving various roles in the organization within information technology, analytics, clinicians, ancillary providers, and executives. For each role, there are questions that fall under the domains to guide discussions

Table 30.3 Interview Questions Used to Guide Organizational Analytic Capabilities Discussion

Role	Domain	Question
Chief executive officer	People	How does the organizational chart demonstrate that analytics is valued as a competitive advantage?
	Process	How is population health analytics represented in the organizational strategic plan? How is the executive level supporting analytics?
	Results	What value does analytics provide to the organization? How are data treated as an asset within the organization?

(continues)

Table 30.3 Interview Questions Used to Guide Organizational Analytic Capabilities Discussion *(continued)*

Role	Domain	Question
Chief analytics officer	People	What are the priorities for hiring analytic staff in terms of mix of skills, knowledge, and experience over the next 6 months to 1 year?
		How do you ensure a diverse workforce?
		What types of policies are in place for flexible work arrangements and staff growth and development?
		Describe the culture in analytics and in the entire organization.
	Process	How do you promote interdisciplinary and collaborative work processes?
		What are the guiding principles for work prioritization and project management?
	Results	What value does analytics provide to the organization? How is it measured? How do you ensure an executive-level understanding?
Analytics team members	People	How would you describe the work culture in your analytic department? In the departments on which you depend? And with your stakeholders (recipients of your work)?
		Who do you go to when you have challenges in certain aspects of your work? Technical, contextual?
		Would you recommend working here, specifically in analytics, to one of your colleagues in another organization?
		What are some areas you would like to improve on as an analyst?
	Process	What types and numbers of data sources do you use for analyses?
		How do you collaborate with others in the organization?
		What are some challenges you face in your daily work?
		How are analytic projects managed?
		Discuss an analytic project you have completed in terms of the data sources used, the level of data preparation, gleaning input from others in the organization, the methods applied, the results, and the way in which the results were shared with and received by stakeholders.
		Which types of analytic methods do you use—for instance, means, percentages, counts, or other statistics?
	Tools	Which analytic tools do you use on a daily basis?
		Which analytic tools are you striving to learn more about?
		What are your challenges and accomplishments in your tool utilization?
	Results	Discuss some of the pertinent findings from your analyses that have impacted decision-making.
		Who do you share your reports and dashboards with in the organization?
		What do you see as areas of growth for the analytics department?

Providers and clinical and social work staff	People	How do you interface with analytic staff?
		How do you inform the analytic work products you use?
	Process	What types of analytics are used in your workflow?
		What types of work-arounds do you need to incorporate into your workflow?
		What are the metrics for which you are responsible or accountable?
	Tools	How do you access analytic results and the metrics you need to do your work?
	Results	What value does analytics provide to your work?
Finance (CFO)	People	What are the analytic roles and responsibilities in the finance department?
		How do financial analysts collaborate with clinical and population-focused analytics in the organization?
	Process	Is population health part of your strategic plan? How?
		What are some challenges you have with analytics?
	Results	What value does analytics provide to your work?
Information technology (IT) (CIO)	People	What are the roles in IT that support analytic infrastructure?
		What are some current joint projects between IT and analytics?
		How do IT staff interface and work collaboratively with other departments in the organization?
	Process	What challenges do you see with analytics? Population health analytics?
		How is population health analytics incorporated into the IT strategy?
	Results	How do you describe the value of analytics to IT and to the organization as a whole?

© ForestVue Healthcare Solutions.

surrounding the organization's capabilities. These questions mainly focus on the role of analytics in the organization, the current state, population health considerations, organizational challenges, and strategic planning. The questions serve as a guide to discussion, and the expectation is that the interviewer will probe into responses as needed to gain valuable insights.

Conclusion

The organizational assessment of population health analytic capabilities is grounded within the basic *structure*, *process*, *outcome* framework and the more specific *people*, *process*, and *technology* format used in process improvement and information technology disciplines. Important components for assessment include people, organizational culture, strategic planning and executive engagement, data sources and structure, processes supporting analytic workflow, processes used for data management, analytic methods, analytic tools, and the value of analytic capabilities. Components are assessed using electronic survey instruments, direct observation, and stakeholder interviews. Information from the assessment culminates in a set of results that can be used to establish baseline capabilities, determine strategic objectives and tactics, measure milestone achievements over time, and benchmark capabilities in similar organizations.

Study and Discussion Questions

- Why is it important to assess organizational capabilities for population health analytics?
- Considering the domains for assessing organizational capabilities, what is the importance of each?
- Why is it important to understand organizational culture and its impact on analytic capabilities? What are some personal experiences with organizational culture?

- Create a basic plan for assessing organizational analytic capabilities for population health?
    - What are the components?
    - What are the objectives?
    - What is the time line?
    - How will it be executed within the organization?
    - What will the resulting report look like? How will it be disseminated?

Resources and Websites

National Association of Health Data Organizations (NAHDO): https://www.nahdo.org/

Healthcare Data and Analytics Association: https://www.hdwa.org/

Center for Healthcare Innovations: https://www.careinnovations.org/

Health Information Management and Systems Society (HIMSS) Analytics: https://www.himssanalytics.org/

The Data Warehouse Institute (TDWI): https://tdwi.org/Home.aspx

The Data Governance Institute: http://www.datagovernance.com/

References

Basu, S., Phillips, R. S., Phillips, R., Peterson, L. E., & Landon, B. E. (2020). Primary care practice finances in the United States amid the COVID-19 pandemic. *Health Affairs, 39*(9). https://www.healthaffairs.org/doi/full/10.1377/hlthaff.2020.00794

Brown, B. (2010). The gifts of imperfection: Let go of who you think you're supposed to be and embrace who you are. Almohreraladbi.

Donabedian, A. (1980). Basic approaches to assessment: Structure, process, and outcome. In *Explorations in quality assessment and monitoring, Volume I*. Health Administration Press.

Gilbert, M., & Jones, M. (2019). 2019 CIO agenda: A healthcare providers perspective. Gartner. https://www.gartner.com/en/doc/450304-a-healthcare-providers-perspective

Hagan, A., Graves, C., Kinsella, D., & Gerhardt, W. (2019). Shifting into high gear: Health system analytics have a growing strategic focus. Deloitte. https://www2.deloitte.com/us/en/insights/industry/health-care/health-system-analytics-growing-strategic-focus.html

Inmon, W. H. (1999). *Building the operational data store* (2nd ed.). John Wiley & Sons.

Panneerselvam, J., Liu, L., & Hill, R. (2015). Requirements and challenges for big data architectures. In B. Akhgar, G. B. Saathoff, H. R. Arabnia, R. Hill, A. Staniforth, & P. Saskia Bayer (Eds.), *Application of big data for national security* (pp. 131–139). https://doi.org/10.1016/b978-0-12-801967-2.00009-4

Preston, E. (2020, July 19). During Coronavirus lockdowns, some doctors wondered: Where are the preemies? *The New York Times*. https://www.nytimes.com/2020/07/19/health/coronavirus-premature-birth.html

Prodan, M., Prodan, A., & Purcarea, A. (2015). Three new dimensions to people, process, technology improvement model. *Advances in Intelligent Systems and Computing, 353,* 481–490. https://doi.org/10.1007/978-3-319-16486-1_47

Reiners, B. (2020). Types of diversity in the workplace you need to know: A guide to 34 unique diversity characteristics. Built In. https://builtin.com/diversity-inclusion/types-of-diversity-in-the-workplace

Rosenbaum, S. (2010, October). Data governance and stewardship: Designing data stewardship entities and advancing data access. *Health Services Research, 45*(5), 1442–1455. https://doi.org/10.1111/j.1475-6773.2010.01140.x

Schein, E. H. (2010). *Organizational culture and leadership* (4th ed.). Jossey-Bass.

Schlegel, K., & Buytendijk, F. (2018, May 15). Create a centralized and decentralized organizational model for analytics. Gartner Research. https://www.gartner.com/en/documents/3875403/create-a-centralized-and-decentralized-organizational-mo

Scott, T., Mannion, R., Davies, H., & Marshall, M. (2003, June). The quantitative measurement of organizational culture in health care: A review of the available instruments. *Health Services Research, 38*(3), 923–945. https://pubmed.ncbi.nlm.nih.gov/12822919/

Shemla, M. (2018, August 22). Why workplace diversity is so important, and why it's so hard to achieve. Forbes. https://www.forbes.com/sites/rsmdiscovery/2018/08/22/why-workplace-diversity-is-so-important-and-why-its-so-hard-to-achieve/#103b017e3096

Sylvia, M. (2020). Introduction to population health analytics. In *Population health management learning series*. ForestVue Healthcare Solutions.

Thomas, G. (n.d.). *The DGI data governance framework.* https://datagovernance.com/

University of Chicago Medicine. (2016). *Strategic and sustainability planning for population health collaborative 2.* https://www.healthit.gov/sites/default/files/strategic_and_sustainability_planning_for_population_health_collaborative.pdf

U.S. Equal Employment Opportunity Commission. (n.d.). Who is protected from employment discrimination? https://www.eeoc.gov/employers/small-business/3-who-protected-employment-discrimination

CHAPTER 31

Building a Team Culture for Population Health

Ines Maria Vigil, MD, MPH, MBA

Coming together is a beginning, staying together is progress, and working together is success.

—Attributed to both Henry Ford (n.d.)
and Edward Everett Hale (n.d.)

EXECUTIVE SUMMARY

Analytics to support population health cannot be developed properly without a team-based approach. Solutions built in isolation or from one person's expertise often cannot be generally applied to populations or scaled. Building a team for population health analytics is essential to ensure the success of the solution. However, simply putting several people together and calling them a *team* is not enough. Several best practices must be applied to build a high-performing and effective team to support population health activities.

To develop a population health team that strives for excellence, the importance of the team must be understood. Each team member must be able and willing to sacrifice individual gain for the gain of the team, the work product, and the population served. A synergy among team members, along with an understanding of each other's strengths and weaknesses, is necessary to develop effective solutions to support population health management and analytics.

This chapter covers the importance of a team and its application to population health management and analytics, how to model the population health team, the importance of a team charter to support population health analytics, and the necessary structure of a team to build and scale population health solutions. This chapter also introduces the *PopHealth Troika* (PHT), which stems from the Russian term for a sleigh pulled by a team of three horses; it is often used to describe a group of three people working together toward a common goal (*Oxford Dictionary*, 2020a). The PHT provides a method for identifying the right team members, setting clear roles and expectations, realizing each team member's potential, building trust, creating shared understanding, and practicing open communication to transform the way health care is delivered to achieve extraordinary results. Several sample tools are detailed in this chapter to support a team-based approach to propagating a culture of population health.

LEARNING OBJECTIVES

At the end of this chapter, the learner will be able to:

1. Explain the importance of a team-based approach to the success of population health management and analytics.
2. Describe the process of population health team development and the PopHealth Troika (PHT).
3. Apply the PHT to population health projects going forward.
4. Deploy various techniques to elicit understanding across team members regarding respect, diversity, equality, perception, and bias and how such understanding informs team performance.

Introduction

Teams are important to developing solutions in health care. High-performing teams exist throughout health care and are needed to ensure proper care is delivered with speed and accuracy. The best example of a high-performing team in health care is a hospital code team. Clinical staff working in hospitals are trained to respond to patients in severe physical distress as designated by a code. The first person in the room to recognize the patient in distress calls a code to alert various clinicians nearby to respond immediately. What follows is a coordinated set of lifesaving activities between the first, second, and third persons to respond; the set is tailored to the patient's cause of distress (MC Hospital Simulation Lab, 2011). A clinical responder does not know whether they will be the first, second, or third clinician to respond to the patient's distress, but what is clear is the job expected of the person who is first, and how that is delineated from the job of the persons who are second and third to respond. This clarity is rooted in the application of coordinated training, defined skill sets, relevant expertise, and a clear understanding of how the team works, communicates with one another, and coordinates activities and respective contributions. True teamwork is realized in clearly delineated roles and responsibilities, clearly defined tasks that are rooted in best practice, and the understanding of one another amid an urgent time frame and a need for definitive accuracy. The importance of teams and their relevance to health care is outlined in this chapter.

How a team is modeled is also important to consider when building a population health team. Many models for high-performing teams exist and can be applied in healthcare settings with exceptional results. This chapter reviews a few models that have been applied with great success by authors in this text, and across varying healthcare organizations spanning the United States, including Tuckman's model, the Orange Revolution, and Clifton's StrengthsFinder (Gallup, 2020; Gostick & Chester, 2010; Tuckman, 1965).

One of the most important considerations for a population health team is identifying the members that make up the team. Many methods exist for selecting and implementing a performance-improvement team, and none is perfect (Deblois & Lepanto, 2016; Knapp, 2015; Shortell, Blodgett, Rundall, & Kralovec, 2018). Note that adaptations to the population health team will likely occur as the content and work inherent to addressing the changing health of populations over time and across diverse demographics changes. Much like the description of the high-performing hospital code team previously referenced, a process is needed to adequately support and sustain population health management and analytics. The *PopHealth Troika* (PHT), developed and tested by the authors of this text, introduces a method to seamlessly bring together team members with the required expertise, relevant experience, and necessary skills to build a high-performing population health management and analytics team.

An obvious but often overlooked component of building a team for population health is introducing team members to one another.

This chapter explores various tactics that can be applied to encourage team members to show courage and vulnerability and thus quickly build trust and a willingness to invest in one another's successes and learnings. Assessing individual team members' emotional intelligence, how to convey and resolve conflict, and hold themselves and other team members accountable to the goal and their performance are key to the success of building a population health team.

The population health team charter is another essential element to building an effective and high-performing population health team. Elements of the population health team charter includes setting clear expectations in writing, ground rules for understanding one another, working together, communication, holding each other accountable, and other team operational functions.

The Importance of a Team

Health care is complex, and solutions to address the rising cost of providing high-quality health care to populations that generates improved health outcomes are often multifaceted. Frequently, a combination of different areas of expertise, experience, and skill sets are needed to appropriately understand the complexity of health and to develop solutions that improve health and make healthcare delivery more affordable for populations (Borek & Abraham, 2018; Clarke, Bourn, Skoufalos, Beck, & Castillo, 2017; Shea, Turner, Albritton, & Reiter, 2018). A team-based approach in population health is necessary to ensure diversity of thinking, to develop comprehensive interventions, and to add rigor to the technical aspects of surveillance, monitoring, and evaluation.

Striving for Excellence

The pursuit of excellence is a common attribute of clinical training and an expectation of clinicians in practice. Clinicians are held to a high standard to perform their duties with confidence and without errors, often making decisions in a silo or based on their singular experience and knowledge base. However, when approaching care of populations, a singular person striving for excellence is not enough. Population health management and analytics requires a multidisciplinary approach, where multiple key individuals are needed to comprehensively asses the population from different perspectives, different methods and analytics techniques must be applied to the data in the analysis of opportunity and measurement, and multiple care teams are responsible for delivering interventions. Alignment, striving for excellence but not perfection, and momentum are all important attributes of a high-performing population health team.

Alignment is key to striving for excellence in a team, and it is important when selecting a team to first ensure alignment of the goals and objectives. If the goals and objectives are not understood by all team members or there is misalignment among team members on the importance of certain goals and objectives, then the team will be unable to function cohesively and the project will suffer. Alignment on how the work will be completed is the second factor to striving for excellence in a team. Any one member of the team can quickly derail a project, and nothing can ruin a good idea faster than a poor implementation. It is important to develop a plan of action and communication for all team members to clearly understand their roles and expected contributions. Misalignment among team members is a common pitfall and can be detrimental to the results.

In some instances, striving for excellence can be confused with striving for perfection. The population health process is complex and needs an atmosphere in which ideas can be exchanged freely, mistakes can become learnings, and creating a culture of asking the right questions is favored over a culture of getting the right answer. It is vital that perfect not be the enemy of good (Ratcliffe, 2020) and that the team has a mutual understanding of what good enough looks like to take action. Built into the population health process are agile methods to monitor progress and make changes, allowing for corrections to be made along the way (Patel, 2017). More information on the agile methods and process feedback can be found in Chapter 2, "Guiding Frameworks for Population Health Analytics."

Momentum, derived from the Latin word *movimentum* and meaning "to move" (*Oxford Dictionary*, 2020b), is one of the most important attributes to have in a population health team-based approach. Having momentum matters to maintain progress, team member engagement, and the perseverance to solve for unforeseen challenges along the way. Momentum in teams can be generated through ongoing recognition of top performers, developing a project time line and protecting the team's time to do the work, and constant communication and reinforcement of the team's goals (Borek & Abraham, 2018; Gostick & Chester, 2010; Teamwork, 2016).

Promoting Teams versus Individuals

For a team to be successful, a collaborative mindset must be in place. An interdisciplinary team-based approach to quality improvement and patient safety has been studied extensively in health care, and the lessons from these healthcare settings can be applied directly to population health (Borek & Abraham, 2018; Clarke et al., 2017; Ferguson, 2008). A 2015 study by Hekmat and colleagues of attitudes toward team-based work in hospitals demonstrated that a few key factors had the most significant contribution to healthcare workers' attitudes toward team-based work—namely, mutual support (using one's own talents to help others) and responsibility (being accountable to the task or duty assigned) (Hekmat, Dehnavieh, Rahimisadegh, Kohpeima, & Jahromi, 2015). Mutual support, responsibility, effective communication, and collaboration are all critical elements to achieving a high-performing team.

Several researchers have discovered a significant discrepancy of attitudes and perceptions toward teamwork among members of healthcare teams (Carney, West, Neily, Mills, & Bagian, 2010; Makary et al., 2006; Thomas, Sexton, & Helmreich, 2003). In one study, nurses had a different assessment of effective teamwork than their physician counterparts when participating in the same team with the same common goals, tools, and clinical setting. This study is a reminder that the perception of teamwork may not always be clear and mutually understood by each team member. It is important to recognize and foster a culture where individual opinions matter in a team and understanding that perceptions are reality until proven otherwise.

Promoting a team culture of collaboration and trust requires individuals to leave siloed attitudes behind and embrace the idea that success can be achieved only through a diversity of thought, experiences, and knowledge. Doing so can improve decision-making, increase team member engagement, generate more ideas, increase productivity, and improve mutual understanding. Population health is inherently relational, and its success is highly dependent on a network of population health work teams coming together to develop solutions that any one individual would be incapable of accomplishing alone.

Modeling the Team

Modeling a high-performing population health team requires that all team members know exactly the roles and responsibilities of themselves and every other team member during every step. In addition, if any problems or misunderstanding occur, it is important to build in a process to address any challenges quickly and efficiently. Several models exist for how to model a high-performing and results-oriented team, all of which are directly applicable to health care, especially population health. Selected below are examples of Don Clifton's belief in the importance of teams to recognize and collectively play to their respective strengths and acknowledge their weaknesses. These can be found in Clifton's StrengthsFinder, Tuckman's model for team development, and the Basic 4 attributes of a team from the Orange Revolution (Gallup, 2020; Gostick & Chester, 2010; Tuckman, 1965).

Clifton StrengthsFinder

The Paul Myers quote, "Focus on your strengths instead of your weaknesses, on your powers instead of your problems" is a wonderful summary of the concepts introduced in Clifton's StrengthsFinder (Tew, 2015). The Strengths-Finder is a set of assessment questions aimed at measuring personal talent in individuals; it was originally developed in the 1990s by educational psychologist Donald Clifton and later adopted by Gallup, a global analytics and organizational consulting services firm. StrengthsFinder 2.0 by Tom Rath (Gallup, 2020) provides an updated version of Donald Clifton's original ideas and can be applied to both individuals and teams to identify areas of strength and weakness, with a focus on helping people and teams leverage 34 of the most common areas of talent to achieve success.

Examples of areas of talent outlined in StrengthsFinder 2.0 include *analytical, communication, discipline, futuristic, ideation, relator*, and *strategic*. These and others are all critical elements of a successful population health team. This type of assessment enables individual contributors to recognize and describe their strengths. When paired with colleagues whose strengths are complementary but not overlapping or competitive, the assessment can produce phenomenal team dynamics and performance.

Tuckman's Model

In 1965, Bruce Tuckman first described the team model of forming, storming, norming, and performing. According to Tuckman, the phases outlined in **Figure 31.1** are essential to team growth, shared responsibility when tackling tough challenges, solution architecting, planning work, and getting results (Tuckman, 1965).

The first stage in this model is described as *forming* and is highly applicable to developing population health teams. This stage is described as team members getting to know one another, and most often it represents a new team coming together for the first time. In this stage, the team will most likely experience excitement, anticipation, anxiety, and optimism. It is important in this

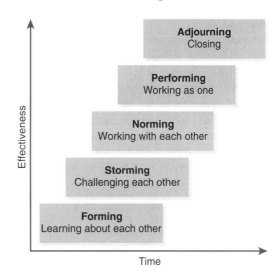

Figure 31.1 Tuckman's Team Development Model.

Data from Tuckman, B. W. (1965). Developmental sequence in small groups. *Psychological Bulletin, 63*(6), 384–399. https://doi.org/10.1037/h0022100

stage of population health team development that adequate time is allowed for team members to share their experiences, skill sets, and motivation. This will create a bond among team members that will later be invaluable when mutual support from one another is needed.

The second stage of this model is *storming*, and it happens to every population health team at some point during the project time line. In this stage, reality sets in for the population health team, and assumptions about members' capabilities, expertise, and dedication can often be questioned. It is not uncommon in this stage for communication gaps, anxiety, frustration, and conflict to arise. This stage is unavoidable and should be anticipated by the leader of the team. Early recognition of this stage and early intervention with a restating of the goals, why each team member was selected, and reinforcement that ideas and solutions are better when generated together will help move teams from storming to the next phase.

Norming is the third stage in Tuckman's model and represents a shift in the way group members work together to tackle the presented challenge. Leaders of population health teams can encourage this stage by sharing goals and recognizing and rewarding team cohesion. The need for team members to compromise, make trade-offs, and mutually accept shared decisions is common in this stage.

The fourth stage of the model is *performing*. Population health teams really hit their stride in this stage, and members are described as working cohesively, freely exchanging ideas, showing trust in one another, and striving for excellence with a focus on results. This stage best represents the original intent of a team and can produce quite extraordinary results.

An additional step to the original Tuckman's model of group development was added by Mary Ann Jensen and Bruce Tuckman: *adjourning* (Tuckman & Jensen, 1977). This is particularly applicable to the development of population health teams because different populations will be identified to need different skill sets, areas of expertise, and business acumen. As part of the adoption of a culture of population health and data-driven decision-making, individuals will likely participate in a number of team-based projects and activities, each time coming together with a new and different set of people, each with their own unique characteristics and contribution. The team leader will need to develop a set of expectations and process steps for what happens when the teams change and people are reassigned, as well as how the work will continue. This stage is characterized by separation anxiety, questions of what comes next, unease in transitioning to other teams, a desire to stay with their original team, and dissatisfaction at not being able to continue to work in the same way with the same people.

The Tuckman model of group development can be applied to a recent population health example, the COVID-19 pandemic response. For many healthcare organizations around the world, COVID-19 came as a surprise, and hospitals and ambulatory care centers found themselves unprepared to adequately respond to the quickly spreading virus and the potential need for intensive care for patients with severe symptoms (Kim, 2020; Rutayisire, Nkundimana, Mitonga, Boye, & Nikwigize, 2020). Teams across the world were brought together quickly—including clinicians, government officials, data scientists, and technologists—to identify, stratify, predict, intervene, and monitor the spread of the disease, its clinical characteristics, and its health and financial impacts on society. As a result, these teams of clinical, business, and analytical and technical resources from different industries rapidly performed population health analysis, developed diagnostic and antibody tests and testing protocols, and worked to develop potential vaccines and treatments. These teams likely experienced the stages that Tuckman describes in his model, and those teams that successfully moved to the *performing* stage, likely by partnering with nonhealthcare industries, are now developing a scientific and technologically innovative response to the virus to stay its spread and severity (Li et al., 2020; Wosik et al., 2020).

The Orange Revolution

A second model that is directly applicable to the practice of population health and developing population health teams theorizes that successful teams set goals that are laudable, they invest in one another's success, they embrace risk, monitor progress and results, and they overcome challenges, and weave together compelling stories that convey their process and work product.

The Orange Revolution by Gostick and Chester identifies five key attributes of high-performing and culture-transforming teams that includes goal setting, communication, trust, and accountability. Recently, recognition was added because of its importance in maintaining the momentum of a culture-changing team. (Gostick & Chester, 2010)

Throughout the book, the authors acknowledge that teams think creatively and possess answers to problems that single persons alone cannot derive, that collaboration in teams allows for compensation of one another's weaknesses, and that teams must possess a broad base of knowledge and a commitment to excellence to be successful. Similar to Tuckman's model of group development, goal setting emphasizes the importance of setting clear expectations and quantifiable and behavioral goals for the team. Quantifiable goals are described as numeric in nature and represent a desired result. Behavioral goals include a set of behaviors or tasks that meet the quantifiable goals when taken (Gostick & Chester, 2010).

Setting quantifiable goals are especially applicable to population health analytics, because often it is the data that are most desired to be used to inform decisions on what the challenge is to solve, who the population is for intervention, and what information will be needed to monitor an intervention and measure results. In addition, the behaviors of freely sharing ideas, engaging in the team's activities and dialogue, and aligning the work with individuals' strengths and skill sets are paramount to developing a robust population health solution.

Constant and effective communication is a strong contributor to building effective teams. It is important for teams to avoid surprises by sharing individuals' expectations and thoughts of the project and of one another (Gostick & Chester, 2010). In population health teams, each team member is expected to contribute a specific expertise and have the necessary skill set to do so. Personal competency, requisite skill set, and the individual contribution to a bigger picture goal are all characteristics of a highly skilled individual contributor and ensure a place on the team. However, the ability and willingness of an individual to communicate frequently and successfully with others while problem-solving is identified in this model as having significant impact to the team's performance and overall results.

> [High-performing teams use] communication to identify problems, freely share ideas, pass on useful tidbits of information to co-workers, take time to listen to team member ideas and concerns, ask for input and assistance, give help as requested even when outside of their duties, become vulnerable, compromise when necessary, take ownership of mistakes, take thoughtful risks, refrain from talking about absent coworkers, respond

promptly to team member requests, and proactively share information. (Gostick & Chester, 2010)

Trust is critical to any project's success, and this is true for population health teams. Having the proper requisites of skills, experience, and expertise is necessary when striving for excellence, and adding trust of one another in a team will ensure that information is sought after and shared across team members and that mutual support is both given and received. A best practice is the tactic of debriefing after the application of a set of decisions. Transformational teams will often review previous decisions for learnings, analyze challenges to prevent future occurrences, and talk through miscommunications to acknowledge potential barriers to progress and create an environment of trust and accountability (Gostick & Chester, 2010).

Demonstrating accountability in a team goes beyond individuals' completion of their respective duties. When working in a team, accountability allows team members to count on one another, hold open debates, and strive for excellence together. We cannot overemphasize the need for team members to demand openness of one another when one is struggling or needs help, that each team member be accountable to the shared goals, and that team members hold one another to a high standard of performance (Gostick & Chester, 2010). This is applicable to population health teams in that power dynamics and hierarchies inherently exist in the practice and administration of health care. These dynamics can lead to unchecked assumptions and misunderstandings when forming the population health team (Gleddie, Stahlke, & Paul, 2018; Liberati, Gorli, & Scaratti, 2016). It is vital to ensure that each team member knows his or her respective role and expected contribution and that team members are accountable for creating a team culture of openness, respect, and equal contribution.

Best practices for leaders and team members when providing recognition include keeping encouragement positive, providing in-the-moment feedback, and the importance of cheering wins publicly and together as a team (Gostick & Chester, 2010). In population health teams, different people with different motivations are brought together to solve a complex healthcare challenge. It is important to recognize the small wins that serve to progress the work and provide a more robust solution. The team should spend time recognizing and rewarding desired behaviors both from a team dynamic perspective (such as timeliness, engagement, idea sharing, and challenging one another) and an effort perspective (such as commitment to the work, bringing one's best to the work, problem-solving, and getting results). High-performing and effective population health teams support, recognize and appreciate one another along the road to results. **Figure 31.2** summarizes the concepts in this section.

The thoughtful selection of talents in team members, the development of a team environment that fosters and guides norming and storming that leads to results, and the creation of a culture of trust, accountability, and recognition through goal setting and communication are all important attributes of a population health team. The concepts, best practices, and tools outlined by Rath, Tuckman, Gostick, and Elton inform a team-based model for changing the culture of a healthcare organization toward population health and analytics known in this textbook as the PopHealth Troika (Daniel & Davis, 2015; Gostick & Chester, 2010).

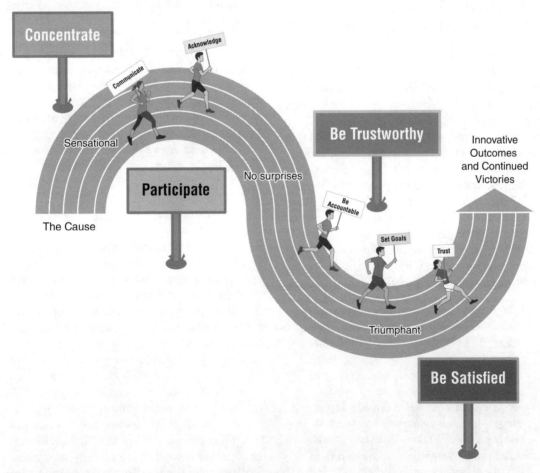

Figure 31.2 Characteristics of Breakthrough Teams.

Forming the Team: The PopHealth Troika

The work of population health is often achieved through project work. Success in population health projects is best achieved on a team-based approach through a series of PopHealth Troika (PHT) team triads, each comprising an analytic, clinical, and business lead. Derived from the Russian word *troika* (*Oxford Dictionary*, 2020a)—a sleigh pulled by a team of three horses—the term is often used in management and administration to describe a group of three people working together toward a common goal. In this way, the population health team works toward a common goal, innovating and learning with one another to develop solutions to some of health care's most complex challenges.

The PHT is essential to achieving success in population health management and provides a method for identifying the right team members, setting clear roles and expectations, realizing each team member's potential, building trust, creating shared understanding, and practicing open communication to transform the way health care is delivered to achieve extraordinary results. Each analytical, clinical, and business leader brings a unique and special set of knowledge, experience, and skills to population health projects. Together, a symbiosis occurs in which benefits are realized when the product the team is working toward is greater than anything that could be accomplished if individuals were working on the same project separately and individually (Sylvia, 2020). Details on the roles, responsibilities, and characteristics of greatness of each leader are included in **Tables 31.1**, **31.2**, and **31.3** and are provided as a guide to leaders interested in using teams to promote a culture of population health in healthcare organizations.

Forming an effective population health team requires significant up-front leadership,

Table 31.1 The Clinical Lead	
Role	<ul><li>Share understanding of the clinical evidence base, clinical workflows, and patient, personal, and familial patient experiences.</li><li>Brainstorm potential barriers as they relate to clinical information and processes.</li><li>Identify leading and lagging clinical indicators for monitoring and results.</li><li>Propose clinical interventions.</li><li>Review analyses, inferences, and conclusions for clinical relevancy, feasibility, level of clinical effort required, and clinical time line to results.</li><li>Propose clinical process and outcomes measures for success.</li></ul>
Responsibilities	<ul><li>Team leadership (as opposed to directorship)</li><li>Clinical leadership and representation</li><li>Point of contact for other clinical subject matter experts (SMEs)</li><li>Intervention design</li><li>Communication with other clinicians</li></ul>
Characteristics of Greatness	<ul><li>Inclusiveness</li><li>Creative thinking and ideation</li><li>An inquisitive approach</li><li>Curiosity</li><li>Ability to make decisions with imperfect information</li><li>Ability to focus work of self and others</li><li>Excellence in collaboration and communication</li></ul>

Reproduced from Sylvia, M. (2020). Assembling the population health team. In *The population health management learning series*. ForestVue Healthcare Solutions.

Table 31.2 The Business Lead

Role	<ul><li>Share understanding of the business's objectives, strategies, initiatives, operations, workflows, and personal and familial patient experience.</li><li>Brainstorm potential barriers as they relate to the business's administration of strategies, operations, and clinical interventions.</li><li>Identify leading and lagging business indicators for monitoring and results.</li><li>Align existing business strategies and initiatives with the proposed clinical interventions.</li><li>Propose new business strategies and initiatives.</li><li>Review analyses, inferences, and conclusions for business relevancy, feasibility, level of business effort required, and time line to results.</li><li>Propose business process and outcomes measures for success.</li></ul>
Responsibilities	<ul><li>Business leadership and representation</li><li>Point of contact with other business SMEs</li><li>Develop strategies, project time lines, milestones, and road map.</li><li>Years 1, 3, and 5—strategic thinking and planning</li><li>Develop communication plan, cadence, updates, and expectations.</li></ul>
Characteristics of Greatness	<ul><li>Strategic thinking</li><li>Business acumen</li><li>Financial acumen</li><li>Creative thinking and ideation</li><li>An inquisitive approach</li><li>Curiosity</li><li>Ability to make decisions with imperfect information</li><li>Ability to focus work of self and others</li><li>Excellence in collaboration and communication</li></ul>

Reproduced from Sylvia, M. (2020). Assembling the population health team. In *The population health management learning series*. ForestVue Healthcare Solutions.

Table 31.3 The Analyst and Engineer Lead

Role	<ul><li>Share understanding of the existing data, infrastructure, skills, process, limitations, availability, and personal and familial patient experience.</li><li>Brainstorm potential barriers as they relate to the data assets, sources, infrastructure, processing speed, privacy and security, and data quality and integrity.</li><li>Identify relevant leading and lagging indicators for identification, stratification, predicting, prescribing, monitoring patterns, and results.</li><li>Articulate what data are (1) available, (2) available but need additional support to be applied for the named use, (3) not available but can be obtained, and (4) not available and cannot be obtained.</li><li>Ideate ways to obtain data that are not available but can be obtained. This is often needed with new or proposed clinical interventions and business strategies or initiatives.</li><li>Review project plan for relevancy to data and analytics (not all decisions need data to be made), feasibility (now, later, or never), level of effort required, type of skill required, and time line to initial prototype and final deliverable.</li></ul>

	▪ Propose data elements and variables that can be used to monitor clinical and business process and outcomes measures for success (direct, proxy, trend, indicator).
Responsibilities	▪ Data and analytic leadership and representation ▪ Point of contact with other data and engineer SMEs ▪ Develop projects, time lines, milestones, road maps for data that are (1) available, (2) available but need additional support to be applied for the named use, (3) not available but can be obtained, and (4) not available and cannot be obtained. ▪ Develop projects, time lines, milestones, road maps for analytic prototypes, models, dashboards, and reports. ▪ Develop templates and tracking mechanisms to obtain data that are not available and can be obtained. Often needed with new or proposed clinical interventions and business strategies or initiatives.
Characteristics of Greatness	▪ Strategic thinking ▪ Business acumen ▪ Financial acumen ▪ Data acumen ▪ Diverse analytic skill set ▪ Courageous communication ▪ Creative thinking and ideation ▪ An inquisitive approach ▪ Curiosity ▪ Ability to make decisions with imperfect information ▪ Ability to focus work of self and others ▪ Excellence in collaboration and communication

Reproduced from Sylvia, M. (2020). Assembling the population health team. In *The population health management learning series*. ForestVue Healthcare Solutions.

support, and investment of time. Without a clear vision, expectations, adequate support, and training, a newly formed team left to its own devices can quickly appear ineffective and derail any initiative.

Introducing the Team

The literature well documents the benefits and challenges associated with managing a multidisciplinary and diverse team to develop technically and socially complex solutions (Carney et al., 2010; Clarke et al., 2017; Green, Oeppen, Smith, & Brennan, 2017; Makary et al., 2006; Manges, Scott-Cawiezell, & Ward, 2016; Moss & Maxfield, 2007; Thomas et al., 2003). Earlier in this chapter, Tuckman's model of group development was introduced to assist leaders of population health teams in understanding the process

of engagement and the interrelationships that teams typically experience. If the team dynamics of forming, storming, norming, performing, and adjourning can be anticipated and recognized by members of the team or by others, then leaders can assist teams in quickly recovering from any dysfunction that may result from the storming phase (Tuckman, 1965).

Conflict and Conflict Resolution

When forming a population health team, such as a the PopHealth Troika, it is important to alert team members that difficult conversations will occur and then provide them with the tools and language to challenge one another respectfully.

One tactic that can be deployed to prepare a team for interpersonal challenges or conflict

---

Table 31.4 **Facilitate a Dialogue to Address Interpersonal Conflict**

Ask the team to think of an example of a team or relationship you were involved with that experienced a conflict.

> Allow time for anyone who is willing to describe his or her example to the team.
>
> Follow the examples shared with the following questions to prompt discussion among the team.

- How did the individuals in the example recognize the conflict?
- How did they choose to acknowledge the conflict to one another, if at all?
- What could they have done to resolve the conflict?
- What was done to resolve the conflict if resolved?

Use elements from the discussion to brainstorm how to develop a process or mutual understanding among team members of how challenges and conflict will be addressed in the project.

> Follow the discussion with a recording of the mutually agreed-on process the team will use to address and resolve challenges and conflict throughout the project.
>
> Include the recorded process in the team's charter to be used as a reference and reminder for the team.

---

can occur when first introducing team members to one another. The leader can facilitate a brainstorming session on conflict and conflict resolution, with each team member providing an example of a team or person they were involved with when they experienced conflict (see **Table 31.4**). The leader can then prompt the tasks and questions outlined in Table 31.4 to elicit a dialogue among team members and ultimately develop a process for how the team will address challenges and conflict when they arise during the project.

Challenges and conflict can also arise from differences of opinion on what ideas or solutions are best and where the team should focus its efforts and resources. This type of conflict is heightened when additional project stressors are present such as an aggressive time line or limited resource. When more ideas are generated than can be acted on by the team, a decision prioritization matrix can be helpful, such as the University of Illinois's Solution Prioritization Matrix, an adaptation from Pande, Neuman, and Cavanaugh, *The Six Sigma Way Team Fieldbook* (2002; see also University of Illinois, 2015). Essentially, all ideas are documented and scored on a gradient against decision factors that are important to the organization and the project's success. In population health, common decision factors can include the following:

- the ease or difficulty of implementing the solution, program, or intervention;
- the likelihood of being accepted by the users of the solution, program, or intervention;
- whether or not the solution addresses the root cause of the challenge (interim versus permanent);
- the time frame within which results will be achieved or value realized (short-term versus long-term);
- the clinical, financial, and business impacts; and
- the implementation and maintenance costs.

Solutions are scored higher if they are generally easy to implement, likely to be adopted into practice, have a high impact, and are relatively low cost or low risk. Solutions with the highest scores can be moved forward by the team, with each team member firmly understanding the criteria for decision-making, having a voice in the decision, and achieving agreement with the results.

Vulnerability and Courageousness

Vulnerability as defined by the *Oxford Dictionary* as "the quality or state of being exposed to the possibility of being attacked or harmed, either physically or emotionally" (Oxford Dictionary,

2020c). In this traditional definition, being vulnerable can be misperceived as having a weakness; in a group dynamic, it can leave an individual feeling afraid that others will observe or judge a comment or contribution in a way that makes him or her feel exposed or embarrassed. However, when applying vulnerability to a group setting in the context of mutual support of individual team members, vulnerability can be the act of opening oneself up to criticism and being honest about one's fears and reservations. Vulnerability can be perceived as a strength in population health teams and can be leveraged to identify gaps in skills and capabilities that can highlight for the team and the leader the need to close those gaps to improve the solution. When team members are vulnerable with one another, which can be uncomfortable, they can be seen by one another as genuine and willing to trust that their exposure to each other is in good faith (Brown, 2018). Vulnerability in the context of openness and willingness to show flaws can be a powerful motivator to the team overall, particularly when motivating other team members to assist in closing any gaps identified.

Courageousness is defined by this same dictionary as "not deterred by danger or pain, brave" (*Oxford Dictionary*, 2020d). Courageousness in the setting of a population health team is doing what one believes to be the true and right thing to do regardless of any external forces that may be pushing in an opposite direction. It is also the ability to not let the fear of criticism stop an individual from being vulnerable and the willingness to proceed despite the fear of failure or judgment. Courageousness in a team can also be uncomfortable, particularly when there is a perceived or actual power dynamic or hierarchy. The possession of emotional and internal strength to take a risk that may not bring success or to ask help from other team members can bring forward an improved solution that would not have otherwise been developed.

The demonstration of both vulnerability and courageousness are needed in the development and fostering of teams working together to solve complex population health challenges.

It will be important for leaders to encourage individuals to show vulnerability and courageousness with the goal of delivering a solution that achieves excellence. One tactic for ensuring that these principles are incorporated is to consider including them as guiding principles in the team charter, with more information provided on guiding principles and team charters in the following section.

Supporting Each Other's Learning

Building the necessary skills to promote successful team performance is required in population health, The recommended PHT is a deliberate compilation of individuals with specific skill sets, knowledge, and experience that will inevitably place team members as both experts and novices. It is important for leaders of these teams to recognize this and put into place safeguards that allow team members to learn while performing.

According to Eduardo Briceño, cofounder and chief executive officer of Mindset Works (a company that promotes organizational cultures of ongoing learning and growth), effective individuals and teams periodically incorporate both learning and performing into their daily practice. Briceño states that when the goal is to improve, individuals place themselves in a learning zone characterized by taking on activities that have not yet been mastered and expecting to make mistakes along the way. This is in contrast to when the goal is to perform, where the individuals place themselves in a performance zone characterized by executing on mastered activities and minimizing mistakes along the way. Briceño concludes that the more time individuals and teams spend in the learning zone, the more improvement can be achieved and directly applied to performance. In addition, building skills in the performance zone can be applied as feedback when in the learning zone, thereby creating an individual's feedback loop (Briceño, 2017).

Relating the learnings from Briceño to forming and developing population health teams, it is key to create the expectation for learning by building in time for conversations among team members on their respective knowledge bases, where they feel their knowledge and expertise is strong, and where it can be improved upon. Protect project time for team members to dedicate themselves to a learning zone and follow time in the learning zone with time to document how to connect the learning to improving overall performance and results.

Guiding Principles

Guiding principles help teams understand how the groups will work, with whom they will interface, and what is important to the team. These principles guide all circumstances, irrespective of changes in goals, strategy, or time lines. They create a team culture in which there is common understanding of what is important to be successful. The guiding principles are developed by each group at the onset of the project's start and adhered to throughout the project's duration. Documenting the principles in a team charter can also solidify the information for reference.

Selecting principles for how the group will work includes decisions on whether the group will meet and communicate in person, online, or via email; how the meetings will be run; what the work is anticipated to be from start to finish (what does "done" look like); and how the team will track and communicate progress. Examples of items to assist in selecting guiding principles include the following:

- Interactions
  - To be scheduled as needed or as a regularly scheduled meeting series
  - In person, online, or email (if in person—meeting location and reserved space)
  - Daily, weekly, monthly, or quarterly cadence
  - Standing or sit-down huddle, working meeting, or touching base
  - Opening remarks, story, or reflection
  - Review of the previous meetings minutes, progress, or assignments

- Communication
  - Record keeping (meeting minutes, recordings, or status reports)
  - Follow-ups, next steps, action items
  - Team member and nonteam member assignments
- Role, Responsibility, and Accountability
  - Expectations of oneself and others
  - Expectations of the responsibilities of oneself and others
  - Evaluation of one's own learning and those of others
  - Evaluation of one's performance and those of others
  - Overall progress toward achieving the desired results

Principles that guide who the team will interface with include documenting a list of anticipated resources the team has access to or will need to complete the project. Anticipating the resources required will provide the team leader time to prepare and secure the resources to have them ready for the team when needed. When interfacing with one another and with others outside of the team, it is important to establish and communicate the expectations for that interface such as how much time to dedicate, which team meetings may be required versus optional, what their role or contribution is to the result, and how to be made aware of any and all results. To understand what or who may be needed for the project to be successful, consider outlining the high-level steps of the project from beginning to end and chart them on a calendar or time line, noting the times during the project when additional resources or expertise may be needed.

Additional principles for the population health leaders and teams to consider including in the documented project charter is the team's stated purpose, goals to achieve, how value is defined, and thoughts on timeliness, quality, quantity, and achievement. It is important for the principles to honor all ideas that come from the team and represent a collaborative and mutually agreed-on list of guiding principles to be referenced by the team throughout the project.

Ground Rules

Ground rules are basic principles that the team recognizes may become challenging or limiting or create potential issues. Team members must understand and be invested in what motivates and is important to each team member. Doing so allows team members to recognize when another team member needs help, to provide feedback, or listen to their concerns. Developing strong relationships is key to developing a strong team dynamic.

Ground rules also shape how meetings will be conducted and ensure processes run smoothly, including who may participate and how decisions will be made. Documenting ground rules solidifies team expectations and can be adjusted as needed. Examples of ground rules include the following (NPD Solutions, n.d.):

- We treat each other with respect.
- We intend to develop personal relationships to enhance trust and open communication.
- We value open dialogue.
- We will give and receive feedback in a constructive manner.
- Each person will come prepared to all meetings.
- For continuity, team members are expected to attend team meetings.
- If a team member is unavailable, then he or she should have a designated, empowered representative attend in his or her place or will be briefed to understand the status of the progress.
- Meetings will start promptly on time. All members are expected to be on time. If members are late because of extenuating circumstances, they must catch up on their own.
- One person talks at a time; there are no side discussions.
- We emphasize open and honest communication; there are no hidden agendas.
- We depersonalize discussion of issues; no attacks on people.
- We will listen, be nonjudgmental, and keep an open mind on issues until it is time to decide.
- We encourage asking "questions of clarification" and avoid asking "questions of attack."

Running the Team(s)

Previously, the PopHealth Troika was introduced as a method to create a diverse and effective population health team. To truly transform health care through the application of population health methods and principles, multiple teams imbedded across the healthcare organization are needed. Developing multiple PHT teams and integrating them across the organization is an effective way to propagate population health management and data-driven analytics.

Running one team requires discipline and focus. Running multiple teams simultaneously while promoting a new way of thinking and working requires resolve and resiliency. Simultaneously forming, developing, and running multiple population health teams representing various domains of expertise, disciplines, and areas of focus in a decentralized model can quickly move a healthcare organization forward in its adoption of population health methods and principles to achieve results. It can also quickly lead to chaos without processes in place to organize the work, the teams, and each team's purpose. Referenced throughout this chapter is the population health team charter, an essential element to building a team-based culture to support population health. The importance of the population health team charter is twofold. First, it grounds each team in the basics, saves time, and reduces confusion. Second, it serves as a living iterative document and a reference for the team to consult when enforcing team expectations, dynamics, conflict resolution, guiding principles, and ground rules.

A population health team charter is created and adopted by the team within the first few team meetings. It should be revisited frequently during the project time line as a reminder to the team of its existence and to enforce the guiding principles and ground rules set by the team. It can be revised as needed. Elements of the population health team charter include *setting in writing* clear expectations, ground rules for understanding one another, working together, communication, holding each other accountable, and other team operational functions. The following shows an example of a population health team charter (Duffy & Moran, 2011; Institute for Healthcare Improvement, 2018). See **Table 31.5**.

Table 31.5 Population Health Team Charter Detail

Forming the Team	
1	*Date and Charter Version*
Value	The team charter is an iterative document that will change over time. Save versions for review after the project is complete.
Example	January 20, 2021: Version 1.0
2	*Project or Problem to Solve*
Value	Team alignment on the problem is the most important aspect of the project for the team to reach mutual agreement and to solve the overall project's purpose.
Example	Reduce hospital admissions in patients with advanced congestive heart failure.
3	*Team Name*
Value	Creating a team bond is an important aspect of team development. Encourage creativity in this element.
Example	Team bravehearts
4	*Team Sponsor or Leadership Committee or Task Force*
Value	Connecting the work to key leaders is important to give and receive feedback, provide needed support and resources, and connect the project to strategic initiatives that drive value for the organization.
Example	VP, Cardiovascular Division, ABC Hospital System.
5	*Team Leader*
Value	Designating a team leader is important to secure one point of contact for sharing communications, project status, and coordinating nonteam resources.
Example	Cheryl Rivera, Manager of Operations for Cardiovascular Health at ABC Hospital System
6	*Team Members and their Skills, Expertise, and Content Area Experience*
Value	Having a written record of team members and their respective skills, expertise, and content area experience can be used when making team assignments, participating in the learning zone, and highlighting any gaps that may be needed to make the project successful.

Example	1. Donald Margolis, MHA, Manager of Operations for Cardiovascular Health at ABC Hospital System
	    a. Degree in healthcare administration.
	    b. Previously worked as an emergency medical technician (EMT).
	    c. Experienced in emergency department, hospital-based medical critical care unit, and cardiovascular step-down unit.

2. Cheryl Rivera MD, MPH, Attending Physician and Division Chief Cardiovascular Health at ABC Hospital System
   a. Degree in clinical medicine, residency in internal medicine and cardiology, board certification in cardiothoracic vascular surgery.
   b. Degree in public health.
   c. Experienced in emergency department, inpatient adult care delivery, advanced heart failure, transplant.
3. Sam Cooper, Data Scientist, Population Health Analytics at ABC Hospital System
   a. Degree in biostatistics and data science.
   b. Previously worked in the banking industry.
   c. Experience in biostatistical modeling, predictive modeling, machine learning.
   d. Experience working with clinical and financial data from health plan, care-delivery systems, and social determinants.

Introducing the Team	
7	**Process to Identify and Resolve Conflict**
Value	Inter- and intrateam dynamic conflict and difficult decision-making will occur in teams working to solve complex challenges. A process to address and resolve conflict will save both time and improve team performance.
Example	The team will work to resolve the conflict in a meeting or in a breakout from an existing meeting and will not let the conflict go unresolved for more than one meeting. Members will treat each other with respect and will be clear and truthful about what is really bothering them and what they want to change. Team members will be willing to take responsibility for their behavior and be willing to compromise.
8	**Learning Zone Opportunities**
Value	Bringing new teams together assumes different baselines of knowledge exist and creating learning opportunities for the team and for individuals improves performance and results.
Example	Each team member will keep a list of ongoing topics for the purpose of learning that connect to improving results. Ten percent of the team's time will be dedicated to learning and will focus on the collective list of topics.
9	**Guiding Principles**
Value	Guiding principles memorialize in writing the desired expectations for team behavior, dialogue, interaction, and performance; it can reduce confusion.
Example	Team meetings will occur once every two weeks, start on time, and follow an agenda dictated by the project plan and time line. To respect other's time, advance notice of one week must be given if a team member cannot attend; this allows for alternative communication or to reschedule the meeting. Team members are expected to come prepared to each meeting, having completed the assignment before the next meeting. Team members will work to resolve the conflict in a meeting or in a breakout from an existing meeting and will not let the conflict go unresolved for more than one meeting, will treat each other with respect, and will be clear and truthful about what is really bothering them and what they want to change. Team members will be willing to take responsibility for their behavior and be willing to compromise. The team leader will communicate all updates and will defer to individual team members for follow-up or clarification if needed. The team will review the team charter, project plan, and project time line monthly to ensure progress is being made and adjustments are well-documented.

(continues)

Table 31.5 **Population Health Team Charter Detail** *(continued)*

Introducing the Team	
10	**Ground Rules**
Value	Ground rules save time and standardize the team members' expectations. They can overlap with guiding principles and outline the expectations for when the team is working together, whether in a work session or a meeting.
Example (Solutions, 2019)	■ Team members will be on time and prepared for meetings. ■ Team members will be engaged and avoid distractions such as multitasking and nonproject-related email. ■ Team members will make points succinctly and be mindful of the time for others to speak. ■ Decisions will be summarized and documented. ■ Action items will be assigned and are expected to be completed before the next meeting.

Population Health-Improvement Project Details	
11	**Population Health Project Improvement Goal**
Value	Answers to the following questions align the team's understanding of the scope of the project and the goal to achieve: (1) What is the magnitude and impact of the problem to solve? (2) What level of improvement is expected to be made? (3) Is the improvement to the root cause or an interim solution?
Example	Within 1 year, reduce hospital admissions by 10% in patients with advanced congestive heart failure presenting to the hospital with fluid imbalance.
12	**In Scope**
Value	Provides a focus for the team on the task at hand.
Example	■ Adult patients with an existing diagnosis of advanced congestive heart failure. ■ Patients who are currently patients of providers (general or specialty) who have privileges at ABC Hospital System. ■ Patients who are identified as not having existing primary care providers and in need of medical homes. ■ Readmissions.
13	**Out of Scope**
Value	Provides a focus for the team on what is not part of the project.
Example	■ Patients with noncongestive heart failure. ■ Patients who do not regularly seek care from ABC Hospital System providers. ■ Inpatient admissions in patients with advanced congestive heart failure not resulting from fluid imbalance.
14	**Stakeholders and End Users**
Value	This is an important step to understanding all of the relevant persons, departments, divisions, and organizations that are impacted by the problem to solve or who can offer assistance to the project team in the form of support, resources, and tools or technology.

Example	<ul><li>Cardiovascular division chief and staff, ABC Hospital System.</li><li>Emergency department staff, ABC Hospital System.</li><li>Primary care medical group, ABC affiliated provider group.</li><li>Home health care group, ABC ancillary care group.</li><li>Population health analytics department, data and analytics division, ABC Hospital Group.</li></ul>
15	**SMART Objectives**
Value	Organizes the work and provides direction for the team with goals that are designed to be specific (S), measurable (M), achievable (A), relevant (R), and time bound (T).
Example: Centers for Disease Control and Prevention (2017)	By December 20, 2020, ABC Hospital System will experience a decrease in admissions because of fluid imbalance in patients with advanced congestive heart failure from 45% to 35% by connecting them to same-day urgent care at ABC Cardiology Outpatient Clinic.
16	**Measures of Success**
Value	Anticipating the measures of success help to quantify and qualify the goals of the project by identifying ways to measure progress toward the goal.
Example	Decrease in ABC Hospital System admissions. Increase in urgent care visits at ABC Cardiology Outpatient Clinic.
17	**Tactics**
Value	Breaking the project objectives into tactics helps the team develop hypotheses to test and assists in assigning work to specific team members.
Example	<ul><li>Evaluate reasons why patients with advanced congestive heart failure go to the emergency room.</li><li>Evaluate reasons why providers send their patients with advanced congestive heart failure to the emergency room or directly admit them to ABC Hospital System.</li><li>Understand how fluid imbalance can contribute to symptoms that warrant evaluation in an emergency or inpatient care setting (also can be considered a learning topic for the team).</li><li>Identify ways to monitor fluid imbalance symptoms of patients at home.</li></ul>
18	**Project Time Line**
Value	Tracking performance and project milestones provides transparency to leaders of the team's activity and progress and helps the team stay on track and on time.
Example	January 20, 2020: Team kickoff meeting and first project assignments. February 1, 2020: First working team meeting. February 20, 2020: First project milestone met; review assignment deliverables, etc.
19	**Anticipated Constraints and Barriers**
Value	Anticipating constraints and barriers can help identify areas of focus when problem-solving, identify areas of concern among team members, and raise awareness to the leader of where assistance may be needed.

(continues)

Table 31.5 Population Health Team Charter Detail   *(continued)*

Population Health-Improvement Project Details	
19	*Anticipated Constraints and Barriers*
Example	■ Individual team member time constraints. This project is in addition to completing day-to-day job activities, and individual team members may be pulled away to address urgent matters. ■ Depending on the number of patients included for evaluation, there may not be the needed sample size for the results to be statistically significant and the project may need more evaluation time.
20	*Resources (Required, Optional, and Needed)*
Value	Identification of required, optional, and needed resources is key to coordinating resources for the project and allows for sufficient time for the optional and needed resources to be secured.
Example	Required: Team members Optional: SMEs and project sponsor to be determined Needed: Electronic health record data warehouse and database access, IT resource to develop patient-tracking method
21	*Project Milestones*
Value	Project milestones provide a transition from one phase of the project to another, urging progress to be made by the successful completion of tasks or objectives throughout the course of the project.
Example	a. Team members understand the project goal, their specific role, and their expected contribution. b. The team understands the problem to solve, has developed learning topics to deepen understanding, and has its first project assignment. c. The team has developed a workflow that maps the experience of patients with advanced congestive heart failure in their use of emergency and inpatient services at ABC Hospital System. d. The team has identified the attributes of patients who are most likely to use emergency and inpatient services at ABC Hospital System to alleviate symptoms and seek care. e. Etc.
22	*Communication Plan*
Value	A communication plan supports alignment across team members, stakeholders, and leadership and provides a road map for expected communications from the team.
Example	A check-in with the project sponsor will occur monthly, and updates will be provided both orally and in written format at that time. Communications will be delivered by the team leader and will include information on team dynamics, progress toward goals and the time line, any actions that need to be taken, and resources that may be needed in the next project phase.
23	*Status Updates*
Value	Status updates are needed to provide specific information on a current situation regarding a team member, intervention, or project.

| Example | ■ A recent loss of a pharmacist SME (left company for another job opportunity) has placed the proposed pharmacy intervention on hold. Anticipate a replacement to be identified within 2 weeks. |
| | ■ Because of unforeseen circumstances beyond the team's control, the project will be placed on hold for 2 months so team members can be triaged to address recent COVID-19 pandemic activity. |

Reproduced from Sylvia, M. (2020). Assembling the population health team. In *The population health management learning series*. ForestVue Healthcare Solutions.

Pitfalls to Avoid When Forming, and Running a Team Culture for Population Health

Throughout this chapter, the advantages of applying a team-based approach to promote population health and data-driven analytics are shared. Too often in health care and particularly in team-based health care, teams are not set up for success. The team members are asked to come together without a clear purpose, a problem to solve, and unclear of their specific roles and responsibilities and those of their team members. The following quote conveys the negative impact a lack of purpose can have on a team.

> [In] the absence of a defined overarching reason for being [shared purpose], members come up with their own agendas. The resulting mishmash of competing personal goals places teammates at cross purposes, triggers rivalries and turf wars, and can even prompt co-worker sabotage. In the most extreme cases, people desert their teams, either by leaving physically or by checking out mentally

and emotionally. (Gostick & Chester, 2010)

When forming population health teams, it is vital to the success of the team that the items outlined in the previous population health team charter are mutually derived and understood by the team members and the project sponsor. The more time spent ahead of the project kickoff to clearly articulate the problem to be solved will prevent additional time spent during the project reconciling misunderstandings and resolving confusion. Early recognition of common pitfalls of teams allows the team leader and project sponsor to intervene and align. Patrick Lencioni's book *The Five Dysfunctions of a Team* (2010) outlines common problems teams experience that negatively impact performance and effectiveness.

Lencioni further recommends that the team dysfunctions outlined in **Figure 31.3** be addressed starting from the left to the right of the arrow, noting that a general lack of trust prevents team members from taking risks or asking for or being receptive to help. As noted previously in this chapter, it is important to outline a process for identifying and resolving conflict. Conflict is a normal part of teams and their work (storming, constructive criticism,

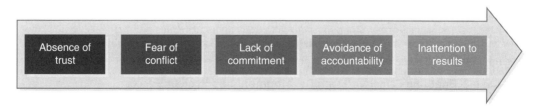

Figure 31.3 The Five Dysfunctions of a Team.

Data from Lencioni, P. (2010). *The five dysfunctions of a team: A leadership fable.* John Wiley & Sons.

Table 31.6 **Additional Attributes of Dysfunctional Teams**

■ Resistance to working in a team	■ Strong personalities
■ Fear of the unknown	■ Fear of ownership
■ Comfort with the status quo	■ Fear of reprisal
■ Personal or hidden agendas	■ Competitiveness
■ Cynicism	■ Placing blame
■ Miscommunication	■ Disparity
■ Gossip and drama	■ Hierarchy

Data from Gostick, A., & Chester, E. (2010). *The Orange Revolution: How one great team can transform an entire organization.* Free Press; Lencioni, P. (2010). *The five dysfunctions of a team: A leadership fable.* John Wiley & Sons. https://doi.org/10.1108/k.2011.06740aae.002; Tuckman, B. W. (1965). Developmental sequence in small groups. *Psychological Bulletin, 63*(6), 384–399. https://doi.org/10.1037/h0022100

feedback), and managing conflict effectively can produce improved results. Lack of commitment and accountability are detrimental to team success. One team member can cause significant disruption in the team's ability to commit to the work, follow through on assignments, and meet critical deadlines. It is important to clearly articulate project milestones and success measures. Failing to do so can lead team members to devise their own personal goals for the project's success and can miss the mark on the original intent of the project.

Additional pitfalls to identify early and avoid are listed in **Table 31.6**.

Applied Learning: Use Cases for a Team-Based Approach for Population Health Analytics

Use Case 1: Creating a Population Health Center of Excellence

You are a leader in a nationally based care-management healthcare company. You have been asked to integrate population health methods and their applications into the existing company's care-management suite of products and services. You are asked to select and lead a population health team, utilize the team's skill sets and experience to create a center of excellence in population health for the company, and identify opportunities for new revenue and improved health outcomes along the way. In researching best practice, you come across a 2009 paper published in *Research Technology Management* by Lisa Daniel and Charles Davis (2015) that studies the characteristics of a high-performing research and development team in a highly competitive industry that defines this team as a "collection of highly trained technical and scientific experts from diverse sources to work collectively and simultaneously on complex technological projects where the demands for rapid development create an intensely challenging environment." You see many similarities between your task of developing a high-performance team to create a center of population health excellence and best practice for the company and the information in this publication, and you are interested in applying the learnings from this publication and others to develop your team and center. What are some of the learnings from this publication that can be applied to developing population health teams, and what other elements do you consider essential to the success of your new team and the company?

Use Case 2: Enabling Effective Team Development and Project Success

The application of Tuckman's model of group development in a clinical setting was highlighted in "Maximizing Team Performance: The Critical Role of the Nurse Leader," (Manges, Scott-Cawiezell, & Ward, 2016) including the challenges inherent in bringing a group of highly independent and successful individuals together to accomplish a common goal through a standardized process to improve patient safety called TeamSTEPPS. This research study proposes several leadership strategies and keys to success to enable effective team development and project success. Describe some of the leadership strategies, behaviors, and keys to success found in this study.

Now think about a team experience you have had in the past and reflect on that experience to answer the following questions:

1. Was the team and project successful? Why or why not?
2. What leadership strategies were or were not in place to guide the team to success?
3. Was the team effective (drive results) and efficient (productive, timely)?
4. What were some of the keys to success that enabled the team to be effective?
5. Describe some tactics and behaviors that will make you more effective in your team-based work.

Conclusion

The complexity of achieving the Triple Aim's mission and goals through a population health approach necessitates a multidisciplinary, orchestrated team approach. Advantages of a team-based approach include enabling a team to tackle challenges that an individual alone cannot solve, the ability for teams to compensate one another's strengths and weaknesses, and the synergy and diversity that teams with different perspectives, knowledge, experience, and skills bring together. This chapter outlines how to create a safe space for team members to simultaneously innovate and learn, set clear performance goals, define the scope of work and stick to it, and challenge one another's assumptions with respect and improve performance and results.

Formation of multiple PopHealth Troika teams can simultaneously propagate population health management and data-driven analytics across an organization to transform care delivery and improve health outcomes. Tools that assist in identifying and managing team conflict, guiding principles, and ground rules for effective meeting management can all be included in the team's population health team charter, along with the team's purpose, project details, and progress. Taking the time to organize the team, the work, and the resources will set up the team and the project for success.

Study and Discussion Questions

- In what ways do team dynamics support or deter project success?
- From your experience, what additional strategies or tactics not included in this chapter would further support the development of a team culture for population health?
- What are some of the pitfalls of not supporting teams in their development and maturity?

Resources and Websites

Centers for Disease Control and Prevention (CDC). (n.d.) *Evaluation guide: Writing SMART objectives*. Atlanta, GA: CDC, Division for Heart Disease and Stroke Prevention. https://www.cdc.gov/dhdsp/docs/smart_objectives.pdf

Farris, G. F., & Cordero, R. (2002, November). Leading your scientists and engineers. *Research-Technology Management, 45*(6), 13–25. https://www.researchgate.net/publication/233665973_Leading_Your_Scientists_and_Engineers_2002

Grossman, S. (1997). Managers at work: Turning technical groups into high-performance teams. *Research-Technology Management, 40*(2), 9–11. https://doi.org/10.1080/08956308.1997.11671111

H&CS Workforce Council. (2013). Guide: Developing a population health project plan. https://www.checkup.org.au/icms_docs/182812_8_GUIDE_Developing_a_Population_Health_Project_Plan.pdf

Hoyt, J., & Gerloff, E. A. (1999). Organizational environment, changing economic conditions, and the effective supervision of technical personnel: A management challenge. *Journal of High Technology Management Research, 10*(2),

275–293. https://doi.org/10.1016/S1047-8310(99)00014-0

MeetingSift. (2020). The 10 ground rules for meetings. http://meetingsift.com/ground-rules-for-meetings/

Reagans, R., & Zuckerman, E. W. (2001). Networks, diversity, and productivity: The social capital of corporate R&D teams. *Organization Science, 12*(4), 502–517. https://doi.org/10.1287/orsc.12.4.502.10637

References

Borek, A. J., & Abraham, C. (2018, February 15). How do small groups promote behaviour change? An integrative conceptual review of explanatory mechanisms. *Applied Psychology. Health and Well-Being, 10*(1), 30–61. https://doi.org/10.1111/aphw.12120

Briceño, E. (2017). How to get better at the things you care about. https://www.ted.com/talks/eduardo_briceno_how_to_get_better_at_the_things_you_care_about?language=en

Brown, B. (2018). Dare to lead: Brave work, tough conversations, whole hearts. https://daretolead.brenebrown.com/

Carney, B. T., West, P., Neily, J., Mills, P. D., & Bagian, J. P. (2010, June 9). Differences in nurse and surgeon perceptions of teamwork: Implications for use of a briefing checklist in the OR. *AORN Journal, 91*(6), 722–729. https://doi.org/10.1016/j.aorn.2009.11.066

Clarke, J. L., Bourn, S., Skoufalos, A., Beck, E. H., & Castillo, D. J. (2017). An innovative approach to health care delivery for patients with chronic conditions. *Population Health Management, 20*(1), 23–30. https://doi.org/10.1089/pop.2016.0076

Daniel, L. J., & Davis, C. R. (2015). What makes high-performance teams excel? *Research-Technology Management, 52*(4), 40. https://www.tandfonline.com/doi/abs/10.1080/08956308.2009.11657578

Deblois, S., & Lepanto, L. (2016, March). Lean and Six Sigma in acute care: A systematic review of reviews. *International Journal of Health Care Quality Assurance, 29*, 192–208. https://doi.org/10.1108/IJHCQA-05-2014-0058

Duffy, G. L., & Moran, J. W. (2011). Applications and tools for creating and sustaining healthy teams. https://bibliovirtual.files.wordpress.com/2011/05/applications_and_tools_for_creating_and_sustaining_healthy_teams.pdf

Ferguson, S. L. (2008, April). TeamSTEPPS: Integrating teamwork principles into adult health/medical-surgical practice. *Medsurg Nursing: Official Journal of the Academy of Medical-Surgical Nurses, 17*(2), 122–125. https://pubmed.ncbi.nlm.nih.gov/18517173/

Ford, H. (n.d.). Coming together. . . . Good Reads. https://www.goodreads.com/quotes/118854-coming-together-is-the-beginning-keeping-together-is-progress-working

Gallup. (2020). Strengthsfinder 2.0 from Gallup and Tom Rath: Discover your clifton strengths by Don Clifton. https://www.gallup.com/cliftonstrengths/en/strengthsfinder.aspx

Gleddie, M., Stahlke, S., & Paul, P. (2018, December 30). Nurses' perceptions of the dynamics and impacts of teamwork with physicians in labour and delivery. *Journal of Interprofessional Care*. https://doi.org/10.1080/13561820.2018.1562422

Gostick, A., & Chester, E. (2010). *The Orange Revolution: How one great team can transform an entire organization.* Free Press.

Green, B., Oeppen, R. S., Smith, D. W., & Brennan, P. A. (2017, March 23). Challenging hierarchy in healthcare teams—Ways to flatten gradients to improve teamwork and patient care. *British Journal of Oral and Maxillofacial Surgery, 55*, 449–453. https://doi.org/10.1016/j.bjoms.2017.02.010

Hale, E. E. (n.d.). Together—one of the most inspiring words in the. . . . Quotes of famous people.

Hekmat, S., Dehnavieh, R., Rahimisadegh, R., Kohpeima, V., & Jahromi, J. (2015). Team attitude evaluation: An evaluation in hospital committees. *Materia Socio Medica, 27*(6), 429–433. https://www.researchgate.net/publication/286524348_Team_Attitude_Evaluation_an_Evaluation_in_Hospital_Committees

Institute for Healthcare Improvement. (2018). QI project charter. http://www.ihi.org/resources/Pages/Tools/QI-Project-Charter.aspx

Kim, T. (2020). Improving preparedness for and response to Coronavirus disease 19 (COVID-19) in long-term care hospitals in Korea. *Infection & Chemotherapy, 52*(2), 133. https://doi.org/10.3947/ic.2020.52.2.133

Knapp, S. (2015, October 12). Lean Six Sigma implementation and organizational culture. *International Journal of Health Care Quality Assurance, 28*(8), 855–863. https://doi.org/10.1108/IJHCQA-06-2015-0079

Last, S. (2019). Five models for understanding team dynamics. Technical Writing Essentials. https://pressbooks.bccampus.ca/technicalwriting/chapter/understandingteamdynamics/

Lencioni, P. (2010). *The five dysfunctions of a team: A leadership fable.* John Wiley & Sons. https://doi.org/10.1108/k.2011.06740aae.002

Li, L.-q., Huang, T., Wang, Y.-q., Wang, Z.-p., Liang, Y., . . . , Wang, Y. (2020, March 12). COVID-19 patients' clinical characteristics, discharge rate, and fatality rate of meta-analysis. *Journal of Medical Virology, 92:* 577–583. https://doi.org/10.1002/jmv.25757

Liberati, E. G., Gorli, M., & Scaratti, G. (2016, February). Invisible walls within multidisciplinary teams: Disciplinary boundaries and their effects on integrated care. *Social Science and Medicine, 150,* 31–39. https://doi.org/10.1016/j.socscimed.2015.12.002

Makary, M. A., Sexton, J. B., Freischlag, J. A., Holzmueller, C. G., Millman, E. A., Rowen, L., & Pronovost, P. J. (2006). Operating room teamwork among physicians and nurses: Teamwork in the eye of the beholder. *Journal of the American College of Surgeons, 202*(5), 746–752. https://doi.org/10.1016/j.jamcollsurg.2006.01.017

Manges, K., Scott-Cawiezell, J., & Ward, M. M. (2016, May 19). Maximizing team performance: The critical role of the nurse leader. *Nursing Forum, 52*(1), 21–29. https://doi.org/10.1111/nuf.12161

MC Hospital Simulation Lab. (2011). Code Blue team: Roles and function. Montgomery College.https://www.montgomerycollege.edu/_documents/academics/departments/nursing-tpss/code-blue-team-roles-and-function.pdf

Moss, E., & Maxfield, D. (2007, March–April). Crucial conversations for healthcare: How to discuss lack of support, poor teamwork, and disrespect. Part II of III. *Professional Case Management, 12*(2), 112–115. https://doi.org/10.1097/01.PCAMA.0000265346.54891.1c

NPD Solutions. (n.d.). Team groundrules. https://www.npd-solutions.com/groundrules.html. ©2019 DRM Associates.

Oxford Dictionary. (2020a). Troika—defined. Lexico.com. https://www.lexico.com/en/definition/troika

Oxford Dictionary. (2020b). Momentum—defined. Lexico.com. https://www.lexico.com/definition/momentum

Oxford Dictionary. (2020c). Vulnerability—defined. Lexico.com. https://www.lexico.com/en/definition/vulnerability

Oxford Dictionary. (2020d). Courageous—defined. Lexico.com. https://www.lexico.com/en/definition/courageous

Pande, P. S., Neuman, R. P., & Cavanaugh, R. R. (2002). *The Six Sigma Way Team Fieldbook: An Implementation Guide for Process Improvement Teams.* McGraw Hill.

Patel, D. (2017). Why perfection is the enemy of done. Forbes. https://www.forbes.com/sites/deeppatel/2017/06/16/why-perfection-is-the-enemy-of-done/#59efba884395

Ratcliffe, S. (Ed.). (2020). Concise Oxford Dictionary of quotations. https://global.oup.com/academic/product/concise-oxford-dictionary-of-quotations-9780199567072?cc=us&lang=en&

Rutayisire, E., Nkundimana, G., Mitonga, H. K., Boye, A., & Nikwigize, S. (2020, June 11). What works and what does not work in response to COVID-19 prevention and control in Africa. *International Journal of Infectious Diseases, 97,* 257–269. https://doi.org/10.1016/j.ijid.2020.06.024

Shea, C. M., Turner, K., Albritton, J., & Reiter, K. L. (2018). Contextual factors that influence quality improvement implementation in primary care: The role of organizations, teams, and individuals. *Health Care Management Review, 43*(3), 261–269. https://doi.org/10.1097/HMR.0000000000000194

Shortell, S. M., Blodgett, J. C., Rundall, T. G., & Kralovec, P. (2018, October). Use of Lean and related transformational performance improvement systems in hospitals in the United States: Results from a national survey. *Joint Commission Journal on Quality and Patient Safety, 44*(10), 574–582. https://doi.org/10.1016/j.jcjq.2018.03.002

Sylvia, M. (2020). Assembling the Population Health Analytics Team. In Population Health Management Learning Series. Charleston, SC: ForestVue Healthcare Solutions.

Teamwork. (2016, July 25). Four ways to gain momentum and trust as a team. https://www.teamwork.com/blog/4-ways-gain-momentum-trust-team/

Tew, R. (2015, June 5). Focus on your strengths instead of your weaknesses, on your powers instead of your problems. Live Life Happy. https://livelifehappy.com/life-quotes/focus-on-your-strengths-instead-of-your-weaknesses/

Thomas, E. J., Sexton, J. B., & Helmreich, R. L. (2003, March). Discrepant attitudes about teamwork among critical care nurses and physicians. *Critical Care Medicine, 31*(3), 956–959. https://doi.org/10.1097/01.CCM.0000056183.89175.76

Tuckman, B., & Jensen, M. (1977, December 1). Stages of small-group development revisited. *Group & Organization Management.* https://journals.sagepub.com/doi/10.1177/105960117700200404

Tuckman, B. W. (1965). Developmental sequence in small groups. *Psychological Bulletin, 63*(6), 384–399. https://doi.org/10.1037/h0022100

University of Illinois. (2015). Solution prioritization matrix how-to guide. https://www.uillinois.edu/common/pages/DisplayFile.aspx?itemId=407095

Wosik, J., Fudim, M., Cameron, B., Gellad, Z. F., Cho, A., Phinney, D., Curtis, S., Roman, M., Poon, E. G., Ferranti, J., Katz, J. N., & Tcheng, J. (2020). Telehealth transformation: COVID-19 and the rise of virtual care. *Journal of the American Medical Informatics Association, 27*(6), 957–962. https://doi.org/10.1093/jamia/ocaa067

CHAPTER 32

Skills Assessment of Population Health Analysts

Elizabeth McCormick, MBA

Ideas don't make you rich. The correct execution of ideas does.

—Felix Dennis (Courtesy of the Literary Executors of the Felix Dennis Estate)

EXECUTIVE SUMMARY

As the healthcare industry continues its transformation to value-based payment, population health analytics are essential to providing actionable insights using data derived from individual patients and aggregated into populations. With fundamental success in population health tied to understanding the intersection of costs and clinical outcomes, the analyst's role and analytics as a discipline are at the center of making a population health approach work. Analysts are at the center of providing data and insights that allow healthcare organizations to take required action. Turning data into actionable information is what good analytics is all about: unlocking data to drive meaningful, sustainable change.

Given that analytics and analysts are central to success, an organization must identify, develop, and retain the talent needed to support this work, commonly using job descriptions and skills assessments to manage this critical function. Skill assessments allow an understanding of staff capabilities and identify gaps where training is needed to maximize the growth and potential of individuals and get the work done.

The process of creating an effective skills assessment starts with identifying the skills needed to be successful and then hiring and developing staff according to those criteria. Although there is a great deal of published literature on the use and value of skills assessments in the hiring process—also called *talent selection*—there is little written on the application of a skills assessment to create internal project teams and even less on how a skills assessment may be applied to the population health analyst role and in the formation of population health analytic teams.

A skills-assessment tool and management process applies to and benefits both the analyst as well as the organization. In today's marketplace, skills formation and effective utilization of skills has become a competitive necessity. Similar to the well understood and documented business value that skills assessment provides to talent selection, application of a skills assessment for existing employees allows employers to build the right teams for successful outcomes. In both talent selection and talent placement, making the wrong decision is extremely expensive. Putting that into specific context for analytics projects, business analytics returns $9.01 for every dollar spent (Nucleus Research, 2019). With that amount of financial impact on the line, organizations must create analytic teams that have the skills to deliver on desired goals.

LEARNING OBJECTIVES

At the end of this chapter, the learner will be able to:

1. Define the desired population health analytic skill set.
2. Describe the concept of a skills assessment and learning levels.
3. Explain the application of a skills assessment in your organization for increased performance.

Introduction

Skills assessments are designed to provide a best practice methodology for measuring and understanding workforce skills. The process supports an effective skills-management practice, and the value is delivered through aligning a company's most important asset, its people, with its ability to deliver meaningful and targeted outcomes.

Skill is most simply defined as the ability to do something and is the application of individual knowledge and experience within certain environmental stimuli (Wikipedia, n.d.). Certain skills are expected of analysts based on their job function and role, and these skills are ideally outlined in their job description. As part of the evaluation of skills mastery, the organization measures, reports, and maintains skills-assessment data that result in a repository of information that can be used to refine the skills the organization requires from analytic roles in population health.

This chapter will focus on three areas of the skills-assessment process: (1) defining the components of a skills-assessment framework and process, (2) identifying the domains of skills that support population health analytics, and (3) showing how skills assessments can be implemented for success within organizations.

A Skills-Assessment Framework

Creating a simple yet effective skills assessment is a five-step process as outlined in **Table 32.1**.

Table 32.1 Process for Developing a Skills Assessment

Step	Benefit
1. Define list of skills	Focuses on the needs of the organization or team and provides transparency to staff on the skills required
2. Group skills by content area or job function	Improves focus and applicability
3. Define level of performance	Sets criteria and allows data comparability across individuals and teams
4. Analyst self-assessment of skills	Empowers analysts to reflect on skills attainment and acknowledge areas of opportunity and growth
5. Leader review with analyst	Reveals discrepancies in perception; allows opportunity to create growth and development plan

The first three steps of the process are focused on creating the tool itself, determining the skills, groupings, and performance levels. The last two steps are more focused on implementing the tool, collecting data, and identifying areas for analysts' growth and development.

Step 1: Defining Skills

The first step in creating a skills assessment is skill identification. This starts with the job description. It is generally accepted practice that organizations classify skills across multiple domains that are required for proper job function and success in the workplace.

Skills are assigned to individuals based on their job function and reflect what the organization requires from the job. The job description for a population health analyst typically includes general indicators of job function in the form of statements like the following:

- "Design population health data sets for purposes such as modeling, production, or mining."
- "Interpret population health data studies to uncover data sources or new uses for existing sources."
- "Develop prototypes, proofs of concept, algorithms, predictive models or custom analysis."
- "Apply statistical computer languages like Python and SAS to varied data sets."
- "Demonstrate familiarity with machine-learning techniques and advanced statistical concepts."

- "Ability to code in multiple languages."
- "Work with key stakeholders in different functional areas to identify analytic solutions for individuals and populations."

The job description will generally not address how actions are driven by specific skills or what skill proficiencies are needed for the job. That is the role of a skills assessment. It is critical that those closest to the work be involved in the formation of the skills assessment, starting with skill identification; doing so prevents the organization from assessing a long list of irrelevant competencies that add time, cost, and no value, and the action creates immediate buy-in and relevance for the tool and process that will guide their professional development and their performance review in some cases.

Step 2: Grouping Skills

Skills are commonly represented in three domains: technical, business, and interpersonal (commonly called *soft skills*). For purposes of this chapter, we will use these domains to group skills into an organizing framework for constructing and successfully applying a proper skills assessment. A technical skill is typically one that is closely related to a specific content domain and job role (research, analysis, modeling). Interpersonal skill is generally applicable across all content domains and multiple roles (communication, problem solving, collaboration). Business skills are focused on the knowledge of the industry and how the organization operates (its function and capabilities). **Tables 32.2A**, **32.2B**, and **32.2C**

Table 32.2 Technical, Business, and Interpersonal Skills

(A) Technical Skills

Skills Category	Description	Example Use in Population Health Analytics
Data management	Query and retrieve data from warehouses, perform calculations, make queries more efficient, code parameters for data quality standards.	■ Create, integrate, update, and delete data resulting in analysis-ready data sets. ■ Assess data quality.

(continues)

Table 32.2 Technical, Business, and Interpersonal Skills *(continued)*

(A) Technical Skills

Skills Category	Description	Example Use in Population Health Analytics
Reporting	Work with end users to define and refine reporting needs and requirements. Define denominators and numerators in data terms. Interpret and validate reporting results and troubleshoot issues.	■ Provide frontline staff members with data needed to manage their workload. ■ Provide management reporting.
Analysis	Ability to access and manipulate databases using querying and analytic software. Ability to interpret, understand and contextualize data for use in business reporting as an end user. Collaborate with stakeholders to understand the clinical and business question asked of the data. Design analysis plan and collect and structure data for analysis. Apply appropriate analytical techniques using optimal tools. Interpret and validate analytic results and troubleshoot issues.	■ Ask relevant and appropriate questions of the data. ■ Extract pertinent insights from data. ■ Execute analytics in support of the population health process.
Modeling	Apply mathematical techniques to create a model that estimates future outcomes or unknown values based on historical data, future expectations, other indicators. Apply mathematical and statistical techniques to create linear and logistic regression-based predictive models. Apply techniques to create machine-learning, pattern-based predictive models. Apply simulation and other relevant techniques to create prescriptive models. Apply model validation techniques and interpret results appropriately.	■ Development and validation of risk-prediction and prescriptive models. ■ Assessment of and ability to compare and contrast vendor-based risk-prediction and prescription models.
Visualization	Present data using appropriate charts, graphs, and tables and understand types of visualizations.	■ Packaging the data insights to increase transparency, clarity, and actionability. ■ Delivering results in way that is best received by the particular audience.

(B) Business Skills		
Skills Category	**Description**	**Example Use in Population Health Analytics**
Operations	The ability to place analytic results in the context of workflow and translate analytic products into operational workflow to enable successful outcomes, value, and sustainability. Linking clinical and other operational workflow to data flow. Recognizing and troubleshooting discrepancies between workflow and data flow. Integrating analytic products into clinical and operational workflow. Developing a sustainability plan for analytic products.	■ Incorporating operational considerations into population health analytic process. ■ Operationalizing analytic products like risk-prediction models and monitoring metrics.
Compliance and ethical principles	Involves following rules and regulations around data use and applying ethical principles when performing analytic techniques and interpreting results. Comply with contractual agreements for data use. Identify ethical considerations and concerns in analytic results. Recognize unintended consequences when using analytic results to develop interventions.	■ Identify ethical and compliance concerns when working with data and managing issues appropriately.
Finance	Appropriately interpret financial data points related to costs and utilization. Apply risk-adjustment techniques. Determine number needed to treat. Determine cost savings and return on investment for interventions. Validate and troubleshoot cost and utilization analytic results.	■ Link health determinants to health cost and utilization outcomes to identify cost drivers. ■ Risk-adjust outcomes. ■ Determine the value of population health interventions. ■ Develop monitoring metrics with performance targets.

(C) Interpersonal Skills		
Skills Category	**Description**	**Example Use in Population Health Analytics**
Communication	Communication includes speaking, listening, and writing. It is the ability to present data to different audiences through various media channels and information technologies.	■ Collaborate as part of the clinician, analyst, business team to achieve analytic results in the population health process. ■ Disseminate and effectively present results of population health analyses.

(continues)

Table 32.2 Technical, Business, and Interpersonal Skills *(continued)*

(C) Interpersonal Skills

Skills Category	Description	Example Use in Population Health Analytics
Critical thinking	Critical thinking is represented in 12 distinct areas: analysis, identification and assessment of a problem, information seeking, questioning, and reflection, conceptualizing, evaluating, interpreting, predicting, reasoning, and synthesizing (Alexander, 2014).	■ Sifting through noise in data to identify important areas of focus. ■ Creating insights from data. ■ Making clinical and business recommendations based on analytical findings.
Problem solving	The ability to handle difficult situations and complex business challenges and identify solutions.	■ Identifying solutions to complex data issues. ■ Managing conflicting findings and recommendations. ■ Determining the what and how of measurement.

Data from Sylvia, M. (2020). Assessing population health analyst skills. In *Population health management learning series.* ForestVue Healthcare Solutions.

delineate the skills categories within each domain and provide examples of their typical use in population health analytics.

Beyond required data and analytic skills taught in most graduate-level programs, specific skills have proven valuable if not essential for effective performance on a population health analytics project and team. Most of these skills are learned on the job during such projects. **Table 32.3** describes the content areas for skill sets that are specific to analysts working in population health. Analysts should be able to demonstrate varying levels of competency in each skills content area. Chapters 30 and 31 provide illustrations of how and when these skills are applied to drive successful outcomes for population health projects.

Table 32.3 Skills Specific to Population Health Analytics

Skills Content Area	Description
Person-centric analytics	An analytic approach that uses people as the denominator (see Chapters 2 and 13)
Data sources and context	The multiple sources of data used for population health analytics along with the use and application of data contextualizers and data input tools (see Sections 2 and 3)
Epidemiologic principles	Surveillance techniques applied to person-centric data (see Chapter 20)
Risk adjustment	Statistical techniques to account for bias in the results of healthcare-related metrics (see Chapter 21)
Risk prediction, regression-based methods	Applying mathematical techniques to data for predicting an adverse outcome using logistic and linear regression (see Chapter 22)

Risk prediction, pattern-based methods	Applying data mining in databases and using machine learning, clustering, and classification methods to identify patterns in data with the goal of preventing adverse outcomes (see Chapter 23)
Run charts, statistical process control, benchmarking	Using principles of statistics to create measures of variation that allow distinguishing between common cause and special cause variation (see Chapter 24)
Big data analytics	Large, multisource, multivariable data sets meeting the five V's: volume, veracity, velocity, variety, and variability
Evidence-based practice	The conscientious, explicit, and judicious use of current best evidence in making decisions about the care of patients and populations (see Chapter 2) (Sackett, Rosenberg, Gray, Haynes, & Richardson, 2007)
Ethical principles	Applying ethical principles to the use of population health data (see Chapter 34)
Social determinants of health	Using data points that reflect the social determinants of health in population health analyses (see Chapter 7)

Data from Sylvia, M. (2020). Assessing population health analyst skills. In *Population health management learning series*. ForestVue Healthcare Solutions.

Step 3: Defining Performance Levels

Once skills are identified and grouped by category or job function, the next step of the skills-assessment process is assigning levels of performance and descriptions for success at each level. For each skill, there is a continuum of proficiency ranging from novice to expert. A common approach to defining performance levels along the continuum is using a five-point Likert scale such as:

1. basic understanding or knowledge,
2. functional knowledge and can do basic tasks with assistance,
3. independent function and knowledge,
4. advanced experience or knowledge, and
5. expert-level experience or knowledge.

Providing a fixed, universal numerical rating scheme provides the organization with a standard methodology for measuring ability that can apply to all staff and all skills. This approach creates a level playing field. Using a standard scoring method allows data to be combined, compared, and manipulated in multiple directions. This

flexibility is practical only if the standard rating scheme is consistently applied.

Next, each skill or competency must include a description to measure success for each level of performance. The descriptions must be specific and relatable to the actual work that occurs, so the descriptions should be developed with input from those who are to be measured as well as the leaders who are validating the work. **Table 32.4** shows an example of one competency defined over five levels of proficiency.

Step 4: Analyst Self-Assessment

At this point in the process, the skills assessment is designed with skills organized by content areas; now it needs to be organized into a data-collection tool. Although a paper mechanism of collection would suffice, data are best collected in an electronic format so that baseline skills can be established and progress can be tracked. In house database tools such as Microsoft Access or external survey tools like SurveyMonkey are ideal for this type of data collection and tracking. An electronic survey tool collects the opinions of employees

Table 32.4 Skills Leveling Example

Skill	Description	Level 1	Level 2	Level 3	Level 4	Level 5
Data sources and structure	Familiarity with the use and application of data contextualizers and data inputs	Can articulate the source needed to answer a question about a data input	Distinguishes between data inputs and articulates appropriate uses for each	Becomes an expert in at least one data source or contextualizer and uses it appropriately and regularly	Becomes an expert in two or more data sources or contextualizers and uses them appropriately and regularly	Trains and provides mentorship for using data sources and contextualizers in which expertise is achieved. Continues to expand expertise.

Data from Sylvia, M. (2020). Assessing population health analyst skills. In *Population health management learning series*. ForestVue Healthcare Solutions.

based on their experience and knowledge of each other, themselves, and the work environment.

Measuring skills subjectively is the easiest and fastest way to achieve results that are assumed to be reasonably accurate because individuals know their own level of ability and can cite specific examples of performance that support their own proficiency rating. Another benefit to collecting data via self-assessment is that it encourages the individual to reflect on their own performance, progress, and learning, and it promotes individual responsibility and ownership of personal development.

The data-collection tool should clearly state the purpose and importance of the assessment. The survey instrument should be constructed with the inputs from the first three process steps. Skills are outlined by category, and each skill is defined with specific descriptions across the performance levels. Each question should allow space for individuals to provide examples that support their self-ranking.

Using an electronic survey tool allows the organization to collect, store, and report information easily, and it offers leadership a way not only to review the individual's performance but also to compare that across a group of individuals or drill down on specific skills.

Step 5: Leader Review with Analyst

Leaders should review analysts' self-perceptions and seek to understand gaps between analyst ratings and their own. Ideally, the leader also indirectly solicits input from the analyst's peers and through observation of the analyst's work products. These actions support proper feedback and goal setting. Leaders should meet with staff individually to review results soon after the analyst completes the self-assessment to keep the dialogue fresh and relevant. If a leader identifies someone who does not meet the skill requirements, then the common next step is to create a personalized development plan with action steps that will help them close their performance gaps. Leaders should use the output of the skills assessment to set baseline skills attainment, track analysts' growth and development, create individual staff development plans, place the right people on the right projects, and form the best and most successful teams. In addition, the aggregated results across the entire analyst team can be used to promote departmental and organizational skills improvement plans.

Benefits of Skills Assessment

The benefits of a skills assessment are relevant at the individual, team, and organization levels. Proper use and application of a skills assessment will increase likelihood of goal achievement.

- *Individual*: The skills assessment provides analysts with insight into their own competencies, their valuable contributions, and their own learning needs. Depending on their role and project and team needs, this insight helps individual analysts define their role on the team and communicate expectations for their performance.
- *Team*: The skills assessment allows team leadership to compare the desired results of the teamwork to the skills necessary for accomplishing these results, thus facilitating delineation of roles and responsibilities. With this information, team leaders can identify where necessary skills are present and the gaps. If a critical skill is missing on the team, then actions can be taken to accommodate for the gaps.
- *Organization*: When teams use resources appropriately, projects are executed with success and result in the achievement of organizational goals. The assessment of competencies and gaps informs strategic investments in human resources, refinement of policies and procedures, a focus on learning and development, and an understanding of expectations for what can be accomplished with existing staff (Sylvia, 2020).

Additional Resources to Build a Population Health Analytic Skill Set

In early 2015 the Association for Community Health Improvement began the work of identifying competencies related to population health. This work took form over several years with contributing organizations and industry professionals coalescing around a set of desired skills related to the core competencies of public health. These competencies are designed for health professionals (e.g., hospitals, health systems, public health, health care) "engaged in assessment of population health needs and development, delivery, and improvement of population health programs, services, and practices. This may include activities related to community health needs assessments, community health improvement plans, implementation of community-based interventions, and coalition building" (Association for Community Health Improvement, 2019).

This body of knowledge can be used to guide population health workforce development efforts, including the creation of training, workforce development and training plans, academic curricula, job descriptions, performance objectives, tools, and other resources to support the activities and growth of population health professionals.

The TRAIN Learning Network is a national network providing training opportunities for professionals working to improve the public's health. Its developers have designed content to accompany this competency set in two areas:

1. The social determinants of health (SDOH) training plan provides an overview of the SDOH, supporting learners in developing knowledge and skills to describe fundamental aspects of SDOH, explain social contexts and effects of SDOH on specific populations, and apply SDOH knowledge to design targeted interventions for improving public health.
2. The health equity learning bundle provides frontline professionals with knowledge to better understand health equity and approaches that can help address related challenges (TRAIN Learning Network, 2019).

Conclusion

The business case for creating a process of skill identification, measurement, and development related to analytics roles within a population health team or approach cannot be undersold. According to Gartner, "by 2023, data literacy will become an explicit and necessary driver of business value, demonstrated by its formal inclusion in over 80% of data and analytics strategies and change management programs" (Rollings & White, 2020).

This chapter provided a framework for designing and implementing a skills assessment, defined the skills of the population analyst, as well as contextualized how a skills-assessment tool can be used by individuals and leaders to drive organizational success.

Study and Discussion Questions

- Why is it important to define, assess, and measure analytical skill sets?
- What is essential to understanding skill development and job performance?
- How can skill assessments add value in your organization?
- How are analytical skills and population health skills related to one another?

Resources and Websites

The Skills Base Competency Framework: https://www.skills-base.com/competency-framework

Public Health Foundation: About the Core Competencies for Public Health Professionals: http://www.phf.org/programs/corecompetencies/Pages/About_the_Core_Competencies_for_Public_Health_Professionals.aspx

Society for Human Resources Management: https://www.shrm.org/about-shrm/Pages/default.aspx

References

Alexander, M. E. (2014). Critical thinking in public health: An exploration of skills used by public health practitioners and taught by instructors. Georgia State University https://scholarworks.gsu.edu/epse_diss/101

Association for Community Health Improvement. (2019). Competencies for population health professionals.

Nucleus Research. (2019, January 28). Investing in analytics returns $9.01 per dollar spent. https://nucleusresearch.com/research/single/investing-in-analytics-returns-9-01-per-dollar-spent/

Rollings, M., & White, A. (2020, March 4). Build a data-driven enterprise. Gartner Research. https://www.gartner.com/document/3981770?ref=solrAll&refval=252272924

Sackett, D. L., Rosenberg, W. M. C., Gray, J. A. M., Haynes, R. B., & Richardson, W. S. (2007). Evidence based medicine: what it is and what it isn't. 1996. *Clinical Orthopaedics and Related Research, 455*(7023), 3–5. https://doi.org/10.1136/bmj.312.7023.71

Sylvia, M. (2020). Assessing population health analyst skills. In *Population health management learning series*. ForestVue Healthcare Solutions.

TRAIN Learning Network. (2019). Welcome to the TRAIN Learning Network. https://www.train.org/main/welcome

Wikipedia. (n.d.). Skill defined. https://en.wikipedia.org/wiki/Skill

CHAPTER 33

Clinical Workflow Transformation

Ron Parton, MD, MPH

Ines Maria Vigil, MD, MPH, MBA

Transforming clinical workflow so that our healthcare system optimizes care for "every single one."

—Ron Parton

EXECUTIVE SUMMARY

According to many involved in healthcare analytics, developing and implementing population-based systems that transform clinical workflow and optimize care for defined populations will require the following (Bodenheimer, Ghorob, Willard-Grace, & Grumbach, 2014; Margolius & Bodenheimer, 2010):

- leadership and cultural transformation,
- population and panel management,
- proactive care teams,
- clinical workflow enhancement and care plan optimization, and
- measurement of outcomes and continuous improvement.

Generally, existing healthcare systems were developed to treat acute health conditions and acute presentations of chronic health conditions. Systematic change to the way health care is delivered is required to apply population health methods to address all aspects of care, including improved patient experience, health outcomes, and healthcare cost (Institute for Healthcare Improvement, n.d.). Whether the goal is to improve the quality of care for an attributed primary care panel of patients, achieve improved health outcomes for patients with advanced congestive heart failure, or identify a cost-effective way of treating patients with chronic back pain, the basics of population health improvement are the same: define the population, support panel management, create the evidence-based guideline or clinical pathway, assign the care team, develop the optimal workflow, measure the outcomes, and provide feedback for continuous improvement (Allen et al., 2014). Adopting population health improvement as a basic methodology and paradigm for designing our clinical systems also requires new data and analytic methods and information technology to support this work (Torres et al., 2014).

LEARNING OBJECTIVES

At the end of this chapter, the learner will be able to:

1. Describe the common elements and building blocks of clinical workflow transformation.
2. Discuss the key issues, resource requirements and constraints, information technology functionality, and data and analytics that can impact clinical workflow development.
3. Understand the application of population health concepts and methods to clinical workflows to transform healthcare services.

Introduction

The journey to transform the current U.S. healthcare system from one that is oriented to acute care for individuals to a system that continuously improves longitudinal care for the entire population is challenging, long, and complex. Optimizing care for "every single one" requires fundamental and transformative changes, including creating clinical workflow and proactive care teams that are supported by information technology and analytics (Allen et al., 2014). The building blocks of a clinically transformed approach to support population health are (Bodenheimer et al., 2014; Wagner, 2019):

- define a population and process for panel management;
- assign a proactive care team with roles, accountabilities, and incentives;
- design and implement a workflow or care plan for ensuring evidence-based medicine; and
- measure outcomes and provide continuous feedback for improvement.

Many examples exist of healthcare systems that have embraced population health measures and are now on the path to cultural and clinical transformation. This transformation cannot happen overnight, and organizations seeking to achieve results using this method must examine and reengineer current processes, workflows, the clinical evidence base, and team design to be successful. This chapter highlights examples of how organizations have incorporated best practice steps to transform the way healthcare services are delivered to a population.

Defining Population Health Clinical Workflow Transformation

The Clinical Workflow Center defines clinical work and clinical workflows as the following:

> Clinical work—Actions performed by clinicians to assess, change, or maintain the health of a patient.

> Clinical workflow—The directed series of steps compromising a clinical process that (1) are performed by people or equipment and computers and (2) consume, transform, [or] produce information [such as clinical outcomes]. (Clinical Workflow Center, n.d.)

Many population health clinical workflows exist and are part of how clinicians practice currently, such as routine screening, prevention, and early detection of many cancers. Primary care providers also use preventive and population health guidelines and workflows to promote vaccines and prevent communicable infectious disease such as pneumonia. In general, these protocols are applied one patient visit at a time, introducing large variation in the ways care is delivered from clinician to clinician, practice to practice, and health system to health system (Shrank, Rogstad, & Parekh, 2019). Even when there is common agreement on how to take care of common chronic illnesses such as diabetes or hypertension, there is huge variation in patterns of use with prescription drugs, testing, patient education, visits, medical costs, and clinical outcomes (Schwartz, Jena, Zaslavsky, & Mcwilliams, 2019). Although there will always be some variation in the practice of medicine, there remains opportunity to optimize care for populations by using population health analytics to identify subpopulations that will benefit from standardized clinical pathways and proactive healthcare management provided by integrated care teams (Boston Consulting Group [BCG], 2015).

Leadership and Cultural Transformation

Population health management and analytics requires a different approach when delivering healthcare services to patients. Population health seeks to address the total cost and quality of care with a proactive approach to health optimization as opposed to a status quo reactive approach of symptom management and procedure-based care. At a system level, the way care is delivered becomes a fundamental building block to successful management of populations. Several considerations need to be clearly articulated to implement a population health approach, and few considerations rise to the level of importance of transforming clinical workflow.

Population health management aims to improve the health of all patients served by a care system or clinical practice. To facilitate organizational transformation from encounter-based care to population health improvement, leaders must be fully engaged in the process of change management, embrace proactive team-based care and create concrete, measurable goals and objectives. The culture of the system and practices must also transition toward performance measurement and continuous outcomes improvement (Johnson, 2017). Healthcare systems must create staffing models that support integrated proactive care teams, prioritize resources, redesign medical records and integrate new information technologies, implement and integrate new care management systems, and align performance payment systems (Margolius & Bodenheimer,

2010; Wagner, 2019). Clinicians must embrace evidence-based care and adopt decision support tools and systems that can support evidence-based decision-making at the point of care (Torres et al., 2014).

Goals for Improvement

Healthcare systems across the United States are prioritizing the hiring of population health leaders and adopting population health-improvement methods to accomplish their business goals. It will be important for these systems to define their specific goals and create initiatives to accomplish and measure their success. Examples of common system goals that population health analytics can support include but are not limited to the following:

- Improve the value of the care provided, including improved Medicare five-star quality rating system performance (Centers for Medicare and Medicaid Services [CMS], n.d.-a).
- Improve the financial results for Medicare Advantage plans or optimize financial performance in shared savings and performance-based contracts, including the CMS Innovation Center's direct contracting model options (CMS, n.d.-b).

Population heath methods paired with integrated care-delivery teams that are aligned and rewarded can help systems meet their clinical and financial goals.

Performance and Aligning Incentives

Many performance-based contracts and programs sponsored by commercial and government payers have prescribed measures and improvement goals specified in their contracts. Provider organizations participating in performance-based contracts are required to adhere to these requirements and report progress toward results. For provider-led organizations working with multiple payers and multiple contracts, the patient populations, time frames, clinical conditions, provider networks, measure definitions, and payment models likely differ and require dedicated resources to monitor and optimize results.

The challenge healthcare delivery systems participating in performance-based contracts face is in a one-size-fits-all model of delivering care. Care teams typically follow established care pathways and clinical workflows to ensure that care is uniform and based in clinical best practice. As such, care is not typically provided differently across the care teams attributed patient panel or by payer contract type. However, opportunities exist to provide care differently to reduce care variation without negatively impacting care quality. A high degree of variation is common in practice and in costs for health conditions where multiple treatment options exist. For example, for severe back pain, treatment options range from rest and pain medications to physical therapy and ultimately to surgery. Depending on the type of clinician initially sought after for treatment, the likelihood of having surgery can be more than five times that of other providers, with no inherent improved outcome of alleviated back pain and improved function for the patient. Where multiple treatment options exist, the most costly option does not always yield the best result, which can significantly impact the total cost of care for a selected population (BCG, 2015).

In general, most healthcare organizations are supportive of improving care for all their patients. However, not all improvements impact financial contract performance. Best practice methods have been shown to remove variation in healthcare delivery, which often results in an overall reduction of profit (Berwick, 2019). Improved health outcomes in patients under fee-for-service payments may cause a net decrease in revenue as reductions occur in unnecessary hospitalizations, emergency room (ER) visits, testing, prescription drugs, and procedures. An example of this challenge was described in 2011 when Intermountain Healthcare in Utah embarked on a population health initiative to reduce overall healthcare costs by targeting and reducing unnecessary variations in care. The focus of this initiative was to reduce cost by improving quality in low-risk pregnant women by reducing the total number of elective induced labors, thereby reducing the total number of unplanned cesarean section procedures and avoiding unnecessary intensive care admissions of newborns. Through robust monitoring of data, providers were able to manage care more effectively for their patients and avoid an estimated $50 million in unnecessary procedures, imaging, labs, and prescription drugs for both moms and their newborn babies. Under the current pay-for-procedure healthcare financial reimbursement model, the estimated savings from this initiative was achieved by reducing hospital-based procedures and treatment and thereby hospital revenue (James & Savitz, 2011). It is important for government agencies and payers to conduct robust financial modeling and planning to understand the impact the transformation from pay for procedure to pay for value will have on existing healthcare organizations and work together to balance the timing and transition to new clinical models and programs to avoid any unintended negative impact to communities from significant financial strain to hospitals that continue to provide needed care.

Risk and Performance-Based Care Models

Many healthcare systems have shared savings or upside–downside risk corridors or full-risk contracts with commercial or government payers (CMS, n.d.-b). Some healthcare delivery systems own insurance companies and integrate care delivery with the management of care (Becker's Hospital Review (2015). In the face of increasing scrutiny of the total cost of medical care and how to optimize value, developing a plan to manage risk and achieve performance in a way that benefits communities will be required. Development of population health programs, care teams that use evidence-based guidelines or care pathways, initiatives to reduce medical cost, and supporting measurement and analytics is an effective strategy for these systems to fulfill the promise of value-based contracting for health care and prevent or manage the health risks of a population.

Change Management and Transformation

Leading an organization toward high-value care and population health management can be daunting. It is important not to try to do this alone. Creating a steering group that can serve as a guiding force and collaboratively create a vision or road map for the system, highlight the organizational imperatives, identify and prioritize resources, communicate the urgency for change, achieve quick wins, and track progress against milestones or goals can be an important critical success factor.

Population and Panel Management

An individual patient may have multiple health conditions, varying levels of physical and behavioral function, and one or more social determinants of health, and he or she may be assessed to be at higher or lower levels of risk for the development of comorbid conditions or complications of their conditions compared to other patients in the practice. Addressing the needs of every patient and across patients is challenging, time consuming, and complex. In the *Annales of Family Medicine*, Altschuler and colleagues (2012) estimated that 21.7 hours per day were needed to provide all of the necessary preventive, chronic, and acute care for an average-sized patient panel of 2,500 patients per physician. The same article showed that the same patient panel size can be managed in a reasonable amount of time when standardized workflows and team-based care for chronic disease management and prevention are utilized. In contrast, direct primary care providers are finding success and balance with average panel sizes of 900 patients and advocate for an approach in which fewer patients means more time per patient to provide care (Alexander, Kurlander, & Wynia, 2005). Multiple models exist to define panel size within a practice and optimize both the process and delivery of care to these patients, which will help to simplify, standardize, and improve clinical effectiveness over time (Altschuler, Margolius, Bodenheimer, & Grumbach, 2012; Doherty 2015).

An individual patient may also be listed in multiple subpopulations within the panel and identified for one or more interventions to improve health and lower cost. Each of these subpopulations will be defined by a set of identification criteria used to create a registry of patients. Thomas Workman (2013) defined the patient registry as a "set of standardized information about a group of patients who share a condition or experience" that can be queried by analysts at a point in time and requires tracking mechanisms to account for patients added to or deleted from the registry. Everyday patients who meet criteria such as the newly diagnosed are added to the registry. Patients may be removed from the registry because of a cure for their diagnosis or they may become sicker and require different care such as hospice or assignment to a different care team, or move away or die. Panel management is the monitoring of the registry for each subpopulation over time and the development by the care team of care plans for each patient guided by the evidence based workflows selected to benefit specific subpopulations and integrated across the subpopulation to form one comprehensive and evidence-guided population health management plan (see Chapter 20 for more information about registries).

Proactive Care Teams

Building and engaging care teams to proactively manage a panel of attributed patients is a core building block of population health management. Whether a two-person team in a small practice or a large integrated team in a healthcare system, all members of the care team must share accountability for improving the health, quality of care, cost, and patient experience of the patient panel. A high-performing team, aligned incentives, and a focus on driving results in the form of improved outcomes will reinforce the culture of population health and continuous improvement. Several prerequisites are needed to proactively manage a panel of attributed patients and are outlined in the following (Allen et al.,

2014; Margolius & Bodenheimer, 2010; Shirey, White-Williams, & Hites, 2019; Texas Medical Association, n.d.; Wagner, 2019):

- adopt evidence-based guidelines, workflows, and decision support tools;
- define roles and responsibilities of each care team member;
- assign accountabilities to roles and level of autonomous decision-making;
- auto-assign care team member tasks using clinical algorithms and technology; and
- implement a system for task reminders, development of care plans, adherence to evidence-based workflows, and scheduling daily huddles.

Consistent application of these prerequisites over time helps drive the systematic transformation toward adoption of population health management and supporting a new clinical model of care. More information on building an effective team to support population health management and analytics is available in Chapter 31, "Building a Team Culture for Population Health."

Evidence-Based Guidelines, Workflows and Decision Support

Although the development, implementation, and maintenance of evidence-based guidelines, care pathways, and decision support tools are beyond the scope of this book, be aware that care teams are guided by this critically important work. Tracking the degree to which a patient's care adheres to evidence-based guidelines is a common quality process measure for a subpopulation. In addition, many population health interventions implement these best practices and guidelines, and ongoing tracking and performance measurement is necessary to quantify clinical effectiveness and create the data needed to continuously improve. Additional information on evidence-based population health interventions and decision support tools are available in Chapter 8, "Grouping, Trending, and Interpreting Population Health Data for Decision Support";

Chapter 27, "Analytics Supporting Population Health Interventions"; and Chapter 28, "Monitoring and Optimizing Interventions."

Role Delineation and Accountability

Managing and creating oversight of proactive care teams is complex because the roles, responsibilities, and accountabilities for each care team may differ slightly from practice to practice. These can vary even within the same system because of resource availability and constraints, geography, clinic size, and staffing patterns. Care team members might be specific to a team, such as a medical assistant or nurse practitioner, or they might be spread across multiple teams such as a clinical pharmacist, social worker, or behavioral health therapist. Hoff and Prout (2019) define the benefits of team-based care delivery as improving care experience and providing care continuity. They also stress the importance when working in a team to have a focus on role delineation for team members to understand who is doing what. It is also important to clearly delineate who in the team is accountable for what and empower team members to make decisions appropriate for their roles.

Above all, the leader is responsible for continuously reinforcing the meaning and purpose of population health and continuous quality improvement. Role delineation, empowerment, decision-making, and accountability cannot be successful if team members do not understand the fundamental principles of how and why population health is a different model of care from the traditional healthcare model of reactive or acute care. A recent *Health Care Management* article describing the contextual factors influencing quality-improvement activities concluded the following:

> Successful [quality improvement, QI] implementation requires effective collaboration within cross-functional teams [and] healthcare workers in primary care settings should strive to create a strong teamwork climate, reinforced by

opportunities for staff in various roles to discuss QI as a collective. (Shea, Turner, Albritton, & Reiter, 2018)

Note that implementing population and role-based task management, shared care plans, oversight of care team operations, care team messaging, and team-based monitoring of sub-populations may not be adequately supported by standard electronic health records and may require additional technology to support.

Patient Engagement and Longitudinal Interaction

Sustained patient engagement is a fundamental requirement to achieve effective proactive care and self-management. Population health interventions that focus on self-management to prevent disease or improve health outcomes associated with increasing severity of disease require patient engagement. Proactive care teams developing care plans require a level of engagement from not only patients but also primary, specialty, and allied health professionals to be successful. Dominique Van de Velde and colleagues (Van de Velde et al., 2019) outline a concept of engagement and self-management in chronic conditions that include the following:

- "person-oriented attributes" such as active participation in the care plan and process, accountability, and responsibility for the process of care, and the ability to cope with adversity in a positive way;
- "person-environment-oriented attributes," including partnering with the patient to provide personalized information about the condition, its progression, treatment options, and tactics to manage risk factors and disease, taking into account the patient's needs, preferences, social support, and priorities; and
- "[summarizing] attributes: self-management" is defined by a patient's commitment to life-long behavior change and personal skill building that includes medical, personal, and emotional management.

Technology is available to care teams to enable sustained patient engagement via tele-communication, remote surveillance, remote engagement, and intervention. The products in this area continue to develop and evolve beyond the electronic health record, primarily created to support the documentation and billing of encounter-based clinical care. The future promise of telehealth and face-to-face video visits, digital messaging, remote monitoring, group chat, videoconferencing, and other forms of asynchronous and synchronous digital connectivity offer alternatives to in-office care. The application of these technologies was clearly demonstrated as a necessity during the recent COVID-19 pandemic and proved to be viable options for engaging patients to manage chronic conditions and prevent the spread of the COVID-19 disease (Wosik et al., n.d.).

Using Analytics to Drive Proactive Team-Based Care

A fundamental component of population health is the continuous monitoring and analyzing of workflows, processes and clinical experience, and financial outcomes. This monitoring provides the care team timely and continuous feedback for improvement over time. Examples of categories of measurement include the following:

- cost;
- utilization;
- quality of clinical care;
- patient preferences and experience;
- patient and care team engagement;
- adherence to evidence-based guidelines, care pathways, and adoption of healthy behaviors;
- social determinants of health;
- referrals to specialists and allied healthcare professionals;
- utilization of healthcare services; and
- total cost of care.

All of these categories can have positive or negative results, and any improvements or sustained success entirely depends on how well the interventions are implemented and measured. A key element to success in population health analytics is the development of short, intermediate, and long-term goals and targets with a clear articulation of success. This allows for analysts to create trends in the data over time and can be used to compare progress across populations and provider practices to help proactive care teams drive results. More detailed information on monitoring interventions and the analytic requirements needed to be successful is available in Chapter 31, "Building a Team Culture for Population Health Monitoring," and throughout this book.

Clinical Workflow Enhancement and Care Plan Optimization

The cornerstone of clinical transformation is developing subpopulation-specific registries that are supported by evidence-based workflows and task management that integrates into a comprehensive individualized care plan for each patient. Assigning care team members to each task outlined previously and creating a culture of shared accountability will drive results. Information, messaging, and medical record technology can help facilitate the creation of care team attributed registries. Along with integrated workflow, task management, and care plans, technology will enable care teams to communicate, monitor, and accomplish their work and achieve their goals.

Development and Implementation

Clinical workflows and care plans need to support both individual subpopulations and specialties as well as multiple subpopulations and specialties. Creating processes for clinical input, accountability, and ongoing management and maintenance of these workflows, care pathways, and care plans will be challenging and require strong clinical leadership and continuous organization-wide support. In addition, clinical evidence changes rapidly over time, and having standardized change management processes in place will help keep workflows, care pathways, and care plans up-to-date and effective.

Information Technology Support

Whereas electronic health records (EHRs) have been shown as more beneficial than not in supporting population and public health, significant gaps exist (Kruse, Stein, Thomas, & Kaur, 2018). To support population health management to optimize clinical workflows and care plans, the ability to support the following is required:

- ability to view and administer workflows or care pathway;
- administrate and manage tasks, including tracking, accountability, reminders, and flags; and
- message care teams and patients, particularly if telehealth or telemonitoring is used.

Designing and implementing information technology that integrates with or is embedded within EHRs to support population healthcare teams will likely define best practice among high-performing healthcare systems. For integrated care teams to be efficient and effective, senior team leaders must work closely with the business and analysts to manage and measure performance on both productivity and outcomes. Along with dedicated information technology support, care teams can be empowered to lead cycles of operational improvement and clinical transformation. For more information on EHRs, see Chapter 6, "Electronic Medical Record Data for Population Health Analytics."

Measuring Outcomes and Continuous Improvement

Analytics, monitoring, and reporting of subpopulations are important for ongoing panel management and creating an environment of continuous improvement. This information is needed by the care team to project resource needs, analyze possible cause-and-effect relationships, and then determine the effectiveness of care plan interventions. Other measurements include integrating analytics with data from interactive remote monitoring systems that contain self-reported data from patients that are needed to ensure timely follow-up and prevent unnecessary ED and hospital admission events. Examples of self-reported measurements that are monitored remotely include blood glucose, blood pressure, daily symptoms, activity, and nutrition. This information helps the care team monitor its patients' progress and make continuous assessments of the patient's status and needs. The ability to collect and capture this ongoing information, including clinical and social interventions is important for the ability to measure the effectiveness of the care team's work.

Data Integration and Analytics

Data Integration and analytics may be among the most critical and challenging functions for healthcare systems to master going forward to support effective population health management. The data sources that healthcare systems need for analyzing the populations they serve are detailed in Sections 2 and 3 of this textbook and include multiple EMRs, insurance medical and pharmacy claims, care-management systems (including workflow, decision support), digital connectivity systems (including telehealth, remote monitoring), financial and administrative systems, customer relationship management systems, public health, quality monitoring, and many more. Integrating this information across time in ways that accommodate the variance in definitions, time frames, and values is highly complex and summarized in Chapter 12, "Development of a Data Model," and Chapter 13, "The Population Health Data Model," along with more detailed information throughout this book.

Risk Assessment, Risk Adjustment, and Social Determinants

Because of the dynamic changes that happen to populations over time, there will be daily changes to individual risk assessments, risk adjustment, social determinants, clinical and functional assessments, and biometrics. The details of how to define these are covered in Chapter 7, "Social and Behavioral Data"; Chapter 21, "Risk Adjustment"; Chapter 22, "Predictive and Prescriptive Analytics"; and Chapter 23, "Advanced Analytic Methods." Variables that have dynamic algorithms in how they are measured are complex and require dedicated resources for operational planning and management.

Assessment, Monitoring, Surveillance and Outcomes

One of the most important reasons to adopt effective population health management strategies is developing the ability to systematically measure health outcomes and value over time and link this to ongoing continuous improvement. For each subpopulation that is defined, an operational plan is needed for measurement, to handle ongoing changes that might occur in definitions and changes to algorithms, to handle the timing of additions and deletions to that population, surveillance for changes (hospitalizations, medication changes, new scientific evidence, remote monitoring, new comorbidities), assessments (daily symptoms, functional status, severity), social determinants, procedures, and more. This operational plan and handbook for each subpopulation is extremely important to identifying, understanding, and measuring all the variables that can impact an analysis of effectiveness and outcomes. Surveillance is also important for triggering clinical workflow and interventions. Chapter 20, "Epidemiologic Methods"; Chapter 25, "Assessing Populations"; Chapter 26,

Applied Learning: Case Study

Use Case 1: Studying Clinical Transformation: CMS Innovation Center Direct Contract Model

The alternative payment model from the Centers for Medicare and Medicaid Innovation Center and sponsored in the Quality Payment Program (CMS, n.d.-b) is a voluntary payment model option for healthcare organizations providing care for Medicare fee-for-service beneficiaries. The model aims to reduce cost and enhance the quality of care and incorporates a combination of lessons learned from previous public and private healthcare markets. This model is intended to allow healthcare organizations to transform the way health care is delivered by transforming the way it is reimbursed in a value-based contract. The model allows for more attention to be placed on managing complex, chronic conditions and includes a set of outcomes-based quality and experience measures. Under the direct contracting model, a healthcare organization can offer enhanced benefits and services.

You are the leader of your healthcare organization and are considering participating in this contracting model with CMS. You would like to apply population health management and analytics to this population to be successful in this risk-sharing alternative financial model. What are some of the questions you need to have answered to understand how population health management and analytics can help you be successful in this model?

Use Case 2: Studying Clinical Transformation: CMS Comprehensive Primary Care Plus (CPC+)

The Centers for Medicare and Medicaid (CMS) is studying population heath and care incentive models for primary care based on the review of the literature and experience of previous innovation programs. The CMS-sponsored Comprehensive Primary Care Plus (CPC+) program (CMS, n.d.-a) aims to enable primary care practices to care for their patients the way they think will deliver the best outcomes and to pay them for achieving results and improving care. CPC+ is an advanced primary care medical home model that rewards value and quality by offering an innovative payment structure to support the delivery of comprehensive primary care. CPC+ seeks to improve quality, access, and efficiency of primary care. Practices in both tracks will make changes in the way they deliver care, centered on key Comprehensive Primary Care functions (Sessums, Mchugh, & Rajkumar, 2016):

1. access and continuity,
2. care management,
3. comprehensiveness and coordination,
4. patient and caregiver engagement, and
5. planned care and population health.

You are the person in charge of developing the operations and management plan for participating in this program. Which of the preceding functions would you focus on, what interventions might you consider, and what are examples of metrics you would use? What are some challenges you might encounter along the way?

"Targeting Individuals for Intervention"; Chapter 28, "Monitoring and Optimizing Interventions"; and Chapter 27, "Analytics Supporting Population Health Interventions," provide detailed information on measuring health outcomes over time to support population health.

Conclusion

Organizations that can create strong and effective leadership for clinical transformation will begin to demonstrate improved clinical quality, health experience, population outcomes, and value. Open integrated care systems that embrace innovation and learning, adopt new population health clinical workflow and interventions, systematically measure their performance against goals, and adopt a culture of continuous improvement using care teams will ultimately differentiate themselves with better value and effectiveness.

Developing the standardized clinical workflow that helps care teams with their work will be partly based on the ability to tailor the information technology and analytics to subpopulations and integrate these microsystems with the overall clinical work so that care plans and the role-based task management needed to administer these care plans integrate with primary and specialty care efficiently and effectively.

Study and Discussion Questions

- How does the concept of population health fit into the framework for U.S. health care today?
- What are some of the basic building blocks for population health management and population health workflow?

- What are some of the current gaps in electronic health records and information technology that are barriers to care teams in optimizing care for their patient panels and subpopulations?

Resources and Websites

Useful resources for examples of clinical workflow transformation include:

Clarifire. (n.d.). Transforming care through the implementation of workflow. https://www.eclarifire.com/clinical-workflows-in-healthcare.aspx

Quality Payment Program. (2019). Alternative payment models in the quality payment program as of November 2019. https://qpp-cm-dev-content.s3.amazonaws.com/uploads/733/2019%20Comprehensive%20List%20of%20APMs%20Nov%206.pdf

Sensmeier, J. (2004, December). Transform workflow through selective implementation. Nursing Management. https://nursing.ceconnection.com/ovidfiles/00006247-200412000-00016.pdf

References

Alexander, G. C., Kurlander, J., & Wynia, M. K. (2005). Physicians in retainer ("concierge") practice: A national survey of physician, patient, and practice characteristics. *Journal of General Internal Medicine, 20*(12), 1079–1083. https://doi.org/10.1111/j.1525-1497.2005.0233.x

Allen, A., Des Jardins, T. R., Heider, A., Kanger, C. R., Lobach, D. F., McWilliams, L., Polello, J. M., Rein, A., Schachter, A. A., Singh, R., Sorondo, B., Tulikangas, M. C., & Turske, S. A. (2014, June 5). Making it local: Beacon communities use health information technology to optimize care management. *Population Health Management, 17*(3), 149–158. https://doi.org/10.1089/pop.2013.0084

Altschuler, J., Margolius, D., Bodenheimer, T., & Grumbach, K. (2012). Estimating a reasonable patient panel size for primary care physicians with team-based task delegation. *Annals of Family Medicine, 10*(5), 396–400. https://doi.org/10.1370/afm.1400

Becker's Hospital Review. (2015, September 17). 100 integrated health systems to know. https://www.beckershospitalreview.com/lists/100-integrated-health-systems-to-know.html?em=ines_vigil@yahoo.com&oly_enc_id=7987D0253156B2R

Berwick, D. M. (2019, October 7). Elusive waste: The Fermi paradox in US health care. *Journal of the American Medical Association, 322*(15), 1458–1459. https://doi.org/10.1001/jama.2019.14610

Bodenheimer, T., Ghorob, A., Willard-Grace, R., & Grumbach, K. (2014, March 14). The 10 building blocks of high-performing primary care. *Annals of Family Medicine, 12*(2), 166–171. https://doi.org/10.1370/afm.1616

Boston Consulting Group. (2015, September 15). The practice variation opportunity for health care payers. https://www.bcg.com/publications/2015/health-care-payers-providers-insurance-practice-variation-opportunity-for-health-care-payers.aspx

Centers for Medicare and Medicaid Services. (n.d.). Part C and D performance data. http://go.cms.gov/partcanddstarratings

Centers for Medicare and Medicaid Services. (n.d.-a). Comprehensive primary care plus. CMS.gov. https://innovation.cms.gov/innovation-models/comprehensive-primary-care-plus

Centers for Medicare and Medicaid Services. (n.d.-b). Direct contracting model options. CMS.gov. https://innovation

.cms.gov/innovation-models/direct-contracting-model-options

Clarifire. (n.d.). Clinical workflows in healthcare: https://www.eclarifire.com/clinical-workflows-in-healthcare.aspx

Clinical Workflow Center. (n.d.). Workflow & process definitions. https://www.clinicalworkflowcenter.com/resources/workflow-process-definitions

Doherty, R. (2015, December 15). Assessing the patient care implications of "concierge" and other direct patient contracting practices: A policy position paper from the American College of Physicians. *Annals of Internal Medicine, 163*(12), 949–952. https://doi.org/10.7326/M15-0366

Hoff, T., & Prout, K. (2019, July–September). Physician use of health care teams for improving quality in primary care. *Quality Management in Health Care, 28*(3), 121–129. https://doi.org/10.1097/QMH.0000000000000216

Institute for Healthcare Improvement. (n.d.). The IHI Triple Aim. http://www.ihi.org/Engage/Initiatives/TripleAim/Pages/default.aspx

James, B. C., & Savitz, L. A. (2011). How Intermountain trimmed health care costs through robust quality improvement efforts. *Health Affairs, 30*(6), 1185–1191. https://doi.org/10.1377/hlthaff.2011.0358

Johnson, P. (2017, April 11). A 5-step guide for successful healthcare data warehouse operations. HealthCataylyst. https://www.healthcatalyst.com/a-five-step-guide-to-healthcare-data-warehouse-operations

Kruse, C. S., Stein, A., Thomas, H., & Kaur, H. (2018). The use of electronic health records to support population health: A systematic review of the literature. *Journal of Medical Systems, 42*(11). https://doi.org/10.1007/s10916-018-1075-6

Margolius, D., & Bodenheimer, T. (2010, May). Transforming primary care: From past practice to the practice of the future. *Health Affairs, 29*(5), 779–784. https://doi.org/10.1377/hlthaff.2010.0045

Schwartz, A. L., Jena, A. B., Zaslavsky, A. M., & Mcwilliams, J. M. (2019). Analysis of physician variation in provision of low-value services. *JAMA Internal Medicine, 179*(1), 16–25. https://doi.org/10.1001/jamainternmed.2018.5086

Sessums, L. L., Mchugh, S. J., & Rajkumar, R. (2016). Medicare's vision for advanced primary care: New directions for care delivery and payment. *Journal of the American Medical Association, 315*(24), 2665–2666. https://doi.org/10.1001/jama.2016.4472

Shea, C. M., Turner, K., Albritton, J., & Reiter, K. L. (2018). Contextual factors that influence quality improvement implementation in primary care: The role of organizations, teams, and individuals. *Health Care Management Review, 43*(3), 261–269. https://doi.org/10.1097/HMR.0000000000000194

Shirey, M. R., White-Williams, C., & Hites, L. (2019). Integration of authentic leadership lens for building high performing interprofessional collaborative practice teams. *Nursing Administration Quarterly, 43*(2), 101–112. https://doi.org/10.1097/NAQ.0000000000000339

Shrank, W. H., Rogstad, T. L., & Parekh, N. (2019). Waste in the US health care system: Estimated costs and potential for savings [Special communication]. *Journal of the American Medical Association, 322*(15), 1501–1509. https://doi.org/10.1001/jama.2019.13978

Texas Medical Association. (2019, September). Five best practices for more effective use of ambulatory electronic health records to manage chronic disease. *Texas Medicine*. https://www.texmed.org/Template.aspx?id=51418

Torres, G., Swietek, K., Ubri, P. S., Singer, R., Lowell, K., & Miller, W. (2014). Building and strengthening infrastructure for data exchange: Lessons from the Beacon communities. *Journal for Electronic Health Data and Methods, 2*(3), 9. https://doi.org/10.13063/2327-9214.1092

Van de Velde, D., De Zutter, F., Satink, T., Costa, U., Janquart, S., Senn, D., & De Vriendt, P. (2019). Delineating the concept of self-management in chronic conditions: A concept analysis. *BMJ Open, 9*(7). https://doi.org/10.1136/bmjopen-2018-027775

Wagner, E. H. (2019). Organizing care for patients with chronic illness revisited. *Milbank Quarterly, 97*(3), 659–664. https://doi.org/10.1111/1468-0009.12416

Wagner, E. H., Austin, B. T., & Von Korff, M. (1996). Organizing care for patients with chronic illness. Milbank Quarterly. https://pubmed.ncbi.nlm.nih.gov/8941260/

Workman, T. A. (2013, September). Engaging patients in information sharing and data collection: The role of patient-powered registries and research networks [Internet]/ National Center for Biotechnology Information. https://www.ncbi.nlm.nih.gov/books/NBK164514/

Wosik, J., Fudim, M., Cameron, B., Gellad, Z. F., Cho, A., Phinney, D., Curtis, S., Roman, M., Poon, E. G., Ferranti, J., Katz, J. N., & Tchengo1, J. (n.d.). Telehealth transformation: COVID-19 and the rise of virtual care. *Journal of the American Medical Informatics Association*. https://www.ncbi.nlm.nih.gov/pmc/articles/PMC7188147/

CHAPTER 34

Ethical Principles for Population Health Analytics

Martha Sylvia, PhD, MBA, RN

Civilizations are driven by technology but defined by Humanity.

—Courtesy of Gerd Leonhard

EXECUTIVE SUMMARY

The very nature of using data to understand characteristics of whole populations and segments of populations based on these characteristics, the determination of who will and who will not be recipients of healthcare benefits and interventions, and the measurement of the effect of interventions on health-related outcomes, the quality of health care delivered, and the cost efficiency in which they are achieved begs the need for an ethical framework to guide the work of population health analytics. It is estimated that by 2023, 60% of organizations with more than 20 data scientists will require a professional code of conduct incorporating ethical use of data and artificial intelligence (AI) and more than 75% of large organizations will hire investigators in AI behavioral forensics and privacy and customer trust specialists to reduce risk (Jones, Hare, & Buytendijk, 2019). When deep in the analysis of data and working to derive insights from person-centric data, it is easy to see individuals as points represented in the data and forget that they are our relatives, friends, colleagues, and fellow humans. Intentionally addressing the ethical aspects of population health analytics brings analytic insights back to the driving force for why population health matters: to improve the health of populations.

LEARNING OBJECTIVES

At the end of this chapter, the learner will be able to:

1. Define ethics and their importance for population health analytics.
2. Identify ethical principles used in health care and relevant to population health analytics.
3. Analyze ethical domains applicable to population health analytics.
4. Compare and contrast existing ethical codes of ethics and conduct.

Introduction

Although other healthcare and data-focused disciplines have established ethical principles and codes of ethics, population health analytics (PHA) currently has no code of ethics. Population health analytics makes data readily available at the person level to make inferences about the factors impacting health outcomes, determine which health interventions are best suited to healthcare needs in the aggregate, predict adverse outcomes, and make decisions about allocation of healthcare resources. Data-driven decision making in population health is plagued by restrictions in data availability at the person level, which limits the ability to understand the complexity of problems in health care, ensure the inclusion of diverse subgroups of populations, and measure a constellation of health determinants in addition to those that are clinical in nature. For these reasons, it is important to be intentional in addressing ethical concerns in PHA. This chapter focuses on the application of ethical principles to population health analytics.

Why Focus on Ethics?

At the culmination of population health analyses lies individuals who are impacted by the results of the conclusions that are revealed. The most important reason for focusing on ethics in PHA is that those individuals are impacted in terms of the trajectory of their illness, the ability to get support for improved outcomes, the treatments they are prescribed, their ability to access care, and more. A focus on ethics can also decrease the cost of compliance for healthcare organizations because there is less misconduct and misconduct is more likely to be reported. In addition, employees are more satisfied working in healthcare organizations where their work is framed within ethical principles, which results in lessened employee turnover. Patients will also desire to access healthcare services at organizations where it is evident that ethics are a priority (Buytendijk, Lee, & Howard, 2020).

Defining and Differentiating Ethics

When discussing ethics, many terms are used in the same context. It is important, however, to differentiate ethics from these other terms that fall into a similar realm.

- *Laws* are the system of rules that regulate the actions of the members of a country or community and are enforced through penalties (*Oxford Dictionary*, 2020a). Health law is focused on the health of individuals and populations, the provision of health care, and the operation of the healthcare system (World Health Organization, 2016).
- *Regulations* are rules or directives made and maintained by an authoritative body (*Oxford Dictionary*, 2020b).
- *Policies* are a course of action for following laws and regulations.
- *Contracts* are written or spoken agreements enforceable by law (*Oxford Dictionary*, 2020c).
- *Compliance* centers around following rules and regulations in healthcare delivery and payment focusing on the prevention, detection, collaboration, and enforcement of rules and regulations (Troklus & Vacca, 2016).

All of these terms have common elements in that they are enforceable by some type of authoritative body and there can be penalties associated with not adhering to laws, regulations, policies, and contracts. Compliance departments and programs often act as authoritative sources in healthcare organizations with the ability to recommend and sometimes determine penalties. Beyond compliance departments, federal, state, and local laws and regulations are enforceable with fines and even jail time in some situations. For instance, violations of the Health Insurance Portability and Accountability Act range from $100 for an unknowing civil violation to a maximum of $1.5 million for willful neglect and imprisonment for criminal penalties.

Ethics

Ethics is philosophical and focused on right and wrong or *moral* concepts. The terms *morals* and *ethics* both address right and wrong, with morality focused more on a personal perspective and ethics representing the standards of "good" and "bad" (Britannica, 2020). Applying these definitions in health care, organizations, governments, and most entities have a mission and vision and a set of principles or values by which they operate. These can be considered the morals of the organization or healthcare entity. Clinical, actuarial, and other disciplines working in health care are usually bound to a *code of ethics*. Together, the healthcare entities' morals and the disciplines' codes of ethics meld into the ethical principles within which people working in health care are guided and health care is delivered. This is different from laws, regulations, policies, contracts, and compliance programs in that ethics are not enforceable and punishable in and of themselves. However, deviance from ethical codes and principles can lead to or result in infractions to laws and regulations.

Unintended Consequences

As they apply to PHA, unintended consequences are unexpected outcomes or results of any type of analytically derived actions; these can occur as a result of a lack of consideration for ethics in healthcare analytics. For instance, an analysis determined that if children with disabilities, living in an inner city, accessed care at certain facilities, the cost of providing that care would be lower and the quality outcomes would be the same, so an insurance benefit structure was put in place to transfer healthcare services to those other facilities. However, an examination of the results 6 months later revealed that the children who were sent to the other facilities did not receive recommended services. As it turns out, the location and hours at the other facilities made access extremely difficult for families to make and keep appointments.

Unintended consequences are a particular challenge in population health analytics because often the data are extremely limited in terms of what can and cannot be measured. For example,

a health plan using claims data to inform benefit design may not understand the social factors determining why certain subgroupings are disadvantaged by certain benefit policies. An intentional effort can be made by analytic leaders to raise awareness and identify areas of concern for unintended consequences by building this focus into analytic work processes. Identifying potential areas of unintended consequences and setting a plan for monitoring those consequences is a beneficial addition to analytical results.

Ethical Principles

A set of ethical principles forms the foundation for ethical codes of conduct for healthcare-related disciplines. These principles form the basis for decision-making in health care and are referenced in the development of ethical codes of conduct and principles within disciplines whose professionals work in health care. These first four principles are central to biomedical ethics:

1. *beneficence*—a group of norms related to lessening or relieving harm, providing benefits, and balancing benefits against risks;
2. *nonmaleficence*—avoiding the causation of harm;
3. *autonomy*—the respect and support of self-governing, independent decisions; and
4. *justice*—a group of norms related to the fair distribution of benefits, risk, and costs (Beauchamp & Childress, 2019).

Other ethical principles applied in health care include:

- *fidelity*—the building and preservation of trust between patients and professionals in health care;
- *veracity*—telling the truth to patients regardless of how the clinician thinks that truth will be perceived; closely linked to the principle of autonomy; and
- *confidentiality*—is concealing information that is considered to be private and disclosed to others out of necessity or a need to know (Gelling, 1999).

Ethical principles in health care may stand in opposition to personally held beliefs, values, and morals. For instance, as part of their personal value systems, individuals may prescribe to the philosophy that people should be told what is best for their health and, once a person is made aware of what is best, should comply with those best prescribed practices. This philosophy is referred to as *paternalism* and can be in conflict with the principle of *autonomy*. An approach that respects the principle of autonomy might start with informing a person of the best practices for their health, which then leads to a dialogue about the best practices in comparison to the individual's goals for his or her own health and culminates in a plan of care that considers both perspectives.

Application of these ethical principles in practice is challenging as they cannot be universally applied, and they are not encountered in isolation when dealing with challenging decisions in health care. For instance, in applying the principle of veracity when delivering the news of a difficult prognosis, the level of truth-telling may be counterbalanced using the principle of nonmaleficence if it is known that a person may have deleterious physical or mental impacts from knowing certain aspects of the details or prognosis.

What is important is the awareness of these ethical principles and recognition of when there is an ethical conflict. Further, it is important to understand that these ethical principles form the basis of codes of conduct and ethics for professions working in health care.

Domains of Ethics Relevant in Population Health Analytics

With the explosion of healthcare data and the multiple ways in which they are now being used to inform decision-making and determine care delivery in health care, frameworks and guidelines are being introduced and developed in data-focused domains to support ethical practices. Some of these unfolding ethical domains are described here.

Digital Ethics

Digital ethics is an emerging field that addresses the use of digital methods to interact online or electronically and constitutes the "systems of values and moral principles for the conduct of electronic interactions among people, organizations, and things" (Buytendijk et al., 2020). It includes norms that are dedicated to ensuring that the autonomy and dignity of users is respected when two parties interact online or electronically and prescribes how the two parties should behave and responsibly conduct transactions when using a digital format (Terrasi, 2019).

Although the evolution of digital ethics applies across industries and disciplines, it is directly applicable to population health when framed in the context of *digital health*, which encompasses digital technologies related to health and medicine. The utility of digital health aligns closely with the population health process in that its intent is to monitor, prevent, screen, diagnose, and treat health-related issues (Brall, Schröder-Bäck, & Maeckelberghe, 2019). Digital health includes software and technologies that

> assist in diagnosis, treatment options, storing and sharing health records, and managing workflow and is critically reliant on analytics in its ability to allow patients to make better informed decisions about their health and provide new options for facilitating prevention, early diagnosis of life-threatening diseases and management of chronic conditions outside of traditional care settings. (U.S. Food and Drug Administration [FDA], 2017, p. 1)

According to the FDA, the scope of digital health includes mobile health, health information technology, wearable devices, telehealth and telemedicine, and personalized medicine.

At the crux of digital health are health-related data, which have been described as a cycle in which patient-generated data from devices and other patient-focused transaction data are collected. Data are then analyzed and insights and actions are derived by clinicians and analysts.

Finally, the data are returned to devices and systems, eventually providing patients with information regarding their health status and how to manage it and clinicians with a recommended course of action (Vayena, Haeusermann, Adjekum, & Blasimme, 2018). This cycle requires careful thought and consideration for ethical concerns. Areas of focus, attention, and concern at the intersect of digital health and digital ethics are multidimensional and include:

- equitable access to digital health services in terms of affordable technical equipment as well as individuals' ability and capacity to interact with e-health tools;
- upholding privacy and security of person-level data;
- establishing ownership of data in terms of who owns the data, who is custodian of the data, data collectors, users of the technology, governments, and sharing between organizations;
- development of trust with patients and collaborating healthcare organizations related to transparency, data management, and data control;

- understanding and assigning accountability for the ways in which data are used to inform decision-making and interventions;
- ensuring that the autonomy, dignity, and freedom of choice for patients is maintained, for instance, in honoring patient preferences for communication and interaction with providers;
- equalizing the balance of power between patients, devices, and providers; and
- challenges in managing informed consent because of the complexity in communicating risks and benefits, the multiple transactions of data points, and velocity at which digital data is generated (Brall et al., 2019; Vayena et al., 2018).

The complexity of digital ethics cannot be understated and is expressed in this summary of themes as a word cloud under the umbrella of medically related digital ethics in **Figure 34.1**. The larger the font size of the word, the greater the inclusion of that theme in the domain of digital ethics.

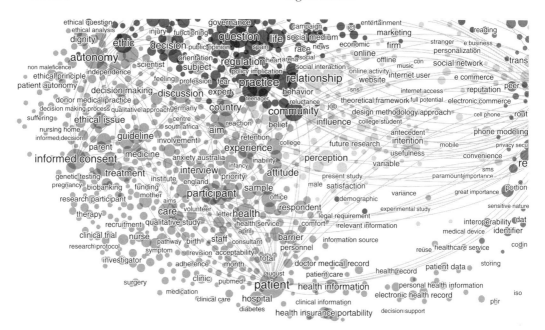

Figure 34.1 Medical Ethics Cluster of Digital Ethics Themes.

Mahieu, R., van Eck, N. J., van Putten, D., & van den Hoven, J. (2018). From dignity to security protocols: A scientometric analysis of digital ethics. *Ethics and Information Technology, 20*(3), 175–187. https://doi.org/10.1007/s10676-018-9457-5

Artificial Intelligence Ethics

A component of the field of digital ethics, artificial intelligence ethics address the moral imperatives associated with using machine-learning techniques to simulate intelligent behavior (see Chapter 23, "Advanced Analytic Methods," for information about AI and machine learning). Unlike digital ethics, which has been an afterthought for organizations or addressed mainly when unintended circumstances have emerged, ethical discussions are occurring before and during implementation of AI across industries (Buytendijk, Sicular, Brethenoux, & Hare, 2019). However, in health care, AI policy and ethical guidelines are lagging behind the application of AI techniques with a lack of clarity around AI's role in patient care, the role of providers in AI development, the adjustments needed for provider education, and the ability to weigh the risks and benefits of AI in healthcare delivery (Rigby, 2019). Ethical areas of concern for AI include those that are pertinent to digital ethics but also have components that are unique to the purpose of AI, which is to mimic human intelligence.

Bias

Perhaps the most important area of concern and one that is difficult to address is the potential for bias in AI models and algorithms. Recall from Chapter 23 that machine learning uses existing data to train models to make predictions or decisions in the current or a future time period. The data that are used in that training have to be carefully scrutinized for bias that can happen in a variety of ways, one of which is when the data used to train a model do not represent the population in which the model will be applied; these data are referred to as "unrepresentative" (Reddy, Allan, Coghlan, & Cooper, 2020). Typical machine-learning programs attempt to maximize prediction accuracy with the training data, which means that if a particular group of individuals appears more frequently than others in the training data, the program will optimize for those individuals because overall accuracy is boosted (Zou & Schiebinger, 2018).

For example, a health insurer may want to predict the likelihood of an admission to identify members at high risk of an admission for an intervention to prevent admissions. One approach might be to pool all of its members across all insurance plans to get the largest training data set possible to predict admissions. However, if the health plan has 50% of its membership in a Medicare Advantage (MA) plan, 20% in employer self-funded plans, and 30% in Medicaid, then the training data set and model to predict admissions will be biased toward the characteristics and predictors of people in the MA plan, with higher morbidity and more complexity of conditions. The result is that if the model is applied in practice, targeting and selection of high-risk participants for the intervention will be mainly from the MA plan, which poses a dilemma when funding for the intervention is equally provided from all three plans with the expectation that admissions will be prevented across all of the plans.

The problem of underrepresentation is more of a concern when demographic and health determinant factors that are known to cause health disparities are not well represented in training data sets. For instance, differences in readmission rates are known to be impacted by gender, insurance policy type, and race (Chen, Szolovits, & Ghassemi, 2019). In another example, African Americans are known to have disproportionately higher rates of diabetes and hypertension, and heart disease, which are conditions known to cause worse complications for anyone who contracts COVID-19. In addition, African Americans have higher incidence of COVID-19 (Moore et al., 2020). Machine-learning models used to predict incidence, prevalence, and poor outcomes of people with COVID-19 that do not account for these health disparities would produce inaccurate predictions and treatment algorithms and miss the mark for prevention activities.

Transparency and Trust

One main concern of both providers and patients using AI models in health care is the ability to understand "why" a person is predicted as having or not having a specific diagnosis or outcome or is selected or not selected for a certain intervention. The complexity of AI algorithms makes it extremely difficult to relay which factors and the weight of each factor that result in a certain conclusion. This inherent lack of transparency of AI models can lead to a lack of trust in their use by providers. In addition, the situation of the so-called black box or proprietary methods leads to challenges in the ability of healthcare organizations to validate AI models and guarantee their safety in healthcare decision-making (Reddy et al., 2020). See Chapter 8, "Grouping, Trending, and Interpreting Population Health Data for Decision Support," for additional limitations of proprietary methodologies and lack of transparency of models.

For example, often in population health management, the result of running a machine-learning model is a list of patients who are "eligible" for intervention. This list is given to clinicians who are expected to intervene. When there is no triggering event for intervention, like a hospitalization or emergency department visit, the conversation between the clinician and the supposedly "eligible" patient becomes more difficult when the triggering event is the identification of eligibility from a machine-learning algorithm that says the patient is "expected to have a hospitalization" in the next year. The clinician needs to understand more about the reason for the prediction to have a meaningful conversation with the patient that can result in "engagement" in the intervention. In addition, the clinician needs to prioritize clinical actions for admission prevention.

Preventing Harm

The U.S. healthcare system has a unique challenge in that the desire for profit in healthcare organizations can conflict with the goals of improving health quality and outcomes. This can lead to AI algorithms that place the goals of profit above the goals of improving patient outcomes. For instance, AI algorithms could be used to influence patients with higher complexity of illness to certain types of health plans, or they could be used to sway patients toward certain healthcare providers to drive the profits of one healthcare organization over another, regardless of whether these choices are in patients' best interest or produce the best quality and outcomes (Char, Shah, & Magnus, 2018).

Data Ethics

Data ethics is a newly introduced branch of ethics built on the foundation of computer and information ethics, which study and evaluate moral problems related to (1) data, including data generation, recording, curation, processing, dissemination, sharing, and use; (2) algorithms, including AI, machine learning, and robots; and (3) associated practices, including responsible innovation, programming, hacking, and professional codes. The focus of data ethics is on the interactions among hardware, software, and data; the content and nature of computational operations; and the challenges of data science (Floridi & Taddeo, 2016). What sets data ethics apart from digital and AI ethics is that it broadly considers the journey of data from generation to insights and the processes that make it available for analytics. For example, some unique aspects of data ethics are understanding data provenance, ensuring data quality, and using consumer and social media data responsibly.

Data Provenance

Data come from multiple sources in population health and are generated at multiple transactional points between clinicians and patients. *Data provenance* refers to an understanding of where data come from and whether that data source is reliable and trustworthy (Hand, 2018). For instance, in one care-management program, race and ethnicity data were available from self-report at the person level and collected by the state in which the associated Medicaid plan was administered; the same data were also entered by the care manager after interaction with the Medicaid member. After it was discovered that a few care managers were not asking members their race and ethnicity but instead inferred their races based on their own perceptions, the care-management data were no longer considered reliable and trustworthy.

Data Quality Assurance

Because the use of healthcare data in deriving insights and opportunities, determining distribution of healthcare benefits and offerings, and making conclusions about patients in healthcare delivery are usually done without patients' consent or ability to validate and clarify their own data points, there is an expectation that data quality-assurance activities be ethically sound (Wade, 2007). For example, if an analysis to determine whether a person has diabetes uses diagnoses on laboratory claims, this often results in a false assignment of a diagnosis because in the particular case of laboratory claims, diagnoses are coded because they are being "ruled out" by the lab test, not necessarily because the patient has the condition. Data quality assurances would ensure that laboratory claims are not used to identify patients with diabetes.

Use of Consumer and Social Media Data for Healthcare Analyses

Consumer-generated data include individual lifestyle or behavior data generated by an individual's engagement in a nonclinical commercial, participatory, or social activity (Granger et al., 2019). Examples include retail purchases, frequented websites and search activities, and social media platform posts and responses. With the increasing availability of consumer data and improved methods for matching at the person level, consumer data sources are progressively easier to acquire and link to clinically generated data. The ethical principles involved in using consumer data for healthcare analytics are the same as those for other areas of ethical consideration, with a particular focus on:

- violations of patient privacy and autonomy,
- disrupted trust in the patient–provider relationship,
- overemphasis on individual responsibility for health, and
- exclusion, marginalization, or discrimination of individuals or populations (Granger et al., 2019).

Codes of Ethics and Codes of Conduct

Given the vastness of the field of PHA and that it represents the convergence of many disciplines, multiple and varied guidance for ethical decision-making exist and are referred to as *codes of ethics*; where they govern action, they are referred to as *codes of conduct*. Because there are no codes specific to population health analytics, **Table 34.1** describes a representative set of codes of ethics and conduct that are useful in PHA. This is not an exhaustive list, but it seeks to identify the relevant principles across codes that individual practitioners and organizations conducting PHA can use to tailor their own ethical decisions and actions.

Table 34.1 Ethical Codes Relevant to Population Health Analytics

Code or Framework	Principles, Components or Elements	Reference or Link
American Health Information Management Association (AHIMA) Code of Ethics	The AHIMA Code of Ethics is focused on the right to privacy for consumers, confidentiality, and information disclosure. The tenants of the code are focused on the informaticist putting others before themselves; protecting personal health information; the appropriate and accepted uses of health information; the advancement of the profession as a whole; and the accurate representation of one's credentials.	AHIMA (2019)

American Medical Informatics Association Code of Ethics	I. AMIA members should involved in patient care should recognize that patients and their loved ones and caregivers have the right to know about the existence and use of electronic records containing their personal healthcare information, and have the right to create and maintain their own personal health records and manage personal health information using a variety of platforms including mobile devices.	Goodman et al. (2013)
	■ Not mislead patients about the collection, use, or communication of their healthcare information.	
	■ Enable and—as appropriate, within reason and the scope of their position and in accord with independent ethical and legal standards—facilitate patients' rights and ability to access, review, and correct their electronic health information.	
	■ Recognize that patient-provided [or] generated health data, such as those collected on mobile devices, deserve the same diligence and protection as biomedical and health data gathered in the process of providing health care.	
	■ Advocate and work as appropriate to ensure that protected health information (PHI), personally identifiable information (PII), and other biomedical data are transmitted, acquired, recorded, stored, maintained, analyzed, and communicated in an appropriately safe, reliable, secure, and confidential manner, and that such data management is consistent with applicable laws, local privacy and security policies, and accepted informatics standards.	
	■ Never knowingly disclose PHI, PII, or biomedical or health data in violation of legal requirements or accepted local confidentiality practices, or in ways that are inconsistent with the explanation of data disclosure and use to the patient. AMIA members should understand that inappropriate disclosure of biomedical information can cause harm, and so should work to prevent such disclosures. AMIA members should avoid acquiring data through means that run the risk of, or fail to prevent, inappropriate disclosure. Likewise, even if an action does not involve disclosure, one should not use—or through negligence permit the use of—patient information and data in ways inconsistent with the stated purposes, goals, or intentions of the patient or organization responsible for these data, except as appropriate for public health, previously approved and communicated research uses, or reporting as required under the law.	
	II. Key ethical guidelines regarding colleagues. AMIA members should:	
	■ Endeavor, as appropriate, to support and foster colleagues' and/or team members' work, in a timely, respectful, and conscientious way to support their roles in health care [or] research and education.	
	■ Support and foster the efforts of patients to be actively involved in the collection, management, and curation of their health data.	

(continues)

Table 34.1 Ethical Codes Relevant to Population Health Analytics (continued)

Code or Framework	Principles, Components or Elements	Reference or Link
	■ Advise colleagues and others, as appropriate, about actual or potential information or systems issues (including system flaws, bugs, usability issues, etc.) that negatively affect patient safety, privacy, data security, or outcomes or could hinder colleagues' ability to delegate responsibilities to patients, other colleagues, involved institutions, or other stakeholders. ■ If a leader, an AMIA member should: • Be familiar with these guidelines and their applicability to their practice, unit, or organization. • Communicate as appropriate about these ethical guidelines to those they lead. • Strive to promote familiarity with, and use of, these ethical guidelines. III. Key ethical guidelines regarding institutions, employers, business partners, and clients (called here collectively "employers"). AMIA members should: ■ Understand their duties and obligations to current and former employers and fulfill them to the best of their abilities within the bounds of ethical and legal norms. ■ Understand and appreciate that employers have legal and ethical rights and obligations, including those related to intellectual property. Understand and respect the obligations of their employers and comply with local policies and procedures to the extent that they do not violate ethical and legal norms. Consider the trade-offs that occur with the configuration and use of technologies (e.g., decision support systems) before implementation, and monitor and manage results when the optimal approach is unclear. ■ Inform the employer and act in accordance with ethicolegal mandates and patient rights when employer actions, policies, or procedures would violate ethical or legal obligations, contracts, or other agreements made with patients. Maintain a safe and high-quality environment even while implementing innovation, recognizing that all changes in a complex adaptive environment generate unanticipated consequences and potential harm. IV. Key ethical guidelines regarding society and regarding research (intentionally removed details of this aspect because ethical principles related to research are not the focus of this topic) V. General professional and ethical guidelines. AMIA members should: ■ Maintain competence as informatics professionals.	

	<ul><li>Obtain applicable continuing education and be dedicated to a culture of lifelong learning and improvement.</li><li>Recognize technical and ethical limitations and seek consultation when needed, particularly in ethically conflicting situations.</li><li>Contribute to the education and mentoring of students, junior members, and others, as appropriate.</li><li>Promote a culture of inclusivity in their work and professional conduct.</li><li>Strive to encourage the adoption of informatics approaches supported by adequate evidence to improve health and health care; and to encourage and support efforts to improve the amount and quality of such evidence.</li><li>Be mindful that their work and actions reflect on the profession and on AMIA."</li></ul>	
International Accountability Foundation Unified Ethical Framework for Big Data Analysis	<ul><li>"Purpose: Before any type of big data analysis, there should be an understanding of its purpose.</li><li>Beneficial: Both the discovery and application phases require an organization to define the benefits that will be created by the analytics and should identify the parties that gain tangible value from the effort. The act of big data analytics may create risks for some individuals and benefits for others or society as a whole. Those risks must be counter-balanced by the benefits created. Data scientists, along with others in an organization, should be able to define the usefulness or merit that comes from solving the problem so it might be evaluated appropriately. The risks should also be clearly defined so that they may be evaluated as well. If the benefits that will be created are limited, uncertain or if the parties that benefit are not the ones at risk from the processing, those circumstances should be taken into consideration, and appropriate mitigation for the risk should be developed before the analysis begins.</li><li>Progressive: Because bringing large and diverse data sets together and looking for hidden insights or correlations may create some risks for individuals, the value from big data analytics should be materially better than not using big data analytics. If the anticipated improvements can be achieved in a less data-intensive manner, that less intensive processing should be pursued. One might not know the level of improvement in the discovery phase. Yet, in the application phase, the organization should be better equipped to measure it. This application of new learnings to create materially better results is often referred to as innovation. Organizations should not create the risks associated with big data analytics if there are other processes that will accomplish the same objectives with fewer risks.</li></ul>	Information Accountability Foundation (2015)

(continues)

Table 34.1 Ethical Codes Relevant to Population Health Analytics (continued)

Code or Framework	Principles, Components or Elements	Reference or Link
	■ Sustainable: All algorithms have an effective half-life—a period in which they effectively predict future behavior. Some are very long, others are relatively short. The half-life of an insight affects sustainability. Big data analysts should understand this concept and articulate their best understanding of how long an insight might endure once it is reflected in application. Big data insights, when placed into production, should provide value that is sustainable over a reasonable time frame. Considerations that affect the longevity of big data analytics include whether the source data will be available for a period of time in the future, whether the data can be kept current, whether one has the legal permissions to process the data for the particular application, and whether the discovery may need to be changed or refined to keep up with evolving trends and individual expectations. ■ Respectful: Respectful relates directly to the context in which the data originated and to the contractual or notice related restrictions on how the data might be applied. The United States Consumer Privacy Bill of Rights speaks to data being used within context. Big data analytics may affect many parties in many different ways. Those parties include individuals to whom the data pertains, organizations that originate the data, organizations that aggregate the data and those that might regulate the data. All of these parties have interests that must be taken into consideration and respected. ■ Fair: Fairness relates to the insights and applications that are a product of big data, while respectful speaks to the conditions related to, and the processing of, the data. United States law prohibits discrimination based on gender, race, genetics, or age. Yet, big data processes can predict all of those characteristics without actually looking for fields labeled gender, race, or age. The same can be said about genotypes, particularly those related to physical characteristics. Section 5 of the United States Federal Trade Commission Act prohibits unfair practices in commerce that are harmful to individuals not outweighed by countervailing benefits. Big data analytics, while meeting the needs of the organization that is conducting or sponsoring the processing, must be fair to the individuals to whom the data pertains. The analysis of fairness needs to look not only at protecting against unseemly or risky actions but also at enhancing beneficial opportunities. Human rights speak to shared benefits of technology and broader opportunities related to employment, health, and safety. Interfering with such opportunities is also a fairness issue. In conducting this fairness assessment, organizations should take steps to balance individual interests with integrity."	

Data Science Oath	¨I swear to fulfill, to the best of my ability and judgment, this covenant:	National Academies Press (2018)
	■ I will respect the hard-won scientific gains of those data scientists in whose steps I walk and gladly share such knowledge as is mine with those who follow.	
	■ I will apply, for the benefit of society, all measures that are required, avoiding misrepresentations of data and analysis results.	
	■ I will remember that there is art to data science as well as science and that consistency, candor, and compassion should outweigh the algorithm's precision or the interventionist's influence. I will not be ashamed to say, "I know not," nor will I fail to call in my colleagues when the skills of another are needed for solving a problem.	
	■ I will respect the privacy of my data subjects, for their data are not disclosed to me that the world may know, so I will tread with care in matters of privacy and security. If it is given to me to do good with my analyses, all thanks. But it may also be within my power to do harm, and this responsibility must be faced with humbleness and awareness of my own limitations.	
	■ I will remember that my data are not just numbers without meaning or context, but represent real people and situations, and that my work may lead to unintended societal consequences, such as inequality, poverty, and disparities due to algorithmic bias. My responsibility must consider potential consequences of my extraction of meaning from data and ensure my analyses help make better decisions.	
	■ I will perform personalization where appropriate, but I will always look for a path to fair treatment and nondiscrimination.	
	■ I will remember that I remain a member of society, with special obligations to all my fellow human beings, those who need help and those who don't.	
	■ If I do not violate this oath, may I enjoy vitality and virtuosity, respected for my contributions and remembered for my leadership thereafter. May I always act to preserve the finest traditions of my calling and may I long experience the joy of helping those who can benefit from my work."	

Applied Learning: Use Cases

The following use cases are derived from real experiences in using data for population health analytics. Consider these use cases in terms of the use of data to develop insights and make recommendations for population health initiatives. For each use case, respond to the following questions:

■ What ethical principles are important to consider?
■ What aspects of the provided ethical codes or frameworks are helpful to guide decision-making and action?
■ What gaps are there in the ethical guidance that would further help to address ethical concerns?
■ What are the next steps to address ethical concerns?

(continues)

Applied Learning: Use Cases   *(continued)*

Use Case 1

A large employer group is looking for ways to incentivize employees and their dependents to be healthier. The group is willing to offer an incentive to employees and dependents of as much as 20% of benefit costs. They have come to your PHA team to ask for an analysis and recommendations for how to structure the benefit, determine eligibility for the benefit, and what the improved health outcomes would be if implemented. The human resources benefit manager at the employer group has a particular interest in managing obesity as he personally has been on a successful weight-loss journey for two years, deeply understands the health concerns around obesity, and observes that many employees seem to be overweight. Your PHA team is excited to be working on such an important initiative and really want to do a great job with the analysis and recommendations.

You approach the analysis as a population assessment to understand the health determinants that are driving quality, utilization, and cost outcomes in the population of employees and their dependents. You start with an inventory of the data sources available to perform the analysis and summarize them as follows:

- Administrative medical and pharmacy claims data are available for all employees and their dependents over the past year. The data include information about all of the medical services and prescription drugs provided as well as basic demographic information, including age, gender, and home address.
- Self-reported health risk assessment data have been collected for only 45% of employees (not dependents). The data have self-reported information, including age, gender, race, ethnicity, mental and physical health conditions and symptoms, height, weight, nutritional intake, exercise habits, smoking status, and readiness to change.
- Laboratory data including hemoglobin A1c levels for employees and dependents with diabetes for the past year.

With this information, answer the preceding set of questions.

Use Case 2

A large health plan has funded an end-of-life intensive intervention that includes primary care services in the home, a personal assistant to help with daily activities, and a nurse case manager to ensure ongoing assessment of clinical needs and care coordination. The program is sustainable when it meets its goal of reducing avoidable and nonlife-sustaining end-of-life costs that are often realized when patients spend their last days hospitalized and receive multiple lifesaving tests, procedures, and treatments. Enrollment in the program is currently based solely on provider referrals, and there is concern over the low number of patients enrolled in the program. Your PHA team has been requested to build a predictive model that will be used to identify and target appropriate candidates for this program. The outcome predicted will be death in the next year and is available for training the model. Input variables for the model are available from administrative medical and pharmacy claims data and lab data.

With this information, answer the preceding set of questions.

Conclusion

Ethical philosophy focuses on right and wrong moral concepts and is differentiated from laws and regulations in that ethics are mostly self-regulated as opposed to being enforced by external bodies. However, ignoring ethical principles is not without consequences, as a lack of ethical principles and guidance leads to issues with compliance, following regulations, and even breaking laws in health care, and can also result in poor organizational performance in terms of keeping high-quality employees and in gaining and maintaining patients' trust and confidence. Unintended consequences are related to ethical considerations in that they are unanticipated and undesired results of analytic process and must be intentionally identified and monitored.

Without its own ethical framework, set of principles, or code of conduct, PHA must rely on the guidance set forth by other similar domains. The good news is that there are ethical principles and codes of conduct that exist in similar fields that can be applied to population health analytics. These ethical principles provide guidance for the spectrum of data-management activities, data sources used for analyses, the appropriateness of questions asked of the data and the ability to answer them using data, the analytic methods applied to data, the interpretation of findings, the impact to the individuals represented by the data, the importance of upholding ethical standards to analytic disciplines, and more. With this knowledge and set of resources, population health analytics can realize its potential in truly improving the health of multitudes of individuals.

Study and Discussion Questions

- Why is it important to consider ethical principles when executing population health analytics?
- Consider the ethical codes provided in Table 34.1. What resonates with your work or the work you plan to do in the future?

- What are the challenges to addressing ethical considerations related to population health analytics in healthcare organizations?
- How can ethical considerations become part of the ongoing processes used in population health analytics?

Resources and Websites

World Health Organization—Global Health Ethics: https://www.who.int/health-topics/ethics#tab=tab_1

National Center for Ethics in Healthcare, U.S. Department of Veterans Affairs: https://www.ethics.va.gov/resources/addl_ethicsresources.asp

American College of Healthcare Executives—ACHE Code of Ethics: https://www.ache.org/about-ache/our-story/our-commitments/ethics/ache-code-of-ethics

Gerd Leonhard's Digital Ethics Page: www.futuristgerd.com

Center for Digital Ethics and Policy—Loyola University of Chicago: https://www.digitalethics.org/resources

References

American Health Information Management Association. (2019). AHIMA code of ethics. https://bok.ahima.org/doc?oid=105098#.YBMEIOgzbIX

Beauchamp, T. L., & Childress, J. F. (2019). *Principles of biomedical ethics* (8th ed.). Oxford University Press.

Brall, C., Schröder-Bäck, P., & Maeckelberghe, E. (2019, October 3). Ethical aspects of digital health from a justice point of view. *European Journal of Public Health, 29* (Suppl. 3), 18–22. https://doi.org/10.1093/eurpub/ckz167

Britannica. (2020). Ethics. https://www.britannica.com/topic/ethics-philosophy

Buytendijk, F., Lee, B., & Howard, C. (2020, January 27). Digital ethics: What every executive leader should know. Gartner Research. https://www.gartner.com/en/documents/3980162/digital-ethics-what-every-executive-leader-should-know

Buytendijk, F., Sicular, S., Brethenoux, E., & Hare, J. (2019, July 11). AI ethics: Use 5 common guidelines as your starting point. Gartner Research. https://www.gartner.com/en/documents/3947359/ai-ethics-use-5-common-guidelines-as-your-starting-point

Char, D. S., Shah, N. H., & Magnus, D. (2018, March 15). Implementing machine learning in health care—Addressing ethical challenges. *New England Journal of Medicine, 378*(11), 981–983. https://doi.org/10.1056/NEJMp1714229

Chen, I. Y., Szolovits, P., & Ghassemi, M. (2019). Can AI Help Reduce Disparities in General Medical and Mental Health Care? *AMA Journal of Ethics, 21*(2), 167–179. Retrieved from www.amajournalofethics.org

Floridi, L., & Taddeo, M. (2016, December 28). What is data ethics? *Philosophical Transactions of the Royal Society A: Mathematical, Physical and Engineering Sciences, 374*(2083). https://doi.org/10.1098/rsta.2016.0360

Gelling, L. (1999, May 26). Ethical principles in healthcare research. Nursing Standard, *13*(36), 39–42. https://doi.org/10.7748/ns1999.05.13.36.39.c2607

Goodman, K. W., Adams, S., Berner, E. S., Embi, P. J., Hsiung, R., Hurdle, J., Jones, D. A., Lehmann, C. U., Maulden, S., Petersen, C., Terrazas, E., & Winkelstein, P. (2013, January). AMIA's code of professional and ethical conduct. *Journal of the American Medical Informatics Association, 20*(1), 141143. https://academic.oup.com/jamia/article/20/1/141/728741

Granger, D. E. L., Skopac, D. J. S., Mbawuike, S. U., Levin, A. T., Dwyer, D. S. J., Rosenthal, D. A. S., & Humphreys, J. A. (2019, July). An ethical framework for the use of consumer-generated data in health care. Mitre. https://www.mitre.org/publications/technical-papers/an-ethical-framework-for-the-use-of-consumer-generated-data-in-health

Hand, D. J. (2018, September 17). Aspects of data ethics in a changing world: Where are we now? *Big Data, 6*(3), 176–190. https://doi.org/10.1089/big.2018.0083

Information Accountability Foundation. (2015, March). Unified ethical frame for big data analysis: IAF Big data ethics initiative, Part A [Draft]. https://b1f.827.myftpupload.com/wp-content/uploads/2020/04/IAF-Unified-Ethical-Frame.pdf

Jones, L. C., Hare, J., & Buytendijk, F., (2019, July 31). *Digital ethics by design: A framework for better digital business.* Gartner Research. https://www.gartner.com/en/documents/3953794/digital-ethics-by-design-a-framework-for-a-better-digita

Mahieu, R., van Eck, N. J., van Putten, D., & van den Hoven, J. (2018, June 27). From dignity to security protocols: A scientometric analysis of digital ethics. *Ethics and Information Technology, 20*(3), 175–187. https://doi.org/10.1007/s10676-018-9457-5

Moore, J. T., Ricaldi, J. N., Rose, C. E., Fuld, J., Parise, M., Kang, G. J., Driscoll, A. K., Norris, T., Wilson, N., Rainisch, G., Valverde, E., Beresovsky, V., Brune, C. A., Oussayef, N. L., Rose, D. A., Adams, L. E., Awel, S., Villanueva, J., & Westergaard, R. (2020, August 21). Disparities in Incidence of COVID-19 among underrepresented racial/ethnic groups in counties identified as hotspots during June 5–18, 2020—22 states, February–June 2020. *MMWR. Morbidity and Mortality Weekly Report, 69*(33). https://doi.org/10.15585/mmwr.mm6933e1

National Academies Press. (2018). *Data science for undergraduates: Opportunities and options* [Consensus study report]. Author. https://doi.org/10.17226/25104

Oxford Dictionary. (2020a). Law—defined. Lexico. https://www.lexico.com/en/definition/law

Oxford Dictionary. (2020b). Regulation—defined. Lexico. https://www.lexico.com/en/definition/regulation

Oxford Dictionary. (2020c). Contract—defined. Lexico. https://www.lexico.com/en/definition/contract

Reddy, S., Allan, S., Coghlan, S., & Cooper, P. (2020, March). A governance model for the application of AI in health care. *Journal of the American Medical Informatics Association, 27*(3), 491–497. https://doi.org/10.1093/jamia/ocz192

Rigby, M. J. (2019). Ethical dimensions of using artificial intelligence in health care. *AMA Journal of Ethics, 21*(2), 121–124. https://journalofethics.ama-assn.org/article/ethical-dimensions-using-artificial-intelligence-health-care/2019-02

Terrasi, J. (2019, April 10). What are digital ethics? Lifewire. https://www.lifewire.com/what-are-digital-ethics-4587289

Troklus, D., & Vacca, S. (2016). *HCAA compliance 101* (4th ed.). Health Care Compliance Association.

U.S. Food and Drug Administration. (2017). *Digital health innovation action plan.* Author. https://www.fda.gov/media/106331/download

Vayena, E., Haeusermann, T., Adjekum, A., & Blasimme, A. (2018, January 16). Digital health: Meeting the ethical and policy challenges. *Swiss Medical Weekly, 148*, w14571. https://doi.org/10.4414/smw.2018.14571

Wade, D. (2007). Ethics of collecting and using healthcare data. *BMJ, 334*, 1330–1331.

World Health Organization. (2016). Health laws. Author. http://www.who.int/health-laws/legal-systems/health-laws/en/

Zou, J., & Schiebinger, L. (2018). AI can be sexist and racist—It's time to make it fair. *Nature, 559*(7714), 324–326. https://doi.org/10.1038/d41586-018-05707-8

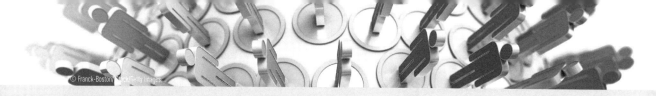

Index

Note: Page numbers followed by *f* or *t* represent figures or tables respectively.